Anesthesiology Core Review

Part One: BASIC Exam

Anesthesiology
Core Review
Part One: BASIC Exam

Brian S. Freeman, MD
Associate Professor of Clinical Anesthesia
Residency Program Director
Department of Anesthesiology
Georgetown University School of Medicine
Washington, DC

Jeffrey S. Berger, MD, MBA
Associate Professor of Anesthesiology
Residency Program Director
Department of Anesthesiology & Critical Care Medicine
The George Washington University School of Medicine & Health Sciences
Washington, DC

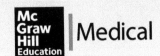

New York   Chicago   San Francisco   Athens   London   Madrid   Mexico City
Milan   New Delhi   Singapore   Sydney   Toronto

Anesthesiology Core Review—Part One: BASIC Exam

1 2 3 4 5 6 7 8 9 0   QVS/QVS   19 18 17 16 15 14

ISBN 978-0-07-182137-7
MHID 0-07-182137-6

The book was set in minion pro by Cenveo® Publisher Services.
The editors were Brian Belval and Christina M. Thomas.
The production supervisor was Rick Ruzycka.
The illustration manager was Armen Ovsepyan; the illustrator was Electronic Publishing Services.
Project management was provided by Sandhya Gola, Cenveo Publisher Services.
The cover designer was Anthony Landi.
Quad Graphics Versailles was printer and binder.

This book is printed on acid-free paper.

Library of Congress Cataloging-in-Publication Data

Freeman, Brian S., author.
    Anesthesiology core review / Brian Freeman.
        p. ; cm.
    Includes index.
    ISBN 978-0-07-182137-7 (paperback : alk. paper)—ISBN 0-07-182137-6 (paperback : alk. paper)
I. Title.
    [DNLM: 1. Anesthesia—Examination Questions.   2. Anesthetics—Examination Questions.   WO 218.2]
    RD82.3
    617.9'6076—dc23
                                                                            2014003623

McGraw-Hill Education books are available at special quantity discounts to use as premiums and sales promotions, or for use in corporate training programs. To contact a representative please visit the Contact Us pages at www .mhprofressional.com.

To my son Alexander (BF)

To Rachel and my girls, Talia, Jessica, and Naomi: your support means so much and I love you.
To Dr. Berrigan, and the faculty and residents at GW: you inspire me each day to find new ways to improve,
both programmatically and personally. Thank you for the encouragement, and the high standard
that you set on a daily basis. And to Dr. Freeman: I cannot imagine a better coauthor,
program director colleague, or friend. (JB)

Contents

PART **III**

ORGAN-BASED SCIENCES 331

PART **IV**

SPECIAL ISSUES IN ANESTHESIOLOGY   535

Contributors

Nima Adimi, MD

Resident
The George Washington University School of Medicine
& Health Sciences
Washington, DC

Taghreed Alshaeri, MD

Resident
Detroit Medical Center/Wayne State University School of
Medicine
Detroit, MI

Kelly Arwari, MD

Assistant Professor of Anesthesiology
University of Arizona College of Medicine
Tucson, AZ

Daniel Asay, MD

Clinical Instructor of Anesthesiology
The George Washington University School of Medicine
& Health Sciences
Washington, DC

Caleb A. Awoniyi, MD, PhD

Adjunct Clinical Associate Professor of Anesthesiology
University of Florida Health Science Center
Gainesville, FL

Adam W. Baca, MD

Resident
The George Washington University School of Medicine
& Health Sciences
Washington, DC

Sami Badri, MD

Resident
The George Washington University School of Medicine
& Health Sciences
Washington, DC

Jamie Barrie, MD

Resident
Georgetown University School of Medicine
Washington, DC

Rohini Battu, MD

Resident
The George Washington University School of Medicine
& Health Sciences
Washington, DC

Shawn T. Beaman, MD

Associate Professor of Anesthesiology
University of Pittsburgh School of Medicine
Pittsburgh, PA

Lisa Bellil, MD

Instructor of Clinical Anesthesia
Georgetown University School of Medicine
Washington, DC

Jeffrey S. Berger, MD, MBA

Associate Professor of Anesthesiology
The George Washington University School of Medicine
& Health Sciences
Washington, DC

Michael J. Berrigan, MD, PhD

Seymour Alpert Professor and Chair, Anesthesiology
& Critical Care Medicine
The George Washington University School of Medicine
& Health Sciences
Washington, DC

Gabrielle Brown, MD

Resident
The George Washington University School of Medicine
& Health Sciences
Washington, DC

Michelle Burnett, MD

Associate Professor of Clinical Anesthesia
Georgetown University School of Medicine
Washington, DC

Eric Chiang, MD

Resident
The George Washington University School of Medicine
    & Health Sciences
Washington, DC

Sandy Christiansen, MD

Resident
Georgetown University School of Medicine
Washington, DC

Catherine Cleland, MD

Resident
The George Washington University School of Medicine
    & Health Sciences
Washington, DC

Hiep Dao, MD

Instructor of Clinical Anesthesia
Georgetown University School of Medicine
Washington, DC

Marianne D. David, MD

Assistant Professor of Anesthesiology
The George Washington University School of Medicine
    & Health Sciences
Washington, DC

Kerry DeGroot, MD

Assistant Professor of Clinical Anesthesia
Georgetown University School of Medicine
Washington, DC

Matthew de Jesus, MD

Instructor of Clinical Anesthesia
Georgetown University School of Medicine
Washington, DC

Joseph Delio

Medical Student
The George Washington University School of Medicine
    & Health Sciences
Washington, DC

Mehul Desai, MD, MPH

Director, Spine, Pain Medicine & Research
Metro Orthopedics & Sports Therapy
Silver Spring, MD

Tricia Desvarieux, MD

Assistant Professor of Anesthesiology
The George Washington University School of Medicine
    & Health Sciences
Washington, DC

Nina Deutsch, MD

Assistant Professor of Anesthesiology
Children's National Medical Center
The George Washington University School of Medicine
    & Health Sciences
Washington, DC

Lorenzo De Marchi, MD

Associate Professor of Clinical Anesthesia
Georgetown University School of Medicine
Washington, DC

Christopher Edwards, MD

Assistant Professor of Anesthesiology
The George Washington University School of Medicine
    & Health Sciences
Washington, DC

Brian S. Freeman, MD

Associate Professor of Clinical Anesthesia
Georgetown University School of Medicine
Washington, DC

Lakshmi Geddam, MD

Resident
The George Washington University School of Medicine
    & Health Sciences
Washington, DC

Ramon Go, MD

Resident
The George Washington University School of Medicine
    & Health Sciences
Washington, DC

Mandeep Grewal, MD

Resident
The George Washington University School of Medicine
    & Health Sciences
Washington, DC

Matthew Haight, DO

Assistant Clinical Professor of Anesthesiology
University of California San Francisco School
    of Medicine
San Francisco, CA

Medhat Hannallah, MD

Professor of Clinical Anesthesia
Georgetown University School of Medicine
Washington, DC

Katrina Hawkins, MD

Assistant Professor of Anesthesiology & Critical Care
  Medicine
The George Washington University School of Medicine
  & Health Sciences
Washington, DC

Kumudhini Hendrix, MD

Assistant Professor of Clinical Anesthesia
Georgetown University School of Medicine
Washington, DC

Anna Katharine Hindle, MD

Assistant Professor of Anesthesiology
The George Washington University School of Medicine
  & Health Sciences
Washington, DC

Jason Hoefling, MD

Instructor of Clinical Anesthesia
Georgetown University School of Medicine
Washington, DC

Elizabeth E. Holtan, MD

Instructor of Clinical Anesthesia
Georgetown University School of Medicine
Washington, DC

Amanda Hopkins, MD

Research Assistant
The George Washington University School of Medicine
  & Health Sciences
Washington, DC

George Hwang, MD

Instructor of Clinical Anesthesia
Georgetown University School of Medicine
Washington, DC

Adrian M. Ionescu, MD

Resident
Georgetown University School of Medicine
Washington, DC

Christopher Jackson, MD

Assistant Professor of Anesthesiology
The George Washington University School of Medicine
  & Health Sciences
Washington, DC

Kuntal Jivan, MD

Assistant Professor of Clinical Anesthesia
Georgetown University School of Medicine
Washington, DC

Sonia John

Medical Student
The George Washington University School of Medicine
  & Health Sciences
Washington, DC

Christopher Junker, MD

Assistant Professor of Anesthesiology & Critical Care
  Medicine
The George Washington University School of Medicine
  & Health Sciences
Washington, DC

Alan Kim, MD

Instructor of Clinical Anesthesia
Georgetown University School of Medicine
Washington, DC

Brian A. Kim, MD

Resident
The George Washington University School of Medicine
  & Health Sciences
Washington, DC

Howard Lee

Medical Student
The George Washington University School of Medicine
  & Health Sciences
Washington, DC

Neil Lee, MD

Assistant Professor of Anesthesiology
The George Washington University School of Medicine
  & Health Sciences
Washington, DC

Victor Leslie, MD

Resident
Georgetown University School of Medicine
Washington, DC

Choy R. A. Lewis, MD

Assistant Professor of Anesthesiology
The George Washington University School of Medicine
  & Health Sciences
Washington, DC

Jonah Lopatin, MD

Resident
Georgetown University School of Medicine
Washington, DC

Jeannie Lui, MD

Resident
The George Washington University School of Medicine
    & Health Sciences
Washington, DC

Tatiana Lutzker, MD

Assistant Professor of Anesthesiology
The George Washington University School of Medicine
    & Health Sciences
Washington, DC

Amir Manoochehri

Medical Student
The George Washington University School of Medicine
    & Health Sciences
Washington, DC

Christopher Monahan, MD

Assistant Professor of Anesthesiology
The George Washington University School of Medicine
    & Health Sciences
Washington, DC

Gregory Moy, MD

Clinical Instructor of Anesthesia
The George Washington University School of Medicine
    & Health Sciences
Washington, DC

Joseph Mueller, MD

Instructor of Clinical Anesthesia
Georgetown University School of Medicine
Washington, DC

Joseph Myers, MD

Associate Professor of Clinical Anesthesia
Georgetown University School of Medicine
Washington, DC

Vinh Nguyen, DO

Instructor of Clinical Anesthesia
Georgetown University School of Medicine
Washington, DC

Eric Pan, MD

Acting Assistant Professor of Anesthesiology
The University of Washington School of Medicine
Seattle, WA

Ronak Patel, MD

Resident
The George Washington University School of Medicine
    & Health Sciences
Washington, DC

Alex Pitts-Kiefer, MD

Resident
Georgetown University School of Medicine
Washington, DC

Raymond A. Pla, Jr., MD

Assistant Professor of Anesthesiology
The George Washington University School of Medicine
    & Health Sciences
Washington, DC

Jeffrey Plotkin, MD

Associate Professor of Clinical Anesthesia & Surgery
Department of Anesthesiology
Georgetown University School of Medicine
Washington, DC

Chris Potestio, MD

Resident
Georgetown University School of Medicine
Washington, DC

Steven W. Price, MD

Resident
Georgetown University School of Medicine
Washington, DC

Michael Rasmussen, MD

Fellow
Stanford University School of Medicine
Palo Alto, CA

Srijaya K. Reddy, MD, MBA

Assistant Professor of Anesthesiology
Children's National Medical Center
The George Washington University School of Medicine
    & Health Sciences
Washington, DC

Elvis W. Rema, MD

Assistant Professor of Anesthesiology
The George Washington University School of Medicine
    & Health Sciences
Washington, DC

Mona Rezai, MD

Resident
Georgetown University School of Medicine
Washington, DC

Camille Rowe, MD

Resident

The George Washington University School of Medicine
& Health Sciences

Washington, DC

Jason Sankar, MD

Assistant Professor of Anesthesiology

The George Washington University School of Medicine
& Health Sciences

Washington, DC

Michael J. Savarese, MD

Resident

The George Washington University School of Medicine
& Health Sciences

Washington, DC

Hannah Schobel, DO

Instructor of Clinical Anesthesia

Georgetown University School of Medicine

Washington, DC

Douglas Sharp, MD

Assistant Professor of Anesthesiology

The George Washington University School of Medicine
& Health Sciences

Washington, DC

Marian Sherman, MD

Assistant Professor of Anesthesiology

The George Washington University School of Medicine
& Health Sciences

Washington, DC

Rachel Slabach, MD

Instructor of Clinical Anesthesia

Georgetown University School of Medicine

Washington, DC

Karen Slocum, MD, MPH

Resident

The George Washington University School of Medicine
& Health Sciences

Washington, DC

Todd Stamatakos, MD

Resident

Georgetown University School of Medicine

Washington, DC

Jessica Sumski, MD

Resident

The George Washington University School of Medicine
& Health Sciences

Washington, DC

Johan P. Suyderhoud, MD

Professor and Vice Chairman

Georgetown University School of Medicine

Washington, DC

Mohebat Taheripour, MD

Assistant Professor of Clinical Anesthesia

Georgetown University School of Medicine

Washington, DC

Sarah Uddeen, MD

Resident

The George Washington University School of Medicine
& Health Sciences

Washington, DC

Rishi Vashishta, MD

Resident

University of California San Francisco School
of Medicine

San Francisco, CA

Sudha Ved, MD

Professor of Clinical Anesthesia

Department of Anesthesiology

Georgetown University School of Medicine

Washington, DC

Andrew Winn

Medical Student

Georgetown University School of Medicine

Washington, DC

Eric Wise, MD

Resident

Department of Anesthesiology

University of Pittsburgh School of Medicine

Pittsburgh, PA

Seol W. Yang, MD

Assistant Professor of Anesthesiology

The George Washington University School of Medicine
& Health Sciences

Washington, DC

John Yosaitis, MD

Georgetown University School of Medicine

Washington, DC

Darin Zimmerman, MD

Assistant Professor of Anesthesiology

The University of Maryland School
of Medicine

Baltimore, MD

Preface

The year 2014 marks the beginning of a new phase in board certification for anesthesiology residents. Previously, all residents had to pass one written and one oral examination, both taken after the completion of residency training. Now the American Board of Anesthesiology has increased the stakes. The Part I examination has been split into two written examinations: "Basic" (administered at the beginning of the third postgraduate year) and "Advanced" (administered the summer after graduation). Anesthesiology residents who are unable to pass the "Basic" examination will not be allowed to finish their training.

Understandably, a brand new, high-stakes examination in the middle of residency training will create much stress and anxiety. This is where *Anesthesiology Core Review* comes in. The organization of this two-volume review book conforms to the newly revised content outline issued by the American Board of Anesthesiologists for the "Basic" and "Advanced" examinations. Each chapter succinctly summarizes key concepts for each topic from the new content outline.

This review book should serve as the "core" of your study preparation. As program directors with many years of board examination advising experience, we recommend supplementing *Anesthesiology Core Review* with multiple-choice practice questions, keyword reviews, and references to major anesthesiology textbooks. Space is provided throughout this book to add notes from other sources.

Anesthesiology Core Review represents the successful collaboration between the two academic anesthesiology departments located in our nation's capitol: Georgetown University and George Washington University. Together we challenge you to recognize your assets and deficiencies, work collaboratively, and use this book to pass the new ABA BASIC Examination with flying colors!

Best regards for a productive career in this dynamic specialty,

Brian S. Freeman, MD
Jeffrey S. Berger, MD, MBA
Washington, DC

Anesthesiology Core Review

Part One: BASIC Exam

Topographical Anatomy as Landmarks

Joseph Mueller, MD

The utilization of topographical anatomic landmarks to assist anesthesiologists during procedural care includes a multitude of regional nerve blocks, interventional pain procedures, neuraxial techniques, and vascular access cannulation. Specialty care for regional and interventional pain medicine relies greatly on a thorough understanding of anatomic relationships to effectively deliver anesthesia and to avoid potential morbidity and mortality.

TOPOGRAPHICAL LANDMARKS ALONG THE VERTEBRAL COLUMN

C6: Chassaignac tubercle

C7: Vertebra prominens, level of stellate ganglion

T1-T4: Cardioaccelerator fibers

T3: Axilla

T4: Nipple line

T7: Xiphoid process

T8: Inferior border of scapula

T9-L2: Origin of artery of Adamkiewicz in 85% of patients

T10: Umbilicus

T12-L4: Lumbar plexus

L1: Level of celiac plexus

L2: Termination of spinal cord (adults)

L3: Termination of spinal cord (pediatrics)

L4: Iliac crest

L4-S3: Sacral plexus

S2: Posterior superior iliac spine (PSIS), termination of subarachnoid space (adults)

S3: Termination of subarachnoid space (pediatrics)

NERVE BLOCK LANDMARKS

Upper Extremity Blocks

1. **Interscalene**—Mark the sternal and clavicular heads of the sternocleidomastoid (SCM) muscle, the cricoid cartilage, and the clavicle. The needle insertion should be in the interscalene groove at C6 that is posterior to the clavicular head of the SCM and between the anterior and middle scalene muscles.
2. **Infraclavicular**—Mark the coracoid process and the needle insertion is 2 cm inferior and 2 cm medial to the coracoid process.
3. **Axillary**—Palpate or visualize the pulse of the axillary artery and guide the needle through the artery until arterial blood is aspirated. Penetrate further until blood return stops (you have now passed through the axillary artery) then inject anesthetic. This will cover the radial nerve as it is directly posterior to the axillary artery. Withdraw needle and again pass through the axillary artery. Once you exit the artery and are anterior to it, inject again to cover the median and ulnar nerves.
4. **Musculocutaneous**—Typically combined with the axillary approach to ensure lateral forearm anesthesia. Local anesthetic can be injected into the belly of the coracobrachialis muscle, which sits just posterior to the biceps.

5. **Ulnar**—Isolated block can be done at the elbow between the medial epicondyle and olecranon process, medial to the ulnar artery.
6. **Radial**—Isolated block can be done at elbow between the brachioradialis and biceps tendons. A block can also be done at the wrist in the anatomic snuff box between brachioradialis and biceps tendons.
7. **Median**—Isolated block can be done at elbow medial to the brachial artery at the pronator teres muscle. A block can also be done at the wrist between the palmaris longus and flexor carpi radialis tendons.

Lower Extremity Blocks

1. **Femoral**—Below inguinal ligament, insert needle lateral to femoral artery at the level of the femoral crease.
2. **Sciatic**
   a. *Classic posterior approach*—A line is drawn between the greater trochanter of the femur and the PSIS. The needle insertion is 4 cm distal to the midpoint of these landmarks.
   b. *Parasacral approach*—A line is drawn between the ischial tuberosity and PSIS. The needle insertion is 6 cm caudal to PSIS on the drawn line.
   c. *Subgluteal approach*—A line is drawn between the greater trochanter and ischial tuberosity. The needle insertion is 4 cm caudal to midpoint of these landmarks.
3. **Popliteal**
   a. *Posterior approach*—Mark the popliteal fossa crease, tendons of biceps femoris (lateral), and the semitendinosus and semimembranosus muscles (medial). The needle insertion is 8 cm superior to popliteal crease at midpoint between tendons.
   b. *Lateral approach*—Mark the vastus lateralis, biceps femoris, and popliteal crease. The needle insertion is 8 cm above the popliteal crease in the groove between the vastus lateralis and biceps femoris.
4. **Lumbar plexus**—Mark the level of the iliac crest and the midline (spinous process). The needle insertion is 4 cm lateral to midline at the level of iliac crest.
5. **Ankle block**
   a. *Saphenous*—The distal extremis of the femoral nerve. It courses medial to the knee and extends distally and anterior to the medial malleolus at the ankle level. A field block can be done from the medial surface of the tibial tuberosity, at the dorsomedial aspect of upper calf or at the medial malleolus.
   b. *Deep peroneal*—Lateral to the extensor hallucis longus tendon at 1–2 digit webspace.
   c. *Superficial peroneal*—Lateral to extensor digitorum longus tendon.
   d. *Posterior tibial*—Posterior to the posterior tibial artery.
   e. *Sural*—Posterior to the lateral malleolus.

LANDMARKS FOR VASCULAR LINE PLACEMENT

1. The **internal jugular vein** (IJV) cannulation landmark is between the sternal and clavicular heads of the SCM muscle. The IJV is lateral to carotid artery.
2. The **femoral vein** cannulation landmark is medial to the femoral artery at the femoral crease.
3. The **subclavian vein** cannulation landmark is at the midpoint of the clavicle with the needle directed toward the suprasternal notch.

HEAD AND NECK LANDMARKS

1. **Cricothyroid membrane**—Also referred to as the "conus elasticus" or lateral cricothyroid ligament. This membrane is the landmark for a cricothyrotomy procedure in which an incision is made through the skin and cricothyroid membrane between the cricoid and thyroid cartilage tissues. This helps establish a patent airway during certain life-threatening airway emergencies where orotracheal and nasotracheal intubation are not possible.
2. **Thoracic duct**—This lymphatic vessel extends vertically in the chest posterior to the left carotid artery and left IJV at the C7 vertebral level. The duct empties into the junction of the left subclavian vein and left IJV, below the clavicle.

The **trachea** commences at C6 and is composed of "C"-shaped cartilaginous rings that are both lateral and anterior to the tracheal lumen. The posterior trachea is composed of a membranous longitudinal muscular layer. This orientation is a helpful tool for anesthesiologists to orient themselves while performing fiberoptic bronchoscopy.

The first carina divides into the **right and left lungs** via the right and left bronchi near the T5 vertebral level in most patients. The right bronchus divides further into three right lobes (the right upper lobe, the right middle lobe, and the right lower lobe). The left bronchus divides into two lobes (the left upper lobe and the left lower lobe). The pulmonary lobes divide further into bronchopulmonary segments as follows: **right lung** (three in the upper lobe, two in the middle lobe, five in the lower lobe) and the **left lung** (four to five in the upper lobe and four to five in the lower lobe).

CARDIAC LANDMARKS FOR AUSCULTATION

- Aortic valve—Second intercostal space to the right of sternum
- Pulmonic valve—Second intercostal space to the left of sternum
- Tricuspid valve—Fifth intercostal space to the left of sternum
- Mitral valve—Fifth intercostal space at the left midclavicular line

Radiological Anatomy

Joseph Mueller, MD

MRI AND CT

Magnetic resonance imaging (MRI) creates more detailed images of the soft tissues of the human body compared to computed tomography (CT) or X-ray. MRI may produce both two- and three-dimensional images of the human body while it provides excellent contrast between the different soft tissues of the body. MRI is particularly well-suited for imaging the brain, muscles, tendons, nerves, vascular structures, and organs.

1. **Brain and skull**—Diagnostic data may be useful for assessing brain lesions, fractures, hemorrhage, infarction, tumor, hydrocephalus, and/or cerebral edema.
   a. *Epidural hematoma* (Figure 2-1)
   b. *Subdural hematoma* (Figure 2-2)
   c. *Subarachnoid hemorrhage* (Figure 2-3)
2. **Chest**—Diagnostic data may include assessment of fracture, infection, bleeding, tumor, pulmonary emboli, pneumothorax, emphysema, and fibrosis.
   a. *Pulmonary embolus* (Figure 2-4)
   b. *Pneumothorax* (Figure 2-5)

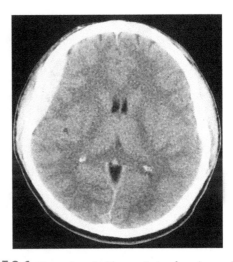

FIGURE 2-1 (Reproduced with permission from Longo DL, Harrison TR, *Harrison's Principles of Internal Medicine,* 18th ed. New York: McGraw-Hill; 2012.)

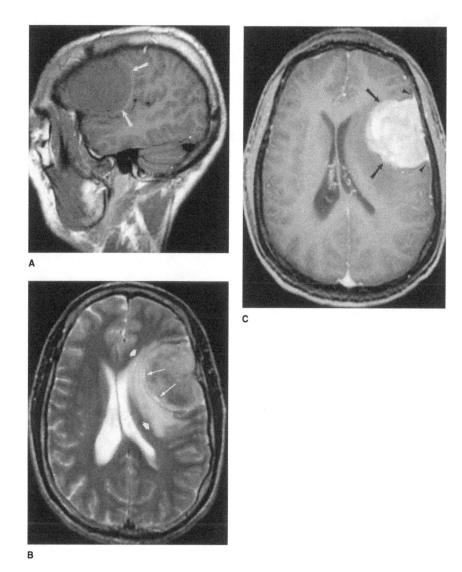

FIGURE 2-2 (Reproduced with permission from Chen MY, *Basic Radiology*, 2nd ed. McGraw-Hill Medical; 2004.)

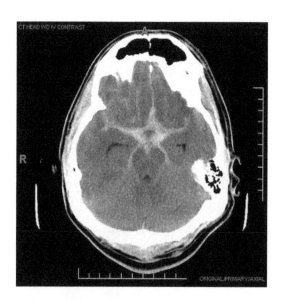

FIGURE 2-3 (Reproduced with permission from Doherty GM, *CURRENT Diagnosis and Treatment: Surgery*, 13th ed. McGraw-Hill Companies; 2010.)

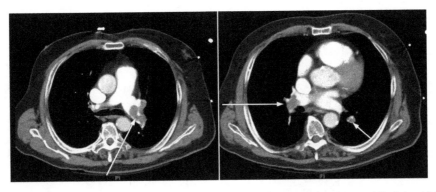

FIGURE 2-4 (Reproduced with permission from Longo DL, Harrison TR, *Harrison's Principles of Internal Medicine*, 18th ed. New York: McGraw-Hill; 2012.)

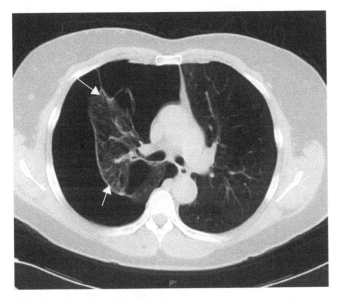

FIGURE 2-5 (Reproduced with permission from Longo DL, Harrison TR, *Harrison's Principles of Internal Medicine*, 18th ed. New York: McGraw-Hill; 2012.)

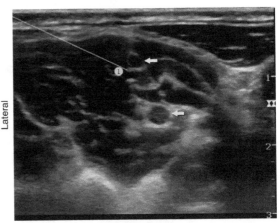

Interscalene brachial plexus

FIGURE 2-6 (Reproduced with permission from Hadzic A, *Hadzic's Peripheral Nerve Blocks*, 2nd ed. McGraw-Hill Professional; 2011.)

ULTRASOUND

Ultrasound may utilize *Doppler* to determine the direction and velocity of blood flow within vascular structures. This is a helpful tool in confirming the presence of venous and arterial vascular structures. Red color represents higher frequency Doppler flows "toward" the probe, whereas blue represents lower frequency Doppler flows "away" from the ultrasound probe.

1. **Nerve blocks**
    a. *Brachial plexus (interscalene)* (Figure 2-6)
    b. *Brachial plexus (supraclavicular)* (Figure 2-7)
    c. *Brachial plexus (infraclavicular)* (Figure 2-8)
    d. *Brachial plexus (axillary)* (Figure 2-9)
    e. *Femoral nerve* (Figure 2-10)
    f. *Popliteal nerve* (Figure 2-11)
2. **Transesophageal echocardiography**
    a. *Transgastric short axis* (Figure 2-12)
    b. *Midesophageal 4 chamber* (Figure 2-13)
    c. *Pericardial effusion* (Figure 2-14)

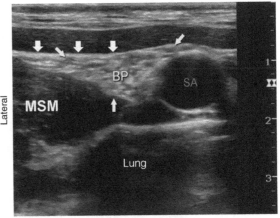

Supraclavicular block

FIGURE 2-7 (Reproduced with permission from Hadzic A, *Hadzic's Peripheral Nerve Blocks*, 2nd ed. McGraw-Hill Professional; 2011.)

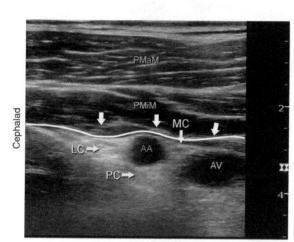

Infraclavicular block

FIGURE 2-8 (Reproduced with permission from Hadzic A, *Hadzic's Peripheral Nerve Blocks*, 2nd ed. McGraw-Hill Professional; 2011.)

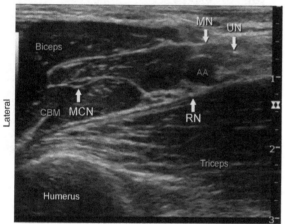

Axillary brachial plexus with anatomical structures labeled

FIGURE 2-9 (Reproduced with permission from Hadzic A, *Hadzic's Peripheral Nerve Blocks*, 2nd ed. McGraw-Hill Professional; 2011.)

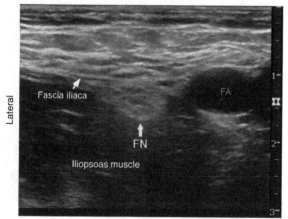

Femoral nerve block

FIGURE 2-10 (Reproduced with permission from Hadzic A, *Hadzic's Peripheral Nerve Blocks*, 2nd ed. McGraw-Hill Professional; 2011.)

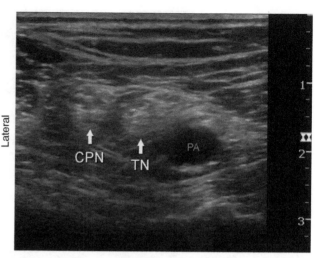

Common peroneal and tibial nerve-3 cm above popliteal crease, labeled

FIGURE 2-11 (Reproduced with permission from Hadzic A, *Hadzic's Peripheral Nerve Blocks*, 2nd ed. McGraw-Hill Professional; 2011.)

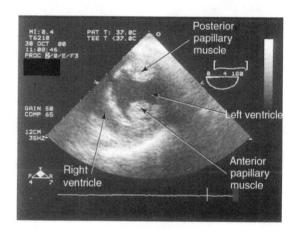

FIGURE 2-12 (Reproduced with permission from Butterworth JF, Mackey DC, Wasnick JD, *Morgan and Mikhail's Clinical Anesthesiology*, 5th ed. McGraw-Hill; 2013.)

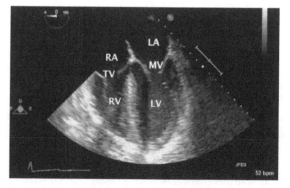

FIGURE 2-13 (Reproduced with permission from Butterworth JF, Mackey DC, Wasnick JD, *Morgan and Mikhail's Clinical Anesthesiology*, 5th ed. McGraw-Hill; 2013.)

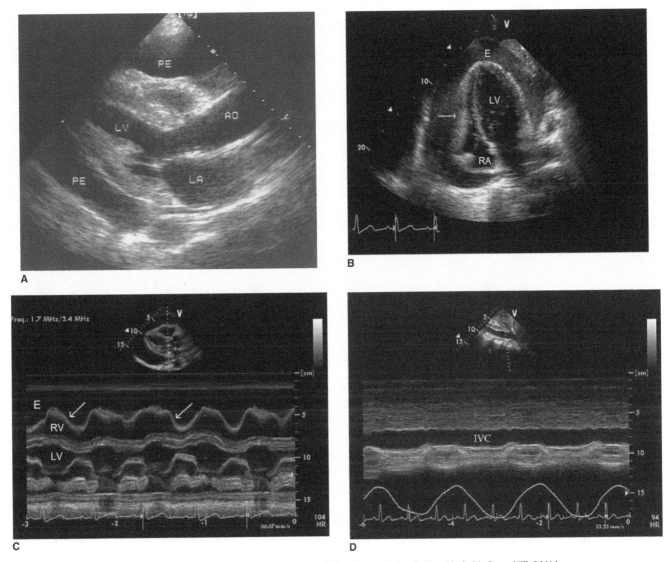

FIGURE 2-14 (Reproduced with permission from Fuster V, Hurst's The Heart, 13th ed., New York: McGraw-Hill; 2011.)

Mechanics

Brian S. Freeman, MD

PRESSURE MEASUREMENT OF GASES AND LIQUIDS

By definition, pressure (P) is the force (F) applied to an object per unit of area (A), such that $P = F/A$. The SI unit of pressure is the pascal (Pa); 1 Pa equals 1 newton of force distributed over an area of 1 m^2. Pressure can also be defined by other units, such as millimeters of mercury (mm Hg), centimeters of water (cm H_2O), pounds per square inch (psi), or atmospheres (atm). These different units are based on the specific way of taking the measurement. For instance, "mm Hg" is the pressure exerted at the base of a 1-mm high column of mercury, whereas "cm H_2O" is the pressure exerted at the base of a 1-cm high column of water at 4°C. To convert among the units, it is useful to start with the pressure of the atmosphere at sea level: 1 atm = 760 mm Hg = 988 cm H_2O = 14.7 psi.

Clinically, gauges are used to display pressure measurements of both gases and liquids. Examples of gauge pressure include central venous pressure, arterial blood pressure, cylinder pressures, and peak inspiratory pressures. Gauges record pressure above or below the existing ambient atmospheric pressure. "Absolute" pressure is the sum of gauge pressure and atmospheric pressure. For example, a full oxygen E-cylinder has a gauge pressure of about 2000 psi. When the gauge pressure reads 0 psi, the cylinder still contains oxygen at ambient atmospheric pressure (14.7 psi). The absolute pressure of this E-cylinder is 2014.7 psi when completely full.

Manometers are the most common systems used to measure pressure. Manometers contain columns of liquid, usually water or mercury, in an open-ended U-shaped tube. Pressure applied to the end not exposed to atmospheric pressure will displace the fluid column. The column adjusts its height until it achieves equilibrium with the pressure difference between the two ends of the tube. The pressure in the column is the product (ρgz) of the height of the column (z), the density of the liquid (ρ), and the force of gravity (g). Manometers work best for measuring pressures that change slowly. The mass of the liquid column yields significant inertia that works against quick changes in height.

Manometers are not helpful in measuring high pressures because the necessary height of the fluid column would be difficult to achieve. Instead, Bourdon gauges are used. These devices are based on the concept that an elastic tube will deflect when subjected to a given applied pressure. Higher gas pressures will uncoil this tube, which causes the pointer to move on the gauge's scale.

PRESSURE REGULATORS

Pressure regulators, also known as pressure-reducing valves, are used in anesthesia machines to lower pressures and regulate the gas supply. Modern regulators have three essential components: a tightly wound spring attached to a diaphragm, which is then connected to a valve controlling the high pressure gas input. These devices are based on the principle that large forces acting on small areas (valve) can be balanced by small forces acting on large areas (diaphragm). Regulators today usually have a preset output pressure that is determined by the spring attached to the diaphragm.

The primary gas source for the anesthesia machine is the hospital pipeline supply from the central oxygen tank. It is usually supplied at a pressure of about 55 psi. The pipeline gauge is located on the pipeline side of the check valve to avoid reflecting any pressure within the machine. To maintain constant flow with changing supply pressures, the anesthesia machine is fitted with pressure regulators for both the pipeline and cylinder supplies. Pipeline pressure is generally preregulated by the first-stage regulator to 45 psi.

The secondary gas source for the anesthesia machine comes from the E-cylinders attached to the yoke assembly. Medical gases in these cylinders (oxygen, air, nitrous oxide) are pressurized to about 2200 psi. Because the anesthesia machine requires lower constant pressures for proper function, a regulator is necessary. There are separate regulators for each gas cylinder. The regulator in the oxygen reserve cylinder reduces pressure from 2200 to 45 psi, whereas that of the nitrous oxide cylinder reduces pressure from 745 to 45 psi. If two reserve cylinders of the same gas are opened at the same time, the cylinder supply gauge will indicate the pressure in the cylinder with the higher pressure.

A secondary function of the pressure regulator is to serve as a check valve to determine the gas source with the highest pressure (cylinder vs pipeline supply). Pipeline supply is of course the preferred gas supply for use by the anesthesia machine (cylinders are for backup). The regulator will shut down cylinder gas supply when pipeline gas supply exceeds 45 psi pressure. The small pressure differential between the pipeline and cylinder gas supplies allows this backup mechanism to occur. For example, if the oxygen cylinder is accidently left open, the higher oxygen pipeline pressure closes the pressure regulator and prevents oxygen from leaving the cylinder. This safety mechanism prevents depletion of the backup E-cylinder when there is still an adequate pipeline gas supply.

"Second-stage" oxygen pressure regulators are present in some contemporary anesthesia machines (Datex-Ohmeda; Datex-Ohmeda Inc., Madison, Wisconsin). These regulators ensure a constant supply pressure to the flow meters even if oxygen supply pressure drops below 45 psi. The second-stage regulator reduces oxygen supply pressure to 14 psi and N_2O supply pressure to 26 psi. Output from the oxygen flow meter is constant when the oxygen supply pressure exceeds the threshold (minimal) value. The pressure sensor shut-off valve of Datex-Ohmeda is set at a higher threshold value (20–30 psig) to ensure that oxygen is the last gas flowing if oxygen pressure failure occurs.

MEDICAL GAS CYLINDERS

Anesthesia machines have cylinders attached for use when the pipeline supply source is not available or if the pipeline system fails. The cylinder most often used by anesthesiologists is the E-cylinder. E-cylinders are also routinely used as portable oxygen sources, such as when a patient is transported between the operating room and an intensive care unit (ICU).

Each medical gas has a critical temperature and pressure that determines its behavior when stored in a cylinder. The critical temperature of a gas is the temperature below which a particular gas enters a liquid phase due to applied pressure. Because the critical temperature of oxygen is −119°C, it cannot be liquified at room temperature, no matter how much pressure is applied. The pressure in a gas cylinder varies with the temperature, the amount of gas remaining, and the state of the contents (gas or liquid). Because the pressure inside an open cylinder will always equilibrate with atmospheric pressure, cylinders are never considered empty.

Some key points on specific medical gas cylinders are as follows (Table 3-1):

1. **Oxygen**—A full E-cylinder of oxygen contains 660 L of oxygen molecules that generate about 2000 psi of pressure. Under high pressures, oxygen will always remain a compressed gas. According to Boyle's law, the pressure in an oxygen cylinder is directly proportional to the volume

TABLE 3-1   Medical Gas Cylinders

	Body Color	Pressure (At Room Temperature) (psi)	Physical State in Cylinder
Oxygen	Green	2000	Gas
Nitrous oxide	Blue	745	Liquid/vapor
Carbon dioxide	Grey	840	Liquid/vapor
Air	Yellow	1800	Gas
Entonox	Blue	2000	Gas
Oxygen/helium (heliox)	Brown	2000	Gas

of gas remaining. Therefore, the pressure gauge can be used to accurately determine how much gas remains in the cylinder. If the gauge reads 1000 psi, the cylinder is approximately half full and contains 330 L of oxygen. If a patient receives 10 L/min flow plus 6 L/min minute ventilation through an endotracheal tube during transport, the cylinder would be depleted in about 21 minutes (330 L/16 L/min). Use of hand ventilation rather than mechanical ventilation can decrease oxygen utilization.

2. **Nitrous oxide**—Unlike oxygen and air, nitrous oxide can be compressed into a liquid form at room temperature (20°C) as its critical temperature is 36.5°C. A full E-cylinder of N_2O contains nearly 1600 L of gas that generates 750 psi of pressure. The majority of the tank is liquid N_2O with a small amount of gaseous N_2O above the liquid. Unlike oxygen, the volume of nitrous oxide cannot be determined from its pressure gauge. The pressure in the cylinder remains constant at 750 psi until all the liquid N_2O has been vaporized. It is estimated that about 20% of the initial volume of gas remains in the cylinder when the gauge finally shows a drop in pressure. To determine how much gas remains in a cylinder of liquefied N_2O, it is necessary to weigh the cylinder and subtract the empty cylinder weight from the total cylinder weight.

3. **Entonox**—Entonox cylinders contain a mixture of nitrous oxide and oxygen in equal parts at a pressure of 2000 psi. This gas is typically self-administered as a means of providing analgesia for dental procedures, labor, and dressing changes. Because the critical temperature of N_2O is 36.5°C, Entonox cylinders are typically stored in environments where the temperature is above 10°C. Below this temperature, a liquid phase could form that contains a much higher percentage of nitrous oxide, leading to the possible administration of a hypoxic mixture.

Flow and Velocity

Brian S. Freeman, MD

DEFINITIONS

The physics of flow underlies the behavior of all fluids. Liquids, such as plasma and crystalloid solutions, and gases, such as oxygen and sevoflurane, are all considered to be fluids. Flow (F) is defined as the *quantity* (Q, mass or volume) of a given fluid that passes by a certain point within a unit of time (t), most commonly expressed in liters per second. This relationship can be expressed by the equation $F = Q/t$. Fluid flow requires a pressure gradient (ΔP) between two points such that flow is directly proportional to the pressure differential. Higher pressure differences will drive greater flow rates. The pressure gradient establishes the direction of flow.

Flow is different than velocity. Velocity is defined as the *distance* a given fluid moves within a unit of time, most commonly expressed in centimeters per second. The flow of a fluid within a tube is related to velocity by the relationship $F = V \cdot r^2$, where V is the mean velocity and r is the radius of the tube.

PATTERNS OF FLOW

There are two types of flow patterns:

1. **Laminar**—Fluids assuming laminar flow contain molecules that move in numerous thin layers or concentric tubes that are known as streamlines. There are no fluctuations. Successive particles within each sheet will pass the same point at the same steady velocity. Although laminar fluid particles move in a straight line, each streamline has a different velocity. Molecules in the center of the flow have the highest velocity, whereas those at the periphery of the tube are almost motionless. Fluids flow in a laminar pattern when they have low flow rates through smooth tubes with large cross-sectional areas, such as at the lung periphery. Laminar flow is directly proportional to the pressure gradient ($F \propto P$). In this linear relationship, according to Ohm's law, resistance (R) serves as a constant such that $F = \Delta P/R$.
2. **Turbulent**—Turbulent fluid flow contains molecules that move in irregular directions due to eddy currents. The disordered nature of turbulent flow increases resistance to flow. Turbulent flow typically occurs when fluid particles move at higher rates but with fluctuations. Unlike laminar flow, turbulent fluids have a nonlinear relationship between flow and pressure. The flow rate is proportional to the square root of the pressure gradient ($F \propto \sqrt{P}$). To increase turbulent flow twofold, the pressure gradient requires a fourfold increase. This is why laminar flow patterns are preferable to turbulent ones. Turbulent fluids are less efficient; they require higher energy to generate the greater pressure differential necessary to achieve an identical flow rate as laminar fluids. For example, if the airflow in the upper airways becomes more turbulent due to an obstruction, the patient will require greater work of breathing to maintain proper gas exchange.

The *Reynolds number* (Re) describes the point at which a fluid transitions from laminar to turbulent flow. This number represents the ratio of the major forces acting on fluid particles: inertial (momentum) forces and viscous (friction) forces. The equation for calculating the Reynolds number is:

$$Re = \rho v d / \eta$$

where, ρ = density of fluid
v = flow velocity
d = orifice diameter
η = viscosity

Re is a dimensionless number with no associated units. Laminar flow occurs with smaller Reynolds numbers (Re < 2000) because of the relatively higher proportion of viscous forces (η). An unstable mixture of both flow patterns exists with Re between 2000 and 4000. Turbulent flow in a straight unbranched tube occurs with larger Reynolds numbers (Re > 4000) due to greater momentum forces. A given fluid will become turbulent if its tube has a large diameter (d), if the fluid is particularly dense (ρ), and especially if a critical velocity (v) has been reached. Turbulent flow is more likely to occur whenever a segment of tube, such as a bronchiole, bends sharply or narrows (increasing velocity) or gives off an orifice (increasing diameter).

The use of heliox therapy illustrates these physical principles. Heliox is a gas mixture usually supplied in cylinders of 80% helium with 20% oxygen (although 70:30 and 60:40 mixtures are available). It is an inert gas with a density less than that of atmospheric air but similar viscosity. Patients with upper airway obstruction or severe reactive airway disease have airflow patterns that are primarily turbulent in nature. Substitution of air with a lower density gas such as heliox reduces the Re and promotes laminar fluid flow. As a result, resistance to airflow decreases, which improves the flow of oxygen. Because of the improved efficiency of ventilation, the patient has a reduced work of breathing. The beneficial effects of heliox should be seen within minutes. Possible clinical applications include upper airway obstruction, asthma exacerbation, postextubation stridor, severe chronic obstructive pulmonary disease (COPD) exacerbations, and croup. However, heliox therapy may not be helpful in patients with supplemental oxygenation requirements because of the inability to deliver fraction of inspired oxygen (Fio$_2$) higher than 40%.

FACTORS AFFECTING FLOW

The Hagen–Poiseuille equation describes the relationship between the variables that affect flow rate (Q) in laminar fluids. The four major factors are the pressure gradient (ΔP), tube radius (r), fluid viscosity (η), and tube length (l).

$$Q = \Delta P \pi r^4 / 8 \eta l$$

1. **Pressure gradient (P)**—Flow is directly proportional to the difference in pressures at two points in the tube. Higher pressures lead to higher flow rates.
2. **Radius (r)**—Flow is directly proportional to the fourth power of the radius. If the diameter of the tube is reduced in half, the flow rate diminishes by one-sixteenth. For example, the flow of intravenous fluids through a 20-gauge catheter (60 mL/min) is less than that of a 16-gauge catheter (220 mL/min). Small changes in the diameter of an endotracheal tube have significant effects on airflow.
3. **Length (l)**—Flow is inversely proportional to the length of the tube. Changing the length is much less significant than changing the radius. Doubling the length will decrease the flow by 50%. For instance, the flow rate through an 18-gauge lumen in a long 15-cm central venous catheter (26 mL/min) is slower than that through a short 18-gauge peripheral intravenous catheter (105 mL/min). For fluid resuscitation, therefore, for a given fluid with the same pressure applied to it, flow is higher through a shorter and wider catheter.
4. **Viscosity (η)**—Viscosity is defined as a fluid's resistance to the motion of a solid due to shearing forces of friction. Flow rate is inversely proportional to viscosity. Fluids with greater viscosity have slower flow rates. In the circulation, higher hemoglobin concentrations will increase blood viscosity and decrease blood flow, leading to a higher risk of thrombosis.

The use of mechanical ventilation illustrates these physical principles. Endotracheal tubes are smooth and straight, which promotes laminar flow and allowing for the application of the Hagen–Poiseuille equation. Smaller endotracheal tubes will significantly reduce air flow because it is proportion to the fourth power of the radius. Ventilators overcome this problem by increasing flow rate to generate the preset tidal volume (if on controlled mechanical ventilation [CMV] or assist control [AC] mode) or preset pressure (if on pressure control [PC] mode). However, a patient breathing spontaneously through a small endotracheal tube will have difficulty generating the necessary higher pressure gradient through their own negative intrathoracic pressure. The work of breathing is increased, which could lead to respiratory fatigue, hypoventilation, and hypoxemia and hypercapnia.

EFFECTS OF FLOW

Fluids flowing in a laminar pattern through a horizontal tube must obey the law of conservation of energy. In this closed system, the sum of all energies (pressure or potential, and kinetic) per unit volume remains constant at all points along the line of flow (Figure 4-1). Mathematically this is expressed in the form of Bernoulli's equation:

$$P_1 + 1/2 \, \rho v_1^2 = P_2 + 1/2 \, \rho v_2^2$$

where P = pressure
ρ = density
v = flow velocity.

If there is a constriction in the tube, kinetic energy increases but the potential energy (pressure) has to decrease to maintain conservation of energy. Therefore, as the velocity of fluid increases at the point of constriction, the pressure exerted by the fluid decreases.

The Bernoulli principle gives rise to the "Venturi effect." When a fluid passes through a tube with varying diameters such as a constriction, the lateral pressure exerted by the fluid drops because of the increase in velocity. The higher flow rates through narrow constrictions can create partial negative or

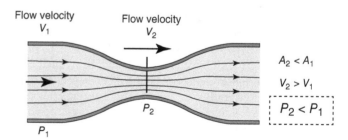

FIGURE 4-1 As the velocity of fluid increases at the point of constriction, the pressure exerted by the fluid decreases.

subatmospheric pressures. Essentially, an opening at the narrow orifice can entrain air or fluid due to the pressure drop at that site. Devices that operate on this principle include nebulizers, Venturi masks, and jet ventilators. In a nebulizer, the high flow of oxygen entrains liquid from a side tube and disperses it in droplet form. Venturi masks deliver supplemental oxygen at varying levels by drawing room air through at a low pressure point at the mask's nozzle due to high flow of 100% oxygen. The nozzle has an adjustable aperture that sets the entrainment ratio and hence the inspired concentration given to the patient. Supraglottic jet ventilation through a catheter or jet needle attached to a suspension laryngoscope also utilizes the Venturi principle to entrain room air.

The Bernoulli principle also explains the "Coandă effect." Because of the higher velocity and lower pressure at a constriction, fluid may adhere to one surface of the constriction causing maldistribution of flow. Accumulation of fluid products may lead to problems such as mucous plugging in the bronchioles or atherosclerotic plaques in the arterial circulation. The result could be unequal distribution of respiratory gases or blood flow that may lead to hypoxemia or myocardial ischemia, respectively.

5

Principles of Doppler Ultrasound

Alex Pitts-Kiefer, MD, and Lorenzo De Marchi, MD

Ultrasound imaging is frequently utilized in modern anesthesiology practice in the context of central and peripheral venous access, placement of peripheral nerve blocks, and echocardiography. Medical ultrasound utilizes longitudinal, mechanically produced high-frequency sound waves to produce a real-time image of tissue.

PRODUCTION OF ULTRASONIC SOUND WAVES

Electrical energy is converted into mechanical waves in an ultrasound probe by a transducer. Most ultrasonic transducers contain artificial polycrystalline ferroelectric materials (crystals), such as lead zirconate titanate, to produce a piezoelectric effect. A voltage is applied to two electrodes attached to the surface of the crystal that creates an electric field resulting in a dimensional change. Serial dimensional changes produce the high-frequency sound waves emitted by the ultrasound probe. The thickness of the piezoelectric element in the probe determines the frequency of the sound waves emitted.

Frequencies of sound waves:

- Infrasound: 0-20 Hz
- Audible sound: 20-20 000 Hz
- Ultrasound: greater than 20 000 Hz (>20 kHz)
- Medical ultrasound: 2 500 000–15 000 000 Hz (2.5-15 MHz)

PROPAGATION AND REFLECTION OF ULTRASONIC WAVES IN TISSUE

Contrasting mechanical properties of tissues in different anatomic structures create interfaces that result in the reflection or echo of ultrasonic waves. A transducer in the ultrasound probe is able to use the same piezoelectric effect as discussed previously to convert the reflected mechanical wave back into electrical energy. The scanner's computer represents the amplitude (strength) of the wave on the ultrasound image by a dot. The interface between tissues with differing mechanical properties, including density and compressibility, will reflect ultrasound waves with a variety of amplitudes, which are represented in the brightness of the dot on the image. The larger

TABLE 5-1 General Echogenicity of Tissues

Hyperechoic (strong reflection)	White dot on imaging	Bone, tendons, ligaments, diaphragm, peripheral nerves, liver angiomas, tumor cells, blood vessels, fibrosis, and liver steatosis.
Hyperechoic (weaker reflections)	Gray dot on imaging	Most solid organs, thick fluid.
Anechoic (no reflection)	No dot on imaging (black)	Cysts, ascites, other fluid-filled regions.

the mismatch is between the two tissues, a concept referred to as impedance mismatching, the larger the amplitude of the echo will be. The ability of a tissue interface to reflect an ultrasonic wave is called echogenicity. The term hyperechogenic or hyperechoic is used to describe tissue interfaces with many echoes. Tissue interfaces that do not produce echoes are said to be anechoic. Two tissues with the same echogenicity that are unable to be depicted separately are referred to as isoechogenic (Table 5-1).

Although some waves are reflected at the interfaces between different tissues, other waves travel deeper into the body and are reflected from deeper structures. The amount of time between the production of the ultrasound wave and its return to the probe is converted to distance (distance = velocity/time; sound travels at 1540 m/s through tissue at 37°C) and is represented on the ultrasound display as depth. The amplitude of the reflected wave and its travel time through tissue is combined to create the ultrasound image.

TRANSDUCER FREQUENCY AND WAVELENGTH

There is a range of ultrasound probes available for a variety of applications. The thickness of the piezoelectric element in the probe determines the frequency of the sound waves emitted. Increasing the frequency of the waves emitted increases the image resolution. However, this decreases the ability of the waves to penetrate the tissue. A probe that produces 12-MHz ultrasonic waves has very good resolution, but cannot penetrate very deep into the body. A probe that emits 3-MHz ultrasonic waves can penetrate deeply into the body, but has a much lower resolution than the 12-MHz probe. Therefore, it is best to select the probe able to produce the highest frequency ultrasonic wave that is able to reach the required depth.

DOPPLER ULTRASOUND

The Doppler effect is the change in frequency of a wave due to relative motion between the wave source and its receiver. This is the audible phenomenon observed when a car races by a stationary observer. When the source of the waves is moving toward the receiver, each successive wave is emitted from a position closer to the receiver than the previous wave. Each wave takes less time to reach the receiver than the previous wave, which results in an increased frequency. Conversely, if the source of waves is moving away from the receiver, each wave is emitted from a position more distant to the receiver and the frequency is reduced.

In medical ultrasound, the Doppler effect is used to measure blood flow velocity. The ultrasound probe is both the source and the receiver. As the ultrasonic wave is reflected by a red blood cell either moving toward or away from the probe, the frequency of the wave will change and the velocity of the blood can be calculated using the following formula:

$$f_d = \frac{2f_o v \cos\theta}{c}$$

where f_d is the frequency shift (also referred to as Doppler shift), f_o is the transmitted frequency, v is the velocity of blood, θ is the angle between the ultrasound beam and the direction of blood flow (referred to as angle of incidence), and c is the speed of ultrasound, which is constant.

Because the vessel/beam angle must be known for the scanner's computer to calculate the blood flow velocity, the ultrasound operator must mark the direction of the vessel axis. An angle of incidence between the ultrasound beam and blood flow of significantly less than 90 degrees is required to achieve good accuracy, which is inversely proportional to the angle of incidence.

The scanner's computer calculates the instantaneous peak velocity for each time interval throughout the cardiac cycle and produces a video and audio representation. The mean of these peak velocities can be calculated from these values. Flow coming toward the probe is represented graphically in a spectral trace above the baseline, whereas flow traveling away from the probe is represented below the baseline. The close-up of the spectral trace above represents velocity on the Y-axis and time on the X-axis. The brightness of each pixel represents the number of red blood cells moving at that velocity at that time. Thus, there are red blood cells moving at different velocities at the same time. The quality of the trace can also be used to diagnose cardiac and peripheral vascular pathology.

COLOR DOPPLER

This imaging mode superimposes areas of color representing blood flow velocities on the two-dimensional ultrasound image. It is common practice for red to represent flow toward the probe/transducer and blue to represent flow away from the probe/transducer. The main advantage of color Doppler is the ease with which vessels can be identified and their patency confirmed.

FURTHER READING

Cosgrove DO. Ultrasound: general principles. In Adam, A, Dixon, A, eds.: *Grainger & Allison's Diagnostic Radiology: A Textbook of Medical Imaging.* 5th ed. New York, NY: Churchill Livingstone; 2008.

6

Properties of Gases and Liquids

Joseph Delio and Jeffrey S. Berger, MD, MBA

Matter in the universe, defined as anything that occupies space and has mass, exists in three phases—gases, liquids, and solids. All substances are made of atoms or molecules that are constantly in motion, although not necessarily seen by the naked eye. This assumption is essential to account for many of the properties of gases and liquids.

Phases are defined as a distinct and homogeneous state of a system with no visible boundary separating it into parts. A conversion from one phase to another is given a specific name and is associated with various standard properties. For example, *condensation* occurs when a substance transitions from a gas to a liquid phase and *vaporization* occurs when a substance transitions from a liquid to gaseous phase.

LIQUIDS

1. **Volume**—Liquids occupy a definitive volume and will take on the shape of the vessel in which they are contained. Unlike a gas, the volume of a liquid does not change much, if at all, as pressure increases. The volume occupied by a given amount of a liquid is much less than that of the corresponding gas at the same temperature, because the constituent particles are much closer together in the liquid phase.
2. **Surface tension**—Surface tension is a unique property of liquids that allows them to assume a shape that has the least amount of surface area. Liquids generally form spherical droplets because spheres are a solid shape with the least surface area per unit volume. Surface tension is created by *Van der Waals' forces*, which are the sum of the attractive or repulsive forces between molecules. Particles in the bulk of the liquid are pulled in all directions by intermolecular forces, whereas particles on the surface are only pulled from molecular forces below, leading to an unbalanced force on the surface of the liquid.
3. **Boiling point**—The boiling point, or vaporization point, of a liquid occurs when its vapor pressure equals the external pressure (ambient pressure) acting on the surface of the liquid. The stronger the intermolecular forces, the lower the vapor pressure and the higher the boiling point. Vapor pressure is created by the pressure exerted on the environment from vapor that is in equilibrium with

its liquid phase. The molar mass of the substance and the intermolecular forces acting on the substance influence vapor pressure. The pressure of the atmosphere at sea level is 1 atm (760 mm Hg), but at higher altitudes, the ambient air pressure is much lower—for example, in Denver the air pressure is approximately 630 mm Hg because it is 1 mile above the sea level. This means that a liquid will boil at a lower temperature in Denver because the vapor pressure has to equal a lower external pressure before boiling compared to the usual 1 atm at sea level.

4. **Cohesive and adhesive forces**—Liquids demonstrate cohesive forces as well as adhesive forces. Cohesive forces are the attraction between a particle and other particles of the same kind such as hydrogen bonding that occurs between water molecules. In contrast, adhesive forces are the attraction between a particle and other particles of a different kind such as the attraction of a water molecule to the inside of intravenous tubing.
5. **Viscosity**—Viscosity is the amount of resistance to flow that a particular liquid has, or a measure of how thick or sticky a liquid is. It can also be thought of as the internal friction of adjacent fluid layers sliding past one another. It is governed by the strength of intermolecular forces and especially by the shape of the molecules of a liquid. Liquids, such as water, that contain polar molecules or can form hydrogen bonds are usually more viscous than similar nonpolar substances. An example is glycerol, $CH_2OHCHOHCH_2OH$, which is viscous due to the length of the molecule and also due to the extensive possibility for hydrogen bonding between molecules. Plasma also has various molecular interactions between its many components, which cause it to have a higher viscosity than water. At about 37°C, plasma is 1.8 times more viscous than water and even higher when one considers the formed elements of plasma such as red cells, white cells, and platelets. Therefore, as hematocrit increases, the viscosity of blood increases as well.

The Poiseuille equation, shown below, is used to determine the resistance of a blood vessel to blood flow, taking into account the viscosity of blood:

$$R = l\eta l/\pi r^4$$

TABLE 6-1   Physical Properties of Inhaled Anesthetics at 20°C

Property	Desflurane	N_2O	Sevoflurane	Isoflurane	Halothane
Formula	CHF_2-O-$CHFCF_3$	N_2O	CH_2F-O-$CH(CF_3)_2$	CHF_2-O-$CHClCF_3$	$CF_3CHClBr$
Boiling point (°C)	22.8		58.5	48.5	50.2
Saturated vapor pressure	700		157	240	244
Odor	Ethereal/Pungent	Sweet	Organic solvent	Ethereal/Pungent	Organic solvent

where R = resistance, η = viscosity, l = length of the vessel, and r = the radius of the vessel. There are numerous conditions where this becomes clinically important. For example, polycythemia occurs when there is an abnormally elevated hematocrit leading to increased blood viscosity. Consequently, the increased resistance requires the heart to work harder in order to perfuse vital organs. On the contrary, patients with anemia have a low hematocrit, have reduced blood viscosity, and reduced resistance to blood flow.

GASES

Inhaled anesthetic gases differ in their physical properties (Table 6-1). In contrast to liquids, gases fill the entire volume in which they are contained, and thus have lower densities than their corresponding liquid phase at the same temperature. Unlike liquids, gases will mix completely and evenly when confined to the same volume. *Pressure*, for gases, is the amount of force exerted on a surface within its volume. Pressure can be measured in the SI unit of pascals (Pa) or atmospheres (atm),

torr, millimeters of mercury (mm Hg), and pounds per square inch (psi). The following demonstrates the equivalent of 1.000 atm in the various other pressure units:

$$1.000 \text{ atm} = 1.013 \times 10^5 \text{ Pa} = 760 \text{ torr}$$
$$= 760 \text{ mm Hg} = 1.934 \times 10^{-2} \text{ psi}$$

The pressure of the atmosphere, or within any enclosed vessel, is exerted in all directions, not just downward. According to the kinetic theory of gases, the pressure of a gas is proportional to the number of molecules present divided by the volume.

Temperature is a measure of the amount of energy of the component particles. As temperature increases, the velocity at which the particles are moving increases proportionally. The standard pressure and temperature (STP) as defined by the International Union of Pure and Applied Chemistry (IUPAC) is 1.000 atm at 273 K (0°C)[5].

A *mole* of gas is simply defined as the amount of gas that will occupy a volume of 22.4 liters at STP.

Gas Laws

Joseph Delio and Jeffrey S. Berger, MD, MBA

KINETIC THEORY OF GASES

When scientists began studying the relationship between pressure, temperature, and volume of gas, they realized that all gases followed the same relationship. There are several gas laws that apply to human physiology.

The *kinetic theory of gases* makes the following assumptions:

1. The molecules in a gas are small and very far apart. The majority of volume that a gas occupies is empty space.
2. Gas molecules are in constant, random motion—just as many molecules are moving in one direction as another.
3. Molecules can and will collide with each other and with the walls of the container. Collisions with the walls account for the pressure created by the gas.
4. When collisions occur, the molecules lose no kinetic energy; that is, the collisions are said to be perfectly elastic. The total kinetic energy of all the molecules remains constant unless there is some outside force that acts on the system.
5. The molecules exert no attractive or repulsive forces on one another except during the process of collision. Between collisions, the molecules move in straight lines.

DALTON'S LAW OF PARTIAL PRESSURES

Dalton's law of partial pressures states that the partial pressure of a gas in a mixture of gases is the pressure that gas would exert if it occupied the total volume of the mixture. Dalton's law is

$$P_x = (P_B - P_{H2O}) \times F,$$

where P_x is the partial pressure of gas X (mm Hg), P_B is the barometric pressure (mm Hg), P_{H2O} is the water vapor pressure at a given temperature (mm Hg), and F is the fractional concentration of gas. For example, the partial pressure of O_2 (P_{O2}) in dry inspired air at 37°C would be calculated as follows:

$$P_{O2} = (760 \text{ mm Hg} - 0) \times 0.21 = 160 \text{ mm Hg},$$

where 760 mm Hg is the atmospheric pressure of dry air at 37°C and 0.21 is the percent oxygen composition of air. We can contrast this with air in the trachea that has been humidified by the nasal turbinates:

$$P_{O2} = (760 \text{ mm Hg} - 47 \text{ mm Hg}) \times 0.21 = 150 \text{ mm Hg},$$

where subtracting 47 mm Hg from the atmospheric pressure of 760 mm Hg corrects for the added water vapor pressure, causing the P_{O2} to be reduced by 10 mm Hg. Inhaled anesthetics will diffuse from the lungs to the blood until the partial pressures in the alveoli and blood are equal.

Dalton went on to further explain that the sum of partial pressures of all gases in a mixture equals the total pressure of the mixture as follows:

$$P_{total} = P_{gas1} + P_{gas2} + ...,$$

where P_{total} is the total pressure of the mixture, P_{gas1} is the partial pressure of gas 1, P_{gas2} is the partial pressure of gas 2, and so on. To calculate the partial pressure of each gas in a mixture, one takes the number of moles of gas and utilizes the ideal gas law, which will be discussed next.

IDEAL GAS EQUATION

The *ideal gas equation*, also known as the combined or general gas law, helps us understand quantitatively the effects of pressure and temperature on gas volume: $PV = nRT$, where P = pressure (mm Hg), V = volume (liters), n = moles (mol), R = the gas constant (0.082 atm L/mol K), and T = temperature (K). It is important to understand that when applying this equation to respiratory physiology, BTPS is used but in the liquid phase, STPD is used. BTPS means at body temperature (37°C or 310 K), ambient pressure (1 atm), and gas saturated with water vapor, whereas STPD means at standard temperature (0°C or 273 K), standard pressure (760 mm Hg), and dry gas.

There are numerous other relationships based on the ideal gas equation:

(1) Charles' law: $V_1/T_1 = V_2/T_2$

This equation can be used to determine the volume or temperature of a given substance while maintaining the pressure constant.

$$(2)\ \text{Boyle's law: } P_1 V_1 = P_2 V_2$$

Similarly, this equation can be used to determine the volume or pressure of a given substance while maintaining the temperature constant. Pockets of trapped gas in the body (ie, the middle ear, paranasal sinuses, intestinal gas, pneumothorax, and gas pockets within monitoring and life support systems) will contract and expand in response to a change in pressure and will follow Boyle's law. For example, doubling the environmental pressure will cause the volume of gas in the middle ear to decrease by half.

$$(3)\ \text{Gay Lussac's law: } P_1 / T_1 = P_2 / T_2$$

This equation can be used to determine the pressure or temperature of a given substance while maintaining the volume constant.

ALVEOLAR GAS EQUATION

The *alveolar gas equation* is used to predict the alveolar P_{O2} based on the alveolar P_{CO2}, and is expressed as follows:

$$Pa_{O2} = PI_{O2} - (Pa_{CO2}/R) + \text{Correction factor,}$$

where Pa_{O2} is the alveolar P_{O2} (mm Hg), PI_{O2} is the P_{O2} of inspired air (mm Hg), Pa_{CO2} is the alveolar P_{CO2} (mm Hg), R is the respiratory exchange ratio or respiratory quotient (CO_2 production/O_2 consumption), and the correction factor is small and usually not taken into account. PI_{O2} is calculated in accordance with Dalton's law of partial pressures:

$$PI_{O2} = FIO_2\ (P_b - P_{H2O}),$$

where FIO_2 is the fraction of inspired oxygen. The respiratory exchange ratio is usually 0.8; however, if the rate of CO_2 production or O_2 consumption change relative to one another, the respiratory exchange ratio will affect the Pa_{O2}. This equation becomes very useful when initiating or monitoring the settings of mechanical ventilation.

HENRY'S LAW

Henry's law is used to determine the concentration of a gas that has been dissolved in a solution: for example, O_2 and CO_2 that has been dissolved in blood, or the concentration of anesthetic in a tissue or the blood. It is important to understand that at equilibrium, the partial pressure of a gas in the liquid phase equals the partial pressure in the gas phase. Henry's law is used to convert the partial pressure of gas in the liquid phase to the concentration of gas in the liquid phase. *Solubility* is the term used to describe the tendency of a gas to equilibrate with a solution, and hence determining its concentration in a solution. *Henry's law* is expressed as follows:

$$C_X = P_X \times \text{Solubility,}$$

where C_X is the concentration of dissolved gas X (mL gas/100 mL blood), P_X is the partial pressure of gas X (mm Hg), and solubility is the solubility of the gas in blood (mL gas/100 mL blood/mm Hg). It is extremely important to recognize that the calculated concentration of gas only takes into account the gas that is free in solution and not in a bound form (ie, gas bound to hemoglobin or to plasma proteins). If the partial pressure of the gas is doubled, the concentration will be doubled as well.

Vaporizers

Sonia John and Jeffrey S. Berger, MD, MBA

Vaporizers are closed containers where the conversion of a volatile anesthetic from liquid to vapor takes place. Modern vaporizers are specific to the particular anesthetic agent and account for temperature and flow to deliver a consistent concentration of agent. The operator controls precise delivery of volatile agent concentration with a calibrated dial.

PHYSICS OF VAPORIZATION

At operating room temperatures, volatile anesthetics exist in both liquid phase and gas phase in vaporizers. The *latent heat of vaporization* is the number of calories required at a specific temperature to convert 1 g of a liquid into a vapor. As the temperature of the liquid decreases, the heat of vaporization necessary for molecules to leave the liquid phase increases. When equilibrium between the liquid phase and vapor phase is reached, vaporization ceases as an equal number of molecules enter and leave the liquid phase.

Specific heat is the calories required for 1 g of a substance to increase by 1°C. Knowledge of the specific heat of an anesthetic agent allows for vaporizers to be designed such that the correct amount of heat can be added to maintain the temperature of the liquid as vaporization occurs. In addition, vaporizer components are designed with a high specific heat to minimize temperature change.

As anesthetic agent molecules collide with each other in the walls of the vaporizer, a pressure is created, known as the *saturated vapor pressure*, which is unique for each volatile anesthetic (Table 8-1). Vapor pressure is independent of atmospheric pressure, but dependent on the physical characteristics of the liquid. Vapor pressure also depends on

TABLE 8-1 Vapor Pressure

Volatile Anesthetic Agent	Vapor Pressure (mm Hg) at 20°C
Halothane	243
Isoflurane	240
Desflurane	681
Sevoflurane	160

temperature such that a decrease in temperature corresponds to lower vapor pressure (fewer molecules in vapor phase). The *boiling point* of a liquid is the temperature at which the vapor pressure equals atmospheric pressure. Cooling the liquid anesthetic is undesirable because it lowers the vapor pressure and, therefore, limits the attainable vapor concentration. Modern vaporizers are temperature compensated.

VARIABLE BYPASS VAPORIZERS

Most vaporizers (Tec 4, Tec 5, SevoTec, Vapor 19.n, Vapor 2000, and Aladin) are considered to have a variable bypass carrier gas flow and a flow-over vaporization method. Not all of the entering gas is exposed to the anesthetic liquid; some gas is exposed whereas the rest bypasses the agent. These vaporizers are agent specific, temperature compensated, and are located outside of the circuit, between the flowmeters and the common gas outlet.

Basic Principles and Components (Figure 8-1)

Variable bypass vaporizers consist of the concentration control dial, the bypass chamber, the vaporizing chamber, the filler port, and the filler cap. The variable bypass vaporizer splits the fresh gas flow into two portions—the first, roughly 20%, going into the vaporizing chamber, where it is saturated with the anesthetic vapor, and the second portion going to the bypass chamber. Subsequently, the gases mix at the patient outlet side of the vaporizer. Ultimately, the concentration of volatile anesthetic delivered to the patient is determined by the concentration control dial, which is given in volume percent for the specific anesthetic agent.

The amount of liquid volatile anesthetic can be approximated from the formula: $3 \times \text{Fresh gas flow (L/min)} \times \text{Volume \%} = \text{Liquid of volatile anesthetic per hour (mL)}$

The filler port is where the liquid anesthetic is poured into the vaporizing chamber. Overfilling or tilting the vaporizer could result in spilling the liquid into the bypass chamber potentially resulting in the vaporizer chamber flow and bypass chamber flow carrying saturated amounts of anesthetic vapor, which could cause an overdose.

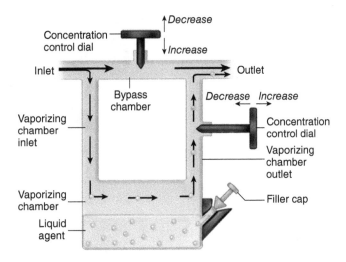

FIGURE 8-1 Generic schematic of agent-specific variable bypass vaporizer. (Reproduced with permission from Barash PG, *Clinical Anesthesia*, 7th ed. Philadelphia, PA: Wolters Kluwer Health/ Lippincott Williams & Wilkins; 2013.)

Flow Rates

The rate of flow affects the vaporizer output especially at rates at the extreme ends of the spectrum. For example, at low flow rates (<0.250 L/min) the output is less than the setting because of the insufficient turbulence generated in the vaporizer chamber to advance the vapor molecules upward. At high flow rates (15 L/min) the output is also less than the dial setting. This is due to the incomplete mixing and failure to saturate the carrier gas in the vaporizing chamber. Furthermore, the resistance characteristics of the bypass chamber and the vaporizing chamber can vary as flow increases, and this ultimately results in decreased output concentration.

Temperature Compensation

The variable bypass vaporizer is temperature compensated because of its temperature-sensitive bimetallic strip or expansion element. The temperature-sensing elements allow increased gas inflow into the vaporizer chamber as the temperature of the liquid anesthetic in the vaporizer decreases. For example, the vapor pressure inside the vaporizing chamber is high in the operating rooms of pediatric patients and burn patients because of the relatively high ambient temperature. In this situation, the bimetallic strip of the temperature-compensating valve leans to the right, decreasing the resistance to flow through the bypass chamber, thus creating more flow to pass through the bypass chamber and less flow to pass through the vaporizing chamber. The bimetallic strip leans to the left in situations when the OR temperature is colder, causing a decrease in vapor pressure in the vaporizing chamber.

Thermally conductive metals, such as bronze or copper, are often used in the production of vaporizers to minimize heat loss, allowing nearly linear output from 20°C to 35°C. In addition, highly conductive metals allow for internal temperature to be maintained uniform.

Intermittent Back Pressure

New variable bypass vaporizers are relatively immune from a process known as the "pumping effect." The pumping effect occurs from intermittent back pressure that results from either positive pressure ventilation or the use of the oxygen flush valve resulting in higher than expected vaporizer output. This effect is more pronounced at low flow rates, low dial settings, and low levels of liquid anesthetic in the vaporizing chamber. It is also increased in rapid respiratory rates, high peak inspired pressures, and rapid drops in pressure during exhalation. However, a smaller vaporizing chamber in newer systems diminishes the pumping effect.

Safety Features

Hazards still associated with variable bypass vaporizers include: contamination, tipping, overfilling, underfilling, simultaneous inhaled anesthetic administration, and leaks. The newer vaporizers, as mentioned before, have built-in safety features such as agent-specific keyed filling devices to help prevent filling a vaporizer with the wrong agent. Furthermore, overfilling is minimized because the filler port is located at the maximum safe liquid level on the side of the machine, and the vaporizer is secured to a manifold on the anesthesia workstation, minimizing tipping. Although there are two to three anesthetic-specific vaporizers present at a time on the anesthetic machine, there is a safety interlock mechanism that ensures that only one vaporizer at a time can be turned on. These considerations have minimized hazards that are associated with variable bypass vaporizers.

Modern variable bypass vaporizers are pressure compensated to account for changes in altitude. They accomplish this by splitting flow at the exit of the vaporizer chamber; consequently, for any percent volume dialed and fresh gas flow delivered, the volume of saturated vapor that leaves the vaporizing chamber is constant. The partial pressure of the anesthetic delivered, the key value for determining anesthetic effect in the brain, is virtually unaffected by the change in altitude.

SPECIAL VAPORIZERS

Desflurane Vaporizer (Tec 6 and D-Vapor)

The vapor pressure of desflurane is 3–4 times that of other contemporary inhaled anesthetics (near 1 atm at 20°C) and it boils at 22.8°C. These factors have necessitated a unique vaporizer design to prevent vaporization at room temperature.

In the Tec 6, the vaporizer has two independent gas circuits arranged in parallel. The fresh gas from the flowmeters enters at the fresh gas inlet, passing through a fixed restrictor (R1), and exits the vaporizer gas outlet. The vapor circuit arises at the desflurane sump, a reservoir of desflurane vapor, which is electrically heated and thermostatically controlled to 39°C, well above its boiling point. The heated sump serves as a reservoir for desflurane vapor. Downstream from the sump is the shutoff valve, which fully opens when the concentration control valve is turned to the on position. Desflurane output can be controlled by adjusting the concentration control valve (R2) which is a variable restrictor. The pressure supplying R1 and R2 are equal and is called the working pressure. The fresh gas flow rate and the working pressure abide by a linear relationship with electronic controls.

The Tec 6 maintains a closed system when filling the anesthetic gas, which allows for filling while in use, and also minimizes spillage.

Desflurane vaporizers will maintain a constant concentration of vapor output by volume percent without pressure compensation. Hence, at high altitude, the partial pressure of desflurane will decrease according to the following formula: Required dial setting (% vol) = Normal dial setting (% vol/vol ×760 mm Hg)/Ambient pressure (mm Hg).

At low flow rates, if the carrier gas is less than 100% oxygen, desflurane vaporizer output is less than expected because it is calibrated with 100% oxygen carrier gas. This is due to the reduction of carrier gas viscosity. Nitrous oxide has roughly 20% lower viscosity than oxygen, so, at low flow rates, the output is lower when nitrous oxide is mixed with oxygen as the carrier gas.

Cassette Vaporizers (Aladin)

Cassette vaporizers are very similar to the variable bypass vaporizers mentioned earlier, in that they are made up of a bypass chamber and a vaporizing chamber. However, this unique system is designed to deliver different inhaled anesthetics.

This system has a permanent internal control unit and an interchangeable color and magnetically coded agent cassette that houses the anesthetic liquid. The bypass chamber houses a fixed restrictor and flow measurement sensors (also in the outlet of the vaporizing chamber). Also unique to this system is that it has an electronically regulated flow control valve located in the vaporizing chamber outlet. The system receives input from the concentration control dial, a pressure sensor, a temperature sensor, and two flow measurement units, one located in the bypass chamber and the other in the vaporizing chamber. It also receives input from flowmeters regarding the composition of the carrier gas. A computer then precisely regulates the flow control valve to attain the desired vapor concentration output.

Also unique to the cassette system is a one-way check valve through which a portion of the gas enters after passing through the inlet of the vaporizing chamber. This valve prevents retrograde flow of the anesthetic back into the bypass chamber, and is crucial when delivering desflurane if the room temperature is greater than the boiling point for desflurane.

Injection Vaporizers (Maquet)

Similar to traditional variable bypass vaporizers it has a graduated concentration knob, keyed fill port with plug and locking screw, and a fill level inspection window. Additionally, it has an on/off switch with a safety lock.

Mixed gas flows into the vaporizer through a regulator valve, which prevents flow into the gas circuit when the ventilator bellows are full. When the bellows are empty, gas flows into the vaporizer when the on/off switch is set to the "on" position. The adjustable throttle valve restricts gas flow in the vaporizer and allows control of pressure by directing excess gas into the liquid reservoir. The gas pressure within the reservoir forces the anesthetic agent through a vaporization nozzle and back into the gas stream. The delivered concentration is mostly independent of the ventilator settings and there is no need for temperature compensation because there is no vaporization of agent.

Uptake and Distribution of Inhalational Agents

Medhat Hannallah, MD

9

BASIC PRINCIPLES

According to Henry's law, gas solubility describes the tendency of a gas to equilibrate with a solution. When a gas comes into contact with a solution, the gas molecules will move into and dissolve in the liquid. Some of the gas molecules will then move back from the liquid phase to the gas phase. At equilibrium, the number of gas molecules moving from the gas phase to the liquid phase will equal the number of molecules moving from the liquid phase to the gas phase. For example, equilibrium exists when arterial blood with a Pao_2 of 100 mm Hg contacts an alveolar gas mixture also with PO_2 of 100 mm Hg (Figure 9-1). There is no net gain or loss of O_2 between the two phases.

The pharmacologic effect of an inhalation agent is determined by the partial pressure of the anesthetic in the brain. At equilibrium, brain partial pressure equals the anesthetic partial pressure in arterial blood. In the absence of transpulmonary shunt, alveolar gases equilibrate with pulmonary capillary and arterial blood gases. The partial pressure of the anesthetic in arterial blood, therefore, will equal its alveolar partial pressure.

According to Dalton's law, the total pressure exerted by a mixture of gases is equal to the sum of the partial pressures of individual gases. By applying Dalton's law, it is possible to calculate the alveolar partial pressure of an inhalation agent: the product of the total gas pressure (atmospheric pressure) multiplied by the fraction of alveolar concentration (FA) of the anesthetic. For example, if the FA of desflurane is 5% and the atmospheric pressure is 760 mm Hg, then the alveolar partial pressure of desflurane will be $760 \times 0.05 = 38$ mm Hg. In the absence of transpulmonary shunt, desflurane partial

pressure in arterial blood and in the brain will also be 38 mm Hg (Figure 9-2).

The partial pressure of a gas in a liquid at a certain temperature is primarily determined by the solubility of that gas in the liquid. Higher gas solubility within a liquid results in lower gas partial pressures. Gas exerts more pressure in a liquid if the gas molecules exist in a free kinetic form within the liquid. Greater solubility means that the gas molecules are more tightly bound to the liquid molecules, resulting in less free, active gas molecules available to exert pressure. This relationship explains the counterintuitive phenomenon that the partial pressure of a highly soluble inhalation agent rises slowly in the blood despite the fact that it is taken up in large quantities by the blood. Despite the fact that there is considerably more dissolved CO_2 than dissolved O_2 in arterial blood, normal $Paco_2$ is 40 mm Hg and normal Pao_2 is

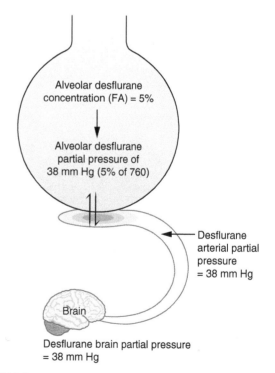

FIGURE 9-2 Desflurane equilibrium across tissues.

Alveolar desflurane concentration (FA) = 5%

Alveolar desflurane partial pressure of 38 mm Hg (5% of 760)

Desflurane arterial partial pressure = 38 mm Hg

Brain

Desflurane brain partial pressure = 38 mm Hg

Gas phase
Atmospheric pressure (760 mm Hg)
O_2 Concentration = 13%
→ Po_2 of 100 mm Hg (13% of 760)
Blood/Liquid phase

Po_2 100 mm Hg

Po_2 100 mm Hg

Equilibrium

FIGURE 9-1 At equilibrium, the partial pressure of O_2 in both the liquid and the gas phases is equal.

100 mm Hg. The reason: CO_2 gas molecules are much more soluble in blood than O_2 molecules.

FACTORS DETERMINING ALVEOLAR CONCENTRATION

The alveolar concentration (FA) of a volatile inhalation anesthetic depends on two primary variables: (1) delivery of the agent to the lungs; and (2) uptake of the agent by the blood (Figure 9-3). In general, the rate of rise of FA increases with a higher rate of anesthetic delivery and decreases with a greater degree of anesthetic blood uptake from the lungs. These factors will have different effects on agents depending on their solubility, such as high blood solubility (eg, ether) versus agents with low blood solubility (eg, desflurane).

Factors Determining the Rate of Delivery of Inhalation Agents to the Lung

A. Alveolar Ventilation

Increased ventilation augments anesthetics delivery to the lungs. This augmentation is greater with ether than with desflurane. With the poorly blood-soluble desflurane FA rises rapidly, irrespective of ventilation because of the minimal blood uptake. Increased ventilation carries only a small additional benefit. With the highly soluble drug ether FA rises slowly, because most of the agent delivered to the lungs is taken up by the blood. Augmentation of ether delivery to the alveoli by increased ventilation compensates for the large blood uptake.

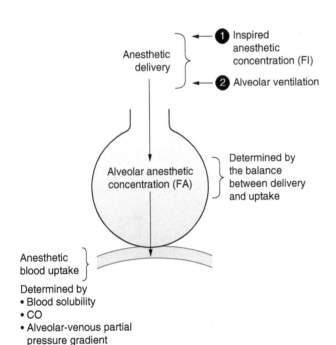

FIGURE 9-3 Factors affecting alveolar anesthetic concentrations.

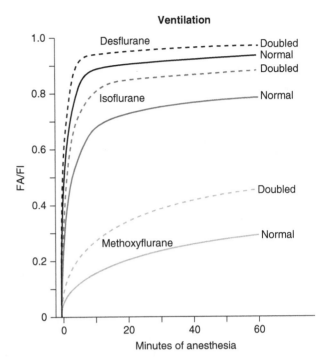

FIGURE 9-4 FA/FI rises more rapidly if ventilation is increased. (Reproduced with permission from Miller RD, *Miller's Anesthesia*, 7th ed. Philadelphia, PA: Churchill Livingstone/Elsevier; 2010.)

Figure 9-4 demonstrates how doubling alveolar ventilation increases the rate of rise in FA/fraction of inspired concentration (FI). The increase is more profound in highly blood-soluble anesthetics (methoxyflurane) and least with the least soluble anesthetic (desflurane).

B. Inspired Concentration

Increasing the FI accelerates the rate of rise of the FA. Overpressurization describes the brief use of higher vaporizer setting than the desired FA to shorten the time needed to reach that target FA. FI is different from the concentration of the agent at the fresh gas outlet of the anesthesia machine since the fresh gas is immediately diluted by the gas in the circuit which is 7–8 liters in volume. The rate at which FI approaches the fresh gas concentration (wash-in time) is greatly influenced by the type of circuit and the fresh gas flow (FGF). Higher FGF leads to shorter wash-in time.

Factors Determining the Uptake of Inhalation Agents by the Blood

A. Solubility

Greater solubility of an anesthetic in blood will lead to a higher rate of blood uptake from the lungs. In the case of highly soluble inhalational agents, the enhanced blood uptake depletes the alveoli of the anesthetics and lowers their FA and partial pressure. The low alveolar anesthetic partial pressure leads to low arterial anesthetic partial pressure. The slow induction with highly soluble anesthetics occurs despite (and because of) their large blood uptake from the alveoli. In contrast, the blood

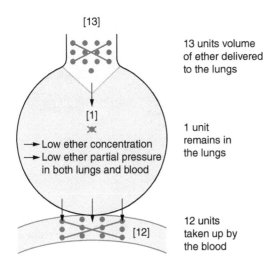

FIGURE 9-5 The low ether partial pressure in the blood occurs because of (or despite) the large blood uptake from the lungs.

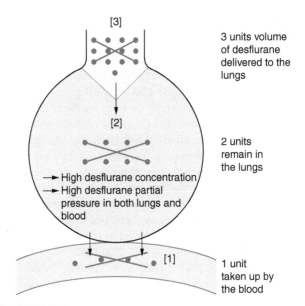

FIGURE 9-6 The high desflurane partial pressure in the blood occurs because of the small blood uptake from the lungs.

uptake of poorly soluble inhalational anesthetics from the alveoli is small. As a result, the FA and partial pressure of these anesthetics rise rapidly. This leads to rapid rise in arterial and brain anesthetic partial pressure and rapid anesthesia induction.

Solubility of inhalation agents in the blood is expressed quantitatively by its blood–gas partition coefficient, which describes the partitioning of the agent between the blood and the alveoli. Older and more highly soluble inhalation agents have high blood–gas partition coefficients. For example, the blood–gas partition coefficient of ether is 12. Therefore, delivery of 13 units volume of ether to the lungs will lead to 12 units taken up by the blood and only 1 unit remaining in the alveoli (Figure 9-5). This large uptake by the blood depletes the lungs of ether, resulting in low ether concentration in the lungs and low ether partial pressure in the lungs, blood, and brain. Since the anesthetic effect of an inhalation agent is determined by its arterial partial pressure, the large blood uptake of ether results in delayed anesthesia induction. In contrast, nitrous oxide and the modern inhalation agents such as sevoflurane and desflurane are poorly soluble in blood. With a blood–gas partition coefficient close to 0.5, delivery of 3 units volume to the lungs will lead to 1 unit taken up by the blood and 2 units remaining in the alveoli (Figure 9-6). This small blood uptake results in rapid rise of the alveolar anesthetic concentration and partial pressure, blood and brain partial pressures, and finally rapid anesthesia induction.

B. Cardiac Output

With higher cardiac output (CO), a greater volume of blood will perfuse the lungs and remove more inhalation anesthetic from the alveoli. This increased uptake decreases the concentration of the anesthetic in the lungs, which ultimately lowers alveolar, arterial, and brain partial pressure, leading to a delay in anesthetic induction. Similar to the effects of ventilation, changes in CO affects the FA of highly soluble agents more than it does the FA of poorly soluble ones. Since most of a

highly soluble drug is taken up by the blood, any significant reduction in CO significantly decreases the blood uptake and increases the alveolar and arterial partial pressures. In contrast, a decrease in CO has minimal effect on the alveolar and arterial partial pressure of a poorly soluble anesthetic since its blood uptake is already minimal. Figure 9-7 demonstrates how doubling CO decreases the rate of rise in FA/FI. The decrease is more profound in highly soluble agents.

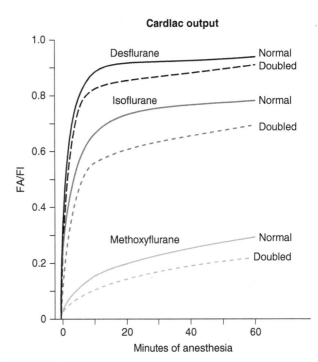

FIGURE 9-7 An increase in CO will decrease alveolar anesthetic concentration by augmenting uptake. (Reproduced with permission from Miller RD, *Miller's Anesthesia*, 7th ed. Philadelphia, PA: Churchill Livingstone/Elsevier; 2010.)

C. Alveolar-to-Venous Anesthetic Partial Pressure Gradient

At the start of induction, the partial pressure of an inhalation agent in mixed venous blood is zero, and its blood uptake from the lungs is maximal. Different body tissues gradually take up the agent from arterial blood, allowing for eventual equilibrium between tissues and blood. As the anesthetic partial pressure in the tissue approaches that of arterial blood, uptake into the tissues gradually decreases. The lower uptake leads to a rise in mixed venous anesthetic partial pressure, a decrease in the alveolar-to-venous anesthetic partial pressure gradient, and a decrease in blood anesthetic uptake from the lungs.

Factors that determine anesthetic uptake into the tissues parallel those that determine blood anesthetic uptake from the lungs: tissue solubility, tissue blood flow, and arterial-to-tissue anesthetic partial pressure difference. Tissue blood flow is the most important of these factors since anesthetic solubility in different tissues (tissue–blood partition coefficient) does not vary widely compared to tissue blood flow. All tissues are, therefore, classified into different groups based on their blood flow:

1. The **vessel-rich group (VRG)**, the brain, heart, splanchnic bed, and liver, comprises less than 10% of the body weight and receives 75% of the CO. The small volume of this group relative to its perfusion leads to its near-complete equilibration within 4–8 minutes.
2. The **muscle group (MG)**, muscle and skin, comprises 50% of the body weight and receives 20% of the CO. It is responsible for most of the uptake beyond 8 minutes and requires 2–4 hours to approach equilibrium.
3. The **fat group (FG)** is relatively poorly perfused but has great affinity for anesthetics, a property that greatly lengthens its equilibration time.

D. Alveolar-to-Inspired Anesthetic Concentration Relationship (FA/FI)

The alveolar anesthetic partial pressure (FA) determines the anesthetic partial pressure in all body tissues, including the brain. Since the inspired anesthetic concentration (FI) determines the FA, the speed of anesthetic induction depends on the rate at which FA approaches FI (Figure 9-8). There are several important take-home points from this relationship, which are outlined below.

- The initial rate rises rapidly for all anesthetics because of the initial absence of uptake. Uptake then increasingly opposes the effect of ventilation driving FA upward.

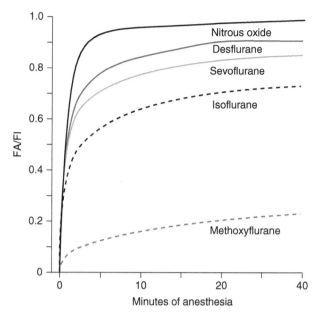

FIGURE 9-8 Rate of rise of FA/FI is faster for more insoluble agents. (Reproduced with permission from Miller RD, *Miller's Anesthesia*, 7th ed. Philadelphia, PA: Churchill Livingstone/Elsevier; 2010.)

Ultimately, a balance is struck between anesthetic delivery to the alveoli and its removal by blood uptake. The height of the FA/FI ratio at which the balance is achieved depends on the anesthetic solubility in blood. Since greater solubility increases uptake, the initial rapid rise in FA/FI is halted at a lower level with more soluble agents. Therefore, the first "knee" of the curve is higher for desflurane than for ether.

- After the first "knee," FA/FI continues to rise at a slower rate. This rise results from the progressive decrease in uptake by the VRG. After about 8 minutes, uptake by the VRG is almost complete, and three-quarters of the CO returning to the lungs contain nearly as much anesthetic as it did when it left the lungs. The resulting decrease in alveolar-to-venous partial pressure difference decreases blood uptake and drives FA upward to a second "knee" at roughly 8 minutes.
- With saturation of the VRG, the MG and the FG become the main determinants of tissue uptake. The very slow uptake by these two groups produces the gradual ascent of the terminal portion of the FA/FI ratio.
- Factors that enhance FA (such as increased ventilation, decreased CO, or low blood solubility) increase the rate of rise in FA/FI. The opposite effect is brought about by factors that tend to lower FA, such as decreased ventilation, increased CO, or high blood solubility.

Concentration and Second Gas Effects

Medhat Hannallah, MD

The concentration and second gas effects are two interesting phenomena that are pertinent in understanding the uptake and distribution of the potent inhalation anesthetics. With the possible exception of nitrous oxide (N_2O), the clinical significance, however, is limited.

CONCENTRATION EFFECT

Increasing the fraction of inspired concentration (FI) of an inhalation anesthetic will more rapidly increase the fraction of alveolar concentration (FA) of that agent. However, increasing the FI will also increase the *rate* at which the FA approaches the FI (FA/FI ratio).

As shown in Figure 10-1, the administration of 65% nitrous oxide produces a more rapid rise in its FA/FI ratio as

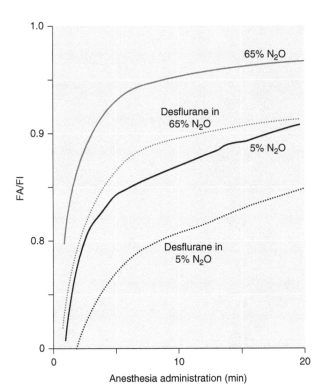

FIGURE 10-1 Concentration (continuous curves) and second gas effect (dashed curves). (Reproduced with permission from Miller RD, *Miller's Anesthesia*, 7th ed. Philadelphia, PA: Churchill Livingstone/Elsevier; 2010.)

compared to the administration of 5% nitrous oxide. To help explain this concentration effect, we will examine the hypothetical scenario of nitrous oxide delivered at 100% FI. Recall that the FA of N_2O is determined by the balance between its delivery to the alveoli and its uptake by the blood. At a hypothetical 100% FI, uptake of N_2O creates a void that draws gas down the trachea to replace the gas taken up by the blood. Because the replacement gas concentration is 100% N_2O, uptake cannot modify the FA. As the FI decreases, blood uptake will be replaced with a lower concentration of nitrous oxide. As a result, the rate at which the FA approaches the FI slows down. Remember that the curve of FA/FI versus time rises more quickly with nitrous oxide than with desflurane despite their nearly equal blood–gas partition coefficients (see Chapter 9, Figure 9-8). Note that in this comparison, N_2O was given at an FI of 70%, whereas desflurane was given in a concentration of 2%. If two agents with identical blood–gas partition coefficients were delivered at identical FIs, their FA/FI ratio would be identical.

This concentration effect has two components:

1. **Concentrating effect**—Consider the administration of 80% (80 volumes per 100 volumes) nitrous oxide to a patient. If 50% of the nitrous oxide is taken up by the blood from the lungs, the remaining 40 volumes will exist in a total of 60 volumes, yielding a concentration of 67%. In other words, the uptake of half the nitrous oxide does not simply halve the concentration because the remaining gases are concentrated in a smaller volume. Now consider the administration of 20% nitrous oxide (20 volumes per 100 volumes) with the same 50% uptake. In this scenario, 10 volumes will be taken up by the blood while 10 volumes remain in the lungs in a total of 90 volumes, yielding an 11% concentration. Therefore, increasing the inspired nitrous oxide concentration fourfold (20%-80%) will increase nitrous oxide FA about sixfold (11%-67%). The higher the FA, the greater the concentrating effect.

2. **Augmentation of inspired ventilation**—As gas leaves the lungs for the blood, new gas at the original FI enters the lungs to replace that which is taken up by the blood. The void created by the uptake of 40 volumes is filled by drawing into the lungs an equal volume of gas containing

80% nitrous oxide. That augmentation of inspired ventilation will result in a final nitrous oxide concentration of 72%.

SECOND GAS EFFECT

During inhalation induction in children, sevoflurane is frequently used together with nitrous oxide to speed up induction. The benefit of using the two agents does not only result from combining the potency of two agents, but also from the fact that nitrous oxide will also increase the rate at which the FA of sevoflurane approaches its FI, the so-called second gas effect.

The factors that are responsible for the second gas effect are similar to those that govern the concentration effect. Figure 10-2A illustrates the scenario where 80% nitrous oxide is given together with 1% of a second gas. The loss of volume associated with the uptake of nitrous oxide concentrates the potent anesthetic. Uptake of 50% of the nitrous oxide increases the second gas concentration to 1.7% (Figure 10-2B). Replacement of the gas taken up by an increase in inspired ventilation

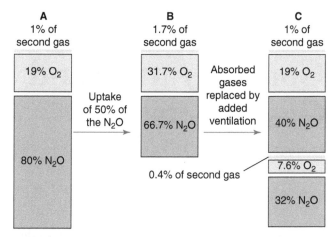

FIGURE 10-2 Second gas effect. (Reproduced with permission from Miller RD, *Miller's Anesthesia*, 7th ed. Philadelphia, PA: Churchill Livingstone/Elsevier; 2010.)

augments the amount of potent anesthetic present in the lung (Figure 10-2C). This phenomenon helps explain why the FA/FI ratio for 4% desflurane rises more rapidly when coadministered with 65% N_2O than with 5% N_2O (Figure 10-1).

Nitrous Oxide and Closed Spaces

Brian S. Freeman, MD

Nitrous oxide is one of the oldest inorganic inhalation anesthetics still used in practice today to achieve unconsciousness. This odorless gas, which can support combustion, is most commonly administered in a concentration of 50%-75% in oxygen. Because it has a minimum alveolar concentration (MAC) value of 104%, nitrous oxide is a weak anesthetic that is typically used as part of a balanced technique with a potent volatile inhalation agent and opioids. Due to the second gas effect, giving high concentrations of nitrous oxide will help increase the alveolar concentration of a second, simultaneously given volatile agent. The solubility of N_2O in blood is very low (blood/gas partition coefficient of 0.47), resulting in faster equilibration of partial pressures between blood and alveolus and rapid induction and emergence.

Compared to other inhalation agents, nitrous oxide has unique physiologic effects. It is neither a vasodilator, nor does it cause hypotension. It is actually sympathomimetic and increases both cardiac output and systemic vascular resistance. In the lungs, nitrous oxide does not inhibit hypoxic pulmonary vasoconstriction, so there may be an increase in pulmonary vascular resistance, especially in patients with known pulmonary hypertension. Unlike other inhalation agents, nitrous oxide has no known effect on uterine contractility and does not cause skeletal muscle relaxation. It has been shown to increase the risk of postoperative nausea and vomiting. It also has mild analgesic properties, with about 30% nitrous oxide by face mask producing the equivalent of 10-15 mg morphine. Prolonged use of nitrous oxide can lead to a megaloblastic anemia. This is because nitrous oxide can oxidize the cobalt atom within vitamin B_{12}, therefore inhibiting vitamin B_{12}-dependent enzymes such as methionine synthetase, which are important for DNA synthesis.

If nitrous oxide is included as part of a balanced general anesthetic, significant amount can enter closed gas spaces within the body. This assumes that the patient is receiving an inspired anesthetic gas mixture consisting of 70% nitrous oxide/30% oxygen. Preoxygenation and denitrogenation of the alveoli will not necessarily remove all the nitrogen molecules from preexisting pockets of air (21% oxygen, 78% nitrogen) in the patient, such as in an obstructed small bowel. Nitrogen is highly insoluble (blood/gas partition coefficient 0.015) and, therefore, is "trapped" in these gas compartments

and does not pass easily from gas to blood. Based on a blood/gas coefficient of 0.47, nitrous oxide therefore is roughly 34 times more soluble than nitrogen. Nitrous oxide will quickly and readily transfer across membranes and enter these closed gas-filled spaces more than 30 times faster than nitrogen will diffuse out of the space proportionally. The transfer of nitrous oxide into these closed air spaces does not influence how quickly it achieves its alveolar partial pressure (FA/FI).

Since the entrance of nitrous oxide into the closed air space is not balanced by an equal loss of nitrogen, a significant increase in volume may result from the entrance of more nitrous oxide molecules. This volume depends on two variables: (1) time; and (2) inspired (then alveolar) concentration of nitrous oxide. At equilibrium, the concentration of N_2O in the closed gas space equals its inspired concentration. A patient breathing 50% inspired nitrous oxide will quickly have a gas space comprised at equilibrium of final 50% N_2O concentration (plus the original oxygen and nitrogen). For this to occur, the gas space volume will double. A higher inspired alveolar nitrous oxide concentration of 75% could even cause a theoretical fourfold increase in volume to have a final N_2O concentration in the gas space of 75% at equilibrium). These relationships can be expressed by the equation $V_F/V_0 = 1/(1 - F_{N2O})$, where V_F is the final gas pocket volume, V_0 is the initial volume, and F_{N2O} is the fraction of N_2O in the inspired gas.

The pathophysiologic significance of these changes depends on the compliance of the walls enclosing the gas space. Highly compliant cavities such as the bowel and the pleural space will experience an increase in volume. Poorly compliant spaces such as the middle ear will have an increase in intracavity pressure. Depending on the space and rate of increase, as well as tissue perfusion, this can be dangerous and lead to poor outcomes. Well-perfused tissues such as the lung can experience an increase in volume quite quickly, whereas less well-perfused tissues such as the middle ear may require a longer period of time to achieve the same increase in volume. The following clinical scenarios are examples in which administration of nitrous oxide is contraindicated.

1. **Intestinal obstruction**—Patients with an acute bowel obstruction or ileus will have air trapped in gas spaces

within the bowel. Administration of nitrous oxide will expand this highly compliant space as N_2O diffuses from the blood into the air space. The volume of air can actually double within 4 hours of giving N_2O. The larger size of the bowel may make the surgery more difficult to complete, and it could even rupture. High intraluminal pressures in the bowel may also significantly decrease perfusion.

2. **Pneumothorax**—The pleural space is a highly compliant compartment. The size of the air pocket within a pneumothorax can double within 10 minutes and even triple within 30 minutes if the patient receives 75% nitrous oxide. The resulting life-threatening tension pneumothorax may significantly decrease cardiopulmonary function.

3. **Vascular air embolus**—Nitrous oxide should be used with caution in surgical procedures which carry a potential risk of air embolism, such as laparoscopy, spine surgery, hip arthroplasty, and posterior fossa craniotomy. Diffusion of nitrous oxide into air bubbles within the blood will increase their size. The expansion of a compliant air embolus in the blood because of N_2O to its final lethal volume can be extremely rapid, occurring within seconds. If an air embolus is suspected intraoperatively, N_2O should be immediately discontinued.

4. **Chronic obstructive pulmonary disease (COPD)**—Patients with significant COPD have large air-filled spaces called blebs within the lung parenchyma. The diffusion of N_2O into these blebs could cause enlargement and possible rupture, leading to an intraoperative pneumothorax.

5. **Laparoscopy**—Nitrous oxide should not be used during laparoscopic procedures such as cholecystectomy. It will diffuse in the lumen of the bowel and cause bowel distension, which can make the operation very technically difficult by distorting the laparoscopic view. It also could serve as a source of combustion.

6. **Intraocular air**—Sulfur hexafluoride (SF6) and perfluoropropane (C3F8) are inorganic gases that can be injected along with air into the vitreous cavity during operations to repair a detached retina. After injection, the gas bubble will expand within 48 hours (SF6 by 2.5 times and C3F8 by 4 times) in the posterior chamber serves to tamponade the retina while adhesions develop, flatten the retina, and promote healing. SF6 will remain in the vitrea for about 10-14 days and C3F8 for 60 days before it is slowly absorbed in the blood. The administration of N_2O can rapidly diffuse into the gas bubble faster than nitrogen will leave and cause a significant increase in intraocular pressure, which

can decrease retinal blood flow, which could cause retinal (central retinal artery ischemia) and optic nerve ischemia. Nitrous oxide should be stopped 10 minutes before any intraocular gas is injected. Although older guidelines recommend avoiding N_2O for 10 days after SF6 and for 28 days after C3F8, the gas bubble may remain in place for more than 2 months in some cases. Therefore, N_2O should be avoided in all subsequent anesthetics until an ophthalmologist certifies that the bubble has been entirely reabsorbed. These patients should have a warning bracelet placed after the operation and only removed once the bubble has been officially certified as being reabsorbed.

7. **Tympanoplasty**—The middle ear is a natural, noncompliant air space. The diffusion of nitrous oxide into the middle ear may increase pressures by 20-50 mm Hg. Normally this is well tolerated because the pressure can be easily vented through the eustachian tube. This could be problematic during reconstruction of the tympanic membrane and the ossicles, especially in patients who have obstructed eustachian tubes due to a history of chronic ear problems. The increased pressures from nitrous oxide diffusion may cause displacement or rupture of the tympanoplastic grafts and adversely affect hearing postoperatively. Most practitioners avoid the use of N_2O during middle ear surgery. If used as part of maintenance, it should be discontinued 15-30 minutes before graft placement, when the middle ear becomes a closed space.

8. **Pneumocephalus**—A gas space can form within any of the intracranial compartments due to neurosurgery, trauma, tumors, or spontaneously. There are reports of pneumocephalus caused by spinal anesthesia and the loss of resistance to air technique of epidural placement. Nitrous oxide can diffuse into this space, enlarge it, and cause a tension pneumocephalus, which is a rare life-threatening emergency. The trapped intracranial air will increase intracranial pressure (ICP), compress the brain parenchyma resulting in delayed awakening from anesthesia and severe neurologic symptoms.

9. **Endotracheal tube cuffs**—The cuff of an endotracheal tube is typically filled with air, creating an air space that is susceptible to rapid expansion by N_2O. Administration of 75% N_2O can double the volume of the cuff within 10 minutes. An increase in pressure on the tracheal mucosa can lead to diminished perfusion. This may also occur in the other cuffs of balloon-tipped catheters, such as Swan–Ganz catheters.

Anesthesia Breathing System: Components

Daniel Asay, MD, and Jason Sankar, MD

Although modern operating room ventilators are typically large and complex, the basic components are fairly simple. Figure 12-1 shows the basic breathing system components: (1) carbon dioxide (CO_2) absorbent; (2) two unidirectional valves; (3) fresh gas inlet; (4) Y-connector; (5) reservoir bag; (6) adjustable pressure-limiting (APL) valve; and (7) low-resistance tubing.

CARBON DIOXIDE ABSORPTION

Carbon dioxide absorbance is vital to preventing hypercarbia with rebreathed tidal volumes. Absorbents remove CO_2 from the circuit's expiratory limb, allowing anesthetic gas to be recycled, thereby making a closed system possible. Soda lime, Baralyme, and Amsorb are the most common substances used for CO_2 extraction.

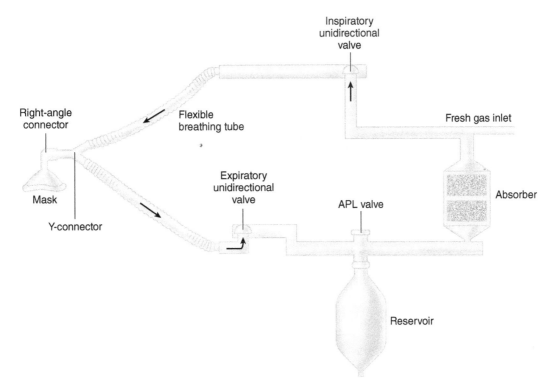

FIGURE 12-1 A circle system. APL, adjustable pressure-limiting (valve) (Reproduced with permission from Butterworth JF, Mackey DC, Wasnick JD, *Morgan and Mikhail's Clinical Anesthesiology*, 5th ed. McGraw-Hill; 2013.)

Soda lime is predominantly made up of calcium hydroxide ($Ca(OH)_2$) with smaller amounts of sodium hydroxide and potassium hydroxide. Silica is added to decrease dust formation. The soda lime reaction is:

$$CO_2 + H_2O \rightarrow H_2CO_3$$
$$H_2CO_3 + 2\,NaOH \rightarrow Na_2CO_3 + 2\,H_2O + Heat$$
$$Na_2CO_3 + Ca(OH)_2 \rightarrow CaCO_3 + 2\,NaOH$$

In the first equation, exhaled CO_2 reacts with water to form carbonic acid. In the second equation, carbonic acid reacts with the hydroxide salts of barium, calcium, potassium, or sodium to form water, heat, and carbonates of barium, calcium, potassium, or sodium. The third equation shows the carbonates reacting with calcium hydroxide to form calcium carbonate and hydroxides of barium, calcium, potassium, or sodium.

As can be seen from the equation, water and heat are produced, adding humidity and heat to the breathing circuit. Soda lime can absorb 23-26 L of CO_2 per 100 g of absorbent. When soda lime absorbent is exhausted, a color change occurs due to a pH-sensitive reaction.

Note: Baralyme is made up of barium hydroxide and calcium hydroxide. Water in Baralyme's structure obviates the need for silica. Baralyme was withdrawn from the US market in 2005.

One of the most important aspects of absorbents is the size of the granules. Smaller granules have greater surface area for absorption, but increased resistance to air flow. Granule size has been carefully engineered to maximize surface area and absorption while minimizing resistance. Typical granule size is 4-8 mesh (ie, will pass through a mesh of 4-8 strands per inch in each axis, or 2.36-4.75 mm).

In addition to CO_2, granules also absorb volatile anesthetics. Dry granules can break down desflurane or isoflurane into carbon monoxide (CO), whereas sevoflurane can be broken down into compound A. These reactions produce extremely high temperatures resulting in absorbent fires. Dessicated absorbent granules, caused by high gas flows over prolonged periods, result in carboxyhemoglobinemia when used for patient care. Compound A has nephrotoxic effects in rat studies, though there has never been confirmed human toxicity. Amsorb is made up of calcium hydroxide lime, which minimizes the formation of compound A and CO.

UNIDIRECTIONAL VALVES

Two unidirectional valves direct gas flow in a typical circle system: one in the inspiratory limb, and the other in the expiratory limb. Forward gas flow opens the valve whereas reverse flow closes it. Incompetence of either the inspiratory or expiratory valve allows rebreathing. Although unidirectional valves do allow lower fresh gas flows (FGFs), they can potentially add to the resistance of the system.

Fresh Gas Entry

In a circle system, fresh gas entry occurs between the absorber and the inspiratory valve. In older ventilators, FGF contributed to tidal volumes, whereas newer ventilators incorporate a decoupling valve, preventing flow during inspiration.

Y-Piece to Connect to the Patient

The Y-piece connects the endotracheal tube (ETT) with the inspiratory and expiratory limbs of the circuit. The Y-piece adds to the mechanical dead space of the circuit; however, Y-piece dead space is negligible compared to total dead space.

Reservoir Bag

The reservoir bag stores O_2 and anesthetic gases. A typical adult bag has a capacity of 2-3 L, though they range from 0.5 L to 6 L. An appropriately sized bag must exceed the patient's inspiratory capacity, allowing a full breath without emptying the bag. A reservoir bag allows the provider to assist or control ventilation, and provides a visual and tactile monitor of spontaneous respiratory effort.

Relief Valve

Also known as the pop-off or APL valve, the relief valve is positioned near the exhalation unidirectional valve. This valve allows exhaled gases and FGF to exit the system when the pressure exceeds the set pressure limit. During spontaneous respirations, barotrauma results from excessive positive pressure buildup due to a closed APL valve over time. An anesthetic gas scavenging system collects any gas exiting the system via the relief valve.

Low-Resistance Interconnecting Tubing

A large diameter minimizes circuit resistance. Corrugations increase flexibility and resist kinks, but they produce turbulent gas flow. Since there is some dispensability to the tubing, it adds to the dead space of the system. However, modern tubing does not distend significantly to affect total dead space.

Anesthesia Breathing System: Safety Features

Lakshmi Geddam, MD, and Jason Sankar, MD

As gas is supplied from a central supply or a cylinder, it passes through a fail-safe valve while traveling toward the flowmeters located in the anesthesia machine. The meters are equipped with a proportioning system and specially designed to prohibit a hypoxic gas mixture from being delivered to the patient. After the meters, the gas enters a manifold or mixing chamber, where it passes through vaporizers and continues to the common gas outlet, and eventually to the patient. Several safety features in the anesthesia breathing system ensure that the patient receives adequate oxygen supply: (1) fail-safe valve; (2) rotameter; and (3) proportioning device.

PRESSURE FAIL-SAFE

This fail-safe device prevents hypoxic mixtures if there is a decreased oxygen supply at the flowmeters' level. A pressure sensor shutoff valve is typically used in Ohmeda anesthetic machines (Datex-Ohmeda, Inc, Madison, WI). This device is present in gas lines supplying all flowmeters except for oxygen and is controlled by the oxygen supply pressure. It does this by interrupting the supply of the other gases if the oxygen supply is reduced to a certain level, usually below 30 psi. That level is the opening threshold pressure for use of the other gases. In a Drager anesthetic machine (Draeger Medical, Telford, PA), there is an oxygen protection device. This is similar to the Ohmeda shutoff valve. The only difference is that as the oxygen pressure is decreased, the other gases decrease proportionally with the opening oxygen threshold pressure of 12 psi. Additionally, an oxygen failure alarm system sounds if oxygen supply falls below a certain value (30 psi).

An oxygen flush valve can provide high flows of oxygen (35-75 L/min) directly to the common gas outlet, bypassing the flowmeters. It is important to note, because of the high pressure, the patient is at risk for barotrauma if oxygen flush is utilized while the breathing circuit is in continuity with the patient's lungs.

ROTAMETERS CONFIGURATION

Flowmeters control gas proportions and gas flow to the common gas outlet. One of the most common types of flowmeters are rotameters, or the variable orifice flowmeters with fixed pressure difference. It adjusts gas flow by means of flow control needle valves and flow tubes. Gas flow enters at the base of a glass flow tube. This glass tube is tapered in that its diameter increases with height. A small metal bobbin or ball rides the gas jet. As the bobbin rises, the space around it, known as the annulus, increases (variable orifice). Greater flow jets are required as the orifice widens to keep the bobbin afloat at that level. The pressure remains constant due to a force counteracting gravity and low flow resistance with a greater annulus. The top of the bobbin or the middle of the ball indicates the flow in liters per minute. Notches are made in the bobbin causing it to rotate centrally with gas flows. There is a wire stop located at the top of the tube that prevents the bobbin from going out of sight. The glass tube is calibrated based on the gas flowing through, its density and viscosity; therefore, it is not interchangeable with other gases. Viscosity is important in low flow states (laminar) and density is important in high gas flows (turbulent).

There may be multiple rotameters for one gas. Typically, it is arranged in series, where the first meter accurately measures low flows (1 L/min) and the other measures up to 10-12 L/min. There is one flow valve that is used. Gas flows from the flow control valve through the first and second tube; the total flow is shown in the second tube. The flow control needle valve is connected to a spindle that will fit into the inlet and turn off gas supply to the flowmeters. A gland, or a washer of compressible material, prevents leakage around the spindle.

Flowmeters are affected by temperature and altitude. As mentioned earlier, the tubes are calibrated to the gas (viscosity and density) at 1 atmosphere pressure and room temperature. A change in temperature has little effect, but a change in altitude will decrease barometric pressure and, therefore, increase flow. In low flow states, viscosity is the key and does not alter much with altitude. In high flow states, density is most important but does depend on altitude. At higher altitudes, the flowmeters will deliver higher flows, but read lower than the actual rate.

The sequence of flowmeters of different gases is important. Oxygen is the most distally positioned because this arrangement decreases the likelihood that leaks proximal to oxygen will result in a hypoxic mixture. If the leak is distal to the oxygen flowmeters, volume, but not concentration, will be reduced. However, a leak in the oxygen flowmeters can result in a lower oxygen concentration, regardless of the arrangement. Gas flow exits into a manifold, or mixing chamber, where it goes through vaporizers and into the common gas outlet.

OXYGEN RATIO AND PROPORTIONING DEVICES

Because of the hazards of administering a hypoxic gas mixture to the patient during anesthesia, machines are equipped with a nitrous oxide to oxygen proportioning device. This system links the two flows to prevent a final inspired oxygen concentration of less than 25%. A gear with nitrous oxide and a gear with oxygen, 14 teeth and 29 teeth, respectively, are connected by a chain. For every 2.07 turns of nitrous oxide flow control spindle, the oxygen flow control rotates once due to the 14:29 teeth ratio. Oxygen flow can be increased independently of nitrous oxide. This allows the control valves to be set independently, but when nitrous oxide is greater than 75%, oxygen is increased to maintain 25% of the gas mixture. This mechanism is used in the Ohmeda system. In the Draeger system, a pneumatic oxygen–nitrous oxide interlock proportioning system limits nitrous oxide based on oxygen flow to prevent a hypoxic mixture, but it does not actively increase the oxygen flow. Proportion systems do not protect against hypoxic mixtures when more than two gases are used, as nitrous oxide and oxygen are the only two gases interlocked.

Anesthesia Breathing System: Physical Principles

Lakshmi Geddam, MD, and Jason Sankar, MD

The anesthesia breathing system is a gas pathway that connects the patient's airway to the anesthesia machine; it extends from the fresh gas inlet to the point where gas escapes, either into the atmosphere or into a scavenging system. The breathing system functions to deliver gas from the anesthesia machine to the patient and to remove carbon dioxide by washout or chemical neutralization. Throughout this circuit, there are many factors that have an impact on the delivery and exit of gases.

RESISTANCE

Breathing circuits have some degree of resistance to flow that causes a pressure drop as gases pass through the tube. This is illustrated through the Ohm's and Hagen–Poiseuille's laws. In Ohm's law, flow (Q) is directly proportional to the pressure (P) difference and inversely related to resistance (R). In Poisseuille's law, the pressure gradient is directly proportional to the length (L), viscosity (v), and the flow rate (V), and inversely proportional to the radius (r) to the fourth power.

$$R = \frac{\Delta P}{Q} \qquad \Delta P = \frac{LvV}{r^4}$$

Two important factors affecting the "airway" resistance are flow rate and the type of flow. Flow can be laminar, turbulent, or, clinically, it is more often a combination of both.

Laminar flow illustrates particles that flow in one direction, parallel to the wall, and down a pressure gradient. Looking at the diameter, the flow is fastest in the center and decreases parabolically due to friction. Resistance is directly related to the flow rate. Poiseuille's law follows laminar flow.

In turbulent flow, particles move in all directions, and the flow rate is the same across the diameter of the tube. The pressure difference will increase to maintain flow, and this, in turn, increases resistance. For turbulent flow, gas density is more important than viscosity, and resistance is directly related to the flow rate squared. Turbulent flow can either be generalized or localized. When laminar flow exceeds a critical flow rate, it becomes generalized, turbulent flow. Localized turbulent flow occurs below the critical flow rate, at constrictions, curves, or other irregularities in the tube.

To reduce resistance, the circuit length should be minimized, diameter maximized, and constrictions, or areas likely to generate turbulent flow, should be avoided.

Resistance will foist strain on the patient if he or she is required to do some, or all, of the respiratory work when on a ventilator. Consequently, resistance in the anesthesia breathing system parallels the work of breathing.

REBREATHING

Rebreathing involves inhaling previously respired gases that may or may not have carbon dioxide removed; inspired gas is a combination of fresh gas and rebreathed gas. The effect rebreathing has on a patient will depend on: (1) fresh gas flow and (2) mechanical dead space.

- *Fresh gas flow* is considered in relation to the minute ventilation. If the flow is greater than the minute ventilation, and the expired gas is appropriately disposed of either in the atmosphere or in a scavenging system, there will be no need or room for rebreathing. However, if the flow is less than the minute ventilation, rebreathing will occur to make up for the volume that is lacking. There is an inverse relationship between fresh gas flow and rebreathing.
- *Mechanical dead space* is defined as the volume in a breathing system occupied by gases that are rebreathed without any change in composition. This should not be confused with anatomical or alveolar dead space—both of which are located within the patient's respiratory tract. Mechanical dead space can vary in its composition depending on if it is from anatomical dead space, alveolar gas, or mixed exhaled gas. If mechanical dead space is derived from anatomical dead space, the dead space will be equivalent to fresh gas but with greater humidity, vapor, and heat. If the mechanical dead space is derived from alveolar gas, it will have similar increased humidity, vapor, and heat. However, the composition will differ in that the anesthetic concentration will be altered, and the oxygen tension will be lower whereas the carbon dioxide tension will be higher. If mechanical dead space is derived from a mixed exhaled gas, it will be a combination of the anatomical and alveolar gas mixtures.

Rebreathing will alter the inspired gas tensions of oxygen, carbon dioxide, and the inhalation anesthetics. Likewise, it will increase heat and moisture retention.

- **Oxygen**—Rebreathing alveolar gas that has lower oxygen tension than fresh gas will result in a decreased inspired oxygen tension.
- **Carbon dioxide**—Rebreathing carbon dioxide will result in increased inspired carbon dioxide tension unless the gases pass through an absorbent or ventilator spill valve (or adjustable pressure limiting-valve). If there is no separation between fresh gas, dead space, and alveolar gas, high flows are required to eliminate carbon dioxide. The optimal level of carbon dioxide varies with the type of ventilation used. Retention during spontaneous ventilation will have a negative effect because the patient will attempt to compensate and increase the minute ventilation, and therefore the work of breathing. However, retention during controlled ventilation may be more desirable as rebreathing can establish normocarbia without hyperventilation while increasing humidification and moisture.
- **Inhalation anesthetics**—Rebreathing of inhalation anesthetics can have varied effects on the patient at different times during the anesthetic window. During induction, when alveolar tension of the anesthetic is lower than fresh gas flow, rebreathing alveolar gas will prolong induction. During recovery, when alveolar tension of the anesthetic is higher than fresh gas flow, rebreathing alveolar gas will slow elimination.

GAS MIXTURES

As the gas leaves the anesthesia breathing machine and travels toward the patient, it may be altered by multiple factors, resulting in a mixture that is different from the original. The factors that modify inspired air include rebreathing, leaks, and air dilution.

If the fresh gas supplied is less than the minute ventilation in conjunction with a leak in the system, negative pressure in the breathing system (spontaneous respirations) can entrain air. This will cause the inspired anesthetic tension to decrease and will result in lighter levels of anesthesia. This is exacerbated by increased ventilation. Deeper anesthesia will depress ventilation, decrease air dilution, and increase anesthetic delivery. If positive pressure is in the system, a leak will not affect the patient because it forces air out rather than in.

Circle and Noncircle Systems

Sudha Ved, MD

CLASSIFICATION OF BREATHING SYSTEMS

An anesthesia breathing circuit is a system of tubing, reservoir bag, and valves used to deliver a precise mixture of oxygen and anesthetic gases from the anesthesia machine to the patient and removal of carbon dioxide. Breathing systems may be best classified in a number of different ways:

- **Open**—Open systems have no valves, tubing, or reservoir bag: for example, insufflation or open-drop ether. In either, the patient has access to atmospheric gases.
- **Semi-open**—A semi-open system has a reservoir such as a breathing bag and there is no rebreathing. For example, a Mapleson circuit or a circle at high fresh gas flow (FGF) (> minute ventilation [V_E]).
- **Semi-closed**—A semi-closed system has a reservoir such as a breathing bag and allows for partial rebreathing. For example, a Mapleson circuit or a circle at low FGF (< V_E), the most commonly used method today.
- **Closed**—A closed system has a reservoir such as a breathing bag and allows for complete rebreathing, and CO_2 is absorbed. For example, a circle with pop-off (adjustable pressure-limiting [APL] valve) valve closed and a very low FGF that equals oxygen uptake by the patient.

Two factors must be considered in the breathing systems:

1. **Dead space**—In the circle systems, the tubing (mechanical) dead space ends at the point where inspired and expired gas streams meet at the Y-connector, resulting in loss of tidal volume (V_T) from the compliance of the distensible corrugated inspiratory and expiratory tubing and from gas compression. The elbow, the heat and moisture exchanger (HME), and the D-lite sensor contribute to real apparatus dead space where part of V_T does not participate in gas exchange. Increasing the dead space increases rebreathing of carbon dioxide. Hence, to avoid hypercarbia in the face of an acute increase in dead space, a patient must increase minute ventilation.

2. **Resistance to breathing**—Resistance is always high with turbulent flow, hence narrow diameter tubing and orifices, sharp bends, increasing circuit length, and eliminating unnecessary valves that produce this should be avoided in the apparatus. Circle system resistance is increased by unidirectional valves, the absorber, and high respiratory rates and tidal volumes.

Noncircle Systems

A. Insufflation

Insufflation is an open system and depending on the respiratory pattern, depth of anesthesia is unpredictable and air entrainment in varying degrees occurs. Ventilation cannot be assisted and fire and toxicity risks exist. Oxygen and/or gases are insufflated over the face during a child's induction or via a catheter/tube placed in the airway, laryngoscope, or trachea during endoscopic procedures or to prevent rebreathing of CO_2 during ophthalmic surgery. One may use spontaneous ventilation (SV) or controlled ventilation (CV) with brief periods of apnea.

B. Open-Drop

No longer used, this open system drips either ether or chloroform onto a gauze-covered mask (Schimmelbusch mask) and as the agent is vaporized there is a lowering of the mask temperature. This results in a drop in rate of vaporization and anesthetic vapor pressure (vapor pressure is proportional to temperature).

C. Draw-Over

Draw-over is a system that uses a nonrebreathing valve, a self-inflating bag, and a vaporization chamber. Ambient air is used as the carrier gas and supplemental oxygen (1-4 L/min) is used to increase fraction of inspired oxygen (FIO_2) to 30%-80%, using an open-ended reservoir tube attached to a T-piece. The devices can be fitted to allow intermittent positive pressure ventilation (IPPV) (continuous positive airway pressure [CPAP] and positive end-expiratory pressure [PEEP]) and passive scavenging. The greatest advantages of the draw-over systems are their simplicity and portability, and may be used in locations and situations in which compressed gases are unavailable (eg, developing countries and battlefields).

D. Unidirectional Valve System

This system with a nonrebreathing valve allows CV and is used primarily with respirators or portable manual resuscitators such as the "Ambu." The valve directs fresh gas to the patient and releases exhaled gas to atmosphere or scavenging system. Other unidirectional valves used with semi-open systems have the disadvantage of increased resistance to breathing, bulkiness, increased dead space, possibility of valve malfunction, occlusion of exhalation port resulting in pneumothorax, or dilution of anesthetic and oxygen concentration, limiting its present-day use.

E. Mapleson Circuits

Mapleson systems are modifications of the Ayre's T-piece, developed in 1937 for the administration of anesthetic gases to infants and young children. The systems are semi-open nonrebreathing or semi-closed partial rebreathing systems (Figure 15-1). The relative location of key components determine circuit performance, amount of CO_2 rebreathing, and dependence on FGF. These components include a face mask, FGF inflow tubing, spring-loaded pop-off valve, reservoir tubing, and a reservoir bag. The Bain circuit, is a modification of Mapleson D where the FGF tubing is inside the reservoir tubing, and in functions it is similar to Mapleson F.

During SV, Mapleson A was the most efficient circuit for CO_2 elimination requiring the least amount of FGF (FGF = V_E) followed by DEF (FGF 2.5 × V_E) and lastly CB (FGF = > 2.5 × V_E) (A > DEF > CB). With CV, the order changes. Now DEF have the lowest FGF (FGF = 2.5 × V_E) requirements to prevent rebreathing followed by BC (FGF > 2.5 × V_E) and then A (as high as 20 L/min) (DEF > BC > A). Mapleson A, B, and C systems are rarely used today.

Variables that dictate the amount of CO_2 rebreathing associated with each system include the fresh gas inflow rate, minute ventilation, mode of ventilation, tidal volume, the respiratory rate, inspiratory-to-expiratory ratio, duration of expiratory pause, peak inspiratory flow rate, volume of the reservoir tube, volume of the breathing bag, ventilation by mask, ventilation through an endotracheal tube, and CO_2 sampling site.

Mapleson systems may be used as transport circuits instead of the "Ambu" bag. They are lightweight, portable, inexpensive, easy to clean, and have the feel of the anesthesia bag. They offer low resistance to breathing and are used in locations and situations in which costly anesthesia workstations are unavailable or their use is uneconomical (eg, developing countries and battlefields, gastroendoscopy and other satellite units).

There are several disadvantages to using Mapleson circuits. The high gas flows are uneconomical and associated with low humidity, heat loss, and increased operating room pollution. Some of these disadvantages are overcome when Bain circuit is used. Scavenging of exhaled gases is possible since the expiratory overflow valve is located away from the patient and CV is possible. The exhaled gases in the reservoir tubing add warmth to the inspired gases by countercurrent heat exchange. The main hazards related to use of the Bain circuit are either an unrecognized disconnection or kinking of the inner fresh gas hose. These problems can cause hypercapnia as a result of inadequate gas flow or increased respiratory resistance, unresponsive to increased V_E. The Pethick test is used to test the Bain circuit: (1) occlude the patient's end of the circuit (at the elbow); (2) close the APL valve; (3) fill the circuit, using the oxygen flush valve; and (4) release the occlusion at the elbow and flush. A Venturi effect flattens the reservoir bag if the inner tube is patent.

Traditional Circle Systems

The traditional circle breathing system invented in 1936 is a unidirectional breathing system with CO_2 absorption allowing for partial or total rebreathing of other exhaled gases. A circle system can be semi-open, semi-closed (the most commonly used version), or closed depending on the amount of FGF.

Numerous variations of the circle component arrangements are possible. However, the components are arranged in a certain way to prevent CO_2 rebreathing, conserve FGF, and allow for recirculation of other expired gases. The major elements are:

- FGF tubing from the anesthesia machine such that FGF cannot enter the circuit between the expiratory valve and the patient;
- inspiratory and expiratory valves to ensure unidirectional gas flows through the corrugated tubing;
- inspiratory and expiratory corrugated tubing;
- Y-piece connector;
- overflow or pop-off valve, also known as the APL valve, located just downstream from the expiratory valve, allowing for preferential elimination of exhaled alveolar gases;
- reservoir bag and ventilator; and
- canister containing CO_2 absorbent.

A 1997 closed claim study found that the breathing circuit was by far the major cause of death or brain damage (39% of all claims), causing a 70% incidence of death or brain damage. The rate of misuse was 3 times higher than pure equipment failure. In the old systems, the APL valve was a major source of leak if not totally closed before initiating ventilation. New workstations use the bag/ventilator selector switch that puts the APL valve outside the circuit and eliminates a source of leak.

Advantages of the circle system include:

- maintenance of relatively stable inspired gas concentrations;
- conservation of respiratory moisture and heat;
- prevention of operating room pollution by adding scavenging systems; and
- the circle system can be used for closed-system anesthesia or semi-closed with very low FGFs.

FIGURE 15-1 Classification and characteristics of Mapleson circuits. (Reproduced with permission from Butterworth JF, Mackey DC, Wasnick JD, *Morgan and Mikhail's Clinical Anesthesiology*, 5th ed. McGraw-Hill; 2013.)

Mapleson Class	Other Names	Configuration[1]	Required Fresh Gas Flows — Spontaneous	Required Fresh Gas Flows — Controlled	Comments
A	Magill attachment	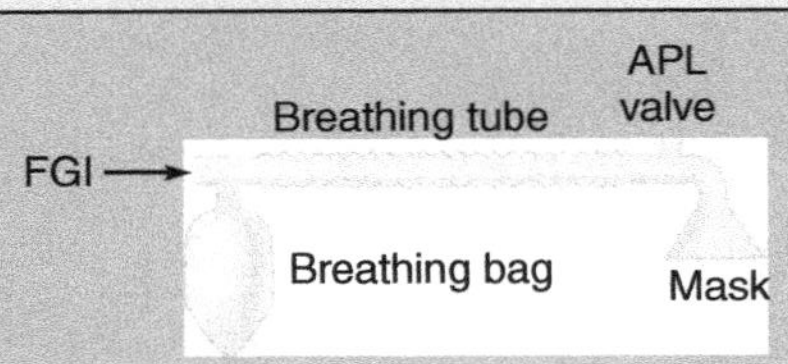	Equal to minute ventilation (≈80 mL/kg/min)	Very high and difficult to predict	Poor choice during controlled ventilaton. Enclosed Magill system is a modification that improves efficiency. Coaxial Mapleson A (Lack breathing system) provides waste gas scavenging.
B			2 × minute ventilation	2–2½ × minute ventilation	
C	Waters' to-and-fro	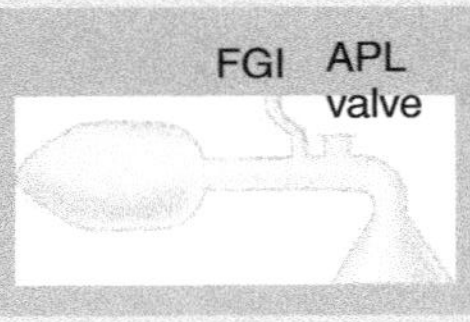	2 × minute ventilation	2–2½ × minute ventilation	
D	Bain circuit	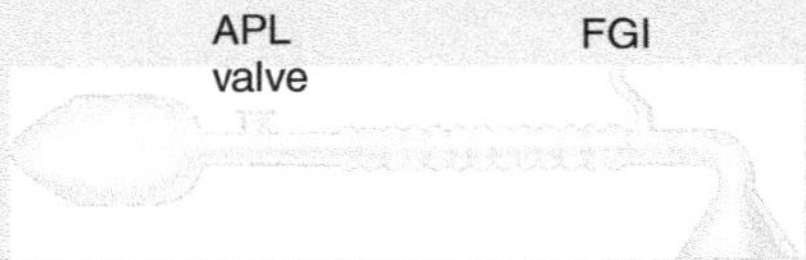	2–3 × minute ventilation	1–2 × minute ventilation	Bain coaxial modification: fresh gas tube inside breathing tube.
E	Ayre's T-piece	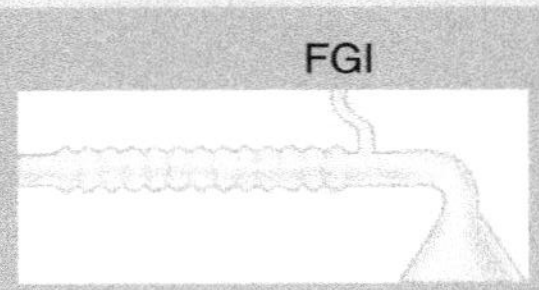	2–3 × minute ventilation	3 × minute ventilation (I:E-1:2)	Exhalation tubing should provide a larger volume than tidal volume to prevent rebreathing. Scavenging is difficult.
F	Jackson-Rees' modification	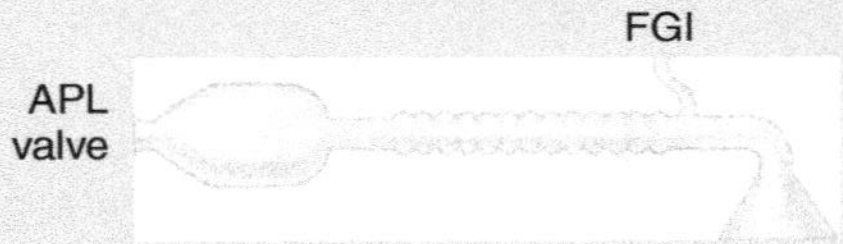	2–3 × minute ventilation	2 × minute ventilation	A Mapleson E with a breathing bag connected to the end of the breathing tube to allow controlled ventilation and scavenging.

[1]FGI, fresh gas inlet; APL, adjustable pressure-limiting (valve).

Disadvantages of the circle system include:

- The circuit is connected to a complex table platform design and checkout procedures are often inadequately performed or not done at all.
- Multiple connections can lead to misconnections, disconnections, obstructions, and leaks leading to hypoventilation and barotraumas.
- Malfunction of the circle system's unidirectional valves can result in life-threatening problems:
  - rebreathing can occur if the valves stick in the open position;
  - total occlusion of the circuit can occur if they are stuck shut; and
  - if the expiratory valve is stuck in the closed position, breath stacking and barotrauma or volutrauma can result.

- Circle system obstruction and failure include manufacturing defects, debris, patient secretions, and particulate obstruction from other odd sources such as albuterol nebulization:
  - obstructed filters located in the expiratory limb of the circle breathing system have caused increased airway pressure, hemodynamic collapse, and bilateral tension pneumothorax.
  - Loss of tidal volume from mechanical dead space and gas compression volumes in the distensible inspiratory and expiratory corrugated tubing.

SUGGESTED READING

Caplan RA, Vistica MF, Posner KL, et al. Adverse anesthetic outcomes arising from gas delivery equipment. *Anesthesiology* 1997;87:741-748.

Portable Ventilation Devices

16

Brian S. Freeman, MD

Portable ventilation devices are essential for patients who require continuous mechanical ventilation during transport to and from the operating room. They are also important tools for providing face mask ventilation during emergency airway management, such as a patient in cardiac arrest. Though the flow of oxygen is usually necessary, these devices do not require electricity or a source of pressurized gas for their function. There are two types of portable manual resuscitators: self-inflating and flow-inflating systems.

SELF-INFLATING SYSTEMS

Self-inflating manual resuscitators are used both in hospital and out-of-hospital scenarios. The primary advantages are the self-inflating nature, portability, and ability to provide room air in the event that oxygen is not available. These systems, however, require an oxygen source to deliver inspired oxygen levels higher than that of room air. They also lack the tactile feel of airway resistance and compliance that can be more easily determined from the anesthesia circle system. Use of these resuscitators may increase the risk of barotraumas due to excessive delivered airway pressure.

There are several self-inflating manual resuscitators on the market. The first product was introduced in 1956 and continues to be the leader even today: the "Ambu bag." Designed by anesthesiologist Henning Ruben, the device received its name based on its components: air-mask-bag unit (AMBU). Although several different manufacturers produce these breathing systems, each of the system shares the following fundamental components (Figure 16-1).

1. **Self-refilling bag**—The self-refilling bag acts as a reservoir for the gas (oxygen and/or air) that is delivered to the patient when manually compressed. Its material has memory-like capability. During expiration, the bag automatically re-expands to its inspiratory position by drawing in gas for the next delivered breath. Because of the semi-rigid nature of these bags, it can be impossible to detect spontaneous breathing. Bag is made of materials such as rubber (silicone, chloroprene, butyl) or polyvinyl chloride (PVC). Most are latex free. Unlike the rubber versions, PVC

resuscitators cannot be steam autoclaved. The typical bag volumes are 1500 mL (for an adult), 500 mL (for a child), and 250 mL (for an infant).

2. **Nonrebreathing valve**—The nonrebreathing valve is designed to release expired gas to the atmosphere and to prevent it from mixing with fresh inspired gas from the self-refilling bag. During inspiration, the valve ensures that the patient will only receive fresh gas from the self-refilling bag.

   The nonrebreathing valve is T shaped and consists of an inspiratory port (directs gas from bag to patient), an expiratory port (directs gas from patient to atmosphere), and a patient port that connects with the artificial airway device. It is a unidirectional valve that closes the expiratory port during inspiration and the inspiratory port during expiration. Manual resuscitators generally use three types of unidirectional valves. Spring valves have a ball or disc attached to a spring that is moved by fresh inspiratory gas to block the expiratory port when the bag is compressed. Duckbill valves open during inspiration to prevent gas from entering the expiratory flow out of the port. Flap valves open during inspiration and close the expiratory port to direct gas flow to the patient. At the end of inspiration, the flap returns to its original position, which allows expired gas to exit through the expiratory port.

   Even if the patient is breathing spontaneously, the administration of oxygen with this system should always be provided with positive pressure support. The nonrebreathing valve is a source of resistance against the patient's inspiratory efforts. Without assistance, work of breathing will increase, leading to patient distress. The patient may also attempt to generate additional negative airway pressure to overcome these transmural pressure gradients, resulting in pulmonary edema.

   Nonrebreathing valves also have the ability to allow attachment of a mechanical positive end-expiratory pressure (PEEP) valve to the expiratory port. Newer resuscitator models have built-in PEEP valves with an adjustable dial.

3. **Fresh gas input and oxygen reservoir**—Self-inflating systems can deliver room air or up to 100% oxygen when connected to an oxygen source. Oxygen is usually delivered into the system through an oxygen reservoir, which are either bags (closed reservoir) or tubing (open reservoir).

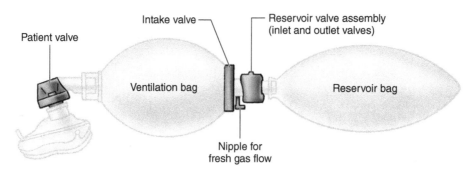

FIGURE 16-1 Basic components of self-inflating resuscitator bags. (Reproduced with permission from Butterworth JF, Mackey DC, Wasnick JD. *Morgan and Mikhail's Clinical Anesthesiology*, 5th ed. McGraw-Hill; 2013.)

Both allow for oxygen accumulation during inspiration and release into the self-refilling bag during expiration. When the volume of oxygen supplied is greater than the volume delivered to the patient, the reservoir bag expands to provide 100% oxygen for ventilation. Adding an oxygen reservoir to the system significantly increases the possible inspired oxygen concentration. The gas inlet to the reservoir is generally located at the other side of the self-refilling bag from the nonrebreathing valve. A pressure relief security valve, placed in between the reservoir and the gas inlet, prevents the bag from being overfilled.

FLOW-INFLATING SYSTEMS

Flow-inflating manual resuscitation devices include certain portable types of Mapleson breathing circuits. These ventilation systems have flaccid bags that do not reinflate after manual compression. Instead, a continuous external flow of gas (usually oxygen) is required to inflate the bag. Once fully inflated, the bag deflates by either manual compression (controlled ventilation) or by direct patient effort (spontaneous ventilation). These devices are primarily used by anesthesiologists and are not typically found in out-of-hospital settings.

Mapleson D (Bain's circuit) and F (Jackson Rees) circuits are the most common portable flow-inflation circuits in use

(see Chapter 15). To the original Ayre's T-piece design, Dr. Rees added a corrugated tube, a fresh gas line at the patient connection, and a small open-ended bag to the end of the reservoir limb. A variable, spring-loaded adjustable pressure-limiting (APL) overflow valve may be added to the distal end of the reservoir bag. Mapleson D circuits have this expiratory APL valve located at the end of the expiratory limb, but operate in the same way as the Mapleson F circuit. Aside from the APL valve, there are no moving components to the system. Dead space and resistance are minimal.

During spontaneous ventilation, the movement of the collapsible bag clearly shows each patient breathe (unlike the rigid Ambu bag). During the inspiratory phase of manual ventilation, the bag is squeezed with the open end of the bag (or APL valve) partially or totally occluded. During exhalation, the open end or APL valve is released to allow the gas in the circuit to leave.

There are some disadvantages to the Mapleson D and F systems. The collapsible bags require an oxygen supply to remain inflated. Rebreathing of expired gases can occur, depending upon the mode of ventilation and state of the APL valve. High rates of fresh gas flow (2-3 times patient minute ventilation) are necessary to prevent rebreathing of bases. If the APL valve is accidently occluded or closed completely, high airway pressures will build, possibly leading to barotrauma.

Absorption of Carbon Dioxide

17

Brian S. Freeman, MD

The absorption of carbon dioxide is mandatory in closed and semi-closed circle breathing systems. The elimination of CO_2 from exhaled gases is achieved through chemical neutralization in transparent canisters containing absorbent granules. The ideal CO_2 absorbent should have high efficiency, low airflow resistance, no toxicity or reactions with inhalation anesthetics, and low cost. Effective carbon dioxide absorption prevents CO_2 rebreathing and the development of hypercapnia.

CHEMISTRY OF ABSORBENTS

There are several types of carbon dioxide absorbents used today. Each type has a different degree of efficiency for CO_2 elimination.

Soda Lime

The components of soda lime are calcium hydroxide (80%), water (15%), and two catalysts: sodium hydroxide (5%) and potassium hydroxide (<0.1%). Some types of soda lime lack potassium hydroxide. Silica is added to make the granules harder and more stable, which reduces alkaline powder formation (which could cause bronchospasm). It has a pH of 13.5. Soda lime absorbs about 19% of its weight in carbon dioxide, hence 100 g of soda lime can absorb approximately 26 L of carbon dioxide.

The ability of soda lime to absorb CO_2 is due specifically to NaOH. The neutralization of CO_2 involves a number of chemical reactions:

(1) $CO_2 + H_2O \rightleftharpoons H_2CO_3$

(2) $H_2CO_3 + 2NaOH\,(or\,KOH) \rightleftharpoons Na_2CO_3\,(or\,K_2CO_3)$
$\qquad\qquad + 2H_2O + Heat$

(3) $Na_2CO_3\,(or\,K_2CO_3) + Ca(OH)_2 \rightleftharpoons CaCO_3 + 2NaOH\,(or\,KOH)$

The first neutralization reaction involves the formation of carbonic acid from CO_2 and water. Then, NaOH (and to a lesser extent, KOH) acts as an activator to speed up the formation of sodium (or potassium) carbonates. Calcium hydroxide reacts with the carbonates within minutes to form calcium carbonate, an insoluble precipitate. In this neutralization reaction, additional sodium (or potassium) hydroxides are regenerated. Some carbon dioxide may also react directly with $Ca(OH)_2$ to form calcium carbonates, but this reaction is much slower. Soda lime is exhausted when all hydroxides have become carbonates.

Amsorb

Amsorb consists of calcium hydroxide lime (70%), water (14.5%), calcium chloride (0.7%), and two agents to improve hardness (calcium sulfate and polyvinylpyrrolidine). Amsorb has half the absorbing capacity of soda lime and costs more per unit. Calcium chloride serves as a moisture-retaining agent to allow for greater water availability. As a result, there is no need for alkali agents like NaOH or KOH. Without these strong monovalent bases, calcium hydroxide lime has fewer adverse reactions associated with the breakdown of inhalation agents (such as the formation of compound A or carbon monoxide [CO]).

Neutralization of carbon dioxide with Amsorb begins with the reaction of carbon dioxide with water present in the granules to form carbonic acid. Carbonic acid then reacts with calcium hydroxide to form calcium carbonate, water, and heat.

(1) $CO_2 + H_2O \rightleftharpoons H_2CO_3$

(2) $H_2CO_3 + Ca(OH)_2 \rightleftharpoons CaCO_3 + 2H_2O + Heat$

Baralyme

Baralyme contains calcium hydroxide (80%) plus barium hydroxide (20%). This less efficient absorbent does not contain any silica for hardening. In the neutralization of carbon dioxide, compared to soda lime, $Ba(OH)_2$ replaces NaOH and KOH in the chemical equations:

(1) $Ba(OH)_2 + 8H_2O + CO_2 \rightleftharpoons BaCO_3 + 9H_2O + Heat$

(2) $9H_2O + 9CO_2 \rightleftharpoons 9H_2CO_3$

(3) $9H_2CO_3 + 9Ca(OH)_2 \rightleftharpoons CaCO_3 + 18H_2O + Heat$

Baralyme was withdrawn from the market in 2005. It has been the agent responsible for breathing system fires in conjunction with the use of sevoflurane.

For all three absorbents, the neutralization of carbon dioxide generates water and heat in an exothermic reaction. The water is helpful for humidifying the fresh gas flows (FGFs). If proper CO_2 absorption is taking place, then the absorbent canister should feel warm to the touch. A canister that feels too hot may indicate excessive carbon dioxide production. If the canister fails to become warm, it is possible that neutralization of carbon dioxide is not occurring.

INFLUENCE OF ABSORBENT GRANULES

The efficiency of carbon dioxide neutralization depends on two factors:

1. **Size of the absorbent granules**—As granule size decreases, the total surface area in contact with carbon dioxide increases, thus improving absorbent efficiency. At the same time, small granules will increase the resistance to gas flow because of the smaller spaces in between the granules. Therefore, the optimal absorbent granule size represents a balance between absorptive efficiency and resistance to airflow through the canister.

   An absorbent's "mesh size" indicates to the number of openings per linear inch in a sieve through which the granules pass. For instance, an 8-mesh screen has eight openings (one-eighth inch each) per linear inch. The soda lime canisters used today are typically between 4 and 8 mesh, a size that optimizes the balance between absorptive surface area and flow resistance.

2. **Channeling**—Channeling of exhaled gases through the absorbent granules can substantially decrease their efficiency. Carbon dioxide absorbent canisters are designed to uniformly distribute expired gas through the granules. However, narrow pathways will inevitably form since the granules are often loosely packed in the canisters. As a result, exhaled gas will flow preferentially through low-resistance areas and, therefore, bypass the bulk of granules. This phenomenon can actually reduce the absorptive capacity of soda lime from 26 L to 10 L of CO_2 absorbed per 100 g absorbent. Channeling can be reduced by gently shaking the canister before use to ensure firm granule packing.

ABSORBENT DESICCATION AND EXHAUSTION

The flow of fresh gases from the bottom to top of the canister through the granules will desiccate the absorbent. Desiccation is a concern because it increases the degradation of inhaled anesthetics. Retrograde gas flow must occur for an extended period of time, usually at least 48 hours, for desiccation to occur.

A number of factors will enhance this flow and increase the degree of desiccation:

- Design and relative resistances of the breathing system components.
- Absence of a breathing reservoir bag.
- Opened adjustable pressure-limiting valve.
- Occlusion of the Y-piece.
- High FGF rates.
- The use of heat and moisture exchangers (HMEs).
- Scavenger suction.

Carbon dioxide absorbents contain organic pH-sensitive indicator dyes that change color when the granules are exhausted. When the absorptive granules are exhausted, lack of CO_2 absorption leads to accumulation of carbonic acid and carbonates. This reduces pH below the dye's critical value (usually 10.3), thus causing a change in the indicator dye color.

Dyes include ethyl violet, ethyl orange, and cresyl yellow. The most common dye is ethyl violet, which changes granule color from white to a vivid purple due to alcohol dehydration. Over time, exhausted granules may return to white despite no recovery in absorptive capacity. However, the dye will become purple again upon reuse. Unlike soda lime, the ethyl violet dye in Amsorb changes from white to purple but does not revert to white again. Due to channeling or degradation from fluorescent light, it is possible for the absorbent to appear white despite a reduced pH and an exhausted absorptive capacity. Because of this lack of sensitivity, the gold standard for assessment of CO_2 elimination is the use of capnometry to detect elevations in inspired carbon dioxide.

COMPLICATIONS ASSOCIATED WITH CO_2 ABSORPTION

Hypercapnia Due to Absorber Malfunction

Hypercapnia is the result of a CO_2 absorber that is either exhausted or experiencing excessive channeling of FGF. It may also be due to the loss of FGF through leaks anywhere in the circuit, which leads to increased dead space and CO_2 rebreathing. Hypercapnia leads to a respiratory acidosis. Significant changes in $Paco_2$ and pH can produce hemodynamic instability, dysrhythmias, increased respiratory rate, and signs of sympathetic nervous system activation (hypertension, sweating, tachycardia). There may also be increased bleeding at the surgical site.

To prevent this problem, the freshness of the absorbent should be checked and if in doubt, the canister should be replaced. It is important to make sure that the soda lime or barium hydroxide lime is packed properly in the canister to avoid any possibility of channeling. Canisters should be fitted onto the canister housing without any circuit leaks that could lead to rebreathing. Ultimately, the measurement of inspired

CO_2 levels is the most important modality. It is recommended to change canisters when inspired carbon dioxide exceeds more than 2-3 mm Hg. The third phase of the capnograph will fail to return to baseline as a result of rebreathing.

Formation of Compound A

Sevoflurane reacts with soda lime absorbent to produce a number of degradation products, the most significant being fluoromethyl-2-2-difluoro-1-(trifluoromethyl) vinyl ether, or compound A. Compound A was found to have dose-dependent nephrotoxicity in rats. In normal clinical use of sevoflurane, levels of compound A can reach the same levels (25-50 ppm) that were found to cause renal injury in rats. However, studies of the actual nephrotoxicity of compound A in humans have had conflicting results. In fact, sevoflurane has been administered with apparent safety for several years.

There are several factors that can contribute to higher levels of compound A in the breathing circuit:

- FGFs <2 L/minute.
- Use of barium hydroxide lime instead of soda lime.
- High concentration of sevoflurane.
- High absorbent temperature.
- Dessicated absorbent canisters.

Current recommendations include the avoidance of sevoflurane in patients with known renal impairment. Fresh gas flows of at least 2 L/min must be maintained and can be used indefinitely. Fresh gas flows between 1 and 2 L/min should not be used for more than 2 minimum alveolar concentration (MAC) hours. Fresh gas flows less than 1 L/min are not recommended at all.

Formation of Carbon Monoxide

Degradation of inhaled anesthetics (desflurane and isoflurane) in the setting of a desiccated absorber has produced rare cases of carbon monoxide (CO) poisoning. Carboxyhemoglobin concentrations can reach 30% or higher. This is primarily the result of prolonged high gas flows which dry out the absorbent. Most reported cases of CO poisoning have been the first case on a Monday morning after the circuit was idle over the weekend. The mechanism is poorly understood. Carbon dioxide absorbers with strong bases like NaOH may extract labile protons from anesthetic molecules, resulting in the production of CO. Newer absorbents like Amsorb lack strong bases so it will not react with volatile anesthetics to produce CO.

The factors which increase the production of carboxyhemoglobin include:

- inhaled anesthetic (desflurane ≥ enflurane > isoflurane >> halothane = sevoflurane);

- type of absorbent (Baralyme > soda lime);
- low FGFs;
- increased absorbent temperatures;
- dry absorbent;
- higher concentrations of inhaled anesthetics; and
- size of patient compared to amount of absorbent (ie, more absorbent and hence more CO exposure per unit of patient mass).

To reduce the risk of CO production, the anesthesia machine should be turned off at the end of the day. Leaving the anesthesia machine on at high oxygen flow rates overnight can dry out the absorbent. The absorbent canister should be changed if FGF is left on over the weekend or overnight. Water may be added to desiccated absorbent to rehydrate. If possible, use products like Amsorb (calcium hydroxide lime) that do not contain strong bases. Maintain a high level of suspicion and check blood carboxyhemoglobin levels when in doubt.

Fire

There have been rare and isolated cases of spontaneous fires in the CO_2 absorbent canister or elsewhere within the circle system. Other reports have detailed incidents of extreme heat without fire. Common features in these reports include the use of sevoflurane anesthesia, Baralyme absorber, and granule desiccation. A chemical reaction between sevoflurane and desiccated Baralyme can produce extreme heat and combustible degradation products (such as methanol and formaldehyde). The added presence of oxygen or nitrous oxide provides the final ingredient for fire.

To prevent this rare but life-threatening complication, providers should:

- Avoid the use of sevoflurane with strong base absorbents like Baralyme.
- Replace any CO_2 absorber that has not been used for an extended period.
- Turn off the vaporizer, anesthesia machine, and FGFs when not in use for extended periods.
- Periodically monitor the temperature in the CO_2 canister.
- Monitor the rate of rise of inspired sevoflurane in relation to the dial setting of the vaporizer (delayed rise or unexpected decrease in inspired levels may be due to extreme canister heat).

If excessive heat in the absorbent canister is evident, the patient should be immediately disconnected from the breathing circuit. The absorbent canister requires immediate replacement. Blood gases with cooximetry should be analyzed to determine any extent of CO poisoning.

Oxygen Supply Systems

Hannah Schobel, DO

Supplemental oxygen, defined as fraction of inspired oxygen (FIO_2) in concentrations greater than 21%, is usually administered to patients throughout the perioperative period. The most common devices utilized in the operating room are attached to the anesthesia work station. Patients arriving in the post-anesthesia care unit (PACU), intensive care unit (ICU), and postsurgical floors will often require oxygen delivery by other means. Upon arriving in the PACU, 20% of patients aged 1-3 years, 14% of patients aged 3-14 years, and 8% of adults will experience arterial oxyhemoglobin desaturation on room air to $SaO_2 < 90\%$.

The goal of oxygen administration is to prevent tissue hypoxia. Supplemental oxygen does not address the cause of hypoxemia, often does not eliminate tissue hypoxia, and may mask hypoventilation. It is one step in the treatment of hypoxemia that is coupled with other interventions such as incentive spirometry, pain control, positioning, and diuresis to insure a good outcome. With the standardization of pulse oximetry in the perioperative setting, administration of supplemental oxygen has increased.

Oxygen delivery systems are categorized as either low-flow or high-flow systems.

Low-Flow Devices

When supplemental oxygen is delivered via low-flow devices, FIO_2 can only be approximated due to the entrainment of room air and variation in minute ventilation. When a patient's minute ventilation exceeds the flow rate, more room air is inspired.

A. Nasal Cannula

Nasal cannulas are the most frequently used device. Flow can be increased from 1 to 6 liters per minute (L/min) after which increasing flow no longer increases FIO_2. With this device, FIO_2 increases approximately 4% above room air (21% FIO_2) per liter per minute increase in oxygen flow. The maximum FIO_2 obtainable with a nasal cannula is 44%.

Humidification of inspired oxygen is necessary to prevent drying of mucous membranes when flows become greater than 4 LPM. The amount of room air inhaled through nose and mouth mixes with supplemental oxygen delivered

via the nasal cannula. Fraction of inspired oxygen decreases as minute ventilation increases (minute ventilation [V_E] = respiratory rate [RR] × tidal volume [Vt]). The actual FIO_2 with nasal oxygen varies with minute ventilation.

FIO_2	Minute Ventilation (L/min)	Oxygen Flow (L/min)
0.60	5	6
0.44	10	6
0.32	20	6

B. Simple Face Mask

Simple face masks are loosely fitted devices that allow entrainment of room air in addition to supplemental oxygen. Flow rates of at least 5 L/min are required for all masks (simple, partial nonrebreather, and nonrebreather) to flush the expired CO_2 from the mask and prevent rebreathing. Like the nasal cannula, each increase in flow by 1 L/min increases the FIO_2 by approximately 4%. With simple face masks, the achievable FIO_2 ranges from 35% to 60%. With these devices, FIO_2 delivery decreases with increased minute ventilation.

C. Nonrebreather Face Masks

The nonrebreather face mask is indicated in clinical situations which require inspired FIO_2 greater than 40%. Oxygen delivery varies from 60% to 90%. The nonrebreather face mask contains an oxygen reservoir (typically 1 L) and one-way valves. The one-way valve allows the patient to exhale CO_2 out of the mask and prevents entrainment of room air. There is also a valve that prevents exhaled gas from entering the reservoir. The reservoir is filled with oxygen at flows between 8 and 15 L/min. The patient inspires concentrated oxygen from the reservoir and a small amount of room air limiting the FIO_2 to 90%. A true nonrebreather would put the patient at risk of suffocation if the O_2 supply became depleted or was unable to fill the reservoir bag. Conventional nonrebreather masks have one of the two one-way valves removed to allow for entrainment of room air in the event of oxygen supply failure. The reservoir must remain one-third to one-half full at all times to allow for tidal breathing of a high concentration of oxygen.

D. Partial Rebreather Face Mask

A partial rebreather mask differs from a nonrebreather mask only with the absence of a one-way valve between the mask and reservoir bag. F_{IO_2} ranges from 60% to 80% and the oxygen flow must be greater than 5 L/min to prevent rebreathing of CO_2. Exhaled gas enters the reservoir bag and is mixed with oxygen. The first 150 mL of exhaled gas enters the reservoir. This portion of expired gas is mainly anatomical dead space and contains very little CO_2. Therefore, the patient rebreathes only a very small amount of CO_2. As expiratory gas flow decreases below the oxygen inflow, exhaled gas no longer enters the reservoir bag, and leaves via the one-way valve in the face mask. Flow must be sufficient to prevent the bag from collapsing during inspiration.

High-Flow Devices

High-flow devices ensure flows that exceed a patient's minute ventilation and deliver a consistent F_{IO_2}. The primary high-flow device is the Venturi mask. This specialized mask mixes oxygen and room air to deliver a controlled F_{IO_2}. It provides a constant and precise F_{IO_2} independent of the patient's minute ventilation. The size of the room air entrainment port determines the F_{IO_2} and varies to provide concentrations of oxygen from 24% to 50%. The larger the port, the more room air is entrained, the lower the F_{IO_2}. Increasing the flow of oxygen will not alter the F_{IO_2} delivered. Oxygen is delivered to mask at a low-flow rate and increases in velocity as it passes through the narrow orifice of the entrainment port. The Venturi mask is most often used in patients with COPD in whom a precise and often low F_{IO_2} is desirable. Humification is unnecessary with Venturi masks due to the large amount of room air inspired by the patient.

19

Waste Gas Evacuation Systems

Matthew de Jesus, MD

The National Institute for Occupational Safety and Health (NIOSH), while unable to define safe levels of exposure, recommends limiting trace gas levels to:

Anesthetic Gas	Maximum Concentration (ppm)
Halogenated agent alone	2
Nitrous oxide alone	50
Combination of halogenated agent plus nitrous oxide	
Halogenated agent	0.5
Nitrous oxide	25

In most cases, the amount to anesthetic delivered exceeds the patient's minimal requirement. Waste gas scavenging systems help to collect and remove excess anesthetic gases that would otherwise contaminate the operating theater. Scavenging is the process by which waste anesthetic gases flowing from the patient circuit are collected, controlled, and evacuated from the workplace, to reduce ambient concentrations of agents or gases. Active scavengers use a vacuum to remove waste gases. Passive scavengers rely on the physical properties of the gases for elimination.

Anesthetic gas contamination occurs via two causes: anesthetic technique and equipment issues. Technical issues include using flows that exceed the scavenging system, poorly fitting face masks and laryngeal mask airways, flushing the circuit, leaving the anesthetic gas on after a case, filling of vaporizers, using uncuffed endotracheal tubes, and use of independent breathing circuits (ie, Jackson Rees). Equipment failures include leaks, disconnections, and malfunctioning scavenging systems.

Scavengers can fail from an obstruction. Valves help a malfunctioning scavenger by protecting from excessive pressures. Open scavenging systems are without valves. Closed systems use either positive or positive and negative pressure relief valves.

SCAVENGING SYSTEM COMPONENTS (FIGURE 19-1)

1. The *Gas Collecting Assembly* receives waste gases from either the adjustable pressure-limiting valve or ventilator relief valve.
2. *Transfer Tubing* carries the waste gases from the gas collecting assembly to the scavenging interface. The ASTM F1343-91 standard requires that the tubing be either 19 or 30 mm to distinguish it from the 22-mm breathing tubing. The tubing should be short and rigid to prevent kinking and occlusion, which can result in back pressure and ultimately barotrauma.
3. The *Scavenging Interface* protects the circuit and ventilator from positive and negative excessive pressures. Open systems are without valves, and stay open to atmospheric pressure. They require an active disposal system. Closed systems use either positive pressure valves or both positive and negative pressure valves.
4. *Gas Disposal Tubing* connects the scavenging interface to the gas disposal assembly. It should be robust as to prevent collapsing.
5. The *Disposal Assembly* is either active or passive, and eliminates the gases to the atmosphere. Active systems use a vacuum to eliminate waste, whereas passive stems rely on the heavier weight of anesthetic gases to force waste through.

WEB SITES

OSHA website section on anesthetic gases. https://www.osha.gov/dts/osta/anestheticgases/index.html. Accessed March 2, 2014.
University of Florida Virtual Anesthesia Machine Simulation. http://vam.anest.ufl.edu/. Accessed March 2, 2014.

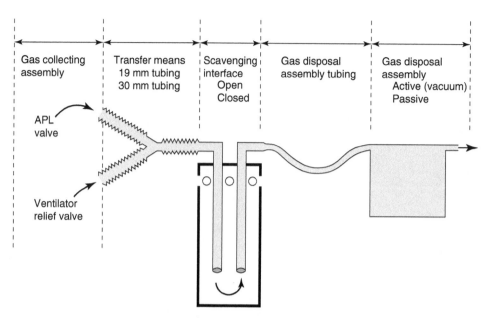

FIGURE 19-1 Components of a scavenging system. (Reproduced with permission from Barash PG, *Clinical Anesthesia*, 7th ed. Philadelphia, PA: Wolters Kluwer Health/Lippincott Williams & Wilkins; 2013.)

Design and Ergonomics of Anesthesia Machines

Sudha Ved, MD

Administering anesthesia in a complex environment of high technology and new surgical innovations is a risky process where any human or equipment failures can result in serious consequences for the patient. An ergonomic and simplified design of the anesthesia workplace should be regarded as a matter of continual evolvement.

ERGONOMICS

Ergonomics, or human factors engineering, is the scientific study of interactions between humans and other components of a system. The purpose of ergonomics is to promote operational efficiency and to decrease human error. Within anesthesiology, ergonomics promotes patient safety by reducing stress and strain on the user.

The American National Standards Institute and the Association for the Advancement of Medical Instrumentation promote attention to ergonomics during the design of medical instrumentation. To apply ergonomics in the anesthesia work environment, it is useful to have a model of the anesthesia provider at work. The model has three elements (anesthesiologist, equipment, and the patient) and two interfaces (ergonomics and machine design). The areas studied in ergonomics include equipment design, workplace layout, environmental conditions such as lighting, and the related questions of skill acquisition, productivity, and safety. The ergonomics of controls and displays has special relevance as anesthetic technology becomes more complex.

DESIGN OF ANESTHESIA EQUIPMENT

Innovations and Discoveries

Historically, there have been four main technological innovations in the area of anesthesia equipment design (Table 20-1):

1. In the early 1900s, the equipment consisted of small hand-held devices, mainly a folded towel and bottle containing anesthetic agents. Later, the cloth was supported by a wire mask and then to a more complex inhaler combining the mask and bottle as one device.

2. In the 1920s, inhaler technology was integrated into a floor-mounted or portable apparatus, where multiple anesthetic agents could be compressed in cylinders with reducing valves and controlled simultaneously.

3. In the 1930s, the anesthesia machine was enhanced with further advancements such as the Waters' soda lime canister, which was added in a table format.

4. From 1950 to 2000, major new components and safety features were added. These parts included work surfaces and drawers, calibrated vaporizers, common gas outlet, and mechanical ventilators. Integrated monitors and central display data recording was developed in the 1990s. Due to new clinical demands, a complete workstation was developed. By integrating devices for patient monitoring and ventilation, the new design allowed for fresh gas flow, independent ventilation, compensation for circuit leak and circuit compliance, intensive care unit (ICU) modes of ventilation and synchronization, electronic vaporization, and automatic preuse checks.

User Needs

Industry has kept lock step with the needs of the anesthesia provider, patient safety and regulations, and ergonomic design of the anesthesia machine. Ergonomic guided design is an iterative and cyclical process. The schematic design is repeated and refined from overall concept based on the feedback of owners, end users, consultants, and customers, until all the major design flaws have been fixed. Techniques such as task and workflow analysis, site visits to similar facilities, building mock-ups, cognitive or computer-based walkthroughs, and interviews and surveys are used to obtain feedback on the proposed designs.

Fortunately, the most basic workstation components are generally fairly consistent from one platform to another. These basic component systems include what was formerly referred to as the anesthesia machine proper (ie, the pressure-regulating and gas-mixing components), the vaporizers, the anesthesia breathing circuit, the ventilator, the scavenging system, and respiratory and physiologic monitoring systems. Modern anesthesia workstations also incorporate advances in digitization, patient safety, and ancillary equipment requirement

TABLE 20-1   A Chronology of Major Safety Features for the Anesthesia Machine

Years: 1950-1960	Years: 1960-1970
Pin index safety system for medical gas cylinders	Ventilator pressure relief system
Oxygen flush value delivering >35 L/min	Check valve between vaporizer and fresh gas outlet
Temperature- and flow-compensated vaporizers	Gate-style cylinder yokes
Oxygen supply failure system	Ascending–filling ventilator bellows
Oxygen failure protection device	Single-agent vaporizers
Vaporizer interlock system	Key index safety systems for filling vaporizers

Years: 1970-1980	Years: 1980-1990
Ventilator low-pressure disconnect alarm	Antidisconnect fitting on fresh gas outlet
Machine-mounted pipeline pressure gauges	Common manifold for breathing circuit components
Diameter index safety system	Volume disconnect alarm
Minimum oxygen flow	Master switch on/off for machine/patient monitors
N_2O/O_2 proportioning devices	Airway pressure monitoring systems
Recessed oxygen flush button	Cable management arm
Pin index safety system for flowmeter modules	Battery backup for power supply
Oxygen analyzer	

such as electronic medical records, suction, monitors, cables, and phones. The machines rectify the deficiencies of mechanical and electronic devices of the past. The basic features as required by user needs include:

- **Machine size and orientation**
    - Typical anesthesia workstation and medication cart dimensions.
    - Anesthesia machines are generally configured, so the patient attachments (ie, the breathing circuit) are located on the left-hand side of the machine.
    - The anesthesia machine is best positioned to the right side at the head of the OR table, or in a less desirable location behind the anesthesia provider.
    - In some surgical procedures, the anesthesia machine may be located at the patient's side or at the patient's feet.
- **Suction**
    - Suction canister and controls should be located in the anesthesia cockpit within reach and view of the anesthesia provider.

- Height of suction canister should be below the level of the surgical table (to decrease effect of hydrostatic pressure).
- **Monitor, computer, phone**
    - Access to patient data in the Electronic Medical Record in real time.
    - Access to "help" materials (Internet, etc) in real time.
    - Wired and/or wireless access.
    - Portable versus fixed computers with keyboards and mice.
    - Use of alternate screen-pointing devices (touch screens, trackballs, knobs).
    - Glare, spillage, infection control considerations.
    - Food and Drug Administration (FDA) Human Factors Design guidelines.
    - Emergency Care Research Institute (ECRI) resources.
- **Power management**
    - Electrical, phone, network, and compressed gas outlets should be located near the anesthesia cockpit, and not across major pathways into and out of the room. Multiple network ports may be needed, as monitors, anesthesia information systems, hospital Electronic Medical Record, and general intranet and Internet usage may require separate networks.
    - Can be located on the ceiling or on ceiling-mounted "booms."
- **Hose, cord, and cable management**
    - Hoses, cords, and cables on the floor can be a trip hazard, and can interfere with positioning of wheeled equipment.
    - Wheel protectors can be used to push cables away.

Patient Safety and Regulations

One of the major reasons for change in machine design in the past has been led by patient safety. The assembled components designated as a machine is adequate for the task but not for the activity or procedural diversity of tasks. Although these studies raised concerns, the design of modern equipment became directed by regulations, standards, and guidelines. This feature has been maintained by the absence of research that investigates the long-term relationship between the design and user of anesthesia equipment.

Recently there has also been increasing divergence between anesthesia workstation designs from different manufacturers. Standards for anesthesia machines and workstations provide guidelines for manufacturers regarding their minimum performance, design characteristics, and safety requirements. Newly manufactured workstations must have monitors that measure the following parameters to comply with the 2000 standards of the American Society for Testing and Materials:

- continuous breathing system pressure;
- exhaled tidal volume;
- ventilatory carbon dioxide concentration;

- anesthetic vapor concentration;
- inspired oxygen concentration;
- oxygen supply pressure;
- arterial oxygen saturation of hemoglobin;
- arterial blood pressure; and
- continuous electrocardiogram.

To improve patient safety, new designs for the anesthesia machine should prevent human error whenever possible. If human error cannot be prevented, then the system should be designed to prevent such errors from causing injury. All machines should be equipped with monitors and alarms. The anesthesia workstation must have a prioritized alarm system that groups the alarms into three categories: high, medium, and low priority. These monitors and alarms may be automatically enabled and made to function by turning on the anesthesia workstation, or the monitors and alarms can be manually enabled and made functional by following a preuse checklist.

Modern anesthesia delivery systems and workstations contain pneumatic, mechanical, and electronic components that are extremely reliable so that unexpected "pure" failure of equipment is rare in a system that has been well maintained and properly checked before use. Design features of new workstations are based on the following premise and have led to anesthesia machine obsolescence. Criteria for anesthesia machine obsolescence can be absolute, such as lack of essential safety features, presence of unacceptable features, and adequate maintenance no longer possible. Relative criteria include lack of certain features, problems with maintenance, potential for human error, and inability to meet practice needs.

Future Directions

State-of-the-art operating rooms of the future will be configured to accommodate current and future surgical innovations, including digital integration, advanced informatics, telemedicine and video conferencing, intraoperative CT, MRI and angiography, robotics, 3D imaging, and virtual reality and high definition video. The new operating rooms will also incorporate design features that will improve anesthesia workstation ergonomics, including compact anesthesia machines, wireless technology, and modular monitoring systems. All data sources—the hospital information system, laboratory information system, intranet and Internet—will be accessible to anesthesia providers at the point of care.

SUGGESTED READINGS

Boquet G, Bushman JA, Davenport HT. The anaesthesia machine: a study of function and design. *BJA* 1980;52:61-67.

Drui AB, Behm RJ, Martin WE. Predesign investigation of the anesthesia operational environment. *Anesth Analg* 1973;52:584-591.

Martin JL, Norris BJ, Murphy E, Crowe JA. Medical device development: the challenge for ergonomics. *Appl Ergo.* 2008;39:271-283.

Monitoring Neuromuscular Function

Steven W. Price, MD, and Sudha Ved, MD

BASIC CONCEPTS

Neuromuscular blocking drugs (NMBDs) interfere with neural transmission at the neuromuscular junction (NMJ). This effectively produces paralysis, which is advantageous to facilitate conditions for intubation by decreasing the tone of supralaryngeal muscles, inhibiting spontaneous ventilation, improving lung dynamics for mechanical ventilation, and providing proper skeletal muscle relaxation to optimize surgical conditions.

Proper monitoring of the degree and adequacy of neuromuscular blockade is vital in clinical practice. Providing too little neuromuscular blockade can lead to substandard conditions for the surgeon and anesthesiologist alike. Meanwhile, overzealous or inappropriate use of NMBDs could result in delayed extubation or the need for reintubation in the post-anesthesia care unit (PACU) (Table 21-1). In addition to the interference with pulmonary mechanics, residual blockade also depresses the ventilatory response to hypoxia. As NMBDs possess no analgesic or anesthetic properties, the use of NMBDs could also lead to increased intraoperative awareness during general anesthesia. It is therefore important to use anesthetics concurrently with the administration of NMBDs.

Several methods exist to measure the status of neuromuscular blockade (Table 21-2). Clinical signs such as 5-second head lift and the ability to hold a tongue depressor between the teeth represent reliable indication of neuromuscular function to tolerate extubation. However, these clinical signs cannot be elected during the course of anesthesia. The use of peripheral nerve stimulators to produce mechanically evoked responses to electrical stimulation, therefore, remains the best means to accurately determine neuromuscular status. Additionally, it aids in the determination of the adequacy of reversal with acteylcholinesterase inhibitors.

Peripheral nerve stimulation is generally performed by applying superficial electrodes over the distribution of a nerve. A supramaximal stimulus current (50-60 mA) is then delivered along the nerve. The muscular response to the stimulation indicates the degree of blockade at that given time. A supramaximal stimulus is necessary for accurate results; it ensures that a weakened response is not a result of the failure to stimulate all nerve fibers. The ulnar nerve at the wrist is commonly chosen as the peripheral nerve to monitor neuromuscular status. One benefit of monitoring this nerve is that it provides the lone innervation to the adductor pollicis; therefore, response to purely ulnar nerve stimulation can be

TABLE 21-1 Clinical Signs and Symptoms of Residual Paralysis in Awake Volunteers after Mivacurium-Induced Neuromuscular Blockade

Train-of-Four Ratio	Signs and Symptoms
0.70-0.75	Diplopia and visual disturbances Decreased handgrip strength Inability to maintain apposition of the incisor teeth "Tongue depressor test" negative Inability to sit up without assistance Severe facial weakness Speaking a major effort Overall weakness and tiredness
0.85-0.90	Diplopia and visual disturbances Generalized fatigue

(Reproduced with permission from Kopman AF, Yee PS, Neuman GG. Relationship of the train-of-four fade ratio to clinical signs and symptoms of residual paralysis in awake volunteers. *Anesthesiology.* 1997;86:765.)

TABLE 21-2   Clinical Tests of Postoperative Neuromuscular Recovery

Unreliable
Sustained eye opening
Protrusion of the tongue
Arm lift to the opposite shoulder
Normal tidal volume
Normal or nearly normal vital capacity
Maximum inspiratory pressure <40-50 cm H_2O
Most Reliable
Sustained head lift for 5 seconds
Sustained leg lift for 5 seconds
Sustained handgrip for 5 seconds
Sustained "tongue depressor test"
Maximum inspiratory pressure ≥40-50 cm H_2O

(Reproduced with permission from Miller RD, *Miller's Anesthesia*, 7th ed. Philadelphia, PA: Churchill Livingstone/Elsevier; 2010.)

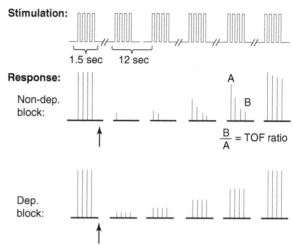

FIGURE 21-1 Pattern of electrical stimulation and evoked muscle responses to TOF nerve stimulation before and after injection of nondepolarizing (Non-dep.) and depolarizing (Dep.) NMBDs (*arrows*). (Reproduced with permission from Miller RD, *Miller's Anesthesia*, 7th ed. Philadelphia, PA: Churchill Livingstone/Elsevier; 2010.)

assessed by adduction of the ipsilateral thumb. Facial nerve stimulation and concurrent observation of the orbicularis oculi muscle is often an alternative when ulnar nerve stimulation is not possible. In fact, orbicularis oculi response does better mirror the blockade status of the laryngeal muscles and the diaphragm than does the ulnar nerve. Median, posterior tibial, and common peroneal are several other peripheral nerves that can be used.

PATTERNS OF STIMULATION

Patterns of mechanically evoked stimulation to create measured neuromuscular responses include single-twitch stimulation, the train-of-four ratio (TOF), tetanus, post-tetanic stimulation and, double-burst stimulation (DBS). They are measured by visual or tactile observation or recorders to evaluate muscular response.

Single supramaximal twitch stimulation is a monitoring technique that measures the strength of a single control twitch at 0.1 (once per second) to 1 Hz (once every 10 seconds), which is elicited before any NMBDs are given. Subsequent twitches are then compared as a ratio to the control. The single-twitch amplitude will begin to decline only once 75% of the receptors are blocked. Therefore, this is a poor technique to assess adequacy of reversal agents. Appropriate surgical relaxation generally requires a single-twitch amplitude of less than 10% of the control. Single-twitch stimulation can be employed with both depolarizing and nondepolarizing NMBDs.

As shown in Figure 21-1, TOF stimulation is a method that delivers four stimuli at 2 Hz (timed 0.5 seconds apart). With partial neuromuscular blockade, the twitch response will fade with progressive stimuli. Greater blockade may inhibit some or all four of the twitches. Therefore, valuable information exists in the number of twitches that are able to be elicited, as well as the TOF ratio if all four twitches are indeed present. The TOF ratio is the ratio of the amplitude of the fourth twitch (T4) to the amplitude of the first twitch (T1). The amplitude of T1 is reduced by 75% when 80% of the receptors are blocked. Meanwhile, absence of the T4 twitch signals an 80% receptor block; absence of T3 signals an 85% receptor block; and absence of T2 signals a 90% receptor block. Recent data show that a TOF ratio greater than 0.9 represents reliable adequate reversal from neuromuscular blockade for extubation. Visual and tactile elicitation of this ratio remains very unreliable; even very experienced anesthesiologists are unable to detect fade at TOF ratios greater than 0.4.

TOF stimulation is less useful for depolarizing NMBDs. When these drugs are given, there will be a stable decrease in amplitude in all four twitches. Therefore, there will be no fade and thus an inaccurate TOF ratio. However, during a phase II block—in which large or repeated doses of depolarizing NMBDs take on nondepolarizing characteristics—fade can be recognized on TOF stimulation.

Tetanus uses a high-frequency stimulus (usually 50 or 100 Hz). It usually is applied for a set time, commonly 5 seconds. In physiologic conditions without any blockade, response is a sustained contraction of the stimulated muscle. However, muscle with any degree of nondepolarizing neuromuscular blockade will demonstrate fade in the contractile strength before the allotted 5 seconds. Sustained contraction indicates a TOF greater than 0.7. Depolarizing block will not demonstrate any fade (in the absence of phase II block), but may show decreased contractility in response to the stimulus. As noted later, neuromuscular fatigue can develop with repeated tetanic testing.

Post-tetanic stimulation response may be useful to measure in cases of intense blockade in which TOF or single-twitch stimulation does not render any response. In these instances, a tetanic stimulus is applied, followed by single-twitch stimulation delivered at 1 Hz. The initial tetanic stimulus will cause a transient increase in the immediately available stores of acetylcholine. This is known as post-tetanic facilitation and will provide a greater likelihood of response to subsequent stimuli. The number of twitches in response to the post-tetanic stimuli correlates with the degree of blockade and can be extrapolated in comparison to other modes of stimulation. For example, when 0.1 mg/kg of vecuronium is given for paralysis, a post-tetanic count of approximately 10 (range 6-16) corresponds to the return of the first twitch in TOF stimulation.

Double burst stimulation (DBS) represents a variation of tetanus. It can be used to appreciably detect small degrees of neuromuscular blockade, even those small enough that would be undetected on TOF stimulation. In DBS, two supramaximal tetanic bursts are fired 750 ms apart. Each burst consists of 50 Hz of impulse for a total of 0.2 ms. Physiologic response in unparalyzed patients would render two contractions of equal magnitude 750 ms apart. However, residual neuromuscular blockade will be clinically evident by a reduction in the contractile strength of the second impulse. The DBS is therefore quantified as the ratio of the second stimulus to the first. However, absence of fade in the manually evaluated response to DBS (and TOF) does not exclude residual neuromuscular blockade. When a manual evaluation of TOF responses is used, fade can only be reliably detected when the TOF ratio is less than 0.4. In contrast, manual assessment of evoked responses to DBS allows for the detection of fade up to TOF ratios of 0.6.

Although each of these techniques employs its own benefits and disadvantages, it is important to recognize that the stimulus frequency affects the response. Single-twitch and TOF stimulation should not be performed more than once every 10 seconds, as progressively diminished responses could be a result of decreased acetylcholine at the NMJ, as opposed to true blockade. Similarly, tetanic stimulation exceeding 50 Hz will cause fade at higher frequencies and overestimate the degree of blockade. Therefore, single-twitch and TOF testing should not be repeated at intervals less than 10 seconds, and tetanic stimulation should be given at physiologic levels of 30-50 Hz and should not be repeated at intervals less than 6 minutes.

RECORDING DEVICES

Because visual or tactile observation is unreliable, there are several methods to measure nerve stimulation objectively:

1. **Mechanomyography** (MMG) is the measurement of evoked muscle tension to nerve stimulation. This is most commonly measured as an isometric contraction in the adductor pollicis in response to ulnar stimulation. A strain gauge transducer and recorder detects a change in tension after applying a preload of 200-300 g resting tension to the thumb, and will record the variable degree of change with each evoked contraction. Measurements are most accurate when the arm and hand are fixed and movement of the thumb is directly along the transducer.

2. **Electromyography** (EMG) is the recording of an action potential during muscular contraction, whether evoked or voluntary. Stimulating electrodes are placed over the peripheral nerve (usually the ulnar). Three recording electrodes are placed; one over the muscle belly, a second over the tendinous insertion of the muscle, and one in a neutral distal site. On stimulation, blockade is determined by the summation of compound action potential generated. Evoked EMG responses usually correlate well with MMG. Although the EMG is easier to assemble than the mechanical recording devices, it is prone to interference and drift. It is therefore unlikely to gain widespread clinical use.

3. **Accelerometry** was developed as a more convenient method of monitoring evoked responses. However, instead of measuring a force, it measures the acceleration of the contraction. In this mode of recording, a piezoelectric ceramic wafer is strapped to the thumb. Stimulation of the adductor pollicis will cause the thumb to move and the attached transducer to produce a voltage, which is proportional to its acceleration, and recorded as a twitch response. Accelerometry has been shown to be comparable to MMG in accuracy.

4. **Kinemyography** (KMG) provides measurement of the evoked electrical response in a film sensor attached to the muscle (thumb), combining both mechanical and electric components into a piezoelectric neuromuscular monitor. Stretching or bending of the flexible piezoelectric film generates a voltage that is proportional to the amount of stretching or bending. Kinemyography may be a valuable clinical tool; however, the values may show wider limits of agreement with accelerometry (AMG) and MMG.

5. **Phonomyography** (PMG) is a relatively new method of neuromonitoring. Low-frequency sounds are generated by contraction of muscles, which are recorded with special condenser microphones. Studies have shown good correlation with AMG, EMG, and MMG; however, it remains to be seen if it will be used clinically.

SUGGESTED READINGS

Hemmerling TM. Brief review: neuromuscular monitoring: an update for the clinician. *Can J Anesth* 2007;54:58 -72.

McGrath CD, Hunter JM. Monitoring of neuromuscular block. *Contin Educ Anaesth Crit Care Pain* 2006;6:7-12.

Monitoring Mechanical Ventilation

Steven W. Price, MD, and Sudha Ved, MD

The goal of ventilation is to generate adequate flow and volume to provide sufficient alveolar ventilation while minimizing the work of breathing (WOB). In mechanical ventilation, it is vital to closely monitor the function of the ventilator system regularly, including the settings, alarms, circuitry, and patient's clinical status.

MONITORING QUALITATIVE CLINICAL SIGNS

- **Respiratory rate**—To detect apnea, set or measured respiratory rate can be measured by airflow sampling, capnography, inductive plethysmography, oscillometry frequency-based changes, ECG, or ventilation acoustics.
- **Physical examination**—Vigilant physical assessment of chest excursion is a necessity for accurate monitoring of mechanical ventilation. Asymmetric chest motion or unilateral breath sounds may indicate pneumothorax, endobronchial intubation, or atelectasis. Paradoxical chest motion can signify flail chest or respiratory muscle dysfunction. Poor synchrony of a patient's breathing pattern with the ventilator's drive may indicate that the ventilator settings are inappropriate or that the patient's depth of anesthesia is too light. Tympanic percussion or tracheal deviation could help diagnose a pneumothorax. Audible endotracheal leaks around the airway cuff indicate insufficient air or a potential cuff rupture.
- **Movement of reservoir bag**—Free and unencumbered movement of reservoir bag during spontaneous ventilation assures a patent airway or early detection of circuit obstruction.
- **Breath sounds**—Continuous auscultation with a precordial or esophageal stethoscope is extremely valuable in detecting disconnects, leaks, airway obstruction by secretions or bronchospasm, and apnea.

MONITORING GAS EXCHANGE

Adequacy of mechanical ventilation can be determined by the ability of the patient to maintain ventilation and oxygenation. Pulse oximetry and capnography are two standard American

Society of Anesthesiologists (ASA) monitors that are utilized for this purpose. Furthermore, arterial blood gas analysis provides significant insight into ventilatory status. A low Pao_2 on an arterial blood gas (ABG) indicates hypoxemia—a dysfunction of the ability to oxygenate arterial blood. A number of ventilator factors can directly affect the Pao_2: chiefly, the Fio_2, positive end-expiratory pressure (PEEP) level, and the patient's lung function. It is important to interpret the Pao_2 as a function of these dependent variables, as a "normal" Pao_2 does not necessarily indicate ideal physiologic pulmonary function.

MONITORING VENTILATORY DRIVE AND BREATHING PATTERN

Dependent upon clinical scenario, mechanical ventilation can be adjusted to provide as much or as little support as necessary. Positive pressure breathing can be categorized by three variables: the *trigger* variable, which initiates the breath; the *limit* variable, which governs the gas delivery; and the *cycle* variable, which terminates the breath. The dependent variable for triggering is *time* in controlled mechanical ventilation modes. Each of these breaths will provide a preset volume or pressure at regular intervals. Cycle time can, therefore, be adjusted based on *volume, pressure*, or *flow*.

Partial ventilator support can also be utilized through pressure support and synchronized intermittent mandatory ventilation modes. In each of these modes, the ventilator will sense the initiation of a breath by the patient and may deliver a set tidal volume or pressure to assist with completion of the breath. Utilization of these modes will optimize respiratory neuromuscular function while limiting the associated WOB. In critically ill patients, partial ventilator support can decrease the need for sedation and paralysis, avoid disuse atrophy of respiratory muscles, and minimize the cardiovascular side effects of mechanical ventilation.

Components of breathing patterns to monitor include:

1. **Tidal volume**—Causes of low tidal volume in pressure preset modes include asynchronous breathing, decreased compliance, increased system resistance, inadequate preset pressure, and gas leak.

2. **Inspiratory flow**—Inspiratory flow is determined by tidal volume/inspiratory time. High flow rates result in high peak airway pressures (P_{peak}). It may not be of concern provided that most of the added pressure is dissipated across the endotracheal tube. Patients may find abrupt bolus of gas uncomfortable and "fight" the ventilator. Low flows prolong inspiratory time and increase the mean airway pressure. Subsequent improvement of oxygenation may occur at the expense of increasing right ventricular (RV) afterload and decreasing RV preload. Low inspiratory flow also decreases expiratory time and predisposes patient to dynamic hyperinflation. Patient may find flow insufficient and begin to "lead" the ventilator, sustaining inspiratory effort throughout much of the inspiratory cycle.

3. **Expiratory flow**—Expiratory flow is determined by tidal volume/expiratory time. Expiratory time is the difference between cycle time and inspiratory time and the principal ventilator-related determinant of dynamic hyperinflation. Expiratory flow cannot usually be set.

4. **Triggering**—Flow/pressure triggering is characterized by sensitivity and responsiveness (delay in providing response). Even with modern sensors there is unavoidable dyssynchrony due to the need for a certain level of insensitivity to prevent artifactual triggering and delay due to opening of demand valves. Strategies to minimize dyssynchrony include: (1) ventilators with microprocessor flow controls often have significantly better valve characteristics than those on older generation ventilators; (2) continuous flow systems superimposed on demand systems can improve demand system responsiveness in patients with high ventilatory drive (but can reduce sensitivity in patients with very low respiratory drive); (3) flow-based triggers are more sensitive and allow responsive breath triggering; (4) small amount of pressure support usually initiates ventilators' initial flow and may help improved response characteristics in CPAP; (5) setting PEEP below $PEEP_i$ may improve triggering in patients with COPD who have an inspiratory threshold load induced by $PEEP_i$.

MONITORING LUNG AND CHEST WALL MECHANICS

Flow–Volume Loops

Flow–volume loops are utilized to measure the rate of airflow as a function of lung volumes. Figure 22-1 illustrates the pathology that exists with various flow–volume loops.

Pressure–Volume Curves

To assess respiratory compliance, pressure–volume (PV) curves can be measured on the ventilator with a constant flow and pressure measurements at various volumes. Mapping of PV curves in patients with acute respiratory distress syndrome and acute lung injury can provide valuable information about lung mechanics and help guide PEEP and tidal volume settings. A *dynamic* PV curve is one that is constructed during gas flow, whereas *static* curves are derived when flow is absent. Plateau (P_{plat}) and peak inspiratory pressures (P_{pk}) are recorded after each breath to allow determination of both static (C_{stat}) and dynamic (C_{dyn}) compliance. Because C_{stat} is calculated by using P_{plat}, it is mainly influenced by chest wall and alveolar elastic recoil; C_{dyn} is derived by using P_{pk}, and therefore takes airway and circuit resistance into account as well.

Airway Pressures

The analysis of pressure versus time during volume-cycled, constant flow with a brief, controlled, end-inspiratory pause provides valuable insight into the mechanics of the respiratory system. The pressure at airway opening (P_{ao}) can be divided into resistive pressure (P_{res}), elastic pressure (P_{el}), and PEEP. The P_{peak} is the sum of P_{res}, P_{el}, and PEEP.

Total PEEP is the sum of extrinsic and intrinsic PEEP. Extrinsic PEEP is generally applied by a ventilator as a strategy to improve oxygenation via alveolar recruitment and decreased atelectasis. More commonly referred to as auto-PEEP, intrinsic PEEP exists when the time available for expiration is shorter than the time required for passive emptying to functional residual capacity. Development of auto-PEEP is more likely to occur in cases of decreased total time per tidal volume (eg, tachypnea), increased expiratory resistance (eg, COPD), or decreased end-inspiratory recoil pressures. Consequently, alveolar pressures will remain more positive than set extrinsic PEEP, and the lung will display a "dynamic hyperinflation" state. In a ventilated patient, dynamic hyperinflation can cause severe hemodynamic consequences due to subsequent increased intrathoracic pressures. These pressures will decrease venous return, decreased preload, and increased right ventricular afterload. Auto-PEEP can be measured with an *end-expiratory hold maneuver* on the ventilator.

P_{peak} represents the maximum respiratory pressure reached at end-inspiration. It expresses the sum of PEEP and both the P_{el} and P_{res} of the system. At a given P_{peak}, an end-inspiratory pause of 0.5-1.5 seconds will occur in the ventilator. This interruption of flow will eliminate the P_{res} in the system. After elimination of resistance, the resultant pressure will represent the P_{plat} with no inspiratory flow. P_{plat} is the sum of the P_{el} and PEEP. P_{plat} is probably a better estimate of peak alveolar pressure than P_{peak}. Based on animal studies and the knowledge that human lungs are maximally distended at a respiratory system recoil pressure of 35 cm H_2O, maintaining P_{plat} of less than 30 cm H_2O is recommended. However, if pleural pressure increases (eg, due to distended abdomen), then P_{plat} will increase without an increase in alveolar pressure.

P_{res} represents the pressure required to generate constant laminar flow in the airways at the initiation of inspiration. The total resistance of the respiratory system is the sum of pulmonary resistance and chest wall resistance. P_{res} of the respiratory system are increased in cases of asthma, acute

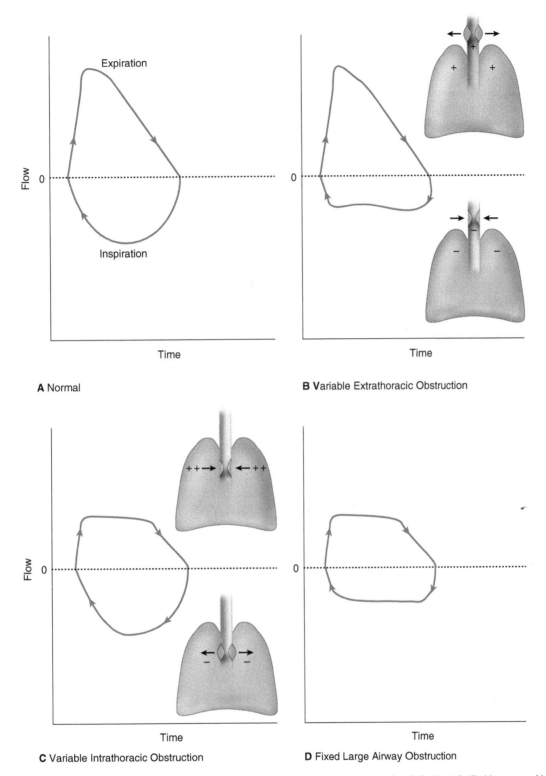

FIGURE 22-1 Flow–volume loops. (Reproduced with permission from Butterworth JF, Mackey DC, Wasnick JD, *Morgan and Mikhail's Clinical Anesthesiology*, 5th ed. McGraw-Hill; 2013.)

cardiogenic pulmonary edema, ARDS, and COPD. However, with very high P_{res} (and, subsequently, high P_{peak}), endotracheal tube obstruction should always be considered in the differential diagnosis.

P_{el} is the difference between the P_{plat} and PEEP ($P_{el} = P_{plat} -$ PEEP). It represents the pressure that is necessary to maintain progressive inflation of the respiratory system. The static compliance and elastance of the respiratory system can be determined by P_{el}. Static compliance can be measured as the ratio of the tidal volume to P_{el}. Elastance is the inverse of compliance. Dynamic compliance, meanwhile, is the ratio of the tidal volume to P_{peak}.

Dynamic and Static Effective Compliance

Calculation of dynamic and static effective compliance may reveal the cause of increased airway pressure. Dynamic effective compliance, which has both compliance and resistance components, is actually a measure of impedance.

Dynamic effective compliance = $(P_{peak} - PEEP)$/delivered tidal volume.

Static effective compliance = $(P_{plat} - PEEP)$/delivered tidal volume.

(Delivered tidal volume = Tidal volume – ventilator compressible volume. PEEP = the higher of intrinsic PEEP [$PEEP_i$] and extrinsic PEEP [$PEEP_e$].)

Dynamic effective compliance is reduced by decreases in lung or chest wall compliance or increases in airway resistance. Static compliance is not affected by resistance (assuming pressure measurement is made when there is no flow). However, respiratory compliance is not solely dependent upon lung mechanics. Chest wall and diaphragmatic distensibility also influence the elastance and compliance of the respiratory system. Abdominal distention, pleural effusions, ascites, decreased muscular tone, recent surgery, position, and binders can all increase pleural pressures. For a given lung volume, increased pleural pressure may decrease respiratory compliance and decrease transpulmonary pressure. Therefore, appropriate interpretation of tidal airway pressures depends on valid intrapleural pressure analysis.

MONITORING RESPIRATORY STRENGTH AND MUSCLE RESERVE

Airway Occlusion Pressure

Airway occlusion pressure (AOP) is often used as an indirect, yet reliable measurement of the respiratory neuromuscular activity. Airway occlusion pressure is the pressure developed at the trachea during the first 0.1 seconds of inspiratory effort against an occluded airway. This measurement can represent a more precise respiratory drive measurement than other measurements since it is relatively independent of modification by respiration machines.

Maximal Inspiratory Pressure

The two most common measures of respiratory muscle strength are the vital capacity and the maximal inspiratory pressure (MIP) or negative inspiratory force (NIF), generated against an occluded airway (normal about -90 cm H_2O). Given the cooperation necessary for vital capacity measurement, MIP tends to be more commonly used in critical care settings. Maximal inspiratory pressure is an isometric pressure optimally measured in a totally occluded airway after 20 seconds or 10 breathing efforts. More negative of MIP is strongly correlated with the ability to tolerate extubation. In fact, MIP less than -20 cm H_2O is a contraindication to extubation.

MONITORING BREATHING EFFORTS

During partial ventilatory support, evaluation of the WOB (WOB = $P \times V$) allows the optimization of support while allowing respiratory muscles to work at their maximal level. This can effectively limit over assistance of the ventilator and overuse of the respiratory muscles. The WOB in ventilated patients will be greater than that in nonventilated patients due to the "iatrogenic" resistance—endotracheal tube, circuit resistances, and inspiratory pressure needed to trigger ventilatory assistance. Work of breathing is normally less than 5% but can be as high as 40% of total oxygen consumption in cases of respiratory compromise. Work of breathing can be estimated in the PV curve by the area enclosed by the curve; the larger the loop, the greater the WOB. Effort and oxygen consumption can also be estimated by the pressure–time product (PTP = $P \times T_i$). The PTP parallels effort more closely than WOB because it includes the isometric component of diaphragm muscle tension that consumes oxygen. Occlusion pressures (P_{100}) measured at the airway has also shown to correlate with the WOB.

SUGGESTED READING

Bekos V, Marini JJ. Monitoring the mechanically ventilated patient. *Crit Care Clin* 2007;23:575 -611.

Monitoring Temperature

Nima Adimi, MD, and Christopher Monahan, MD

It is critical to monitor the effects of anesthetic drugs on core and surface temperatures in an attempt to detect and prevent hypothermia, hyperthermia, and malignant hyperthermia.

TYPES OF THERMOMETERS

The most common thermometers used are thermocouples and thermistors. These electrical systems are efficient, accurate, inexpensive, and disposable. The infrared system used to measure temperature from the tympanic membrane or forehead is largely inaccurate and should not be used.

General Anesthesia

Core temperature monitoring is mandatory for patients undergoing more than 30 minutes of general anesthesia. This monitoring is essential in detecting hypothermia, hyperthermia, and, less commonly, malignant hyperthermia. Although increased temperature is usually not the initial diagnostic sign, a rising core temperature may signify malignant hyperthermia.

Early signs of malignant hyperthermia are tachycardia and increasing end-tidal carbon dioxide.

General hyperthermia can be caused by fever secondary to infection, inaccurately matching blood products, excessive warming, and presence of blood in the fourth ventricle.

Hypothermia is the most common thermal disturbance, and can cause myocardial events like arrhythmias and decreased contractility, wound infections, increased blood loss, and prolonged hospitalization. Intentional hypothermia, however, can be protective against ischemia. It should be noted that 30 minutes after induction, core body temperature decreases 0.5°C to 1.5°C. In most surgical cases, unless hypothermia is indicated, it is important to keep core body temperature greater than 36°C.

Local Anesthesia

Local anesthesia, used for sedation and regional blocks, can frequently cause hypothermia. Local anesthesia does not cause malignant hyperthermia.

TABLE 23-1 Clinical Considerations for Temperature Monitoring Sites

Body Site	Temperature Accuracy	Clinical Correlation
Distal esophagus, tympanic membrane, nasopharynx, and pulmonary artery	Highly accurate core temperature site.	Good for surgical cases with rapid and frequent temperature changes (ie, cardiopulmonary bypass).
Skin surface	Temperature collected is lower than core temperature but can reflect core temperature when adjusted.	Fails to confirm malignant hyperthermia.
Oral, axillary	Reasonably accurate.	Limited when there is extreme thermal disturbance.
Rectal	Moderately accurate, "intermediate temperature," temperature lags behind that measured in core thermal sites.	Lags in cooling patients. Fails to rise in malignant hyperthermia.
Bladder	Accuracy dependent on urine flow.	Low urine output (ie, cardiac surgery) is equal to rectal temperatures. High urine output allows bladder temperatures to equal that of core sites.

TEMPERATURE MONITORING SITES

Measuring the temperature from core thermal sites is necessary, as these regions are well perfused and uniform in temperature. Table 23-1 discusses temperature monitoring sites.

SUGGESTED READING

Insler SR, Sessler DI. Perioperative thermoregulation and temperature monitoring. *Anesthesiol Clin* 2006;24:823-837.

Oximetry

Vinh Nguyen, DO

Pulse oximetry enables continuous monitoring of functional oxyhemoglobin saturation using an accurate, noninvasive and real-time probe. A continuous pulse oximeter reading allows the early warning sign of hypoxia. As a result, the loss of airway patency, potential loss of oxygen supply from the anesthetic machine, or intrinsic shunting can be clinically detected early to prevent any disastrous outcome.

CORE CONCEPTS

The basic principle of pulse oximetry depends on two components: the generation of an arterial pulsatile waveform and the ability to differentiate two different wavelengths. The pulse oximeter emits two light measuring wavelengths, 660 nm (red) and 940 nm (near infrared [IR]), for the calculation of fraction of oxygenated blood ($FHbO_2$) and ultimately oxygen saturation. Oxygenated blood (O_2Hb) absorbed more IR light whereas deoxygenated blood (deoxyHb) absorbs more red light. This phenomenon is generally observed with the naked eye: O_2Hb is seen as red because it scatters the red light more than deoxyHb does. As a result, deoxyHb appears less red because these molecules actually absorb more of the red waveform. Most pulse oximeters also provide plethysmographic waveforms to help distinguish between a true or artificial signal.

PHYSICAL PRINCIPLES

Conventional pulse oximetry uses two waveforms to measure the hemoglobin saturation through tissue bed. Pulse oximetry can be used on the finger, ears, or other skin tissue. The tissue bed is composed of bone, soft tissue, capillary blood that can affect the accurate absorbance reading. To distinguish arterial blood from tissue, most pulse oximetry will distinguish between a nonpulsatile or direct current (DC) component and a pulsatile or alternating current (AC) component. The fixed DC absorbance results from solid tissues, venous and capillary blood, and nonpulsatile arterial blood. The AC component is caused by pulsations in the arterial blood volume. During the AC component, systolic volume expands the arteriolar bed, thus producing an increase in optical path for an increased

light absorbance. Most pulse oximeters assume that arterial blood is the only pulsatile absorber. Each wavelength (660 nm and 940 nm) measures its corresponding AC and DC component. AC component of the wavelength is divided by the corresponding DC component to calculate the absorbance (S): $S_{660} = AC_{660}/DC_{660}$ and $S_{940} = AC_{940}/DC_{940}$. As a result, the pulse oximeter divides the absorbance ratio between the two wavelengths to establish a Red:IR modulation ratio (R):

$$R = \left\{ \frac{AC_{660}/DC_{660}}{AC_{940}/DC_{940}} \right\} \text{ or } \left\{ \frac{\text{Red}}{\text{IR}} \right\}$$

"R-value" is plotted on a calibration curve created by directly measuring arterial blood oxygen saturation (SaO_2) in healthy volunteers. The result is stored in a digital microprocessor. Increased red light absorbance (increased R) is associated with increased deoxyHb, that is, lower SpO_2. Therefore, a normal SpO_2 calls for a low "R-value" ratio. The value of R varies from roughly 0.4 at 100% saturation to 3.4 at 0% saturation. An "R-value" ratio of 1 corresponds to 85% saturation.

CLINICAL APPLICATIONS

Pulse oximeter has been a useful tool to detect hypoxic events but has its limitations. In general, oximeters using finger probe have been the standard placement, but other areas may have greater advantages than the finger probe, such as the bridge of the nose. In particular, the earlobe and forehead may be more superior especially in the setting of shock or hypothermic events. Even with the most accurate probe available, there will be some false reading in certain clinical and medical setting (Table 24-1).

Falsely Normal or High SpO_2 With a Leftward Shift in the Dissociation Curve

The typical pulse oximeter can only measure two existing solute species, O_2Hb and deoxyHb. Any other unknown solute will give a relatively normal or higher SaO_2 but a low percentage of O_2Hb or $FHbO_2$. SaO_2 is defined as $[O_2Hb]/([O_2Hb] + [deoxyHb])$, whereas $FHbO_2$ is calculated as $[O_2Hb]/([O_2Hb] +$

TABLE 24-1   Artifacts Causing a Disturbance in SpO$_2$ Readings

1. Falsely normal or high SpO$_2$ with a leftward shift in the dissociation curve
   - Carboxyhemoglobinemia and methemoglobinemia
2. Falsely normal or high SpO$_2$ with a rightward shift in the dissociation curve
   - Sulfhemoglobinemia
3. Unable to generate an adequate SpO$_2$ waveform
   - Poor perfusion state, that is, shock, hypothermia, etc
   - Arterial compression
4. Falsely low SpO$_2$
   - Intravenous dyes
   - Excessive movement
   - Fingernail polish
   - Severe anemia
5. Not affected by SpO$_2$
   - Fetal hemoglobin
   - Hyperbilirubin

[HHb] + [COHb] + [MetHb] + other]). Carbon monoxide toxicity has a strong avidity for Hb ($240\times$ greater than O$_2$), which causes the formation of carboxyhemoglobin (COHb). Due to the lack of O$_2$ capacity, tissue hypoxia will ensue and cause injury. The COHb levels above 50% are considered lethal to humans. O$_2$Hb and COHb absorb red light while relatively transparent in the IR zone. The pulse oximeter interprets COHb as if it were composed mostly of O$_2$Hb. This can be explained by the instance where a patient with carbon monoxide poisoning does not present with cyanotic skin tone but rather with a bright pink color.

Methemoglobinemia is formed when the heme moiety is oxidized from Fe^{2+} (Ferrous) to Fe^{3+} (Ferric). As a result, methemoglobin (MetHb) impairs oxygen delivery to vital organs and tissues. The lack of ability to bind oxygen and the leftward shift in the dissociation curve are the two mechanisms that impair unloading. Most of the causes of methemoglobinemia include oxidizing chemicals, drugs with nitrites, nitrates, specific local anesthetic, sulfonamides, and others. Similar to COHb, MetHb causes the pulse oximeter to overestimate fractional hemoglobin saturation. Measured by pulse oximeter, MetHb has high absorbance value at both wavelengths and absorbs both equally well measured. As a result, toxicity level (MetHb 20%-40%) will cause the "R-value" to be close to 1 or an SpO$_2$ value of approximately 85%. The high absorbance gives a very dark brown color to blood. This can be analyzed using a co-oximeter and treated with methylene blue in severe cases.

Falsely Normal or High SpO$_2$ with a Rightward Shift in the Dissociation Curve

Sulfhemoglobinemia can cause an erroneous SpO$_2$ reading. The sulfur atom incorporates the porphyrin ring and causes the irreversible oxidation from ferrous (Fe^{2+}) to ferric (Fe^{3+}). Those patients who are at higher risk include those taking a large quantity of metoclopramide, dapsone, nitrates, phenozapyridine, phenacetin, and sulfur compounds (sulfonamides, sulfasalazines). Small amount of toxicity can cause a detectable cyanosis. There is a rightward shift of the normal hemoglobin–oxygen dissociation curve, which is opposite in case of COHb and MetHb. Since sulfhemoglobin (SulHb) has similar absorbance at red and IR light, some investigators have demonstrated an SpO$_2$ of approximately 85%, which can be falsely reported as MetHb. To differentiate between MetHb and SulHb, a new co-oximeter has been developed. The addition of cyanide to blood sample can separate the two, wherein the SulHb toxicity remains but MetHb toxicity disappears. Empirically treating with methylene blue will treat only MetHb but not SulHb.

Unable to Read SpO$_2$ or Poor Pulse Oximeter Waveform

It may be quite common to visualize an inconsistent pulse oximeter waveform, thus rendering it unreliable. The amplitude of the waveform reflects the amount of cardiac-induced systolic volume with the onset of a QRS complex. During a low-amplitude waveform, the minimal difference between AC and DC causes a decrease in signal-to-noise ratio. This is commonly seen in vasoconstriction crisis due to poor perfusion. Such a situation would include hypovolemia or distributive shock, poor cardiac outflow due to cardiac insult, or arrhythmia. The use of significant vasoconstrictor agents can limit peripheral blood flow. A patient with a history of peripheral vascular disease or any occlusion of arterial blood flow (sphygmomanometer or tourniquet) may have inaccurate reading. Furthermore, an increase in ambient room light exposure increases DC signal, limiting the accuracy of the pulse oximeter. Thus, the clinical assessment is important in these scenarios to differentiate the inaccurate reading.

Falsely Low SpO$_2$

The false-low reading of SpO$_2$ can be due to an increase in artificial absorption to red waveform (660 nm) causing a lower-than-normal pulse oximeter reading. The use of nail polish, if blue, green, or black can lower SpO$_2$ by up to 10%. Furthermore, highly opaque acrylic nails do interfere with pulse oximeter readings. This can be avoided by rotating the fingertips 90 degrees to prevent the optical pathway to pass through the nail bed. Intravenous pigmented dyes including methylene blue, indocyanine green, and indigo carmine may cause an inaccurate pulse oximeter value due to the close proximity of its light absorption peak. Since methylene blue (668 nm) is the closest to red light absorption by deoxyHB, this will cause a higher "R-value" ratio, leading to a falsely reduced SpO$_2$ reading. Less red absorption is seen with indigo carmine and indocyanine green, and hence a much smaller decrease in SpO$_2$ reading. Anemia has been widely studied and found to affect SpO$_2$ below a hematocrit of 10% due to the lack of light scattered from the low amount of hemoglobin.

Measuring Blood Gases

Nina Deutsch, MD

Blood gas measurement and analysis is an important diagnostic tool used in both the operating room and intensive care unit. Normally drawn from an arterial blood source, they are performed to assess: (1) acid–base balance; (2) pulmonary oxygenation; and (3) alveolar ventilation.

ACID–BASE BALANCE

Normal arterial blood pH is in the range of 7.35-7.45. Through the Henderson–Hasselbalch equation, pH can be calculated as follows:

$$pH = 6.1 + \log [HCO_3/(0.03 \times Paco_3)]$$

Acid–base disturbances can result in either acidosis (pH < 7.35) or alkalosis (pH > 7.45) and fall into the following categories: (1) metabolic acidosis; (2) metabolic alkalosis; (3) respiratory acidosis; and (4) respiratory alkalosis.

Table 25-1 lists several medical conditions that produce these acid–base disturbances. To maintain acid–base balance within the normal range, the body has three compensatory mechanisms: pulmonary ventilation to control the arterial carbon dioxide ($Paco_2$), renal regulation of the metabolic component (bicarbonate or HCO_3^-), and weak acid buffers. The primary protein buffer is hemoglobin, which takes up H^+ ions when pH decreases and releases H^+ ions when pH increases. With hemoglobin more than 5 g/dL, there is little change in the buffer system with variations in hemoglobin.

In the presence of a metabolic disturbance, the respiratory system will acutely compensate to correct acid–base derangements. For example, in the presence of a metabolic acidosis, the respiratory system will increase ventilation to decrease $Paco_2$, thereby minimizing the change in pH. In the presence of a respiratory disturbance, the renally mediated metabolic component will compensate. However, this compensation requires a more prolonged period of at least 6-12 hours to appear, and only develops fully after several days. A mixed acid–base disturbance commonly occurs in clinical practice since the compensatory mechanisms do not necessarily correct these imbalances immediately or completely.

PULMONARY OXYGENATION

Arterial PO_2 (Pao_2) is dependent on several factors: inspired oxygen concentration, alveolar ventilation, mixed venous oxygen saturation (SvO_2), and ventilation–perfusion (V/Q) matching. As a person ages, there is an expected decrease in Pao_2. A normal Pao_2 for age can be determined by the following equation:

$$Pao_2 = 109 - 0.4(age) \quad (Range: 72\text{-}104 \text{ mm Hg}).$$

To determine the efficacy of pulmonary oxygenation of arterial blood, one must calculate the pulmonary shunt, also known as the A–a gradient, between the alveolar and arterial

TABLE 25-1   Medical Conditions and Their Associated Acid–Base Disturbance

Respiratory Acidosis	Respiratory Alkalosis	Metabolic Acidosis	Metabolic Alkalosis
Respiratory arrest	Fever	Hemorrhagic shock	Vomiting
Opiate overdose	Fear, anxiety	Septic shock	Diuretic use
Sedative drug overdose	Pain	Cardiogenic shock	Citrate (high transfusion)
Asthma exacerbation	Cirrhosis	Ketosis	Nasogastric aspirate
Hypoventilation	Cerebrovascular accident (CVA)	Diarrhea	Licorice
Chronic obstructive pulmonary disease (COPD)		Renal failure	Contraction alkalosis

TABLE 25-2 Causes of Metabolic Acidosis

Elevated Anion Gap Acidosis	Normal Anion Gap Acidosis
Lactic • Shock • Sepsis • Hypoxia • Liver failure	Fistulas (pancreatic)
Ketoacidosis • Diabetic • Alcoholic	Saline (0.9 NaCl) administration
Uremia	Hyperparathyroidism
Formic (methanol ingestion)	Diarrhea
Glycolic (ethylene glycol ingestion)	Carbonic anhydrase inhibitors (eg, acetazolamide)
Toxic ingestion of aspirin	Renal tubular acidosis
Toxic ingestion of iron	Spironolactone

blood oxygen levels. The A–a gradient in a healthy individual is less than 10 mm Hg. This normal gradient exists secondary to physiologic shunting through bronchial and coronary veins that drain deoxygenated blood directly to the left heart as well as normal V/Q gradients in the lungs.

Alveolar PO_2 is determined by the following equation:

$$PA_{O_2} = FI_{O_2}(P_B - P_{H_2O}) - Pa_{CO_2}/0.8,$$

where FI_{O_2} is the fraction of inspired oxygen, P_B is barometric pressure, P_{H_2O} is water vapor pressure, and 0.8 is the respiratory quotient (CO_2 production/O_2 consumption).

If the A–a gradient is normal in the presence of hypoxemia, then the hypoxemia is secondary to either hypoventilation or decreased inspired oxygen concentrations. If the A–a gradient is increased, the hypoxemia is secondary to V/Q mismatch, pulmonary shunt (perfusion of lung that receives no ventilation), or a diffusion barrier. The exact cause of the hypoxemia will still need to be determined.

VENTILATION

A normal Pa_{CO_2} ranges from 36 to 44 torr. In the absence of a metabolic disturbance, measured Pa_{CO_2} below this range is indicative of hyperventilation, whereas a higher Pa_{CO_2} results from hypoventilation. If Pa_{CO_2} changes due to a respiratory cause, one would expect that a 10 torr change in Pa_{CO_2} would change the pH by 0.08 units in the opposite direction. If the change is greater than this, then a mixed metabolic and respiratory component exists.

THE ANION GAP IN ACID–BASE ANALYSIS

The anion gap concept is based on the idea that the addition of 1 mmol of acid to blood will result in the consumption of 1 mmol of HCO_3^-, which is replaced with 1 mmol of acid anion.

The type of substituted anion affects serum electrolytes and has both diagnostic and therapeutic significance. The anion gap can be determined by the following equation:

$$\text{Anion gap} = [Na^+] - [Cl^-] - [HCO_3^-] = 12 \pm 2 \text{ mmol/L}$$

The normal anion gap occurs secondary to normally unmeasured anions such as albumen and phosphate. However, a high anion gap is due to an organic acid. Table 25-2 lists the various types of both gap and nongap metabolic acidosis. An algorithm for blood gas interpretation is depicted in Figure 25-1.

BLOOD GAS TEMPERATURE CORRECTION

Most blood gas machines run samples at 37°C, which will accurately reflect true values so long as the patient temperature is likewise 37°C. As patient temperature changes physiologic changes occur, which introduces errors between machine and patient values. With significantly hypothermic patients, such as during cardiopulmonary bypass or deep hypothermic circulatory arrest, blood gas measurements must be corrected for temperature to reflect actual values.

As temperature decreases, the solubility of O_2 and CO_2 increases, and thereby decreases the Po_2 and Pco_2. Changes in pH also occur. For every decrease in temperature by 1°C, the pH will increase by 0.015 units (Table 25-3). Temperature correction in blood gas analysis occurs when a sample is heated to a temperature of 37°C by the analysis machine. If the patient's temperature is lower than this, elevated H^+ levels, and therefore lower pH, will be recorded relative to the patient's actual values.

pH Stat

pH stat blood gas analysis utilizes a temperature-corrected system and is most commonly used during cardiopulmonary

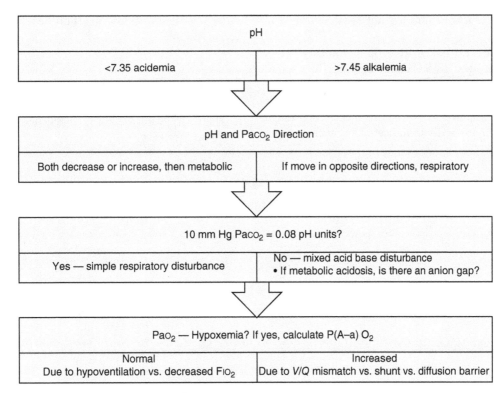

FIGURE 25-1 Algorithm for blood gas analysis.

bypass-induced hypothermia. This system aims at maintaining a constant pH, with a target of 7.4 despite variations in temperature. To achieve this, CO_2 is added to the inspired gases since the temperature correction decreases $Paco_2$ and raises pH. Advantages of this method relate to the increased cerebral blood flow that occurs with increased CO_2 levels. On bypass, this may also allow for faster cerebral cooling and better oxygen delivery with the leftward shift of the oxyhemoglobin dissociation curve. However, there is concern for increased microemboli and loss of autoregulation with pH stat management on cardiopulmonary bypass.

Alpha Stat

During hypothermia, the efficacy of the primary buffers (bicarbonate and phosphate) decreases and amino acids become the most important buffers. Of these, the alpha-imidazole ring of histidine becomes the most effective. Alpha stat analysis maintains the patient's *uncorrected* $Paco_2$ and pH at normal levels.

In this system, as the patient temperature decreases, pH rises (becomes increasingly alkalotic) because less H^+ is dissociated. However, electrochemical neutrality is maintained since equally less OH^- is available. Proponents of this method believe that this is more physiologically normal. Benefits of this method include maintenance of cerebral autoregulation and normal cellular transmembrane pH gradients, protein functioning, and enzyme activity.

Venous Blood Gases

Venous sampling typically is less painful and easier to obtain. As with an arterial blood gas, analysis of pH, Pco_2, and Po_2 is possible. In a venous blood gas (VBG), normal pH is in the range of 7.32-7.42 (approximately 0.03 lower than the arterial). PvO_2 is 40-50 mm Hg (approximately 5 mm Hg greater than in arterial blood), and $PvCO_2$ is 5.7 mm Hg higher than the arterial (46 mm Hg rather than 40 mm Hg). Although the agreement between arterial and venous gases is acceptable in clinical

TABLE 25-3   Effects of Changes in Temperature on Blood Gas Components

	Hypothermia	Hyperthermia	
Pco_2	↓	↑	
PO_2	↓	↑	
pH	↑	↓	0.015 unit/°C

practice in many situations, this has not been confirmed in shock states.

Mixed venous P_{CO_2} taken from the pulmonary artery should differ from Pa_{CO_2} by less than 6 mm Hg. However, in low cardiac output states when blood flow through the dependent tissues is impeded, mixed venous P_{CO_2} may be greatly increased when compared to Pa_{CO_2}. This increased gradient has been used diagnostically to indicate low cardiac output states since tissue acidosis may only be reflected in the mixed venous sample.

SUGGESTED READING

Breen PH. Arterial blood gas and pH analysis: clinical approach and interpretation. *Anesthesiol Clin N Amer* 2001;19:885 –906.

Gas Concentrations: Monitoring and Instrumentation

Sudha Ved, MD

Standards of basic anesthesia monitoring include measurement of adequate inspired oxygen delivery with an oxygen analyzer and continual exhaled carbon dioxide (ETCO$_2$) with capnography.

The oxygen sensor is placed on the inspiratory limb of the anesthesia machine. Blood concentrations and depth of anesthesia is assumed by monitoring expired gas analysis of oxygen, carbon dioxide, and anesthetic agent concentration. Several systems are available to monitor inspired and exhaled oxygen, carbon dioxide, and volatile inhalation agents. These technologies include: (1) electrochemical analysis—polarographic and galvanic cells (O$_2$); (2) paramagnetic (O$_2$); (3) magneto-acoustic (O$_2$); (4) mass spectrometry (O$_2$, N$_2$, CO$_2$, N$_2$O, and gases); (5) Spectral analysis (a) infrared (CO$_2$, N$_2$O, and gases) and (b) Raman scattering (O$_2$, N$_2$, CO$_2$, N$_2$O, and gases); and (6) piezoelectric crystal (quartz) oscillation.

OXYGEN ANALYZERS

Currently, three types of oxygen analyzers are available: polarographic (Clark electrode), galvanic (fuel cell), and paramagnetic. The polarographic and galvanic electrochemical sensors differ in the composition of their electrodes and electrolyte gels. The cathode and anode electrodes are embedded in an electrolyte gel separated from the sample gas by a semipermeable membrane (usually Teflon). As oxygen reacts with the electrodes, a current is generated that is proportional to the partial pressure of oxygen in the sample gas. The components of the galvanic cell are capable of providing enough chemical energy so that the reaction does not require an external power source.

1. **Polarographic**—The electrode has a gold (or platinum) cathode and a silver anode. Unlike the galvanic cell, a polarographic electrode works only if a small voltage is applied to two electrodes. The amount of current that flows is proportional to the amount of oxygen present. The units can provide fast oxygen analysis within 1 minute, but has a higher failure rate compared to the galvanic cell.
2. **Galvanic**—Fuel cell monitors are used on many anesthesia machines in the inspiratory limb. The cell contains a lead anode and gold cathode bathed in potassium chloride. At the gold terminal, hydroxyl ions are formed that react with the lead electrode (thereby gradually consuming it) to produce lead oxide, causing current, which is proportional to the amount of oxygen being measured, to flow. Because the lead electrode is consumed, monitor life can be prolonged by exposing it to room air when not in use. It has a slow response time of 3 minutes but lasts longer. Predictors of galvanic cell exhaustion include underreading of high oxygen concentration, failure to remember calibration, "blipping out," and color changes.
3. **Paramagnetic**—The paramagnetic oxygen analyzer plots oxygen concentration continuously breath by breath as a real-time waveform and displays as an oxygraph. The oxygraphy waveform has four phases similar to capnography, although displayed in a reverse manner. The device gives a digital display of fraction of inspired oxygen (FIO$_2$) and fraction of exhaled O$_2$ (FEO$_2$). Factors affecting the FEO$_2$ include oxygen consumption (VO$_2$) (metabolism), transport (cardiac output [CO]), and delivery (ventilation, FIO$_2$). If the CO is unchanged, the relationship of these factors can be expressed by the equation: VO$_2$ = V_A (FIO$_2$ − FEO$_2$). If VO$_2$ is unchanged, an increase in FIO$_2$–FEO$_2$ difference is the most sensitive indicator of hypoventilation than ETCO$_2$/Paco$_2$ or Pao$_2$, whereas the arterial oxygen saturation (SaO$_2$) is the least sensitive. Sum of alveolar gases remain constant; therefore, any decrease in FEO$_2$ will cause an increase in other gases (slow increase in CO$_2$ and faster rise in N$_2$O). Other very useful clinical uses of oxygraphy include adequacy of preoxygenation (FI–FE difference of 10%); minute changes in flow characteristics help detect airway complications (endotracheal tube kinking and loss of tidal volume) and neuromuscular recovery earlier than capnography; and tracheal jet ventilation.

GAS ANALYZERS

Currently, the most commonly used method for analyzing CO$_2$ and inhaled gases is infrared spectrophotometry with sidestream sampling. Monochromatic infrared spectrometer emits a beam of light with a wavelength of 7-13 μm. The absorption spectrum of inhaled gases is relatively different at this wavelength and automatically identifies the inhaled gases. Polychromatic infrared spectrometer measures concentrations of two anesthetic agents simultaneously. Mass spectrometry and Raman spectroscopy are primarily of historical interest in spite of their capability of additionally monitoring O_2 and N_2. Oxygen does not absorb infrared light and has to be measured by other analyzers mentioned above.

The value of monitoring inhaled gases include using the monitor to assess depth of anesthesia; effects of rebreathing; closed-system anesthesia; and to recognize failure of vaporizers, such as (a) control valve not turned on; (b) calibration error; (c) mislabeled or misfiling of agents; (d) unintentionally leaving the vaporizer in the ON position; and (e) simultaneous running of two agents.

1. **Capnography**—Measurement of $ETCO_2$ concentration is used to confirm endotracheal tube placement, assess the adequacy of ventilation, and guide estimation of arterial carbon dioxide concentration. Capnography comprises the continuous analysis and recording of $ETCO_2$ concentrations in respiratory gases. Although the terms capnography and capnometry are sometimes considered synonymous, *capnometry* suggests measurement (ie, analysis alone) without a continuous written record or waveform. *Colorimetry* (eg, the Easy Cap end-tidal CO_2 detector) provides continuous, semiquantitative $ETCO_2$ monitoring. The pH-sensitive indicator changes color when exposed to CO_2. This device has three color ranges: purple ($ETCO_2 < 3.8$ mm Hg), tan ($ETCO_2$ 3.8-15 mm Hg), and yellow ($ETCO_2 > 15$ mm Hg). Normal $ETCO_2$ is more than 4% so the device should turn yellow when an endotracheal tube is inserted into patients with intact circulation.

   a. **Sidestream gas sampling** is the most commonly used in which gas is withdrawn via a sampling tube near the endotracheal tube and travels to a sample cell within the monitor for analysis. CO_2 concentration is determined by comparing infrared light absorption in the sample cell with a chamber devoid of CO_2. The accuracy of the sample is improved by decreasing dead space ventilation to this tube and increasing the flow rate of aspiration by the machine. Sidestream sampling is prone to erroneous readings secondary to water precipitation in the circuit, which can obstruct flow of gas samples.

   b. **Direct flowthrough** gas sampling can also be performed by allowing expiratory flow to pass directly through an adaptor that uses infrared light to measure gas sample carbon dioxide. These systems have been associated with thermal skin burns, and are generally bulkier and add dead space. Therefore, they are less commonly used in the operating room setting.

   c. **Microstream capnography**—Molecular correlation spectroscopy (MCS) uses laser-based technology to generate infrared emission. The emitter is electronically activated and self-modulated. Unlike the broad spectrum produced by traditional capnography, the MCS creates an emission precisely matching the absorption spectrum of CO_2. Microstream uses breath sampling rate of 50 mL/min, thereby broadening capnography applications for patients of all ages, including neonates and all environments throughout the hospital, including respiratory risk associated with patient-controlled analgesia and sedations for procedures. It also reduces the potential for moisture and humidity obstructing the sample line. It has a small sample cell of 15 μl and a hydrophobic filter in the sampling line preventing liquids from entering the monitor and allowing for oxygen delivery without diluting the sample.

2. **Mass spectrometry**—It is a technique by which concentration of gas particles in a sample can be determined according to their mass–charge ratio. All the positively charged ions generated by passing a gas sample through an ionizer allows ionized particles of differing atomic weights to fall on a magnetized plate and translated to concentrations. Results of identifying different type of particles and concentration of the anesthetic are quickly obtained in fractions of a second. It cannot provide continuous gas monitoring since it has to be shared by different operating rooms and analyzes gases from each room sequentially. Because of the size, expense, and complexity of the system, it is no longer used.

3. **Raman scattering**—The spectrometer emits an intense beam of laser light into a sample of gas. Collision of photon and gas molecules produces unstable vibrational and rotational energy states which causes photons to change and emerge at substantially different wavelengths typical for the particular gas. The light is collected with a system of lens and sent through a monochromator and the Rayleigh scattering is filtered out while the rest of the light is dispersed onto a detector. The Raman light is of low intensity, so it is best measured at right angles to the high-intensity exciting beam. Change in frequency allows the monitor to identify type and concentration of the specific inhaled agent.

4. **Piezoelectric analysis**—The piezoelectric method uses oscillating quartz crystals, one of which is covered with lipid. Volatile anesthetics dissolve in the lipid layer and change the frequency of oscillation, which, when compared to the frequency of oscillation of an uncovered crystal, allows the concentration of the volatile anesthetic to be calculated. Neither these devices nor infrared photoacoustic analysis allows different anesthetic agents to be distinguished. New dual-beam infrared optical analyzers allow gases to be separated and an improperly filled vaporizer to be detected.

Pressure Transducers

Howard Lee and Christopher Monahan, MD

A transducer is any device that converts energy from one form to another. A pressure transducer converts a pressure waveform (kinetic and potential energy) into an electrical signal (electrical energy). Invasive arterial blood pressure monitors measure the constant variation of blood pressure through an arterial catheter connected to fluid-filled tubing, which in turn is connected to a pressure transducer. The arterial pulse pressure is transmitted through a pressurized column of saline into a flexible diaphragm causing the shape of the diaphragm to change. The displacement of the diaphragm is measured by a strain gauge. Strain gauges work based on the principle that the electrical resistance of a wire increases as it extends. When several strain gauges are incorporated into a Wheatstone bridge circuit, the movement of the diaphragm stretches or compresses several wires and alters the resistance of the unit. This process results in the generation of a current and electrical signal. The pressure transducer then sends this electrical signal via a cable to a processor where it is filtered and displayed as a waveform.

RESONANCE AND DAMPING

The physical display of the blood pressure waveform is influenced by resonance and damping. Resonance refers to the amplification of a signal that can occur when a certain force is applied to a system. Every system has a frequency at which it oscillates freely, called the natural frequency. If a force with a similar frequency to the natural frequency is applied to a system, the system will oscillate at maximum amplitude. This phenomenon is called resonance. Resonance produces excessive amplification that distorts the electrical signal, resulting in greater systolic pressure, lower diastolic pressure, and increased pulse pressure. To prevent resonance, it is important for the invasive arterial blood pressure (IABP) system to have a much higher natural frequency than the frequency of the force applied to the system. The natural frequency of the system can be increased by reducing the length of tubing, reducing the compliance of the tubing, reducing the density of the fluid in the tubing, or by increasing the diameter of the tubing.

Like resonance, damping can also alter the signal displayed from a transducer (Figure 27-1). Damping refers to the decrease of signal amplitude that accompanies a reduction of energy in an oscillating system. Increased damping will manifest as a decrease in systolic blood pressure and an increase in diastolic blood pressure. In the pressure transducer system, most damping arises from friction between the tubing and fluid in the tubing. Other factors that decrease energy in the system and cause damping include three-way stopcocks, bubbles, clots, arterial vasospasm, large catheter size, and narrow, long, or compliant tubing. By contrast, an underdamped system can also cause signal distortion. In an underdamped system, the tracing can resemble a resonant system with increased systolic amplitude, and decreased diastolic amplitude.

ZEROING AND LEVELING

For a pressure transducer to read accurately, it must be zeroed and leveled. Zeroing refers to the process of eliminating the impact of atmospheric pressure on the transducer system by closing the system off to the patient, and opening the system to atmospheric pressure. Calibrating the system to zero in this position will eliminate the impact of atmospheric pressure on the system, thus ensuring that the signal generated reflects only the force of the patient's blood pressure.

After the transducer is zeroed, it must be placed at the appropriate level for accurate monitoring. The most common level is that of the heart, but the level of the brain may be used in sitting cases to accurately measure cerebral perfusion. The level of the transducer is important due to pressure exerted by the fluid in the tubing. A transducer that is too low will measure not only the force generated by the patient's blood pressure, but also the hydrostatic pressure generated by the fluid in the tubing that is between the low transducer and heart (or other level being monitored). The pressure generated by the fluid in the tubing can be significant, as the blood pressure is altered by 7.4 mm Hg for every 10 cm in leveling error. Thus, a transducer that is 10 cm below the heart will read 7.4 mm Hg higher than the pressure at the level of the heart.

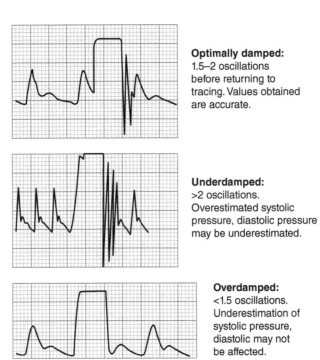

Optimally damped:
1.5–2 oscillations before returning to tracing. Values obtained are accurate.

Underdamped:
>2 oscillations. Overestimated systolic pressure, diastolic pressure may be underestimated.

Overdamped:
<1.5 oscillations. Underestimation of systolic pressure, diastolic may not be affected.

FIGURE 27-1 Square wave flush test with intraarterial blood pressure measurement. During a flush bolus of the catheter tubing, a square wave is observed. The number of oscillations after the square wave at the end of the bolus and prior to returning of the blood pressure tracing may result in an overestimated or underestimated blood pressure. (Reproduced with permission from Tintinalli JE, et al. *Tintinalli's Emergency Medicine: A Comprehensive Study Guide,* 7th ed, McGraw-Hill; 2011.)

SUGGESTED READINGS

Barbeito A, Mark J. Arterial and central venous pressure monitoring. *J Clin Anesth* 2006;24:717-735.

Gilbert M. Principles of pressure transducers, resonance, damping and frequency response. *Anaesth Intens Care Med* 2011;13:1-6.

Noninvasive Blood Pressure Measurement

Vinh Nguyen, DO

The use of noninvasive blood pressure monitoring is critical in any anesthesiology practice. The standards of monitoring, as defined by the American Society of Anesthesiologists, require measurement of blood pressure at a minimum every 5 minutes during an anesthetic procedure. Two types of noninvasive method for arterial pressure measurement can be defined: periodic or continuous sampling using pulse waveform. Periodic sampling techniques provide systolic and diastolic information over a series of heart beats, whereas continuous monitoring provides beat-to-beat measurements and pulse pressure waveform in real time.

PERIODIC SAMPLING

Manual Techniques

Scipione Riva-Rocci first created the occlusive cuff-based method in 1895. The vascular unloading principle was adapted using an external compression pressure against the limb to indirectly collapse the vessel. At this point, equilibrium exists between the external force and the vessel. The compression is released until tension on the wall of the vessel is zero, which equals the transmural pressure that unloads the vessel. Using the Riva-Rocci principle, the detection of opening and closing of artery can be clinically demonstrated by examining skin flushing or by palpating the pulse.

In 1905, Korotkoff adopted the ascultatory method, which is currently the most common approach in clinical practice. The blood pressure cuff is inflated above the systolic blood pressure (SBP), a stethoscope is placed over the brachial artery, and the external compression is slowly decreased. There are five phases of the Korotkoff sounds but clinically only two are important for measurement. Phase 1 will begin as the initial "tapping" sounds correspond to SBP, whereas phase 5 is the end of the muffled sound corresponding to the diastolic blood pressure (DBP). In between, phases 2 and 3 produce progressively changing sound, whereas phase 4 is the beginning of the muffled sound. Although the mean arterial pressure (MAP) is not measured, it can be calculated using SBP and DBP (MAP = 2/3 DBP + 1/3 SBP).

Oscillometric Measurements

Within a pressure chamber, the pressure produced with each heartbeat contains pulsatile variations. The amplitude of each pulsation can vary by changing the chamber pressure. Even with manual measurement, pulsatile variation in an air gauge can be appreciated. Because of this oscillation effect during cuff deflation, it is possible to estimate SBP, DBP, and mean blood pressure. Oscillometry forms the basis of the automated noninvasive blood pressure cuff. The cuff contains an inflatable device with a sensor that measures oscillations electronically. A microprocessor initiates an inflation–deflation sequence, in which the cuff is inflated to a pressure above the previous SBP and then slowly deflated in an incremental manner. The start of rapidly increasing oscillations indicates SBP, whereas DBPs occur when the oscillations quickly slow down. The DBP can be difficult to measure directly because oscillations can still be present even when the cuff is below the actual diastolic value. The maximum oscillation amplitude occurs when the arterial wall is maximally unloaded at the lowest cuff pressure; this corresponds to the MAP (Figure 28-1). Each manufacturer designs their own algorithms to estimate the systolic and diastolic value when oscillations reach 0.5 and 0.66 of the maximum amplitude, respectively.

Sources of Error and Complications

Sampling blood pressure for either the manual or oscillation techniques uses the same cuff, leading to similar problems. The proper cuff size is important for accuracy. Too large cuff size will give erroneously low oscillation readings and falsely low blood pressure, whereas too small cuff size will give falsely higher reading. The ideal cuff width should be approximately 46% of arm circumference. Cuffs must be properly applied especially with a single bladder cuff to compress the vessel against the bony structure. The further away the compression of blood vessel is from the aorta, the more falsely elevated the systolic and falsely lowered the diastolic will be seen. The MAP will remain constant.

Besides cuff complications, patients' diseases or other issues can give an erroneous reading. These problems include

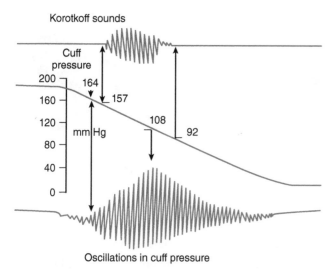

FIGURE 28-1 Noninvasive blood pressure measurement with auscultatory and oscillatory methods. By auscultation, the appearance and disappearance of Korotkoff sounds result in a blood pressure measurement of 157/92 mm Hg. The oscillatory method incorporating an empiric algorithm will measure a similar blood pressure, with the maximal point of oscillation being the MAP of 108 mm Hg. (Reproduced with permission from Tintinalli JE, et al. *Tintinalli's Emergency Medicine: A Comprehensive Study Guide,* 7th ed, McGraw-Hill; 2011.)

patients with vascular disease, dysrhythmias, generalized edema, obesity, and chronic hypertension. Excessive patient movement or surgeons leaning on the cuff can lead to false measurements. Complications associated with frequent sampling can result in extremity discomfort and neuropathy (particularly that of the ulnar nerve) if "stat" mode is left on without a rest period. Intravenous fluid flow or pulse oximeter readings can be interrupted with the blood pressure on the same extremity.

CONTINUOUS SAMPLING

Penáz Technique

In the 1970s, physiologist Jan Penáz examined the idea that pressure exerted by the circulation can be determined by measuring an opposing pressure that prevents disruption. He employed the idea of "volume unloading" with the volume-clamp method. Noninvasive devices that measure blood pressure based on this principle all employ a small air cuff designed to fit around the middle phalanx. The cuff contains photoplethysmography, a built-in light source, and an infrared receiver on the other side. An infrared beam transverses through both

digital arteries and generates a signal proportional to the blood volume of the finger. The signal is used in a feedback loop that causes a rapid inflation or deflation of the cuff to keep blood volume constant and the vessels in a constant state of "vascular unloading." Thus, the principle is that an inflatable finger cuff assesses the arterial pressure by clamping the finger artery to a constant volume by varying the counter pressure, which is then visualized as a pulse pressure wave form. The finger arterial pressure is subsequently reconstructed into a brachial arterial pressure and the signal is sent to an amplifier and displayed similarly to an invasive arterial line.

Arterial Tonometry

These noninvasive devices consist of an external pressure transducer that compress superficial artery against a bony structure. In most cases, the radial artery is targeted. The vessel is compressed until flat but not occluded, otherwise known as the "proper hold-down pressure." A pressure sensor measures arterial blood pressure via contact pressure. It uses a proprietary algorithm that can calculate SBP, DBP, and pulse pressure over the hold range.

Photometric Transit Time

The newest technology to provide a closer relationship to continuous invasive monitoring is the pulse transit time (PTT). This monitor uses the relationship between pulse wave velocity and blood pressure. Two pulse transducers are placed at distal distance from each other. The distance between the peak signal from each sensor is calculated as the delay time between the arterial pulses. Alternatively, PTT can be defined as the time interval between the ECG R-wave and the arrival of the photoplethysmograph waveform at the finger site. The speed at which this arterial pressure wave travels is directly proportional to blood pressure. An acute rise in blood pressure causes vascular tone to increase, which stiffens the arterial wall and shortens the PTT. The changes in blood PTT are transformed into blood pressure measurements using the manufacturer's algorithm.

SUGGESTED READINGS

Chung E, Chen G, Alexander B, et al. Non-invasive continuous blood pressure monitoring: a review of current applications. *Front Med* 2013;7:91-101.

deJong RM, Westerhof BE, Voors AA, van Veldhuisen DJ. Noninvasive haemodynamic monitoring using finger arterial pressure waveforms. *Netherlands J Med* 2009;67:372-375.

Autotransfusion Devices

Anna Katharine Hindle, MD

Autotransfusion techniques reduce the need for allogenic blood transfusion. Patients are transfused with their own blood via either preoperative self-donation or intraoperative blood salvage.

PREOPERATIVE AUTOLOGOUS DONATION

Patients donate their own blood at weekly intervals prior to surgery; patients may donate three or more units prior to elective surgery. Donated blood is stored, often without the need for freezing, and may be used perioperatively to treat anemia. Consideration must be given to the patients' overall medical condition, including hemoglobin and cardiac status. Relative contraindications for autologous donation include severe aortic stenosis, coronary artery disease, low initial hematocrit, and low initial blood volume. Though patients receive their own blood, the use of autotransfusion does not eliminate the chance of human clerical errors that may occur.

Anemia typically limits donation. Erythropoietin and iron supplementation prior to donations effectively increases blood collection; however, these strategies may be expensive. The costs, administrative efforts, potential wasted autologous blood, and resulting anemia must be weighed against the benefits of possibly avoiding allogenic transfusion.

ACUTE NORMOVOLEMIC HEMODILUTION

Two to four units of blood may be withdrawn from a patient early in the operative course, with the withdrawn blood volume replaced with an equivalent volume of crystalloid. Crystalloid is typically substituted for blood in a 3:1 ratio; or colloid replacement can be used in a 1:1 ratio. Hemodynamic monitoring and serial hemoglobin checks during acute normovolemic hemodilution (AHN) confirm tolerance of the procedure as notable blood volume shifts occur. Additionally, care must be taken to ensure that anticoagulant in the collection bags mixes thoroughly with removed blood to prevent clotting. Depending on the patient's medical status, goal of dilution for hematocrit is 27%-33%. Acute normovolemic hemodilution theoretically permits low-hematocrit blood loss during the operation, and patient's own blood may be transfused later, as needed. Since the blood does not leave the operating room, the risk of clerical error is minimized. Few data exist to prove efficacy of the technique. As with preoperative autologous donation (PAD), use of ANH must weigh the effort required to donate and monitor the patient against the theoretical benefits.

PERIOPERATIVE BLOOD SALVAGE

Blood salvage (ie, CellSaver; Haemonetics Corp., Braintree, MA) allows surgical blood loss collection, processing, and transfusion back to the patient. Salvage techniques should be considered for significant blood loss surgical procedures, including cardiac, spinal instrumentation, liver transplant, and trauma surgery. Contraindications include pus or fecal material exposure, amniotic fluid contamination, or certain types of malignant cell exposure during surgery. Additionally, intraoperative salvage should be avoided in patients exposed to antibiotic irrigants or microfibrillar collagen hemostat (Avitene Hemostat [Davol, Warwick, RI]).

Surgical blood loss is collected via suction and anticoagulated as it leaves the surgical field. Collected blood undergoes centrifuge processing to separate red blood cells from other blood components, such as fat, clot, free hemoglobin, clotting factors, and anticoagulants. Spun red cells are washed with saline and collected for possible return to the patient. Modern machines prevent air embolism with design improvements and air alarms.

The most notable blood salvage complication is incomplete blood filtration, resulting in residual heparin or surgical field contamination of salvaged blood. An additional complication is dilutional coagulopathy. Coagulopathy occurs because blood salvage only allows for red blood cells to be transfused. Platelets and clotting factors are removed with the filtration process. The process of intraoperative salvage requires trained personnel and specialized equipment, accounting for its greater expense than other autotransfusion techniques.

Aside from the risks and costs, the benefit of intraoperative cell salvage is its potential to reduce allogenic transfusion requirements during large blood loss operations. Some surgeries, such as cardiac and orthopedic procedures, may produce more postoperative blood loss than intraoperative losses. Collected blood can be filtered and washed for postoperative autologous transfusion in these cases.

Body Warming Devices

Nina Deutsch, MD

Perioperative hypothermia occurs to some degree in all patients undergoing general or regional anesthesia for more than 30 minutes. Hypothermia occurs through several mechanisms:

- **Redistribution**—The initial intraoperative temperature drop is secondary to redistribution of heat from the core to peripheral tissues and is proportional to the gradient between these two compartments. This gradient depends on the room temperature, vasomotor status of the patient, adiposity, and anesthetic drug effects.
- **Radiation**—Radiation is the transfer of heat between two objects that are not in contact. An example of this is the sun warming the earth. The emitted radiation carries the warmth from the warmer object to the cooler object and occurs in the infrared light spectrum. Most heat lost in the perioperative setting occurs through radiation.
- **Convection**—Convection contributes a great deal to perioperative heat loss as well. Convective heat loss is the transfer of heat to moving molecules, such as air or liquid. This depends on the rate of air movement (wind speed), the surface area exposed, and the temperature difference between the object and ambient temperature.
- **Conduction**—Conduction is the transfer of heat between two surfaces in direct contact. It depends on the temperature difference between the two objects and the surface area of the objects in contact.
- **Evaporation**— Evaporative heat loss occurs through the skin and respiratory system and consists of three main components: sweat (sensible water loss); insensible water loss from the skin; respiratory tract and wounds; and evaporation of liquids (ie, skin preparation solution) from the skin. Factors affecting evaporative heat loss include the vapor pressure difference between the body surface and the environment, the relative humidity of the ambient air, the velocity of airflow, and lung minute ventilation.

WARMING STRATEGIES

One of the easiest ways to reduce intraoperative radiant heat loss is to maintain operating room temperature at a sufficiently high level. In adults, 21°C has been reported as the critical ambient temperature to maintain normal esophageal temperatures between 36°C and 37.5°C. However, operating rooms are often kept cooler than this for operator comfort. Several strategies exist, therefore, to achieve and maintain perioperative normothermia. By instituting a multimodal approach, drops in temperature can be minimized. These approaches are divided into three broad strategies.

Passive Insulation

Passive insulation minimizes thermal dispersion by insulating the air layer between covers placed on the patient and the patient's skin surface. Examples of these insulating covers include: surgical draping, cotton blankets, and metalized plastic covers. These devices reduce radiant, convective, and evaporative heat losses, minimizing thermal dispersion by about 30%. Their efficacy is not dependent on the material they are made of, but rather seems to be directly proportional to the covered surface area.

Active Cutaneous Warming Devices—

Forced air warmers are the most commonly used active warming systems in the perioperative period. These consist of an electrically powered heater blower unit that generates airflow to be distributed via a hose into a blanket. The blanket is made of either plastic or paper and can cover the whole body, the upper body, or the lower body. A thermostat allows for air temperature adjustment to fit the clinical situation.

Heat exchange occurs through both convection and reducing the heat loss that occurs through radiation. Heat exchange efficiency improves when there is a higher gradient between the blanket and the body surface and when the blanket covers a larger surface area. Forced air warmers are able to increase central temperature by approximately

0.75°C/hour. However, these systems do have disadvantages. Active prewarming is required to prevent the heat loss that occurs due to redistribution with anesthesia induction, and forced air warming often needs to be recommended in the recovery period. Finally, the potential to increase the infection rate with these systems has not been fully determined.

Resistive heating systems can be in the form of carbon fiber blankets that cover the patient or servocontrolled underbody mattresses. Heat transfer occurs through conductive warming. These electrically heated covers are efficient and often cheaper than forced-air warmers since they can be sterilized and reused. Their efficacy depends on how well the cover contacts the skin surface. They appear to be particularly beneficial in accidental hypothermia treatment and have been found to be as efficient as forced air warmers in the operating room environment.

Circulating water mattresses are placed under the patient to warm their posterior surfaces via conduction. However, their efficacy is often decreased since the majority of heat loss occurs from the larger anterior surface of the body. Furthermore, patient's body weight will compress cutaneous capillaries. This reduced perfusion reduces heat exchange by decreasing the ability of these vessels to dissipate absorbed heat to the rest of the body. Therefore, water mattresses appear to be more effective in pediatric patients, who are lighter in weight and have a higher proportion of skin surface warmed by the device. Newer circulating-water garments that cover both anterior and posterior portions of the body appear to be more effective.

Radiant warmers are placed over the patient and infrared radiation is produced to warm the patient. These are especially useful in pediatric patients when they are uncovered during induction and line placement. Efficacy is dependent on the distance between the device and the patient. However, a minimal recommended distance must be maintained to prevent skin burns. These warmers do not prevent heat loss that occurs by convection. Prolonged use of radiant warmers can actually increase insensible losses.

Internal Warming Systems

Intravenous fluid warming reduces the heat loss that occurs with infusion of room temperature solutions. Infusion of 1 L of crystalloid can decrease the body temperature by 0.25°C. Therefore, intravenous fluids and blood products should be warmed, especially during rapid or massive fluid administration. Studies have shown that even if an intravenous infusion is warmed to 37°C and then exposed to 25 cm of tubing in the ambient air, extremely high flow rates (750 mL/hour) are necessary to maintain the fluid temperature above 32°C. The longer the tubing, the more heat lost from the fluid while in transit from the warmer to the patient. Therefore, the shortest tubing that is practical should be used. Fluid warming, although important in preventing worsening hypothermia, cannot maintain normothermia by itself and needs to be used in combination with other body warming techniques.

Airway heating and humidification—When an endotracheal tube is in place, the epithelial surface area available to warm and humidify inspired gases is decreased. Use of a humidifier minimizes convective and evaporative heat losses from the respiratory tract. There are two forms of humidifiers: ultrasonic heated humidifiers that actively add heat and humidity to the inspired gases; and passive heat and moisture exchange filters (an artificial nose). By heating inspired gases, these devices help maintain normothermia and can reverse hypothermia in surgery. Further benefits of gas humidification include reduction of tracheal damage and bronchospasm, as well as preservation of cilia function. Although these devices have beneficial properties, they are not without some drawbacks. Humidifiers add to the circuit's dead space. This results in hypercarbia that may require adjustments to ventilation. Furthermore, they add to the resistance to gas flow, increasing the work of breathing in spontaneously ventilating patients. Blockage of the circuit and the device can also occur if liquid enters it and is undetected.

Cardiopulmonary bypass (CPB)—CPB actively warms the blood as it passes from the body through a heat exchanger built into the bypass circuit. Though being the most efficient warming device available, CPB is not used for the routine mild hypothermia seen in the perioperative period. Rather, it is used for active cooling and rewarming during cardiac procedures and occasionally to reverse significant hypothermia related to trauma and accidental extreme exposure.

SUGGESTED READINGS

Brauer A, Quintel M. Forced-air warming: technology, physical background and practical aspects. *Curr Opin Anaesthesiol* 2009;22:769-774.

Galvao CM, Marck PB, Sawada NO, Clark AM. A systematic review of the effectiveness of cutaneous warming systems to prevent hypothermia. *J Clin Nursing* 2009;18:627-636.

Putzu M, Casati A, Berti M, et al. Clinical complications, monitoring and management of perioperative mild hypothermia: anesthesiological features. *Acta Biomed* 2007;78:163-169.

Wilkes AR. Heat and moisture exchangers and breathing system filters: their use in anaesthesia and intensive care. *Anaesthesia* 2011;66:40-51.

Mechanical Ventilation: Principles of Action

Darin Zimmerman, MD, and Christopher Junker, MD

Mechanical ventilation utilizes positive-pressure devices to improve oxygen (O_2) and carbon dioxide (CO_2) exchange. There are two main goals of mechanical ventilation: (1) maintain appropriate levels of arterial O_2 and CO_2; and (2) reduce the patient's work of breathing. Mechanical ventilation is a supportive intervention that does not treat the underlying disease process.

INDICATIONS

Positive-pressure ventilation can be administered with an endotracheal tube (ETT) or noninvasively with a mask. Noninvasive management can be used for patients who have a nonobstructed airway, a preserved respiratory drive, and protective airway mechanisms intact. Invasive airway management is required if there is acute airway obstruction, inability to handle secretions, loss of protective airway reflexes, or respiratory failure that is refractory to noninvasive positive- pressure ventilation with persistent hypoxemia and hypercapnia.

GOALS

Mechanical ventilation can be used to ensure a controlled airway for patients who require sedation, such as during surgical procedures, or to tolerate resuscitation and life support. Other goals include oxygenation, minute ventilation (MV) and pH control, and work of breathing reduction.

Oxygenation

Oxygenation is improved by titrating fraction of inspired oxygen (FIO_2), and improving mean airway pressures by adjusting tidal volume (V_T) and positive end-expiratory pressure (PEEP). Control of MV allows for regulation of CO_2 and pH. Depending on the mode of mechanical ventilation selected, an MV can be guaranteed regardless of effort, which is useful for treatment of hypercapnic respiratory failure as well as for maintaining physiologic pH. Mechanical ventilation decreases work of breathing by ensuring adequate V_T,

optimizing inspiratory and expiratory times during respiration to prevent air trapping, and preventing airway collapse.

During mechanical ventilation, V_T, PEEP, and FIO_2 control oxygenation. V_T and PEEP work together by increasing alveolar volume and mean airway pressures. In patients with obstructive airway disease, larger V_T with slower respiratory rate (RR) prevents air trapping. With noncompliant lungs, smaller V_T and faster RR avoid volutrauma and barotrauma. Decreasing FIO_2 minimizes toxicity while also maintaining adequate O_2 saturation (SpO_2).

Positive end-expiratory pressure improves oxygenation by maintaining airway pressures more than 0 cm H_2O during exhalation, preventing alveoli collapse, and improving recruitment of atelectatic areas. PEEP increases functional residual capacity (FRC), which is the volume remaining in the lung after normal exhalation. Closing capacity (CC) is the volume in the lungs at which small airways that do not have cartilaginous support begin to close. If CC exceeds FRC, atelectasis occurs. PEEP increases FRC, preventing atelectasis. Assessment and optimization of volume status prior to increasing PEEP levels avoid reduction in right heart blood return.

Ventilation

Minute ventilation adjustments alter either RR or V_T to regulate CO_2 and pH. Dead space ventilation (V_d) is ventilation in the absence of perfusion. It is gas that does not participate in gas exchange. This can be anatomic within the conducting airways, and can also be physiologic if there is interruption of the alveolar: pulmonary capillary interface. During spontaneous ventilation, blood flow closely matches ventilated lung areas; positive-pressure ventilation alters this relationship, increasing dead space ventilation.

MECHANICAL VENTILATORS

Mechanical ventilation allows physicians to control V_T, mean airway pressure, FIO_2, PEEP, RR, and gas flow. V_T, mean airway pressure, and flow are interrelated by pressure gradients. The volume of gas delivered depends on flow as well as lung compliance. Depending on core goals, one of these independent variables (pressure, flow, or volume) is set by the operator, making the other two variables dependent.

A respiratory cycle is the time from the beginning of one breath until the beginning of the next breath. There are multiple phases during each respiratory cycle, including the start of inspiration, sustained inspiration, stopping of inspiration, and the time between stop of inspiration and start of the next breath during which exhalation takes place.

Trigger variables initiate the respiratory cycle. Time, pressure, flow, and volume can all be used as trigger variables. If the ventilator is triggered by time as its variable, respiratory cycles will begin at preset intervals. The ventilator can also be set to trigger with pressure, volume, or flow based on patient effort. Pressure, volume, and flow triggers are determined based on patient strength, effort, and respiratory mechanics.

Target variables are used to limit or mandate the magnitude of whichever parameters are chosen. They do not cause an end to inspiration, but create a ceiling effect for the variables selected. Pressure, flow, or volume can be used as target variables independently or in combination. Using targets prevents barotrauma and volutrauma by preventing excessive airway pressures and V_T.

CLINICAL USES OF MECHANICAL VENTILATION

Mechanical ventilation strategies vary based on clinical presentation. For example, patients with chronic obstructive pulmonary disease (COPD) will have different goals than patients with hypoxic respiratory failure.

Patients with COPD have obstruction within the airways, limiting their ability to fully exhale. Hypercapnia is present by the time these patients require mechanical ventilation, so ensuring adequate MV is a priority. The second priority is to avoid breath stacking, so that MV is targeted using higher V_T with decreased RR, while avoiding high airway pressures. Setting the inspiration:expiration (I:E) ratio to allow for longer expiratory time, in addition to slowing the RR, permits full exhalation before the next inspiration. Increased flows generate the same V_T during a shorter inspiratory phase. FIO_2 for COPD patients can be titrated to maintain SpO_2 between 88% and 92%.

For hypoxic respiratory failure due to intrinsic lung disease, the priority is oxygenation. Ensuring adequate V_T and PEEP optimizes mean airway pressures, although high FIO_2 requirements persist. Positive end-expiratory pressure recruits alveoli and improves gas exchange, permitting lower FIO_2 to minimize O_2 toxicity. Barotrauma prevention for noncompliant lungs, such as with acute respiratory distress syndrome (ARDS), requires lowering V_T as PEEP levels increase to reduce mean airway pressures. As V_T is lowered, hypercapnia develops because of an increased dead space to V_T (V_d:V_T) ratio. "Permissive hypercapnia" is well tolerated, provided significant acidosis is avoided.

HEART–LUNG INTERACTIONS DURING POSITIVE-PRESSURE VENTILATION

During negative-pressure ventilation (spontaneous breathing), inspiration increases venous return via the superior and inferior venae cavae to the right atrium, increasing right ventricular filling. Blood fills the pulmonary circulation, which acts as a reservoir that reduces blood flow to the left heart. During exhalation, blood is pushed into left-sided circulation from the pulmonary vasculature. In patients with normal volume status, cardiac output (CO) is minimally affected by respiration.

Positive-pressure ventilation reduces blood return and decreases preload during inspiration. At inspiration, positive pressure drives blood out of the heart, increasing arterial pressure. During continued inspiration, preload is decreased. During exhalation, blood pressure decreases along with CO from the decrease in preload. Right ventricular afterload is increased because of high intrathoracic pressure causing a decrease in blood traveling through the pulmonary circulation. This reduction in blood flowing from right-sided circulation to left-sided circulation reduces CO. Optimizing volume status prior to positive pressure ventilation minimizes this effect.

In addition to right heart effects, positive-pressure ventilation impacts left-sided circulation. Afterload is reduced, which improves left ventricular emptying. In addition, positive-pressure ventilation reduces work of breathing.

For patients with congestive heart failure, positive-pressure ventilation reduces right-sided preload, pulmonary vascular congestion, and left heart afterload, thus improving cardiac emptying.

Other changes with mechanical ventilation include: (1) bypass of upper airway and nasopharynx humidification; (2) V_d is increased, requiring increased MV to compensate; and (3) increasing V_T reduces the fraction of V_d, whereas altering RR does not. Gas exchange improves as the V_d fraction is reduced.

ADVERSE EFFECTS

The more days that a patient spends on the ventilator, the more likely they are to develop a ventilator-associated pneumonia (VAP). Barotrauma results from excessive pressures generated during mechanical ventilation; volutrauma results from excessive V_T. Lung-protective ventilation strategies have been developed, which employ low tidal volumes, low inspiratory pressure targets, and aggressive FIO_2 weaning to minimize toxicity while preventing hypoxemia. Barotrauma and volutrauma cause alveolar inflammation and fibrosis, damaging the alveolar:capillary membrane. This leads to poor gas exchange and significant ventilation–perfusion (V/Q) mismatching. Alveolar damage and inflammation may lead to ARDS.

Adjusting PEEP to minimize FIO_2 minimizes O_2 toxicity. Gradual PEEP adjustments account for slow improvement and avoid hemodynamic compromise. As alveolar recruitment takes place and gas exchange improves, F_{IO_2} can be weaned, targeting Spo_2 to be more than 92%. As hypoxemia improves, lowering PEEP slowly avoids derecruitment of alveoli.

Incomplete exhalation prior to the next inhalation causes progressive air trapping, leading to higher alveolar pressure at the end of expiration. This is known as auto-PEEP or dynamic hyperinflation. The causes of auto-PEEP include: short expiratory phase during each breath, high RR, and airway obstruction causing high expiratory resistance and expiratory flow limitations. Auto-PEEP can lead to profound CO reduction and circulatory collapse. It can also cause pneumothorax. Best PEEP is the level that maximizes gas exchange, but minimizes hemodynamic compromise.

SUGGESTED READING

McGee WT. A simple physiologic algorithm for managing hemodynamics using stroke volume and stroke volume variation: Physiologic Optimization Program. *J Intensive Care Med* 2009;24:352.

32

Mechanical Ventilation: Modes

Jeffrey Plotkin, MD

ASSIST/CONTROL VENTILATION

Assist/control (A/C) ventilation, otherwise known as continuous mandatory ventilation (CMV), is a mode that delivers a preset volume or pressure at a specified rate, but allows the patient to trigger an assisted breath at any time (Figure 32-1). The A/C ventilation can be pressure or volume controlled. The machine is set to "sense" the patient's negative inspiratory effort. It is therefore triggered to deliver the preset tidal volume or inspiratory pressure. All delivered breaths, whether mandatory or patient triggered, will be delivered by the ventilator according to the set parameters (volume or pressure). Fraction of inspired oxygen concentration (FIO_2) and positive end-expiratory pressure (PEEP) are also set by the operator and remain the same for every breath delivered (whether mandatory or patient triggered).

The A/C rate is the minimum number of full ventilator breaths the patient will receive. The actual respiratory rate is equal to the A/C rate plus any patient-triggered breaths per minute. If volume control is used, the delivered tidal volume will be constant but the pressure may change with each breath. If pressure control is chosen, the pressure of each delivered breath will be constant but the tidal volume may change.

INTERMITTENT MANDATORY VENTILATION

Intermittent mandatory ventilation (IMV) is a volume control mode that will deliver a preset volume at a preset rate. As with A/C mode, the operator must set FIO_2 and PEEP. In contrast to A/C, if the patient takes a breath on his/her own, the machine will not provide any additional support. In a straight IMV mode, if the patient's breath is "out of sync" with the machine, a set breath could be delivered while the patient is attempting to take a breath. For this reason, synchronized IMV (SIMV)

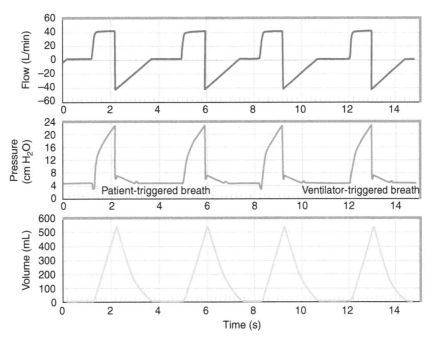

FIGURE 32-1 Assist control ventilation. (Reproduced with permission from Longnecker DE, *Longnecker Anesthesiology*, 2nd ed, New York: McGraw-Hill Medical; 2012.)

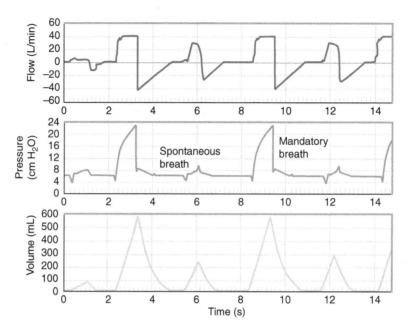

FIGURE 32-2 Intermittent mandatory ventilation. (Reproduced with permission from Longnecker DE, *Longnecker Anesthesiology*, 2nd ed, New York: McGraw-Hill Medical; 2012.)

was developed. In this mode, the ventilator senses the patient's attempts at spontaneous breathing but will not deliver a set breath at the same time. The advantage of SIMV is that the patient may not want or even require the full preset tidal volume with any given spontaneous breath. However, the patient must expend significant energy to take a breath through a full ventilator circuit. To overcome the higher work of breath, clinicians often combine pressure support ventilation (PSV) with SIMV ventilation (Figure 32-2). The combination of SIMV with PSV has proved to be an excellent ventilator weaning mode.

PRESSURE SUPPORT VENTILATION

Pressure support (PS) is an adjunct to mechanical ventilation (Figure 32-3). PS provides pressure assistance to each spontaneous breath. Pressure support used alone (without a mandatory rate) is called PSV. Each PS breath is delivered under positive pressure but triggered and cycled by the patient rather than the ventilator. Along with F_{IO_2} and PEEP, the actual level of PS desired is controlled by the operator. PS reduces the work of breathing for the patient by providing positive pressure during inspiration. The higher the PS setting, the more support

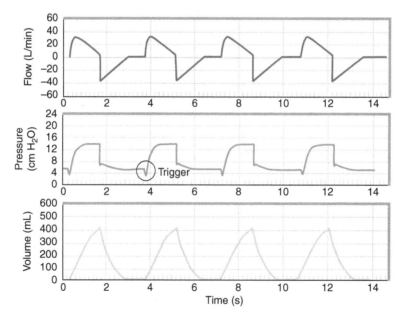

FIGURE 32-3 Pressure support ventilation. (Reproduced with permission from Longnecker DE, *Longnecker Anesthesiology*, 2nd ed, New York: McGraw-Hill Medical; 2012.)

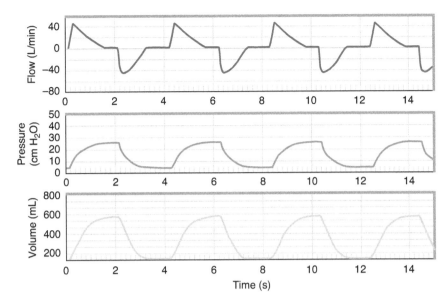

FIGURE 32-4 Pressure control ventilation. (Reproduced with permission from Longnecker DE, *Longnecker Anesthesiology*, 2nd ed, New York: McGraw-Hill Medical; 2012.)

is provided and the less work is required of the patient. The amount of PS required to overcome the resistance of the ventilator circuitry (including a size 8.0-mm endotracheal tube) has been shown to be between 8 and 12 cm H_2O.

The set PS level in conjunction with pulmonary compliance and resistance determines the delivered tidal volume. Tidal volumes will be variable from breath to breath and must be trended to ensure adequacy. Patients will require varying amounts of PS as pulmonary compliance and resistance change. Using this mode in combination with SIMV allows one to wean the number of mandatory breaths until the patient is completely on PSV. Once the PS is down to the desired level, and the patient is breathing with good tidal volumes at an acceptable rate, extubation may be considered. Despite the logical nature of this combination weaning mode, there has never been a definitive study that proves one mode is better than another for weaning.

PRESSURE CONTROL VENTILATION

Conventionally, "pressure control" refers to a type of A/C mode (it is to be kept in mind that there is also an SIMV pressure control mode on some ventilators). In PCV, a pressure-limited breath is delivered at a set rate (Figure 32-4). The tidal volume is determined by the preset pressure limit. This is a peak pressure rather than a plateau pressure limit, which is much easier to measure. The pressure will be constant while the tidal volume varies with each breath. The operator must also keep in mind that the peak pressure generated with each breath will be a combination of the set pressure of each breath added to the set PEEP. The goal of PCV is to limit the peak pressure from exceeding 40 cm H_2O, the level at which the chances of barotrauma significantly increase.

AIRWAY PRESSURE RELEASE VENTILATION

This advanced mode of ventilation is used for the most complicated patients, especially those with severe acute respiratory distress syndrome. Airway pressure release ventilation (APRV) applies continuous positive airway pressure (P_{high}) for a prolonged time (T_{high}) to maintain adequate lung volume and alveolar recruitment (Figure 32-5). There is a time-cycled release phase to a lower set pressure (P_{low}) for a short period of time (T_{low}) where most ventilation and CO_2 removal occurs. It is possible for the patient to take spontaneous breaths while inflated to P_{high}, although these are generally quite ineffective breaths.

All four parameters, P_{high}, T_{high}, P_{low}, and T_{low}, along with FIO_2, are set by the operator. Patients typically require significant sedation and sometimes paralysis to tolerate this mode. Although APRV has been shown to improve oxygenation in patients compared to failure using other modes, there is no evidence showing improvement in overall survival.

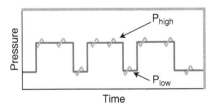

FIGURE 32-5 Airway pressure release ventilation. (Reproduced with permission from Longnecker DE, *Longnecker Anesthesiology*, 2nd ed, New York: McGraw-Hill Medical; 2012.)

Mechanical Ventilation: Monitors

33

Mona Rezai, MD, and Sudha Ved, MD

Mechanical ventilation monitors are designed to continuously measure the characteristics of the inspiration and expiration cycle (ie, respiration). These monitors typically use sensors and electronic circuits to measure and display: (1) volume of air moved (eg, tidal and minute volume); (2) inspiratory and expiratory pressures (eg, mean airway pressure and positive and expiratory pressure); (3) the respiratory rate; and (4) to detect cessation of breathing (apnea). Monitors of mechanical ventilation also test system integrity, such as the presence of system leaks, patient disconnections, and operational verification of chosen setting and alarms.

Ventilatory support begins with pressure, which drives flow, which after integration with time yields volume. These primary variables, along with their transduced signals, generate additional variables, resistance and compliance. By convention, specific variables are tracked and displayed as functions of time (eg, pressure, flow, volume, minute ventilation, end-tidal carbon dioxide). Specific combinations of variables, each of which are time dependent (eg, pressure and volume, and flow and volume), are processed and displayed as loops and displayed breath by breath. The key steps in this process of data management are the transduction of a variable into its electrical equivalent and, then, digitization of that electrical signal. Once a variable (eg, pressure at a specific moment) is transduced and digitized it becomes similar to a picture that can be copied, filed, shared, compared, and manipulated in myriad other ways.

MEASURING GAS FLOW, VOLUME, AND PRESSURE

There are several methods to set or measure gas flow. Flow is actually not easy to measure. Flowing gases in tubes generate velocity and pressure, which can be used to measure the flow indirectly. These spirometers or respirometers are prone to errors caused by inertia, friction, and water condensation. Typically the spirometers are placed proximal or distal to the inspiratory and expiratory valves or at the Y-connector that attaches to the patient's airway.

Velocity and Pressure Flowmeters

Flow may be described as laminar or turbulent. The velocity at which flow turns from laminar to turbulent flow is the critical velocity and is dependent on the radius (r) of the tube, as well as, the viscosity (η), density (ρ), and Reynolds number (κ), a constant specific to the gas. Critical velocity = $\kappa\eta/\rho r$. Volume can be directly measured.

A. Fixed-Orifice Flowmeters

They channel gas through a narrowed conduit. This narrowing increases the resistance to flow dropping the pressure of the gas as it exits. Using Poiseuille's law, the flow of the gas can then be calculated. Flow = $(\pi r^4 \Delta P)/(8\eta L)$, where r and L is the radius and length of the resistor, respectively; η is the viscosity of the gas; and ΔP is the difference in pressure across the resistor. The pressure drop across this resistance is sensed by a differential pressure transducer and is proportional to the flow rate. Disadvantage of a fixed-orifice flowmeter is that it requires different flow sensors for pediatric and adult tidal volumes (D-Lite and Pedi-Lite sensors [GE Healthcare]) since each is linearized and calibrated for specific flow measurements.

A *pneumotachometer*, a type of fixed-orifice flowmeter, is only accurate when the flow is laminar as turbulent flow would drop the pressure of the gas independent of the flow resistor. The Fleisch pneumotachometer is the most common and uses a series of small caliber tubes (mesh) to maintain laminar flow. The system is bulky and not suited for pediatric use.

Turbulent flowmeters are a variation of a fixed-orifice flowmeter. They channel gases through a very high, but known, resistance creating turbulent flow. The flow is then calculated from the difference in the upstream laminar flow and downstream turbulent flow. These turbulent flowmeters are not in common use due to insensitivity at low flows and high resistance at high flows.

B. Variable-Orifice Flowmeters

They similarly use the drop in pressure across a resistor to calculate the flow. However, these flowmeters contain a flap that opens the diameter of the orifice at high flows and narrows it at low flows. By changing the diameter of the conduit, flow can be more accurately calculated at both very high and low flows (eg, V.O.S. sensor [GE Healthcare]).

Pitot tube flowmeter uses a pair of measuring tubes. One tube is placed parallel to the flow of the gas causing an increase in pressure within the sampling tube as gas attempts to flow within the narrower pitot tube (resistor). The other tube is placed perpendicular to the gas flow and measures the baseline pressure within the conduit. Flow is proportional to the difference in pressure between the tubes. A modification of this system places two pitot tubes—one tube facing upstream of flow, whereas the other faces downstream (GE D-Lite and Pedi-Lite sensors). Additionally, the monitor samples gas composition to correct for the density and viscosity of the gas mixture. Flow and pressure of the gas can then be determined in either direction.

Balance-of-Pressure Flowmeters

A. Thorpe Tube

Rotameters contain a bobbin floating in a tube tapered toward the bottom. A Thorpe tube has a constant pressure and variable orifice. Near the bottom of the tube, the walls are closer to the bobbin and low gas flow is sufficient to make it float. As the bobbin rises, the walls are further away allowing a higher flow percentage of gas to escape around the bobbin rather than pushing it up. The bobbin stops rising or falling when the pressure difference above and below it equals its weight. Each tube is calibrated for the specific gas, bobbin, and at a specific temperature. Flow measurements will not be accurate if a different gas is used, if the tube is not vertically aligned, if leaks are present in the tube, if the bobbin sticks to the walls, or if there is debris within the tube.

B. Bourdon Tube

It is commonly used to measure and display the high pressure of gas cylinders. A Bourdon tube has a constant orifice, but variable pressure. Pressure from the cylinder is channeled into a flexible tube that straightens at higher pressures. As the tube straightens at higher pressures or relaxes at lower pressures, a gear which rotates the needle around the display turns. The tube uncoils under the high back pressure making it unsuitable for low-pressure respiratory systems.

Kinetic Energy Flowmeters (Wright Spirometer)

Vane anemometer is one of the earliest devices invented to measure the flow. It utilizes a low-friction turbine device that spins when the gas strikes the blades passing its kinetic energy. The rate of rotation is directly proportional to the rate of flow. Vane anemometers tend not to be as accurate at very high or low flows as more of the gas passes between the blades of the anemometer rather than striking the blades themselves. A limitation of a vane anemometer is inaccuracy during low flow and requires approximately 2 L/min of flow. Modern anemometers use LEDs and silicon photodetectors to overcome this limitation by overreading at lower flows and underreading at higher flows.

Mass and Volume Flowmeter (Volumeter)

Sealed volumeters contain rotating polystyrene valves that rotate in a sealed container similar to a revolving door conducting a large flow of people. Sealed volumeters are more accurate at lower flows than vane anemometers as the energy of the gas flow is better transmitted to the rotating elements.

MEASURING GAS PRESSURES

Circuit and ventilator pressures are usually measured either by the volumeters described above or by solid-state transducers.

Bourdon Pressure Gauge

It is commonly used to measure and display the pressure of gas cylinders. Pressure from the cylinder is channeled into a flexible tube that straightens at higher pressures. As the tube straightens at higher pressures or relaxes at lower pressures, a gear which rotates the needle around the display turns.

Piezoelectric Gauge

It uses any material, such as quartz, that produces an electric charge under compression. This electric current is then calibrated with the system to produce a meaningful signal. Modern anesthesia machines and ventilators make use of a similar system but use specific metals or semiconductors that vary in resistance when placed under pressure. This change in resistance can be measured and transmitted as a pressure signal. This piezoresistive effect allows pressure transducers to be very small and lightweight.

Aneroid Diaphragm Gauge

It is used to measure barometric pressure. It contains a vacuum chamber that is connected by a lever and spindle to the needle on the gauge. As the air pressure increases or decreases the vacuum chamber contracts or expands pushing the needle around the display.

MEASURING RESPIRATORY RATE

Mechanical ventilation monitors also determine respiratory rate by measuring chest wall motion, ventilation acoustics, or directly by sensing the flow of gas.

Air Flow Sampling

Respiratory rate can be derived from the information transmitted by any of the flowmeters described previously. These include vane anemometers, hot-wire anemometers, fixed- or variable-orifice flowmeters, Pitot tubes measuring pressure differences, or by ultrasonic meters. Additionally, respiratory rate can also be calculated from the difference in gas composition between inhaled and exhaled gas. Capnography is the most widely used method. Respiratory rate is calculated from the expiratory rate signaled by an increase in CO_2.

Chest Wall Motion

Inductive plethysmography uses mechanical changes in the chest wall to transmit electrical signals. Bands containing wire coils wrap around the rib cage and abdomen in a dual band configuration. These bands are connected to an oscillator. With increased diameter of the chest or abdomen the bands stretch and the oscillatory frequency changes thus signaling the respiratory effort. In contrast, ECG-based respiratory monitoring makes use of the fact that increased chest wall diameter will increase the resistance of flow of current across the thorax. During inspiration the electrical resistance increases and the QRS axis rotates. Both can be detected by ECG electrodes. The number of times the resistance changes can be measured and a respiratory rate calculated. Techniques that infer respiration from chest wall movement assume that respiratory effort implies actual ventilation and gas exchange, which is an obvious limitation.

Ventilation Acoustics

Acoustic air flow sensors measure the sounds transmitted from gas exchange. These sensors may be incorporated into an adhesive sensor placed on the patient's neck or as part of a nasal cannula that senses the sound of air as it passes into the nasal prongs. A variation of acoustic monitoring uses a facemask lined with pyroelectric polymer that electrically signals the increased temperature from exhaled air.

VENTILATOR SETTINGS AND ALARMS

High Airway Pressure Alarm

The alarm sounds when the peak or plateau inspiratory pressure reaches above a set threshold. Causes of high peak inspiratory pressure include increased airway resistance, a decrease in the patient's compliance, or a malfunctioning machine. In addition to providing the alarm, tidal volume should be pressure limited which will ensure that the patient will only receive part of the preset tidal volume.

A. Plateau Pressures

The plateau pressures reflect static effective compliance. Compliance is defined as the change in volume for a given pressure, $C = \Delta V/\Delta P$. Low compliance implies stiffness and resistance to volume change for a given pressure. A patient's compliance is composed of intrinsic lung compliance and the compliance of the chest wall. Intraoperative changes in compliance include pulmonary pathology (pulmonary edema, pneumothorax), pneumoperitoneum during laparoscopy, right main stem intubation, steep Trendelenburg positioning, or hyperinflation from excessive positive end-expiratory pressure (PEEP) or an obstructed PEEP valve or expiratory port.

B. Peak Inspiratory Pressures

The peak inspiratory pressures reflect dynamic effective compliance and has both compliance and resistance components. The airway in this case refers to the patient's airway from the trachea to the terminal bronchioles or the breathing circuit. Poiseuille's law states for flow through a given conduit $P = 8\eta LQ / \pi r^4$, where P is the pressure, η is the viscosity, L is the length of the conduit, Q is the flow, and r is the radius. Given a constant viscosity of a gas, the pressure will increase if the flow is increased (setting shorter inspiratory time for a given volume), length is increased (using a longer circuit), or the radius is decreased (using a smaller endotracheal tube, secretions within the tube, bronchospasm). Note that the changes in the radius make the largest difference in pressure.

There are other unique machine causes of high peak inspiratory pressures. For instance, a hole in the bellows allows direct transmission of the gas to the patient. Changes in the measured inspired oxygen (either higher or lower depending on whether room air or oxygen is used) should alert the anesthetist to this possibility. During positive pressure inhalation, the positive pressure relief valve of the ventilator may be partially closed (the upper threshold for release of gas is set at the ventilator, similar to the adjustable pressure-limiting [APL] valve). Opening the oxygen flush valve during this period of time will raise airway pressure to the upper set limit of the pressure relief valve. If not for a functioning APL or the ventilator relief valve, opening the oxygen flush valve would subject the patient to 45 psi of pressure, equivalent to approximately 3000 cm H_2O.

The machine protects the patient from high pressure by three primary pressure relief valves: the APL used during spontaneous ventilation; the ventilator pressure relief valve used during machine ventilation; and the scavenging pressure relief valve used continuously. Failure of any of these valves may result in highly transmitted pressure to the patient. If pressure limit is repeatedly exceeded and the cause of high pressure is unknown, or not immediately correctable, patient should be disconnected and manually ventilated while the problem is diagnosed.

Continuing Pressure Alarm

The alarm sounds when pressure is greater than 10 cm H_2O for more than 15 seconds. It signals that gas is unable to exit the system and pressure is gradually building within. This may occur if the ventilator pressure relief valve is stuck, if the oxygen flush valve is activated, if APL is closed above 10 cm H_2O, or if scavenging system outflow is occluded.

Subatmospheric Alarm

The alarm sounds when the pressure within the circuit is negative. The direction of gas flow in this situation may be toward the patient or toward the machine. The former occurs during attempts at spontaneous respiration with inadequate fresh gas flow or against an occluded circuit. Less commonly a gastric tube may have been inadvertently placed in the trachea resulting in suctioning of gas flow. Negative pressure toward the machine may be caused by failure of the negative pressure release valve from a suctioning (active), scavenging system.

Low-Pressure Alarm

The alarm signals when the circuit does not reach a minimum threshold within a specific period of time, usually 15 seconds.

If this threshold is set too low it may not detect significant leaks or partial disconnections. To prevent false negatives, ideally the limit should be set to just under the patient's peak inspiratory pressure. Some machines automatically alter the threshold based on the peak pressure. Of note, low-pressure alarms only signal during positive pressure ventilation and will not signal a circuit disconnection during spontaneous ventilation. Causes of low-pressure alarms include partial or complete disconnection, inadvertent extubation, esophageal intubation, incompetent expiratory valve, cuff leak, or circuit leak. Of note, 70% of all disconnections occur at the Y-piece. Anything that would elevate the pressure above normal positive pressure ventilation may prevent signaling of a disconnection. Some examples include partial extubation, compression, or obstruction of the breathing circuit, a decrease in patient's lung or chest compliance, compression of empty bellows, or the addition of high-resistance component such as a heat and moisture exchanger.

Noninvasive Mechanical Ventilation

34

Brian S. Freeman, MD

Noninvasive positive pressure ventilation (NPPV) is a form of mechanical ventilatory support using a mask instead of an invasive airway device such as an endotracheal or tracheostomy tube. Its use has been increasing in frequency in both intensive care and postanesthesia care recovery units.

Successful use of this intervention requires careful patient selection, proper management of the underlying disease necessitating its use, and continuous respiratory monitoring. Noninvasive positive pressure ventilation can be used as first-line therapy in patients with respiratory insufficiency (eg, exacerbation of chronic obstructive pulmonary disease [COPD]), as a form of weaning from ventilator therapy, and as a bridge support after early extubation. After initiation of NPPV, patients must be closely monitored. Lack of improvement within several hours, intolerance to therapy, or signs of clinical deterioration should prompt a decision for endotracheal intubation. Patients intubated after a failed trial of noninvasive ventilation may spend a longer period of time in the intensive care unit (ICU) on the ventilator.

ADVANTAGES AND INDICATIONS

Noninvasive ventilation has a number of advantages over invasive ventilation, the sum of which may contribute to reductions in ICU length of stay and mortality.

- Reduces the need for endotracheal intubation.
- Reduces the risks of artificial airway complications, such as airway trauma due to laryngoscopy and intubation.
- Reduces the rate of nosocomial infections associated with invasive mechanical ventilation: ventilator-acquired pneumonia, sinusitis, and sepsis.
- Causes less patient discomfort.
- Reduces the need for intravenous sedation.
- Serves as an alternative for patients whose advanced directives prohibit endotracheal intubation (ie, DNI— "Do Not Intubate").

Noninvasive ventilation is best suited as an adjunct to manage pulmonary insufficiency in which the underlying condition responds well to other simultaneous treatments.

Randomized controlled clinical trials have shown that the following indications for NPPV can reduce pulmonary complications, improve mortality rates, and decrease length of stay:

- COPD exacerbation.
- Cardiogenic pulmonary edema.
- Respiratory failure of any etiology (hypercapnia or hypoxemic).
- Respiratory distress in immunocompromised (solid organ and bone marrow transplant) patients.
- Respiratory distress immediately after lung resection, gastric bypass, or upper abdominal surgery.
- Preoxygenation of patients in hypoxemic respiratory failure prior to intubation.

Consideration of noninvasive ventilation begins with a patient who has signs of respiratory distress. These signs include moderate-to-severe dyspnea, tachypnea greater than 24 breaths per minute, and evidence of increased work of breathing (such as pursed-lip breathing or use of accessory muscles). Analysis of arterial blood gases shows respiratory acidosis (pH 7.10-7.35) due to hypercapnia ($Paco_2$ > 40 mm Hg) as well as hypoxemia (Pao_2/Fio_2 < 200 mm Hg). Patients suitable for NPPV must be alert, cooperative, and have an obstructed airway with intact respiratory drive.

DISADVANTAGES AND CONTRAINDICATIONS

Compared to endotracheal intubation, the use of noninvasive modalities for oxygenation and ventilation has several disadvantages:

- May not work effectively due to air leaks from poorly fitting masks.
- Increases aspiration risk.
- Hinders speaking and coughing.
- May cause claustrophobia for the patient.
- Initial fitting and settings are more time- and labor intensive.

Patient selection is essential. Contraindications to the use of NPPV include:

- Cardiopulmonary arrest.
- Impaired level of consciousness or coma.
- Hemodynamic instability or shock.
- Acute myocardial infarction.
- Uncontrolled dysrhythmias.
- Severe facial deformity or trauma.
- Patient intolerance of the mask (agitation, lack of cooperation, claustrophobia).
- High aspiration risk (altered mental status, copious secretions, intractable emesis, impaired cough or swallowing).
- Uncontrollable upper gastrointestinal bleeding.
- Pathologic conditions of the upper airway (epiglottitis, angioedema).
- Extensive head and neck tumors.
- Recent upper gastrointestinal surgery.

No contraindication exists to applying noninvasive ventilation in the postanesthesia care unit. However, there is no evidence that supports its use to either prevent or treat patients with postextubation respiratory distress. In the immediate recovery period, the risk of hypoxemia and hypercapnia increases as a result of upper airway edema due to airway trauma, diaphragmatic dysfunction, and higher respiratory workload. However, NPPV has not been shown to reduce reintubation rates in patients who develop postextubation respiratory distress. In fact, it may even be associated with a higher mortality than immediate reintubation. Noninvasive positive pressure ventilation could increase the risk of aspiration, gastric distension, and wound dehiscence, especially in patients who have just undergone gastrointestinal surgery.

HOW NONINVASIVE VENTILATION WORKS

Noninvasive ventilation requires the use of an external interface to deliver positive pressure ventilation, such as a mask, mouthpiece, nasal pillow, or helmet. The most commonly used devices are face (oronasal) and nasal masks. Oronasal masks provide more effective ventilation. They are preferred for patients who are mouth- or pursed-lip breathers, edentulous, or less cooperative. They may not work well in claustrophobic patients and carry a higher risk of aspiration if the patient has emesis. Nasal masks are generally better tolerated but require a more cooperative patient. They allow the patient to speak, cough, and clear secretions. They are preferred in patients with less severe respiratory insufficiency. However, nasal masks have greater leaks and have limited effectiveness in patients with obstructed nasal airways. For both types of masks, the smallest mask that enables an effective proper fit should be chosen. The straps used to hold the mask in place should be tight enough to prevent leaks but loose enough so that at least one finger can be passed between the face and straps.

The application of positive pressure through the mask has several physiologic effects. Noninvasive positive pressure ventilation splints open the upper and lower airways, reduce the work of breathing, and increases tidal volume. It redistributes extravascular lung water, decreases the ratio of dead space to tidal volume, and thereby improves ventilation–perfusion matching (which reduces shunting). In the postoperative recovery unit, noninvasive ventilation can help prevent the reduction in functional residual capacity and secretion clearance due to pain and residual anesthesia. NPPV can impair the cardiovascular system. Increased intrathoracic pressure can decrease venous return.

Monitoring the patient who is receiving noninvasive ventilation can be time intensive but necessary to determine the likelihood of success. The mask should be evaluated frequently for patient tolerance, air leaks, skin necrosis, and rebreathing of carbon dioxide. Assessment of the patient's mental status and respiratory comfort is important. Physiologic variables to be measured include oxygen saturation, respiratory rate, tidal volume, blood pressure, heart rate, and arterial blood gases. Physical examination of accessory respiratory muscles, paradoxical abdominal breathing, and ventilator synchrony should occur in the first hour of therapy.

Successful noninvasive ventilation should lead to a decrease in the patient's respiratory rate and $Paco_2$ (by >8 mm Hg) and correction of respiratory acidosis (pH > 0.06) within the first 2 hours of a trial of therapy. Predictors of success for NPPV include patients with lower illness severity, intact dentition, younger age, moderate respiratory acidosis (pH 7.25-7.35), high level of consciousness, and fewer mask air leaks. Noninvasive ventilation is more likely to fail for patients with severe illnesses (pH < 7.25, $Paco_2$ > 80 mm Hg), lower levels of consciousness (eg, Glasgow Come Scale [GCS] < 8), poor nutrition, copious secretions, low functional status, and concomitant complications such as shock, acute respiratory distress syndrome, or pneumonia.

MODES OF VENTILATION

The two most common modes of ventilation used to administer NPPV are continuous positive airway pressure (CPAP) and bi-level positive airway pressure (BiPAP). Compared to modes such as assist–control ventilation, they enable good patient comfort and ventilator synchrony. Both modes allow for short-term respiratory support during treatment of the underlying condition. Initial support settings are based on achieving tidal volumes of 5-7 mL/kg, respiratory rates less than 25 breaths per minute, and oxygen saturation greater than 90%. The waveforms seen on the ventilator differ depending upon the type of therapy chosen (Figure 34-1).

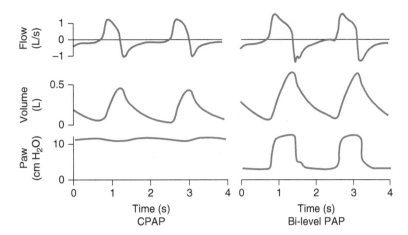

FIGURE 34-1 Tracings of flow, tidal volume, and airway pressure during CPAP and BiPAP. (Reproduced with permission from Antonescu-Turcu A, Parthasarathy S. CPAP and bi-level PAP therapy: new and established roles. *Respir Care*. 2010;55(9):1216-1229.)

Continuous Positive Airway Pressure

This basic level of support provides CPAP throughout the entire respiratory cycle. CPAP helps restore and maintain adequate functional residual capacity, thus improving oxygenation. It is less efficacious for improving ventilation. The typical initial setting is 5-10 cm H_2O.

Bi-level Positive Airway Pressure

This mode provides two levels of support during spontaneous breathing: inspiratory positive airway pressure (IPAP) and expiratory positive airway pressure (EPAP). As the equivalent of pressure support, IPAP improves ventilation by increasing tidal volume and decreasing the work of breathing. The higher initial IPAP setting is 8-10 cm H_2O (recommended maximum 20 cm H_2O). EPAP is the equivalent to positive end-expiratory pressure (PEEP). By preventing alveolar collapse, baseline EPAP helps maintain functional residual capacity and oxygenation. The lower initial EPAP setting is 3-5 cm H_2O (recommended maximum 10 cm H_2O). Management of worsening hypoxemia or hypercapnia should occur by increasing both settings in 2 cm H_2O increments in a 2.5:1 IPAP:EPAP ratio.

COMPLICATIONS

Compared to endotracheal intubation, noninvasive ventilation carries a different set of potential complications:

- Air leaks
- Pressure necrosis of the skin
- Gastric distention
- Aspiration
- Mask intolerance
- Nasal congestion
- Eye irritation
- Nasal bridge ulceration
- Dry mucous membranes
- Thick secretions
- Difficulty using an oral feeding tube

SUGGESTED READING

Boldrini R, Fasano L, Nava S. Noninvasive mechanical ventilation. *Curr Opin Crit Care* 2012;18:48-53.

Operating Room Alarms and Safety Features

Daniel Asay, MD, and Jason Sankar, MD

FIRE SAFETY

Despite eliminating flammable gases such as ether and cyclopropane from operating rooms (ORs), OR fires are just as relevant today as they were when those agents were in use. Fire ignition requires three components, commonly referred to as the fire triad: source, fuel, and an oxidizer. At the molecular level, a fire is a chemical reaction of a fuel plus an oxidizer that produces heat and light. It has been estimated that annually in the United States, there are 50-200 OR fires. To improve patient safety in the OR, the American Society of Anesthesiologists has issued a practice advisory on how to prevent and manage OR fires (Figure 35-1).

An oxidizer is a substance that removes electrons from another reactant. In the OR, the main oxidizers are O_2 and N_2O. Closed or semi-closed breathing systems create oxidizer-rich atmospheres that promote combustion.

Ignition sources are also prevalent in an OR environment. Surgeons often make use of cautery, lasers, argon beams, fiber optic cables, and defibrillator pads. Any of these devices can be the fire source.

The OR fuel sources are common on the surgical drapes, gauze pads, antibiotic preparation solution, dressings, and surgical caps and gowns. There are also many fuel sources emanating from the anesthesiologist's equipment: endotracheal tubes, oxygen masks, nasal cannulae, and suction catheters can readily fuel a fire. Patient hair is another combustible fuel.

Fires cause burn damage and risk damage from fire byproducts. For example, an endotracheal tube on fire produces damaging substances such as carbon monoxide (CO), cyanide (CN), and hydrogen chloride (HCl).

LINE ISOLATION MONITOR

Numerous electrical devices operate in an OR. Electrical power is typically grounded in people's homes but *ungrounded* in the OR. This is accomplished by using an isolation transformer to induce a current via electromagnetic induction between the primary circuit coming from the electrical company and the secondary circuit going to the OR. Consequently, the power going to the OR is isolated from ground. To receive a shock, a person needs to make contact between two conductive materials at different voltages, thereby completing a circuit. Since the power going to the OR has no connection to ground, a person can touch one side of the isolated power system and not receive a shock due to the incomplete circuit.

The line isolation system (transformer and monitor) is designed to protect people from electrocution in the OR by power isolation and continuous monitoring of the isolated power system integrity. It is designed to detect short circuits (or leakage currents) and to alert OR personnel if a piece of equipment is no longer isolated from ground. It does this by monitoring each side of an isolated power system. Modern line isolation monitors (LIMs) are typically set to alarm with a leakage current of 2-5 mA. The LIM detects a *first fault*, such as a broken piece of equipment that became ungrounded or plugged into the outlet. The OR personnel must systematically unplug equipment until the faulty equipment is discovered and the LIM alarm ceases. The OR environment only becomes truly hazardous if a second fault occurs.

GROUND FAULT CIRCUIT INTERRUPTER

The ORs utilize a line isolation transformer and monitor rather than a ground fault circuit interrupter (GFCI) to ensure that vital equipment does not turn off at inappropriate times. All other equipment can be plugged into an outlet utilizing a GFCI. These are the outlets found in most homes to prevent an electric shock in a grounded system. The GFCI monitors both sides of the circuit, ensuring equal flow on both sides. If a person comes into contact with faulty equipment, the GFCI detects an imbalance and stops current passage. Most GFCI outlets detect a 5 mA current difference, offering significant protection.

MICROSHOCK AND MACROSHOCK

Microshock occurs when a current is applied directly to the heart, whereas a macroshock occurs when a much larger current passes through the body, usually via the skin. As noted in the electrical safety chapter (see Chapter 37), 100 µA are

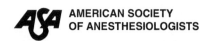

OPERATING ROOM FIRES ALGORITHM

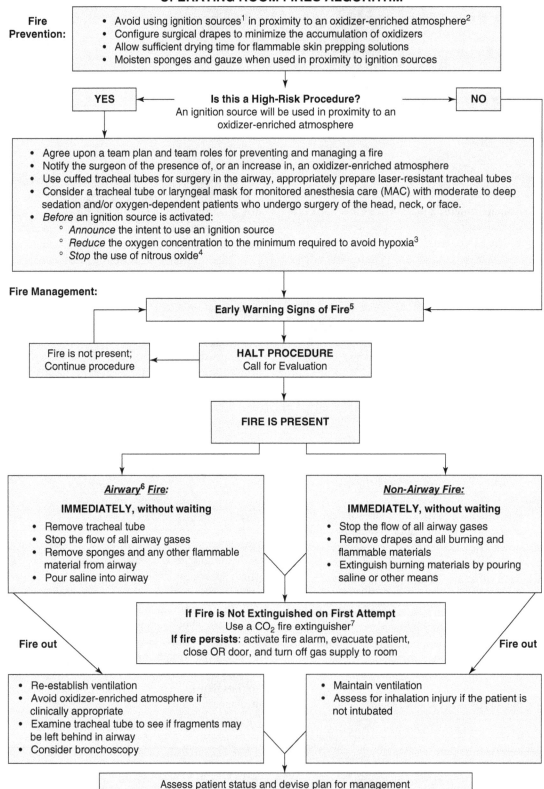

FIGURE 35-1 Operating room fire algorithm. (Reproduced with permission from American Society of Anesthesiologists Task Force on Operating Room Fires. Practice advisory for the prevention and management of operating room fires. *Anesthesiology*. 2008;108(5):786-801.)

enough to cause ventricular fibrillation. Since the LIM will only detect leakage current between 2 and 5 mA, the LIM does not warn of currents in the microshock range.

ELECTROSURGICAL UNIT ALARMS

Electrosurgical units (ESUs), or Bovies, have become commonplace in modern ORs. Both monopolar and bipolar electrosurgery function by completing a circuit. Monopolar electrosurgery disperses its electrical current through the patient to a return electrode, whereas bipolar does not require a patient plate, restricting the current to the immediate area of forceps application. The dispersive electrode has a large surface area to allow the high-frequency current to flow back with low intensity, preventing burns. The electrode also has a monitor to sense tissue impedance that will turn off and which alarms if the plate is applied incorrectly or dislodges during a surgical procedure.

AIR EXCHANGE

The National Institute for Occupational Safety and Health (NIOSH) is a federal agency that has set established criteria for anesthetic gas exposure limits. The criteria recommend the maximum exposure for waste anesthetic gases of 2 ppm for halogenated anesthetic agents when used alone or 0.5 ppm of a halogenated agent with 25 ppm of N_2O.

In addition to scavenging equipment present in the ventilator, ORs require efficient ventilation systems to reduce waste gases. The American Institute of Architects require 15-21 air exchanges hourly with three of those supplying outside air.

SUGGESTED READING

American Society of Anesthesiologists Task Force on Operating Room Fires. Practice advisory for the prevention and management of operating room fires. *Anesthesiology* 2008;108:786-801.

Defibrillators

Brian S. Freeman, MD

BASIC CONCEPTS

During defibrillation, a randomly timed high-voltage electric current is discharged across two electrodes placed on the chest of a patient in cardiac arrest. The purpose of defibrillation is to simultaneously depolarize a large critical mass of myocardium. As a result, nearly all ventricular myocytes will enter their absolute refractory periods, when no action potentials can be generated. Successful defibrillation means that the reentry focus underlying the ventricular dysrhythmia is now either quiescent or eliminated. At this point, the pacemaker with the highest automaticity (such as the sinus or atrioventricular nodes) will take over control of ventricular pacing and contraction with a proper sequence of depolarization and repolarization.

Successful defibrillation occurs when ventricular fibrillation (VF) has terminated for at least 5 seconds following the shock. It is still considered shock success even if the postshock rhythm is nonperfusing, such as asystole, or if hemodynamics remain unstable. The definition of successful defibrillation is independent of resuscitation measures such as return of spontaneous circulation, survival to hospital discharge, and neurologic outcome.

A number of variables can affect the likelihood of terminating VF via an electrical current. Time is perhaps the most important. The probability of successful defibrillation decreases, the longer the patient remains in a pulseless dysrhythmia. Higher success rates have been noted if the underlying cause is ischemic in nature, such as an acute myocardial infarction. Nonischemic causes of cardiac arrest (such as tamponade, tension pneumothorax, pulmonary embolus, hypovolemia, hypoxemia, acidosis, and electrolyte abnormalities) have lower defibrillation success rates. Measures to decrease the transthoracic impedance against an electric current can also improve the chance of successful defibrillation. These methods include applying firm pressure (at least 25 lb) on the paddles, using proper paddle sizes and conductive gel, defibrillating during end-expiration, and using "stacked" shock strengths with a higher frequency.

Ventricular fibrillation and pulseless ventricular tachycardia (VT) are the primary indications for electrical defibrillation. These dysrhythmias are rarely spontaneously reversible and will often deteriorate into asystole if the underlying reentry circuit is not eliminated. Rapid defibrillation is absolutely essential to restore spontaneous circulation promptly and to achieve the best possible neurologic outcome. For pulseless VT, whether monomorphic or polymorphic, the shock must be "unsynchronized" to achieve proper defibrillation, as opposed to electrical cardioversion.

Contraindications to defibrillation include pulseless electrical activity (PEA) and asystole, the two major "nonshockable" cardiac arrest rhythms. A patient with VT who has a pulse and a stable perfusing rhythm should not receive defibrillation. A patient with VT who becomes unstable with evidence of decreased cardiac output should receive synchronized cardioversion. Defibrillation should not be performed if there is any danger to the rescuer or patient. For instance, excessive moisture on the patient's chest could lead to improper current distribution, or a patient lying in a wet environment could increase the risk of electrical injury to the bystanders.

DEFIBRILLATOR UNITS

Members of the "code blue" or resuscitation team should have a solid understanding of the type of defibrillation equipment used. There are different configurations of defibrillator units depending on the specific manufacturer. Most defibrillators today have the capability of such features as performing electrocardiographic (ECG) monitoring, pulse oximetry, sphygmomanometry, cardioversion, and external pacing.

All defibrillator units provide the energy source for the electrical current. The operator will select an energy level (in joules) desired for release during defibrillation by a selection switch. A second charge switch will trigger the flow of current from the unit's battery to the capacitor, where a significant amount of energy is stored in the form of a charge. Activation of the shock control will enable the release of current into the electrodes or paddles that are placed on the patient. Most devices revert automatically into a default unsynchronized mode between shocks to discharge the defibrillation current independently of the ECG rhythm, although this should be verified prior to defibrillation. If electrical cardioversion is necessary, the operator must select the "sync" button to place the unit into the synchronized mode so that the current is only released during the peak of the R-wave of the QRS complex. Defibrillation in the synchronized mode will not discharge a shock because there are no discernible QRS complexes in VF. Both defibrillation and cardioversion charge releases are followed by an easily observable whole body twitch of the patient's muscles.

Defibrillator units are categorized based upon their operational characteristics:

a. Manual defibrillators—These are the most common types found in hospitals. Manual defibrillators require the operator to perform all of the necessary steps: turning on the device, selecting input (quick-look paddles vs patient ECG electrodes), placing the pads on the patient's chest, determining the underlying malignant dysrhythmia, selecting the appropriate energy level, charging the capacitor, checking the mode switch, and delivering the shock by depressing the "shock" controls.

b. Semiautomated defibrillators—These are found in public settings. These automated external defibrillators (AEDs) require fewer decisions by the operator. After turning on the device, the operator follows the voice prompts to attach the electrode pads, presses the "analyze" switch, and then hits the "shock" button if the AED detects and announces a shockable rhythm. The AED is preprogrammed to perform ECG rhythm analysis and to select the energy level delivered.

c. Fully automated defibrillators—These will not only analyze the ECG and diagnose the dysrhythmia, but also automatically discharge the shock. The operator only has to turn the device on and connect the electrodes to the patient. Although some AEDs are fully automated, the best example of fully automated devices is implantable cardioverter-defibrillator (ICD) units.

DEFIBRILLATION ELECTRODES

Electrodes are necessary to place the patient into the circuit with the defibrillation unit. Defibrillator electrodes come in two forms: handheld paddles (often with several control buttons located on the handles) and self-adhesive pads. Both types of electrodes yield comparable defibrillation success rates. Operators should apply significant pressure onto the paddles to lower transthoracic resistance. For adult patients, operators should use the largest electrodes (8-12 cm) that will fit on the chest with overlapping. By decreasing transthoracic impedance at the chest wall, large pads generate a current of optimal density that can terminate fibrillation with minimal damage to the myocardium. Paddles that are too large will divert excessive current to the thorax yielding lower current flow through the heart. Electrodes that are too small for the patient may cause myocardial necrosis.

High resistance to current flow can compromise the amount of current actually delivered to the myocardium, leading to failed shocks. Conductive materials further help to decrease transthoracic impedance. Paddles require the use

of special electrode paste (not ultrasound gel), whereas self-adhesive pads have built-in gel material. Inappropriate use of conductive material can lead to short circuits that can produce sparks, burn the patient's skin, and become a possible explosion hazard. Care should also be taken not to place electrodes directly on top of a transdermal drug delivery patch, such as clonidine or fentanyl. The patch may block delivery of energy from the electrode pad to the heart or cause small burns to the skin. If shock delivery will not be delayed, remove medication patches and wipe the area before attaching the pad.

There are four possible positions for the pads/paddles: anterolateral, anteroposterior, anterior-left infrascapular, and anterior-right infrascapular. Although any of the four pad positions is reasonable and equally effective for defibrillation success, the usual default placement is anterolateral. In this placement, the sternal electrode is placed below the clavicle to the right of the sternum. The apical electrode is placed on the midaxillary line around the fifth or sixth intercostal space.

WAVEFORMS AND POLARITY

Defibrillators deliver electrical currents over a brief period of time to the myocardium with two different waveform technologies: monophasic and biphasic. Each waveform delivery is comparable when it comes to the rate of return of spontaneous circulation, survival to hospital admission, or survival to hospital discharge.

Monophasic

Monophasic defibrillators were the first systems created but are mostly phased out of production. These traditional units deliver a unidirectional (one polarity) flow of current from the apical to sternal electrode. Monophasic damped sinusoidal (MDS) waveforms have a rapid positive increase in current flow to a predetermined peak which then slowly returns to baseline (Figure 36-1). These currents usually resemble a sine wave. Monophasic truncated exponential (MTE) waveforms are currents that return very suddenly to baseline zero flow. The initial shock energy level with either monophasic waveform should be 360 J. Because of the lower success rate

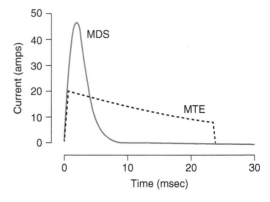

FIGURE 36-1 Monophasic waveforms.

with these defibrillators, subsequent shocks should also have 360 J of energy.

Biphasic

Newer defibrillators release the current output in both directions (positive and negative polarity) between the two electrodes, generating a biphasic waveform. The reversal of current occurs sequentially. Biphasic waveforms have a rapid rise in current flow with a slight plateau followed by an abrupt reversal in current flow at a predetermined time (Figure 36-2). Biphasic rectilinear (BR) waveforms deliver a constant current flow during the first phase (thus reducing potentially harmful peak currents) regardless of patient impedance before reversing polarity and then returning gradually to baseline. The constant current delivery reduces the potential adverse effects of patient impedance on successful defibrillation. Biphasic truncated exponential (BTE) waveforms, originally developed for use in implantable defibrillators, have currents which gradually return to baseline due to the effects of patient impedance.

Biphasic defibrillators require lower energy levels than their monophasic counterparts. Advanced cardiac life support (ACLS) providers should use the manufacturer's recommended device-specific effective waveform energy dose (120 J for BR waveforms; 150-200 J for BTE waveforms). If the manufacturer's recommended dose is not known, the default of 200 J is recommended for the initial shock.

Biphasic waveforms lower the electrical threshold for successful defibrillation. They have been shown to have the same or even better first-shock success rates for VF termination compared to monophasic shocks of the same or higher energy. Clinical outcomes, such as return of spontaneous circulation or survival to hospital discharge, have not been proven superior with biphasic devices over monophasic. However, the lower energies used in biphasic defibrillation may decrease the incidence of myocardial damage and post-shock dysrhythmias. In addition, newer biphasic waveform technology can compensate for transthoracic impedance, thus allowing uniform current delivery.

IMPLANTABLE CARDIOVERTER-DEFIBRILLATORS

Patients with implantable cardioverter-defibrillators (ICDs) should have the antitachycardia function of the device disabled for surgery. Electromagnetic interference from electrocautery could cause the device to inappropriately discharge a shock. Depending on the manufacturer, the defibrillation function may be suspended either by placement of a magnet over the device or by programming.

During the perioperative period, emergency defibrillation may be necessary for a patient with a deactivated ICD. Before attempting external defibrillation, providers should terminate all sources of electromagnetic interference (EMI) and either remove the magnet or consult the appropriate provider to reprogram the device to reestablish antitachycardia therapy. If these measures fail to restore native ICD function, emergency external defibrillation is necessary. But special considerations must be taken when performing external defibrillation on patients with an ICD. Although ICD pulse generators have circuits designed to prevent damage from external electrical surges, current flow through the pulse generator and leads should be minimized. Damage to the circuit could cause propagation of high energy currents from the generator to the electrodes causing significant thermal damage to the myocardium.

Optimal positioning of the defibrillation paddles may prevent adverse ICD effects. Without delaying defibrillation, the pads should be placed as far as possible from the pulse generator (at least 8 cm away). The standard anterior–lateral placement is ideal because this positions the paddles perpendicular to the major axis of the ICD pulse generator and minimizes current flow. Existing ACLS protocols should be followed regarding the clinically appropriate energy output of the defibrillator regardless of the presence of an ICD. The device should be interrogated and the generator and pacing threshold checked by a competent authority immediately postoperatively. Any patient with disabled antitachycardia therapy must be monitored until restoration.

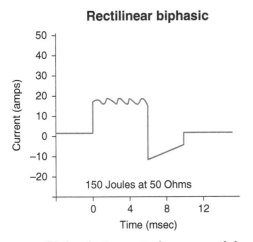

Rectilinear biphasic

150 Joules at 50 Ohms

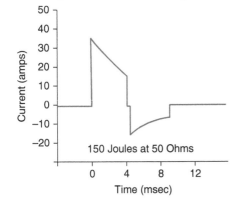

Biphasic truncated exponential

150 Joules at 50 Ohms

FIGURE 36-2 Biphasic waveforms.

COMPLICATIONS OF DEFIBRILLATION

1. Postdefibrillation dysrhythmias can occur, although the incidence is decreasing with the use of low-energy biphasic waveforms. For example, asynchronous shocks can convert pulseless VT into VF. Bradycardia, atrioventricular blocks, and asystole may occur due to vagal discharge or underlying sick sinus syndrome. For these, atropine or emergency transcutaneous pacing may be necessary.

2. Soft tissue injury, such as burns to the chest, can occur if inadequate electrode paste is used between the skin and paddles.

3. Myocardial injury and necrosis may result from total cumulative energy delivered in a short period of time. Transient elevations of the ST segment of the ECG may be seen after restoration of a perfusing rhythm.

4. Pulmonary edema rarely results from transient left ventricular dysfunction.

5. Injuries to the operator can occur if there is contact with the patient. Since most of the defibrillation energy is actually shunted into the thorax rather than the heart, the operator who is touching the patient can receive a shock injury, ranging from pain and paresthesias to burns at the contact site.

SUGGESTED READINGS

American Society of Anesthesiology. Practice advisory for the perioperative management of patients with a pacemaker or defibrillator. *Anesthesiology* 2011;114:247-261.

Link MS, Atkins D, Passman R, et al. 2010 American Heart Association Guidelines for cardiopulmonary resuscitation and emergency cardiovascular care science; Part 6: electrical therapies. *Circulation* 2010;122:S706-S719.

Takata TS, Page RL, Joglar JA. Automated external defibrillators: technical considerations and clinical promise. *Ann Intern Med.* 2001;135(11):990-998.

Electrical Safety

Kumudhini Hendrix, MD

Since anesthesia machines and monitors are electrically powered, it is important to have a good understanding of electricity and electrical safety. Burns, electrocution, and fires are hazards of electricity in the operating room (OR). Morbidity and mortality from electrocution depends on type (direct vs. alternating), amount, pathway, density, and duration of the electrical current.

BASIC CONCEPTS

In electronics, solids are classified as conductors, insulators, and semiconductors. Conductors have loosely bound electrons in their outer shell which can move freely under application of electrical potential. Conductors such as metals, saline, and carbon-containing matter are able to conduct electricity well. Conversely, insulators have tightly bound electrons in their outer shell which do not move freely. Insulators such as rubber, mica, and glass do not conduct electricity well. Semiconductors such as silicon, germanium, and lead behave like nonconductors unless subjected to high temperature.

The three basic quantities in electricity are:

1. **Voltage** (*V*)—Voltage is the electrical force that drives the current. One volt is the potential difference applied to a conducting wire in which 1 A of current flows.
2. **Current** (*I*)—Current is measured in amperes. One ampere, or amp (A), represents the flow of 1 coulomb or 6.24×10^{18} electrons past a given point in the conductor.
3. **Resistance** (*R*)—Resistance, measured in ohms, is the opposition to the flow of current when a voltage is applied. A good conductor will have low resistance, whereas a good insulator will have high resistance.

Ohm's law relates these three quantities in the equation $V = I^*R$. Electrical current must flow in circuits. Electrical safety in the OR focuses on current as the most important variable, and so it is necessary to rearrange Ohm's law into the relationship $I = V/R$. Because of the use of electronic devices in the OR, there is particular concern about current density flowing through an area such as skin.

In the United States, electricity is provided as alternating 60 Hz current based on 120 V with peak amplitude of 150 V. Alternating current is more dangerous than direct current. Lower frequencies cause more morbidity than higher frequency currents. This alternating current can flow across resistors and capacitors. The power company provides two lines—a "hot" lead and a neutral or "ground" lead. The neutral lead is connected to ground at the power company as well as at the point at which the electrical wiring enters the building. There is a third lead known as the "ground wire" that connects the device to return any current leaking from device (known as the "chassis current") back to the ground.

ELECTROCUTION

Current flowing across the thorax can precipitate dysrhythmias such as ventricular fibrillation or asphyxia due to tetany of respiratory musculature. Current that passes in a caudal to rostral axis can render a patient unconscious or cause damage to the spinal cord. The amount of current is also important. One milliampere of current causes tingling sensations or paresthesias, whereas 15 mA of current leads to tetanic contractions of skeletal muscle.

The density of the current is also important. When current enters catheters and intracardiac electrodes (microshock), the current density is high. Therefore, a lower amount of current is needed to cause symptoms. To elicit ventricular fibrillation, 75 mA of current is required via a macroshock, whereas only 10 µA of current is necessary via a microshock.

a. Macroshock—Skin resistance varies from 50 000 ohms (dry) to 500 ohms (wet). As a result, the magnitude of the conducted current will vary from 3 mA for dry skin to 300 mA for wet skin. Three milliampere of current may cause a local burn but is insufficient to elicit ventricular fibrillation. At least 80 mA is needed to cause dysrhythmias. In the OR, a wet patient lying on an electric bed and connected to electric monitors poses a very high risk for electrical hazard. In addition, when under anesthesia, they are unable to respond or withdraw to the current. A line isolation transformer serves as the most effective method to prevent macroshock.

b. Microshock—Microshock occurs when the current is delivered directly to the myocardium through intracardiac electrodes or catheters, such as pacemaker leads or central venous catheters. The current only needs to traverse a small area to cause harm. Therefore, the dysrhythmia threshold current for microshocks is very small—typically around 10 μA. Because intracardiac electrodes have a lower resistance than saline-filled catheters, these electrodes conduct microshocks much more effectively.

LINE ISOLATION TRANSFORMER

The line isolation transformer prevents electrocution by preventing the neutral lead from being grounded. Ungrounding of the neutral lead prevents macroshock since the electrical circuit cannot be completed. Line isolation monitors (LIMs) constantly check whether or not the neutral lead is indeed isolated. The LIM emits an alarm when it detects at least 2 mA current (<75 000 ohms) flowing between the neutral and ground leads.

ELECTROCAUTERY UNITS

Electrocautery units (ECUs) operate at frequencies of 500 000 to 2 000 000 Hz. Although these frequencies are too high to cause cardiac dysrhythmias, ECUs can cause burns. The "grounding pad" is not a pad that grounds the patient; instead, it simply returns the current to the ECU. When ECG leads are placed near the surgical site and distant from the grounding pads, the return current may exit through an ECG lead, resulting in a burn. Grounding pads should not be placed above metallic prostheses to prevent internal burns. Bipolar electrocautery reduces the current dispersion by keeping the current return through one of the electrodes. The ECU units may provide sparks for ignition of fire in the OR. Alcohol-based skin preparations, bowel gas, and drapes provide the fuel. When this mixture occurs in the presence of oxygen, fire ensues.

SUGGESTED READING

Boumphrey S, Angton JA. Electrical safety in the operating theater. *BJA CEPD Rev* 2003;3:10-14.

38

Review of Simple Mathematics

Jason Hoefling, MD

The ability to perform precise mathematical calculations quickly is of paramount importance throughout the course of a clinical career. On a day-to-day basis, the anesthesiologist will compute drug doses, drug concentrations, and various physiologic formulae. Even though most of the calculations should be rote, the following are more complex and close attention should be paid at each step to avoid a miscalculation that could result in patient harm.

BASIC MATHEMATICS

Basic Exponential Function

Exponential function can be used to describe bacterial growth and radioactive decay. The "basic" exponential function is the function $y = a^x$ where a is some positive constant called the base and x is the exponent. For instance, to solve the equation $y = 4^3$ it can be expanded to $y = 4 \times 4 \times 4$ resulting in a y of 64.

Simple Logarithms

In addition to their utility in describing drug half-lives, logarithms are used in the Nernst equation describing the potential across a cell membrane and the Henderson–Hasselbalch equation governing the relationship between pH and pKa.

A logarithm (log for short) is actually just the reverse of the exponential scale. Therefore:

$$\log_a x = y \text{ is the same as } a^y = x$$

In the example $\log_2 8 = 3$, the base is the subscript number found after the letters "log (ie, 2), the argument is the number following the subscript number (ie, 8), and the answer is the number that the logarithmic expression is set equal to (ie, 3).

Common logarithms ($\log_{10} x$) have a base of 10. If a log is written without a base (as $\log x$), then it is assumed to have a base of 10. *Natural* logarithms ($\ln x$) have a base of e which is approximately 2.71828.

Graphing Simple Equations

Linear relationships can be represented in the form $y = mx + b$, where m is the slope of the line and b equals the point where the line crosses the y-axis (y-intercept).

Points are named by an ordered pair such as (4,2) where the first number in an ordered pair is the x-coordinate and the second is the y-coordinate.

To solve the equation and convert it into a graphical format, first select an x-coordinate, then solve the equation yielding a y-value. Repeat this process about 4 or 5 times and then connect the points you have graphed. The line you see will be the graph of a linear equation.

For the equation $y = 2x + 1$:

x	y
0	1
1	3
2	5
−1	−1

Dimensional Analysis

To convert units, multiply by an identity or conversion factor.

$$760 \text{ mm Hg} \times \left(\frac{14.7 \text{ psi}}{760 \text{ mm Hg}} \right) = 14.7 \text{ psi}$$

$$\frac{50 \text{ μg}}{\text{mL}} \times \left(\frac{1 \text{ μg}}{1000 \text{ μg}} \right) = \frac{0.05 \text{ mg}}{\text{mL}}$$

In each example, the fraction is an identity (14.7 psi and 760 mm Hg are equivalent in the formula). Multiplying any quantity by an identity does not change the underlying quantity, but only the label.

Proportions

Proportions are used to determine the answers to questions like "how many mL of 0.75% bupivacaine contains 12 mg?" or "how long will the tank of oxygen last at pressure reading of 200 psi and a flow rate of 6 L/min?"

$$\frac{1\ mL}{7.5\ mg} = \frac{x\ mL}{12\ mg}$$

$$(12\ mg) \times \frac{1\ mL}{7.5\ mg} = \frac{x\ mL}{12\ mg} \times (12\ mg)$$

$$\frac{12}{7.5} mL = x$$

$$x = 1.6\ mL$$

Remember that a full tank of oxygen contains approximately 660 L at a pressure of 2000 psi.

$$\frac{x\ L}{200\ psi} = \frac{660\ L}{2000\ psi}$$

$$x = 66\ L$$

Thus, the tank will last 11 minutes at a flow rate of 6 L/min.

Desired versus Available Concentrations

If you desire 50 mg/mL of remifentanil and have 1 g available, how much diluents are needed?

$$\frac{x\ mL}{1\ g} = \frac{1\ mL}{50\ mg}$$

$$\frac{x\ mL}{1\ g} = \frac{1\ mL}{50\ mg} \times \left(\frac{1000\ mg}{1\ g}\right)$$

$$\frac{x\ mL}{1\ g} = \frac{1000\ mL}{50\ g}$$

$$(1\ g) \times \frac{x\ mL}{1\ g} = \frac{1000\ mL}{50\ g} \times (1\ g)$$

$$x = 20\ mL$$

Epinephrine Concentration

Epinephrine vials are labeled by concentration of a ratio of medication per milliliter. For example, a solution may be labeled as 1:100 000. This concentration represents 1000 mg/100 000 mL or 0.01 mg/mL. It is important to remember that 1 mL of water weighs 1 g.

$$\frac{1\ g}{100\ 000\ mL} \times \left(\frac{1000\ mg}{1\ g}\right) = \frac{1000\ mg}{100\ 000\ mL}$$

$$\frac{1000\ mg}{100\ 000\ mL} \times \left(\frac{0.001}{0.001}\right) = \frac{1\ mg}{100\ mL}$$

$$\frac{1\ mg}{100\ mL} \times \left(\frac{1000\ \mu g}{1\ mg}\right) = \frac{1000\ \mu g}{100\ mL}$$

$$\frac{1000\ \mu g}{100\ mL} \times \left(\frac{0.01}{0.01}\right) = \frac{10\ \mu g}{1\ mL}$$

Percentage Solutions

The percentage of a solution is expressed as the number of grams per 100 mL and represents the parts of drug per hundred. To determine the mg/mL in a solution expressed as a percent, simply move the decimal point one place to the *RIGHT*. For example, a 1% solution has 1 g/100 mL or 10 mg/mL.

CLINICAL FORMULAS

Acceptable Blood Loss

Acceptable blood loss (ABL) is calculated using the estimated blood volume (EBV) as well as the starting hematocrit and the target hematocrit. Estimated blood volume (mL/kg) differs with age and gender: men and children aged 1-2 years (75 mL/kg), women (65 mL/kg), term neonates (85 mL/kg), and premature infants (90 mL/kg).

$$ABL = ((Hct_{original} - Hct_{final})/Hct_{average}) \times EBV$$

Oxygen Concentration

To confirm that your oxygen analyzer is functioning properly, you can calculate the percent composition based on gas flow. For example, to determine the concentration of oxygen when 4 L/min oxygen is combined with 4 L/min air:

$$4000\ mL\ O_2 + (0.21 \times 4000\ mL\ air) = 4840\ mL\ O_2$$

$$\frac{4840\ mL\ O_2}{8000\ mL\ FGF} = 60.5\%\ O_2$$

Alveolar Gas Equation

$$PAO_2 = FIO_2(P_{Bar} - P_{H_2O}) - 1.2(PaCO_2)$$

It is important for physicians to avoid making clinical decisions based on PaO$_2$ alone, without reference to the calculated PAO$_2$. This abbreviated version assumes a respiratory quotient of 0.8 and water vapor pressure in the airways (dependent on body temperature) is 47 mm Hg at 37°C.

Oxygen Delivery and Consumption

The arterial oxygen content (CaO$_2$) is the amount of oxygen bound to hemoglobin plus the amount of oxygen dissolved in arterial blood:

$$CaO_2\left(\frac{mL}{100\ mL\ blood}\right) = (1.39 \times Hb \times SaO_2) + (PaO_2 \times 0.003),$$

where SaO$_2$ is the arterial oxyhemoglobin saturation and PaO$_2$ is the arterial oxygen tension. Normal CaO$_2$ is approximately 20 mL O$_2$/dL.

$$CvO_2\left(\frac{mL}{100\ mL\ blood}\right) = (1.39 \times Hb \times SvO_2) + (PvO_2 \times 0.003),$$

where SvO_2 is the mixed venous oxyhemoglobin saturation and PvO_2 is the mixed venous oxygen tension. Normal venous oxygen content (CvO_2) is approximately 15 mL O_2/dL.

Oxygen delivery (DO_2) is the rate at which oxygen is transported from the lungs into the microcirculation:

$$DO_2\,(mL/min) = Q \times CaO_2,$$

where Q is the cardiac output.

Normal DO_2 is approximately 1000 mL/min.

Oxygen consumption—Oxygen consumption (VO_2) is the rate at which oxygen is removed from the blood for use by the tissues.

Calculation of VO_2 can be performed by rearranging the Fick equation:

$$VO_2\left(\frac{mL\ O_2}{min}\right) = Q \times (CaO_2 - CvO_2)$$

Normal VO_2 is approximately 250 mL O_2/min.

Statistics

Jason Hoefling, MD

Epidemiology is the study of the distribution and determinants of disease. It is based on the assumptions that disease does not occur randomly and that both causal and preventative factors can be identified. The evaluation of both human disease and pharmacological therapy goes through a specific sequence of events. Initially, there is suspicion of influence (eg, environmental, genetic, behavioral, or therapeutic) on an individual or disease. Next, a hypothesis is formed, followed by the systemic collection of data that includes an appropriate comparison group. Statistical analysis of the data will determine whether outcomes associated with the risk factor or intervention are different than outcomes in their absence. Finally, the validity of the statistical analysis is assessed by accounting for chance, biased data interpretation, and the presence of any confounding variables. Only then can judgment be made as to the importance of the risk factor or intervention under review.

DEFINITIONS

- Variables
  - Categorical: values that function as labels rather than as numbers.
  - Continuous: numeric values where the relative magnitude is significant.
- Measures of central tendency
  - Mean—(average) sum of values divided by number of values.
  - Mode—most commonly occurring value.
  - Median—middle value.
  - Standard deviation—"statistical dispersion."
- Probability qualitative expression of the likelihood of its occurrence $\Pr(A) = \frac{\text{times } A \text{ occurs}}{\text{times } A \text{ can occur}}$

MEASURES OF DISEASE FREQUENCY AND ASSOCIATION

Incidence and prevalence are the two basic measures of disease frequency used to qualify disease in a population. Incidence rates are designed to measure the rate at which previously healthy individuals develop the disease within a specific period of time, that is, the number of *new* cases in a population over a period of time. Prevalence rates measure the number of people in a population who have the disease at a given point in time.

$$\text{Incidence} = \frac{\text{Number of new cases}}{\text{Population at risk}}$$

$$\text{Prevalence} = \frac{\text{Number of cases at a given time}}{\text{Population at risk during a given time}}$$

CLASSIFICATION OF STUDY DESIGN

There are many different types of epidemiological study design ranging from observational to interventional. The two basic types of observational studies are the cohort study and the case–control study. The cohort, or prospective, study classifies patients based on the presence or absence of a risk factor and follows them through time to determine when and if they develop disease. Prospective studies have limitations; they take many years to complete and require many subjects leading to high cost and attrition. Since these studies are less susceptible to bias, they can obtain a true measure of incidence, leading to an accurate relative risk.

On the other hand, a case–control, or retrospective, study compares the proportions of patients with various exposures in a group of patients with a disease to a group without the disease. Such a study is most useful for diseases with a low incidence and for a group representative of the general population. These studies are usually performed quickly, easily, and inexpensively. The major limitation of a retrospective study is that the descriptive statistic, odds ratio, is only an estimate of risk. There is potential for significant bias.

Intervention studies, or clinical trials, are similar to cohort studies but distinguished by the fact that exposure status is assigned by the investigator in a randomized, blinded, and controlled manner. Clinical trials are considered the most robust form of investigation because the randomization process controls for factors that may influence the outcome.

ANALYSIS OF INVESTIGATIONAL STUDIES

The findings of most studies are usually presented in a 2×2 table, a tool that serves as a basis for many calculations. The table is populated by classifying each patient using two study-related criteria.

	First Criterion of Classification		Second Criterion of Classification
	Disease	No Disease	Total
Positive	a	b	$a + b$
Negative	c	d	$c + d$
Total	$a + c$	$b + d$	$a + b + c + d$

MEASURES OF ASSOCIATION

Relative risk is a measure of the association between exposure and outcome in a *cohort study*. Using data derived from the 2×2 table, it is expressed as a ratio $\frac{a/(a+b)}{c/(c+d)}$. It quantifies the risk of disease in one group with a factor (eg, gender, age, alcohol usage) compared with a group without such factors. Relative risk does not measure the likelihood of developing disease given a certain exposure. Rather, it measures the benefit conferred by removing an exposure. Although a given factor such as cigarette smoking may have a high relative risk, its prevalence may be high or low. Both relative risk and the prevalence of said attribute determine the effect on the incidence in the population. In a *case–control study,* it is usually not possible to calculate the rate of disease development because patients are selected based on disease status. Therefore, this risk is estimated by comparing the odds of exposures among cases to those among controls. This statistic, the *odds ratio*, is derived from the 2×2 table and expressed as $\frac{ad}{bc}$.

SENSITIVITY AND SPECIFICITY

Sensitivity and specificity are two probabilities used to measure the ability of a screening tool to discriminate between individuals with or without a disease. These measures (sensitivity $= \frac{a}{a+c}$ and specificity $= \frac{d}{b+d}$) are determined by comparing the results of a screening test with those derived from some definitive diagnostic modality. Sensitivity is the ability of a test to give a positive result when the patient actually has the condition (positive in disease). Specificity is the ability of a test to give a negative finding when the patient does not have the disease (negative in health). A reciprocal relationship exists between sensitivity and specificity. An increase in sensitivity occurs at the expense of specificity. In practice, when choosing a diagnostic value for a screening test, sensitivity and specificity are each set to be less than 100%, resulting in very small numbers of false positives and false negatives. Considerations such as disease prevalence, disease latency, and effectiveness of treatment with early diagnosis are important when determining where to set the cut-off point.

STATISTICAL SIGNIFICANCE

The term "statistically significant" is often encountered in scientific literature, yet few clinicians actually understand its meaning. Determination of statistical significance is made by performing a statistical test on the obtained data and then comparing the result to a table of standard values. The concept of statistical significance is important in understanding the results of a study. For instance, there are three possible explanations for a study demonstrating that a new drug is superior to an older one. First, the drug is actually superior. Second, there is another factor accounting for the difference (age, sex, smoking, etc). Third, the result is simply random variation. To prove that the new drug is actually superior we need to eliminate the second and third explanations.

SIGNIFICANCE TESTS

Underlying all statistical tests is a null hypothesis which states that there is NO difference between the two groups being compared. Any difference seen is a result of chance. To reject the null hypothesis (and show a real difference between the two groups), a computed test statistic is compared to a value in a statistical table. The data in the statistical table is based on standard populations and sample sizes. When the test statistic exceeds the critical value, the null hypothesis is rejected and the difference is statistically significant. Any decision to reject the null hypothesis carries some chance of being wrong—the significance level. The ideal significance level has a value of 5%—meaning, there is a 1 in 20 chance that the null hypothesis is true. In addition, many investigators will report the lowest significance at which the null hypothesis could be rejected using the P-value, which expresses the probability that the difference is not due to chance alone. The statement "$P < 0.01$" means that the probability is 1 in 100 that the observed difference is due to chance alone. "$P < 0.001$" implies that there is a 1 in 1000 chance of the observed difference being due to chance. It is important to recognize that the P-value only represents the chances of the null hypothesis being wrong. It does not represent the strength of any differences in study populations. Only the investigators can judge whether these differences warrant any degree of clinical significance. A clinician may interpret a small, statistically significant difference to have no relevance in practice. This is especially true in large studies with small differences between the two patient populations.

ERROR

Type I error, also known as "false positive," involves rejecting the null hypothesis when it is true. In other words, observing a difference when there is none. Type II error, also known as "false negative," involves accepting the null hypothesis when the alternative hypothesis is actually true. This error represents the failure to observe a difference when there is indeed one.

SAMPLING ERROR

The target population is the collection of individuals under study. Since the entire population is seldom available, investigators rely on the information provided by a sample to make generalizations. Sampling error is the difference between the sample results and the characteristics of the general population. There are two factors that must be controlled to reduce sampling error: bias and random variation. There are many types of bias, including investigator and reporting bias.

CORRELATION

Often a scientific study will require a description of the relationship between two variables where one variable influences the other. To describe this relationship, the two variables are plotted on a scattergram that provides a visual representation of the relationship between the two variables. In addition, two statistical techniques called *regression* and *correlation* are used to provide a more quantitative description.

The regression equation is most useful when the study goal is to provide a predictive model. After plotting the data on the scattergram, the *least squares* technique provides the equation for the line of best fit. This equation can then be used to predict y given a certain x.

The correlation coefficient, denoted r, is an index of the extent to which two variables are associated. It can take on values between -1.0 and $+1.0$ depending on the strength of association and the direction of the change in y for a positive change in x.

COMPARISON OF BASIC STATISTICAL TESTS

The following three tests are the most commonly used to determine how likely it is that an observed distribution is due to chance. The differences lie in the type of variable included in the sample and the number of groups being compared.

- Chi-square test
  - Categorical variables.
  - Compares distribution of test results with normal distribution to evaluate independence.
- *t*-test (Student's *t*-test)
  - Continuous variables.
  - Comparing the means of *two* populations.
  - Useful with small samples.
- Analysis of variance (ANOVA)
  - Continuous variables.
  - ANOVA compares the means of *multiple* groups.

SUGGESTED READINGS

Daniel WW, Chad CL. *Biostatistics: A Foundation for Analysis in the Health Sciences.* 10th ed. New Jersey: John Wiley & Sons; 2013.

Hennekens CH. *Epidemiology in Medicine.* Lippincott Williams and Wilkins; 1987.

Hulley S, Cummings S. *Designing Clinical Research.* Lippincott Williams and Wilkins; 1988.

Computerized Patient Records

Jason Hoefling, MD

Electronic health records (EHRs) are essentially digital versions of a patient's paper medical chart. By means of their organization and functionality, EHRs can be powerful clinical and administrative tools. Ideally, an EHR is a dynamic, comprehensive representation of a patient's health. The EHR consolidates medical history, diagnoses, medications, immunization dates, allergies, images, as well as laboratory results. The information captured by an EHR is stored in a relational database with archival and backup capabilities, which supports simultaneous multiuser access. The electronic format is more organized and accurate compared to its paper counterpart resulting in a more efficient delivery of health services. In addition, EHRs offer evidence-based decision support tools for providers that can improve clinical outcomes and patient safety.

The implementation of EHRs in the United States has long been impeded by cost, lack of standardization among vendors, and issues of security and privacy. However, in 2009, the Federal Government began offering incentives to providers to encourage implementation of EHRs. The incentives are in the form of rebates or reimbursements based on a set of criteria called "Meaningful Use." Under Meaningful Use, the Federal Government has defined a complete EHR system as containing four basic functionalities: computerized orders for prescriptions, computerized orders for tests, reporting of test results, and physician notes.

ANESTHESIA INFORMATION MANAGEMENT SYSTEMS

Anesthesia Information Management Systems (AIMS) is a component of the EHR designed to record the entire clinical encounter in both an efficient and comprehensive manner. As technology evolves outside of health care, the AIMS is better able to capture the tremendous amount of physiologic and pharmacological data generated during anesthesia. Multitouch interfaces, faster data retrieval, and intuitive design allow the AIMS to represent the data in a way that facilitate diagnostic and treatment decisions without compromising the anesthesiologists workflow. An AIMS is built within the EHR and synthesizes anesthesia-relevant data pulled from disparate systems, such as laboratory, billing, imaging, communication,

pharmacy, and scheduling. The more complete and less biased documentation facilitates both clinical and management research. Realization of value from the AIMS requires additional expenditures of resources to adapt the system to meet specific institutional requirements.

Although financial benefits are the most attractive to the anesthesia department, there are many other facets of AIMS that can influence the bottom line of a medical system. In terms of actual monetary savings, three important areas of focus are reimbursement, operations management, and cost containment. By utilizing an AIMS the anesthesia department can capture more billable actions, including time units, line placement, and blocks. A more comprehensive billing system can lead to increased charges as well as decreasing the workload on the billing department, resulting in additional savings. By merging operational and clinical systems within a hospital, both staffing and resource management can be optimized. Features such as a real-time whiteboard can help reduce turnover time and predictive algorithms can maximize operating room utilization. Finally, although drug and supply costs are small compared to professional fees, real-time accounting can reduce waste and prevent shortfalls.

BENEFITS AND CHALLENGES

There are a number of intangibles that cannot be quantified monetarily but taken together lead to better outcomes for patients through improved delivery of care. The most obvious benefit to clinicians is the automatic collection of vital signs, so that the anesthesiologist can focus on patient care. Patient safety can be further improved as the AIMS has the ability to provide warnings about drug interactions and appropriate dosing as well as potential issues with transfusion of blood products. One of the greatest advantages of an AIMS is the decision support algorithms that serve to guide providers toward evidence-based best practices. For instance, evaluation with a preoperative algorithm can be used to take histories and suggest laboratory tests that optimize resource utilization and reduce surgical cancellations. In addition, an AIMS can help to ensure that providers comply with quality of care (pay-for-performance) initiatives, such as beta-blocker and antibiotic administration. With the tremendous amount of data available for mining, providers can receive valuable feedback about the quality and safety of the care they deliver. Lastly, the AIMS provides much improved documentation over the paper record, resulting in an accurate, legible representation of the anesthetic given. This has significant value in the area of risk management and can be critical in litigation support.

Implementing an AIMS involves significant investment, both financially and in terms of human resources. A typical AIMS installation will involve both hardware and software that interfaces with the intraoperative patient monitors. The upfront costs include software licenses and extensive hardware needs, such as workstations, input devices and monitors, and network costs. Human costs involve professional systems analysts, implementation experts, and educators as well as user training and loss of productivity during implementation. Ongoing costs include staffing costs for IT professionals, system maintenance agreements and upgrades (hardware and software), as well as the anesthesia information

director's nonclinical time to administer and enhance the system. Electronic health records, and specifically AIMS, add value, promote safety and result in improved outcomes for the patient, clinician, and the hospital.

SUGGESTED READINGS

Dutton RP, DuKatz A. Improvement using automated data sources: the Anesthesia Quality Institute. *Anesthesiol Clin* 2011;29:439-454.

Egger Halbeis CB, Epstein RH. The value proposition of anesthesia information management systems. *Anesthesiol Clin* 2008;26:665-679.

Ehrenfeld JM, Rehman MA. Anesthesia information management systems: a review of functionality and installation considerations. *J Clin Monitor Comput* 2011;25:71-79.

Kadry B, Feaster WW, Macario A, Ehrenfeld JM. Anesthesia information management systems: past, present, and future of anesthesia records. *Mt Sinai J Med* 2012;79:154-165.

Pharmacokinetics

Chris Potestio, MD, and Brian S. Freeman, MD

Pharmacokinetics describes the body's response to administration of a drug, which determines drug absorption, distribution, and elimination. An easy way to make sense of this elusive topic is to think of pharmacokinetics in the simplest terms: drug goes in (front-end kinetics) and drug goes out (back-end kinetics).

"FRONT-END KINETICS"

Absorption

Most drugs in the perioperative period are given intravenously, thus bypassing the pharmacokinetics of absorption. Drugs injected directly into vasculature are not impacted by absorption pharmacokinetics; however, drugs administered by oral administration, transmucosal delivery, transdermal delivery, or tissue injection have variable absorption rates. Even inhaled anesthetics are absorbed through the lungs, typically by very rapid transport. Bioavailability is the relative amount of a drug dose that reaches the systemic circulation unchanged and the rate at which this occurs.

The key concept of absorption is transfer from the depot to the systemic circulation. The depot refers to the organ system where the drug gets deposited: stomach, lung, nerve bundle, transdermal patch, and muscle tissue. This transfer is principally driven by the concentration gradient but can be affected by intrinsic properties of the drug that are specific to the route of administration.

Diffusion for the depot to systemic circulation occurs through a bilipid membrane; therefore, the physical properties of the drug play an important role in the rate of absorption. Small, nonpolar molecules pass easily through a bilipid membrane that contains a large hydrophobic central region and a small hydrophilic surface. Therefore, the pKa of a drug relative to physiologic pH will determine polarity of the molecule. In addition, diffusion of drug across a membrane is directly proportional to the concentration gradient between the depot and the system circulation (first-order kinetics).

The absorption of inhaled anesthetics depends on the blood–gas partition coefficient. This physical property of inhaled anesthetics describes its concentration in the blood compared to that in the alveolar gas at equilibrium. For example, if the concentration of a drug in blood is 10 and its concentration in alveolar gas is 5, its partition coefficient is 2. A high blood–gas partition coefficient means that a large amount of drug must be absorbed before equilibrium occurs. Clinically, this means that it will take longer for the desired effect to be achieved. Partition coefficients are temperature dependent.

Distribution (Protein Binding, Compartmentalization)

Distribution describes the process of dilution from very high concentration at the entry point of the drug (IV site, mucosal lining of the stomach, site of subcutaneous injection, etc) to the relatively low concentration in plasma and other tissues. Distribution of a drug is discussed in terms of *volume of distribution* (V_d), the volume of tissue that the drug "reaches," which can be calculated by the following equation:

$$V_d = dose/concentration$$

Volume of distribution is an intrinsic property of a drug that describes its ability to distribute in the human body. Many drugs that distribute widely throughout the body have volume of distribution that greatly surpasses total body volume. For example, the V_d of propofol is around 5000 L due to its high lipophilicity.

The *central volume of distribution* is calculated by injecting a drug intravenously and then measuring its arterial concentration. It is an elusive concept. In the simplest terms, central V_d accounts for the volume of the lungs, heart, great vessels, and venous volume proximal to the site of injection. Using the V_d equation, we can use central volume of distribution to calculate the initial concentration after bolus injection.

The *peripheral volumes of distribution* describe the drug's solubility in tissue compared to that of plasma. Each tissue group has its own peripheral volume of distribution that is linked to the central compartment via blood flow. This relationship is often described as the "mammillary model," which is descriptive of the smaller chambers feeding off of the large central chamber.

The *volume of distribution at steady state* describes the tissue solubility at steady state and accounts for both central and peripheral volume of distribution.

"BACK-END KINETICS"

Clearance

Clearance, described in units of flow (L/min), is the process of removing drug from a tissue. Clearance can occur either by permanent removal of a drug or by intercompartmental clearance, where the drug moves from plasma to peripheral tissue. Permanent removal typically occurs by hepatic metabolism, tissue metabolism, or renal clearance, although other organs have been implicated in metabolism (ie, propofol is metabolized by pulmonary endothelium on passing first through circulation). Intercompartmental clearance, also known as distribution clearance, describes the transient clearance of a drug from the plasma to peripheral tissue. It is a function of cardiac output, tissue blood flow to the tissue, and capillary permeability to the drug.

Hepatic Metabolism

Most anesthetic drugs are metabolized by hepatic biotransformation. Liver metabolism is discussed in terms of phase 1 reactions (oxidation, reduction, hydrolysis) and phase 2 reactions (conjugation). Oxidation and reduction occurs via cytochrome p450 system, which is a set of enzymes that catalyze metabolism of drugs by many biochemical mechanisms, namely hydroxylation, dealkylation, deamination, desulfuration, epoxidation, and dehalogenation. The P450 enzymes can be induced or inhibited by a long list of drugs. Important inducers include phenobarbital and phenytoin, and important inhibitors include amiodarone and calcium channel blockers.

Conjugation occurs with the help of the P450 system as well. This set of reactions conjoins hydrophobic drug molecules with polar moities (ie, glucuronide) to increase solubility and, therefore, renal clearance. These molecules generated by the liver are typically inactive; however, there are a few important exceptions to this rule. Morphine is metabolized in the liver to form morphine 3-glucuronide (M3G) and morphine 6-glucuronide (M6G). M3G is inactive, but M6G has a mechanism and potency similar to its parent molecule. This concept is particularly important in the setting of renal disease, as the body will be unable to clear this active metabolite. Midazolam also has an active metabolite of equal potency to its parent drug.

In all instances relevant to anesthesia, we assume that the rate of metabolism is proportional to the concentration of the drug. The liver does eventually become saturated and at that point the relationship between rate of metabolism and concentration is no longer linear; however, for practical reasons, the linear relationship is assumed. Because of this linear relationship, we can calculate the rate of metabolism:

$$\text{Rate} = Q\,(C_{in} - C_{out})$$

Rate, in this equation, refers to the rate of metabolism; Q is the blood flow to the liver; and C_{in} and C_{out} refer to the concentration of drug flowing into and out of the liver, respectively.

Another important concept in liver metabolism is the hepatic *extraction ratio*. The liver is not capable of removing the molecule of a drug from the plasma; therefore, we must consider the hepatic *extraction ratio* when discussing clearance. Extraction ratio can be calculated in the following equation:

$$\text{ER} = (C_{in} - C_{out})/C_{in}$$

Clearance, therefore, can be calculated in terms of the extraction ratio:

$$\text{Clearance} = Q \times \text{ER}$$

If a drug has a high extraction ratio (eg, propofol), then clearance depends on Q, the blood flow to the liver. The metabolism of such a drug is said to be "flow limited"; that is, the amount of drug that is metabolized is dependent on the amount of blood flow to the liver. This is an important concept considering that general anesthetics decrease hepatic blood flow. If a drug has a low extraction ratio (eg, alfentanil), blood flow to the liver is a less important determinant of metabolism and the liver's ability to extract drug from the plasma becomes more important. Therefore, if a drug has a low extraction ratio, it is said to be "capacity limited."

Renal Clearance

Renal clearance, although less intricate than hepatic clearance, must also be considered when administering an anesthetic drug. Pancuronium is the only major anesthetic drug that undergoes more than 80% renal excretion; however, most anesthetic drugs undergo partial renal clearance. Therefore, renal disease and factors impacting renal clearance should be considered.

The Cockcroft–Gault equation, variants of which are used to calculate glomerular filtration rate (GFR), provides a good summary of the determining factors of renal function:

$$\text{Creatinine clearance (mL/min)} = (140 - \text{age [yr]} \times \text{weight [kg]})/(72 \times \text{serum creatinine [mg/dL]})$$

Renal function, as per the Cockcroft–Gault equation, is inversely proportional to age. General anesthetics also decrease creatinine clearance.

Tissue Clearance

Whereas the vast majority of anesthetic drugs are metabolized by the liver and/or the kidney, there are a few notable exceptions that are metabolized in other tissues. This type of

TABLE 41-1   Unique Metabolism of Anesthetic Drugs

Type of Metabolism	Location	Anesthetic Drugs
Butylcholinesterase metabolism (formerly pseudocholinesterase)	Plasma	Succinylcholine, mivacurium, 2-chloroprocaine
Nonspecific ester hydrolysis	Muscle and intestine (major contributors)	Remifentanil, atracurium (<50% of total metabolism)
	Lung, liver, kidney, plasma (minor contributors)	
Hofmann degradation	Plasma	Cisatracurium, atracurium (<10%)

metabolism is simply called *tissue clearance* and the major examples are listed in Table 41-1. Exceptions include esmolol, succinylcholine, and remifentanil, which are cleared by ester hydrolysis in tissue and plasma. Pancuronium is excreted unchanged in the urine.

It is important to note that atracurium is metabolized by several different pathways. Although the majority of its metabolism is hepatic, it also undergoes degradation by nonspecific ester hydrolysis and, to a lesser extent, it undergoes Hofmann degradation. This process is a spontaneous elimination reaction that occurs in plasma at physiologic pH and temperature. It is the major metabolic pathway for cisatracurium, which is an isomer of atracurium.

Protein Binding

Many of the anesthetic drugs bind readily to plasma proteins. The major plasma proteins for binding anesthetic drugs are albumin and alpha-1-acid glycoprotein. Protein binding is important to consider, as it has a large impact on the amount of drug that is available to obtain desired pharmacological effect and also the amount of free drug available for clearance. Even for the least potent drugs (ie, those with the highest serum concentrations), the concentration of drug is far less than that of plasma protein. Therefore, protein binding depends only on the concentration of plasma protein and NOT on the concentration of drug. The term *free fraction* describes the ratio of unbound drug to total amount of drug. A free fraction of 1.0 means that 100% of the drug is free in plasma and 0% is bound to protein. It would follow that a drug with a free fraction of 1.0 would not be impacted by changes in plasma protein concentration. Drugs with free fraction less than 1.0 will, of course, be impacted.

It is important to remember that it is the free drug, not the bound drug, which interacts with different systems of the body, including the liver, kidney, and effect site. A decrease in protein binding results in an increase in the concentration of the free form of the drug. Increase in the concentration of free drug will result in increased activity at the effect site (assuming the receptors are not saturated). In addition, a decrease in protein binding results increased uptake by the liver for drugs that are capacity dependent (low hepatic extraction). Lastly, it will lead to increased renal clearance.

Another important consideration is the effect of protein binding on concentration and also volume of distribution. Concentration is a measurement of total drug whether it is bound to protein or not. A decrease in protein binding leads to increased free drug which will equilibrate with peripheral tissue. This will cause a decrease in the total plasma concentration and an artificially decreased volume of distribution.

Pharmacokinetic Models

Pharmacokinetic models help us to understand the pharmacokinetic properties of a drug on a larger scale. It is important to be able to define and understand both exponential models and compartmental models.

To say that a system has zero-order kinetics means that it occurs at a constant rate. The process proceeds at a rate independent of concentration of the drug. The change in the quantity of the drug and the change in time are constant ($dx/dt = $ k). Zero-order kinetics are linear kinetics and the integral of the previous equation can be manipulated to form an algebraic linear expression: $x(t) = x0 + $ k $\times t$. For example, the clearance of ethanol occurs as zero-order kinetics. The human body will clear ethanol at a constant rate no matter the dose. Whether a person has one, four, or eight drinks at a party on a Friday night, they will experience a hangover (ie, the result of acute withdrawal of ethanol from the serum) around the same time on Saturday morning.

First-order kinetics are dose dependent; therefore, the rate of clearance is proportional to the concentration according to $dx/dt = $ k $\times x$. Taking the integral of this equation yields a more complex natural logarithmic equation: $x(t) = x \times e^k t$. This relationship is best appreciated graphically. A drug with low hepatic extraction ratio like alfentanil is metabolized via first-order kinetics. The more the drug is available, the more is extracted and metabolized.

Second- and third-order kinetics are extremely complicated and outside the scope of anesthesia practice.

Each individual drug and each individual organ has its own pharmacokinetic properties, making accurate physiologic pharmacokinetic models incredibly complex and impractical. In their stead, we use compartmental models, which are modeled after physiologic models but with gross simplification. The one-compartment model is the simplest of these and consists of a single volume with a single clearance.

Multicompartment models, specifically three-compartment models, give us a theoretical basis for pharmacokinetics of most drugs. In the three-compartment model, the body is divided into a central compartment (plasma), a rapid equilibrating compartment (vessel-rich tissue like the brain and GI tract), and a slow equilibrating compartment (vessel-poor tissue like fat tissue). For most drugs there are three distinct phases that follow intravenous bolus injection (Figure 41-1). First, there is the "rapid distribution phase" that follows immediately after injection. Prior to the rapid distribution phase, at the moment of injection, 100% of the bolus dose is located in the plasma. The rapid distribution phase refers to the time shortly after injection when this bolus dose quickly proceeds down its concentration gradient to the surrounding tissue. The rapid distribution phase is followed by the "slow distribution phase," where the drug continues to equilibrate with slow uptake tissues, whereas the drug returns to the plasma from rapid uptake tissues due to an "overshoot" into the rapid uptake tissues during the rapid distribution phase. The final phase is the "elimination phase," where the drug concentration decreases in a linear fashion due to the first-order kinetics of elimination.

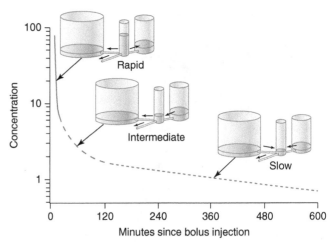

FIGURE 41-1 Graphic representation of three phases of distribution in three-compartment model. (Modified from Youngs EJ, Shafer SL. Basic pharmacokinetic and pharmacodynamic principles. In: White PF, ed. *Textbook of Intravenous Anesthesia*. Baltimore, Williams & Wilkins; 1997.)

Pharmacokinetics of Neuraxial Drug Administration

42

Amanda Hopkins, MD, and Michael J. Berrigan, MD, PhD

A solid understanding of the pharmacology of neuraxially administered drugs is vital to the practice of anesthesiology as it informs the clinician in choosing the proper agents to safely achieve analgesia and anesthesia in a wide variety of settings.

OPIOIDS

Pharmacokinetics of Epidurally Administered Opioids

Epidurally administered opioids must make their way out of the epidural space if they are to reach their site of action in the spinal cord's dorsal horn. Experimental data indicate that there are two main processes that interfere with an opioid's ability to reach the cerebrospinal fluid (CSF) from the epidural space: (1) clearance of the drug into plasma and (2) partitioning of the drug into other tissues. The extent to which these processes affect a drug's distribution is dependent on the drug's lipid solubility. Highly lipid-soluble drugs (ie, fentanyl, sufentanil) reach lower peak concentrations in the CSF compared to hydrophilic drugs (ie, morphine) after deposit into the epidural space. The reason for this is twofold: first, lipophilic drugs more readily partition into the epidural fat, where they remain until they are slowly re-released back into the epidural space; second, since lipophilic drugs more easily traverse vascular walls, they are more rapidly cleared from the epidural space into the plasma. The majority of this vascular clearance seems to occur in the rich capillary network of the dura mater. The ability of epinephrine to reduce the clearance rate of drugs from the epidural space has been attributed to its capacity to reduce dural blood flow.

Administering an opioid into the epidural space does not guarantee a spinal site of action. When very lipophilic opioids (ie, fentanyl) are administered by continuous epidural infusion, they may not produce analgesia by a spinal mechanism. Instead, owing to their tendency to rapidly clear into the plasma, lipophilic opioids can redistribute through the bloodstream to the brainstem, producing unwanted side effects (ie, sedation, respiratory depression).

Pharmacokinetics of Intrathecally Administered Opioids

As in the epidural space, the pharmacokinetics of opioids in the intrathecal space is determined by their lipid solubility. Lipophilic (hydrophobic) opioids tend to move out of the aqueous CSF compartment, primarily diffusing across the meninges and into the epidural fat. Because of this tendency to move quickly out of the CSF, lipophilic opioids have limited bioavailability at spinal cord sites rostral to the site of administration. This explains why lipophilic opioids (ie, fentanyl) are not associated with the delayed respiratory depression seen with hydrophilic opioids (ie, morphine) when given intrathecally. Unlike fentanyl, morphine is able to remain primarily in the CSF, where it gradually spreads toward the brainstem, eventually producing respiratory depression.

Just as administration of an opioid into the epidural space does not guarantee a spinal site of action, placing an opioid into the intrathecal space does not assure a selective spinal mechanism. Although all opioids likely have some degree of spinal action when placed in the intrathecal space owing to their proximity to the spinal cord dorsal horn, lipophilic opioids again tend to redistribute into the plasma, producing systemic side effects at smaller doses than their hydrophilic counterparts. A good example of this is seen when comparing sufentanil (lipophilic) and morphine (hydrophilic). When administered intravenously, sufentanil is about 1000 times more potent than morphine. However, when placed intrathecally, morphine is around 100 times more potent that sufentanil, owing to sufentanil's limited bioavailability at the spinal cord dorsal horn.

LOCAL ANESTHETICS

Uptake

The exact disposition of epidurally administered local anesthetics is still under investigation; however, the factors identified as important in this process are the same as seen in opioids: (1) the drug's lipophilicity (which relates to its potency) and

(2) factors affecting the rate of clearance, such as the local blood flow and the use of additives (ie, vasoconstrictors).

Intrathecal bioavailability of epidurally administered local anesthetics increases with lipophilicity. This contrasts the findings regarding opioids, which indicate that increasingly lipophilic agents tend to exit CSF to epidural fat, decreasing spinal bioavailability. Additionally, increased intrathecal bioavailability after epidural local anesthetic injection has been associated with decreasing meningeal permeability rates. The combined findings that increasingly lipophilic drugs have slower transfer rates yet greater intrathecal bioavailability is counterintuitive, underscoring the complexity of the disposition of local anesthetic agents administered epidurally. One theory to explain this relationship is that increasing lipophilicity is associated with increasing clearance from the epidural space via the vasculature (ie, distribution and clearance are competing processes—the more lipophilic agents are less eliminated in epidural vasculature and are thus more available for eventual transfer into the intrathecal space), but this has not yet been confirmed.

When considering a drug's clearance rate, one factor to consider is that the local anesthetics themselves have various degrees of vasoactivity, with some agents producing vasodilatation (tetracaine > lidocaine) whereas others act as vasoconstrictors (bupivacaine). Presumably, there is a resulting affect on clearance rates via the vasculature.

It is also worth noting that the overall spinal bioavailability of all local anesthetics deposited in the epidural space is low. One study of ropivacaine estimated its intrathecal bioavailability to be approximately 10% after epidural placement.

Distribution

The distribution of local anesthetic solutions within the intrathecal space is determined not only by the dose administered but also by (1) the baricity of the solution and (2) the positioning of the patient. Baricity, a measure of a solution's density relative to that of CSF, is particularly important in determining the extent of anesthetic spread within the spinal compartment.

Hyperbaric solutions, those having greater density than CSF, are made denser by the addition of glucose to the local anesthetic. These solutions are able to achieve considerable spread and are the most commonly used agents. The direction of anesthetic spread is determined both by the contour of the vertebral canal and the position of the patient, with hyperbaric solutions traveling to the most dependent regions of the spine. For example, in a patient lying supine, the kyphoses of the thoracic and sacral spine are in dependent position, with the lumbar lordosis creating a relative high point. The anesthesiologist can then achieve thoracic (T6–T8) spread by administering the anesthetic cephalad to the peak of the lumbar lordosis.

Isobaric solutions have limited subarachnoid spread, as the distribution of these agents is not affected by gravity and CSF itself does not have much net movement. Because isobaric solutions do not travel far from the site of instillation, the local anesthetic concentration remains relatively high, resulting in a more profound motor block and more prolonged duration of action compared to an equivalent hyperbaric local anesthetic solution.

Hypobaric solutions tend to move in a nondependent fashion (ie, they "float up" within the CSF). Hypobaric solutions can be prepared by using sterile water or dilute saline to lessen the baricity of a local anesthetic solution. However, these solutions are very hypotonic, so caution must be taken to avoid putting too much osmotic stress on the neural tissues.

KEY POINTS

- The bioavailability of opioids in the intrathecal and epidural spaces is determined primarily by their lipid solubility, with hydrophilic opioids having greater spinal bioavailability.
- Spinal opioid administration does not guarantee a spinal site of action.
- Epinephrine reduces the clearance rate of drugs from the epidural space primarily by reducing blood flow through the dura mater.
- Hydrophilic opioids (eg, morphine) administered neuraxially can cause delayed respiratory depression, because they have longer mean residence times in the CSF and can migrate rostrally to act in the brainstem.
- The mechanisms governing the bioavailability of local anesthetics in the intrathecal space are complex and still under investigation.
- The three most important factors in determining neuraxially administered spread of local anesthetics are: (1) the baricity of the solution; (2) patient position; and (3) dose of local anesthetic injected.
- Hyperbaric local anesthetic solutions (made hyperbaric by the addition of glucose) achieve considerable spread within the CSF compartment.
- Isobaric solutions tend to stay around the site of subdural administration and thus achieve relatively higher local anesthetic concentrations.
- Hypobaric solutions are nondependent (tend to "float up" in the CSF) and must be used with caution due to their very hypotonic nature.

SUGGESTED READING

Bernards CM. Recent insights into the pharmacokinetics of spinal opioids and the relevance to opioid selection. *Curr Opin Anesthesiol* 2004;17:441-447.

Drug Tolerance and Tachyphylaxis

Rishi Vashishta, MD, and Michael J. Berrigan, MD, PhD

Physiologic tolerance, or desensitization, is well described in clinical pharmacology. It is defined by progressively diminished response to drug at a certain dose following repeated exposure, and requiring increasing dosages to achieve the desired effect on subsequent administrations. Drug tolerance refers to changes in the potency (higher effective dose required), the effectiveness (decreased maximal effect), or both aspects of the drug.

There are four key characteristics of drug tolerance:

1. Reversible, once exposure to the drug is discontinued.
2. Dependent on the dose and frequency of drug exposure.
3. Variable time course and extent of tolerance development between different drugs.
4. Not all drug effects develop the same amount of tolerance.

Physiologic tolerance may also occur in the form of drug resistance, whereby an organism develops resistance to the effects of a substance following exposure. Pathogens are said to be drug resistant when drugs meant to neutralize them have reduced effects.

On a dose–response curve, drug tolerance causes a right shift of the curve, thereby increasing median effective dose (ED_{50}) and requiring greater dosages to achieve similar effects. ED_{50} does not necessarily increase with tolerance and may have serious implications.

TOLERANCE VERSUS DEPENDENCE

Drug tolerance is not equal to drug dependence, although they often coexist and have similar cellular mechanisms. Whereas tolerance requires increasing dosages of a drug to achieve similar effects, dependence is defined as the compulsive need of an individual to use a drug to function normally. Dependence develops in an individual when the brain adapts to continuous, high drug levels and appears to function "normally" at those levels due to functional tolerance. If drug administration is halted, an abrupt decrease in drug levels results in abstinence syndrome or withdrawal reactions that are opposite to

the drug's initial effects (ie, hyperactivity for depressants or hypoactivity for stimulants).

MECHANISMS OF DRUG TOLERANCE

There are multiple mechanisms that explain tolerance to a drug following repeated exposure. It is possible for a single drug to develop more than one type of tolerance. The three major mechanisms responsible for tolerance are:

- *Dispositional (metabolic) tolerance* occurs when repeated use of a drug reduces the amount of that drug available at the target tissue. The underlying pharmacokinetic mechanism involves accelerated drug clearance due to induction of metabolic enzymes from repeated or continuous use of the drug. While this usually takes weeks to develop, the net effect is a shortened half-life and a decreased quantity of drug at the target site. Examples of this phenomenon are seen with alcohol, opiates, and barbiturates.
- *Reduced responsiveness (pharmacodynamic) tolerance* occurs when repeated use of a drug alters nerve cell function (ie, receptor density, intracellular cascade). This type of tolerance takes days or weeks to develop. Chronically increased receptor activation by agonistic drugs results in receptor downregulation (loss of receptors), whereas chronic reduction in receptor activation due to drug antagonism results in receptor upregulation (production of more receptors). Examples of this mechanism of tolerance are seen with alcohol, opiates, amphetamines, benzodiazepines, caffeine, and nicotine.
- *Behavioral (context-specific) tolerance* occurs when repeated drug use reduces its effect in the environment where it is typically administered, but not in other environments. Learned behaviors offset or compensate for drug impairments. Although these learned behaviors develop during repeated drug exposure, they are not due to changes in circulating drug levels. A common example of this is seen with marijuana, where chronic users may function competently despite levels of intoxication that would otherwise incapacitate less accustomed users.

TACHYPHYLAXIS

Tachyphylaxis describes the acute decrease in response to a drug following its administration. It occurs either after initial dosing or after a series of rapid exposures. Although this phenomenon is often referred to as the rapid development of drug tolerance, the underlying mechanism highlights the differences between tachyphylaxis and tolerance. The onset of tachyphylaxis is typically sudden and not dose dependent. The perceived tolerance is caused by neurotransmitter depletion, creating the effect of insufficient drug or reduced receptors. Examples of drugs that commonly exhibit tachyphylaxis are amphetamines, ephedrine, antidepressants (selective serotonin reuptake inhibitors [SSRIs] and tricyclic antidepressants [TCAs]), beta-2-agonists, dobutamine, nitroglycerin, hydralazine, desmopressin, and intranasal decongestants.

CROSS-TOLERANCE

Cross-tolerance is a phenomenon whereby tolerance to one drug produces a similar tolerance to other, chemically related drugs. Cross-tolerance is frequently observed among illicit drug users. For example, heroin-tolerant individuals also exhibit cross-tolerance to morphine and other opiate analgesics. The cross-tolerance typically develops within related drug groups, such as central nervous system stimulants (ie, amphetamine, methamphetamine, cocaine), opiate analgesics (ie, morphine, codeine, fentanyl), or sedatives and hypnotics (ie, benzodiazepines, barbiturates, inhalation anesthetics, alcohol), but it does not develop between these groups. Other examples of drug classes exhibiting frequent cross-tolerance include antibiotics, antivirals, and illicit hallucinogens.

REVERSE TOLERANCE (SENSITIZATION)

Reverse tolerance, or sensitization, occurs when a drug effect increases with repeated administration. Although not fully understood, research in this area focuses on the stimulating effects of drugs such as amphetamines, cocaine, and alcohol. These drugs have been shown to activate the brain's dopaminergic system with each dose, even when low doses are repeatedly administered. Although tolerance to certain effects of a drug may diminish over time if the drug is not administered, sensitization appears to continue long after the drug has been stopped.

44

Drug Termination of Action

Rishi Vashishta, MD, and Michael J. Berrigan, MD, PhD

Exposure to xenobiotics immediately initiates a cascade to remove the foreign compound from the body's circulation. The elimination of many drugs begins with a *first pass effect*, where orally administered drugs absorbed from the gastrointestinal tract into circulation pass through the liver before reaching targeted sites of action. Although the liver and kidneys are used to clear most compounds, other organs, including the skin and lungs, also assist with clearance. In most cases, the drug action terminates by enzyme-catalyzed conversion to inactive (or less active) compounds and/or elimination via the kidneys or other routes. Drug redistribution from the primary site may also terminate the action, although this occurs infrequently.

BIOTRANSFORMATION AND DRUG METABOLISM

Biotransformation is a major mechanism for drug elimination. Most drugs undergo biotransformation to produce more polar metabolites than the administered drug. Excretion of compounds through renal and hepatic systems largely depends on lipophilicity or fat solubility. More lipophilic compounds tend to be reabsorbed back into circulation, either following renal glomerular filtration or through hepatic biliary excretion. Therefore, biotransformation of compounds into more polar (hydrophilic) structures is essential for complete removal of the drug. In addition, decreased drug lipophilicity limits a drug's capacity to redistribute and accumulate in highly lipophilic areas, such as fat or brain tissue.

Many drugs undergo several sequential biotransformation reactions that are catalyzed by specific enzyme systems, primarily in the liver, which may also catalyze the biotransformation of endogenous compounds (ie, steroids). These reactions produce inactive drug metabolites; however, consequences of these reactions include secondary metabolites with increased or decreased potencies, metabolites with different pharmacological actions, toxic metabolites, and active metabolites from inactive prodrugs. The biotransformation of drugs is variable between individuals and is dependent on a multitude of factors, including age, diet, genetics,

liver function, prior administration of the drug, and drug interactions.

Biotransformation reactions are classified into two types: *phase I (nonsynthetic)* and *phase II (synthetic)* reactions. Phase I reactions include oxidations, reductions, and hydrolysis reactions. These reactions typically introduce functional groups (ie, –OH, –SH, –NH$_2$) that serve as active centers for subsequent phase II reactions. Enzymes catalyzing phase I reactions include cytochrome P450, aldehyde dehydrogenase, alcohol dehydrogenase, monoamine oxidase, deaminases, esterases, amidases, and epoxide hydrolase. Phase II reactions are conjugation reactions, involving an enzyme-catalyzed combination of endogenous compounds to functional groups produced from phase I reactions. These reactions utilize energy from "activated" forms of the endogenous compounds (ie, acetyl-CoA, UDP-glucuronate, glutathione). Enzymes catalyzing phase II reactions include glucuronyl transferase (conjugates glucuronyl group), sulfotransferase (conjugates sulfate group), transacylases (conjugates amino acids), glutathione *S*-transferase, acetylases, ethylases, and methylases.

REDISTRIBUTION

Drug redistribution from primary target site to other storage sites, or reservoirs, is another mechanism by which the drug action terminates. Greater lipid solubility results in faster redistribution of drug to reservoirs. The underlying mechanism involves delivery of highly lipid-soluble drug to primary target organs (ie, brain) with high blood flow, where the drug produces the desired effect due to rapid equilibration between blood and organ tissue. Following that, moderately perfused tissues (ie, adipose tissue, muscle) take up drug, thereby decreasing the drug concentration in plasma. As the primary target organs continue to equilibrate with plasma containing progressively lower drug concentrations, the desired effect is rapidly terminated. For example, redistribution occurs with thiopental, which accumulates primarily in the brain as a result of its high lipid solubility and blood flow. Thiopental terminates its action by redistribution to more poorly perfused adipose tissue.

RATE OF ELIMINATION AND CLEARANCE

The rate of elimination can be expressed either in terms of a **half-life** ($t_{1/2}$), the time required for 50% to be eliminated, or a **rate constant** (k_e), the fraction eliminated per unit time. If either value is known, the other may be calculated from the equation:

$$t_{1/2} = 0.693/k_e$$

For most drugs, elimination follows first-order kinetics (exponential), where a constant proportion of the drug is eliminated in a unit of time, depending on drug plasma concentration. In rare cases, drugs may exhibit zero-order kinetics (linear), where a constant amount of the drug is eliminated in a unit of time. Zero-order kinetics is not dependent on drug plasma concentration.

The **total clearance** of a substance is a measure of the sum of all organ clearances, and is defined as the volume of plasma from which the drug is removed in a unit time, expressed in milliliters per minute per kilogram (mL/min/kg). Given the volume of distribution (V_d) of a drug, its clearance may be calculated by:

$$\text{Clearance} = V_d \times k_e$$

DRUG EXCRETION

Drugs may be excreted through urine, feces (from bile), saliva, sweat, tears, milk, and the lungs. Although any of these routes may be clinically important to recognize for a particular drug or as a possible source of unwanted exposure in nursing infants, the kidneys are the primary excretion sites for most drugs. The liver, though an important organ in drug metabolism, has a minor role in drug excretion and comparatively little is known about biliary excretion and enterohepatic cycling of specific drugs.

Renal excretion of a drug combines three separate processes: glomerular filtration, active secretion, and passive reabsorption. Most drugs have low molecular weights and freely filter from plasma at the glomerulus, with the exception of drugs bound to plasma proteins, which are too large to be filtered. In the proximal tubule, drugs may be further secreted into the ultrafiltrate through active transport systems specific for organic acids and organic bases. Finally, as the ultrafiltrate progresses through the renal tubules, reabsorption of unionized, weak acids or bases occurs via passive diffusion. Therefore, **net renal excretion** of drug equals the amount filtered at the glomerulus, plus the amount secreted through active transport mechanisms, minus the amount reabsorbed passively throughout the renal tubule. Renal clearance measures the volume of plasma that is cleared of drug per unit time:

$$\text{Renal clearance} = U \times V/P,$$

where U = concentration of drug per milliliter of urine, V = volume of urine excreted per minute, and P = concentration of drug per milliliter of plasma. Renal clearance values less than 130 mL/min suggest glomerular filtration excretion alone (ie, insulin); clearance values between 130 and 650 mL/min suggest excretion by glomerular filtration, active secretion, and partial reabsorption; and clearance values more than 650 mL/min suggest excretion by glomerular filtration and complete secretion (ie, para-aminohippuric acid). Several factors influence drug excretion, including age (undeveloped mechanisms at birth), concomitant drugs, comorbid diseases, and renal function.

Drug Interactions

Chris Potestio, MD, and Brian S. Freeman, MD

PHARMACEUTICAL INTERACTIONS

The formulation of drugs is often overlooked but may contribute to bioavailability and desired effects. For example, adding epinephrine to a local anesthetic solution gives the solution a much lower pH due to highly acidic commercial preparations of epinephrine. A more acidic solution of local anesthetic results in lower concentration of the ionized, membrane permeable form of the local anesthetic. This equilibrium change decreases tissue penetration and diminishes the desired effect.

Propofol is prepared in a lipid emulsion containing soybean oil and egg phosphatide. This hydrophobic solution stabilizes the propofol molecule, but has several clinical consequences. First, it is a ripe environment for microbial growth; so all propofol syringes must be timed and dated and discarded 6 hours after the sterility of the vial is broken. The second issue related to the propofol emulsion is a concern that it will cause anaphylaxis in those with egg or soybean allergy. This is a controversial issue without strong data to support the risk of anaphylaxis; however, it is prudent to avoid propofol in those with allergy to soy, peanut, or egg so long as a suitable alternative is available. The lipid emulsion of propofol also causes burning when administered in small peripheral intravenous lines (IVs).

The combination of agents in a single intravenous line is another important pharmaceutical interaction. Combination of acidic drugs and basic drugs will form a salt precipitate in the intravenous line. For example, thiopental is acidic and, when mixed with alkaline drugs such as opiates or muscle relaxants, the intravenous tubing may be obstructed by the resulting precipitate.

Carbon dioxide absorbents such as soda lime and Baralyme allow for removal of exhaled carbon dioxide from the ventilator circuit. These compounds are integral to safe mechanical ventilation, but contain strong bases that can degrade volatile anesthetics. All volatile anesthetics can react with the carbon dioxide absorber to produce carbon monoxide, but this reaction occurs most often with desflurane. A concerning byproduct of sevoflurane interaction with carbon dioxide absorbents is the formation of compound A (penta-fluoroisopropenyl fluoromethyl ether) which causes nephrotoxicity in rats. Correlation with nephrotoxicity in humans

has not been established, but this side effect is nonetheless concerning.

PHARMACOKINETIC INTERACTIONS

Uptake

Anesthesiologists often manipulate the interaction between epinephrine and local anesthetic when administered for peripheral nerve blocks. When mixed with local anesthetics prior to local injection, epinephrine causes vasoconstriction of muscle and skin, which decreases systemic uptake and results in longer duration of action for the anesthetic. In a similar mechanism, any agent that changes pulmonary blood flow (vasoactive agents, prostaglandins, phosphodiesterase inhibitors, etc) can alter the ventilation/perfusion (V/Q) ratio, thereby altering uptake of volatile anesthetics. Since volatile anesthetic uptake is directly proportional to pulmonary blood flow, the drug's effect on cardiac output will affect the onset of inhaled anesthetics.

Several medications alter gastrointestinal absorption and must be considered when giving oral medications. Histamine (H2) receptor antagonists (eg, ranitidine) and proton pump inhibitors (eg, omeprazole) decrease acidity of the gastric contents, which will raise the pH and alter the absorption of weak acids/bases. Metoclopramide is a prokinetic that increases gastric emptying time and will decrease gastric absorption.

Distribution

A drug can alter the distribution of another drug by two main mechanisms: (1) increasing or decreasing cardiac output or (2) displacing the drug from protein binding sites.

All medications are reliant on the cardiovascular system to reach their target tissue, but alterations in cardiac output do not significantly change the onset of drugs. The relationship between cardiac output and drug clearance is more clinically relevant.

Two drugs may compete for protein binding, and thus the free fraction of one may be altered by administration of the other. However, these interactions are oftentimes not clinically significant because the number of free binding sites on proteins is much higher than the concentration of the drug itself; therefore, relatively small changes in binding site availability will not alter the distribution of the drug.

Not all pharmacokinetic interactions are unwanted side effects. For example, sugammadex is synthesized specifically to interfere with the distribution of rocuronium. It irreversibly binds to plasma rocuronium and confers a simple, rapid neuromuscular blockade reversal. This pharmacological reversal has led to much promising research, but is not yet available in the United States.

Metabolism

If a drug alters hepatic blood flow, it will decrease metabolism of drugs metabolized in the liver. Examples are vasoactive drugs, such as phenylephrine, ephedrine, and other vasopressors. Volatile anesthetics also affect hepatic blood flow by causing vasodilation and decrease flow through the portal circulation.

The other important way that drugs alter hepatic metabolism is by inhibition and induction of the hepatic cytochrome P450 enzyme system (Table 45-1).

TABLE 45-1 Important Cytochrome (CYP) Inducers/Inhibitors in Anesthesia

Enzyme	Substrate	Inhibitor	Inducer
CYP2C8	Carvedilol	Dihydropyridine calcium channel blockers (nifedipine) antifungals (ketoconazole, fluconazole), gemfibrozil	Rifampin, phenobarbital
CYP2C9	Sulfonylureas, ARBs, warfarin	Antifungals (fluconazole), trimethoprim, amiodarone, zafirlukast	Rifampin, phenobarbital
CYP2D6	Captopril, carvedilol, metoprolol, water-soluble opiates (codeine, oxycodone, hydrocodone)	Amiodarone, SSRIs (fluoxetine, paroxetine)	
CYP3A4	CCBs, ARBs, enalapril, lipid-soluble opiates (fentanyl, alfentanil), benzodiazepines (midazolam)	Antibiotics (clarithromycin, erythromycin), antifungals (itraconazole, ketoconazole), SSRIs, HIV protease inhibitors, grapefruit juice	Rifampin, phenobarbital, rifabutin, phenytoin, St. John's wort, carbamazepine

SSRI, selective serotonin reuptake inhibitors; CCB, calcium channel blockers; ARB, angiotensin receptor blockers

PHARMACODYNAMIC INTERACTION

Direct Receptor Agonism/Antagonism

There are many drugs used specifically for their antagonism effect at receptor sites. For example, naloxone binds to opiate receptors and blocks the effect of narcotics, flumazenil blocks the effects of alcohol or benzodiazepines at the gamma-aminobutyric acid (GABA) receptor, and acetylcholinesterase inhibitors antagonize the breakdown of acetylcholine molecules to overcome a muscle blockade.

Opiate agonist–antagonist compounds (nalbuphine, buprenorphine, butorphanol, pentazocine) are a subset of medications with unique receptor interactions. These drugs are synthesized to act as agonists at the kappa-opiate receptor (KOPr) and antagonists at the mu-opiate receptor (MOR). Buprenorphine is the only medication in this class to act as a partial agonist of MORs, but its effect is blunted compared to that of full opiate agonists such as morphine. The interaction of these drugs with opiates is receptor specific and can lead to peripheral analgesia at the KOPr with diminished euphoria and addictive potential due to antagonism of the mu-receptor.

Physiologic Agonism/Antagonism

Interaction of physiologic effect occurs much more frequently than drug–receptor interactions. In fact, a majority of anesthetic medications alter the effect of other drugs administered. Anesthesiologists use this to their advantage when they practice "balanced anesthetic technique." A balanced anesthetic technique employs several drugs with the same anesthetic properties to avoid toxic levels of any one drug. For example, hypnotics such as propofol or etomidate are often combined with opiates and benzodiazepines for anesthetic induction. The interaction between alfentanil and propofol is synergistic, causing hypnosis at a much higher level than the additive effect of each drug. They work at different receptors, so this interaction occurs on the physiologic level, not the receptor level.

Serotonin syndrome is an important pharmacodynamic interaction that results in high concentrations of serotonin in the central nervous system. At high concentrations, serotonin causes mental status changes, muscle twitching, excessive sweating, shivering, and fever (usually >101.5°F). Drug interactions that can lead to this syndrome include opioids such as meperidine combined with monoamine oxidase inhibitors or selective serotonin reuptake inhibitors (SSRIs). Amphetamines, venlafaxine, linezolid, paroxetine, and bupropion are other drugs that have been implicated in this syndrome.

Inhaled anesthetics are affected by central catecholamine levels; therefore, their effectiveness can be increased or decreased by catecholamine altering drugs, such as amphetamines and ephedrine which increase minimum alveolar concentration (MAC). Ephedrine may not be effective if catecholamine stores are depleted. Clonidine, methyldopa, and reserpine decrease catecholamines, and therefore decrease MAC.

Drug–time interactions are an important tangent from drug–drug interactions. In drug–time interactions, the body's response to the administration of a drug changes over time. For example, nitroprusside administration typically results in tachyphylaxis. Nitroprusside infusion will lead to acute desensitization; therefore, it is often necessary to increase a nitroprusside infusion over time to maintain the desired effect. On a cellular level, nitroprusside infusion leads to repetitive activation of a receptor, which causes intracellular phosphorylation of the receptor that acts as negative feedback to decrease further response. This mechanism occurs at varying degrees in all receptors, both G-coupled protein receptors and second messenger systems. Nitroprusside receptor response is particularly robust and acts as a good example. Receptor desensitization is the mechanism responsible for opiate tolerance.

Drug–time interactions have the opposite effect as well. Long-term antagonism of a set of receptors leads to upregulation of receptors. Therefore, antagonism is withdrawn, the target tissue is sensitized, and an exaggerated response is expected. Beta-blockers are continued in the perioperative period due to concern of sensitization of the sympathetic nervous system due to long-term antagonism.

Another classic example of sensitization concerns nicotinic receptors at the neuromuscular junction leading to receptor sensitivity in patients with spinal cord injury, burns, or prolonged immobilization. The resulting sensitization can cause life-threatening hyperkalemia when depolarizing muscle blockade with succinylcholine is used.

Drug Reactions

Srijaya K. Reddy, MD, MBA

Anaphylaxis is a severe allergic reaction mediated by an antigen–antibody reaction, or type I hypersensitivity reaction. Antigen binding to immunoglobulin E (IgE) antibodies on the surface of mast cells initiates the release of various chemical mediators. These mediators cause specific end organ reactions in the skin, respiratory system, gastrointestinal system, and the cardiovascular system. Clinical manifestations (Table 46-1) of anaphylaxis usually appear within close proximity of exposure to a specific antigen in a previously sensitized person. Death can occur from irreversible shock or loss of airway.

Anaphylactoid reactions resemble anaphylaxis symptomatically, but IgE does not mediate them. Prior sensitization to a specific antigen is not required for anaphylactoid reactions to occur. Though the mechanism of action differs between anaphylactoid and anaphylactic reactions, they can't be clinically indistinguishable.

COMMON TRIGGERING AGENTS

Antibiotics

Antibiotics are the most common cause of anaphylactic reactions in the perioperative setting, with penicillin, cephalosporins, and vancomycin being the main sources. Patients who are allergic to penicillin have a less than 10% chance of cross-reactivity with cephalosporins. If administered too rapidly, vancomycin can cause "red man syndrome," which is caused by histamine release leading to flushing of the skin and hypotension.

Muscle Relaxants

Muscle relaxants also account for a large portion of anesthesia-related drug reactions. Mivacurium and atracurium are associated with anaphylactoid reactions. Although rare, both cisatracurium and rocuronium have been associated with IgE-mediated anaphylaxis. Succinylcholine is generally regarded as the muscle relaxant most likely to cause an anaphylactic reaction. Cross-sensitivity between nondepolarizing muscle relaxants is relatively common.

Local Anesthetics

Allergies to ester local anesthetics are well documented, but the incidence of reactions to amide local anesthetics is rare. A para-aminobenzoic acid (PABA) derivative, methylparaben, is a preservative used in multidose vials of ester local anesthetics. Exposure to methylparaben is usually the cause for adverse reactions to local anesthetics.

Latex

Although it is not a drug per se, latex is a common cause of anaphylaxis in the operating room. Chronic exposure to latex, patients with neural tube defects, and patients undergoing frequent procedures involving the genitourinary tract or repeated bladder catheterization are increased risk factors for latex allergy. The incidence of latex anaphylaxis in children has been reported to be 1:10 000, but the incidence seems to be decreasing as more and more operating rooms move toward a latex-free or latex-safe environment. Anesthetic equipment that may contain latex includes gloves, tourniquets, intravenous injection ports, rubber stoppers on drug vials, blood pressure cuffs, face masks, and even certain endotracheal tubes.

Other Agents

Narcotics, protamine, heparin, blood products, colloids, methyl methacrylate, intravenous contrast, methylene blue, mannitol, NSAIDs, oxytocin, and antiseptics (chlorhexidine, povidone-iodine, etc) should also be considered as potential causes of anaphylaxis or anaphylactoid reactions.

TREATMENT

Treatment of anaphylaxis and anaphylactoid reactions is initially aimed at discontinuing exposure to the offending agent or drug and administering 100% oxygen to the patient.

TABLE 46-1 Clinical Manifestations of Anaphylaxis

Cardiovascular	Hypotension, tachycardia, arrhythmias
Pulmonary	Bronchospasm, dyspnea, cough, pulmonary edema, hypoxemia
Dermatologic	Urticaria, facial edema, pruritis
Gastrointestinal	Vomiting, diarrhea

Generous intravenous fluid boluses (2-4 L of crystalloid) are given to treat hypotension, and epinephrine (0.1 μg/kg IV initially, or 0.1-0.5 mg IV for cardiovascular collapse) can also be administered to treat hypotension or cardiovascular collapse. Secondary therapies for these types of reactions may include diphenhydramine or corticosteroids to reduce the inflammatory response and bronchodilators. Securing the airway with intubation or tracheostomy, or a vasopressor infusion might be required in severe cases. Anaphylaxis usually resolves anywhere from 2 to 8 hours after exposure, depending on the severity and secondary pathology developing from the reaction.

MINIMIZING THE RISKS

In patients with prior allergic reactions to anesthetic agents, latex, antibiotics, or those with predisposing risk factors (youth, pregnancy, history of atopy) for anaphylactic or anaphylactoid reactions, proper preparation is warranted. Ideally, drugs or agents that trigger anaphylaxis or anaphylactoid reactions should be avoided. In certain cases, this is not always possible. For example, intravenous contrast is a frequently used agent that causes anaphylactoid reactions, and it is often used even in the setting of known prior reactions. To prepare these patients, volume status should be optimized preoperatively. Pretreatment with an H_1 and/or H_2 blocker and corticosteroids should also be considered 12-16 hours before planned exposure.

SUGGESTED READINGS

Axon AD, Hunter JM. Anaphylaxis and anesthesia-all clear now? *Br J Anaesth* 2004;93:501-504.

Withington DE. Allergy, anaphylaxis and anesthesia. *Can J Anaesth* 1994;41:1133.

47

Alternative & Herbal Medications

Srijaya K. Reddy, MD, MBA

Herbal medicines are composed of the biologically active components of plants or parts of plants, such as seeds, roots, or flowers, for medicinal purposes. Although herbal medicines have been used for centuries in Chinese and Ayurvedic medicine, their use has dramatically increased for primary health care over the past few years. The World Health Organization estimates that 80% of the people worldwide use alternative and herbal medications as part of their health-care regimen. Awareness of the rising use of these alternative medicines is important to prevent, recognize, and treat potential perioperative problems.

Patients often take a combination of prescription and herbal medications, which can cause adverse reactions in the perioperative period (Table 47-1). Both patients and physicians frequently underestimate the risks associated with drug and herbal medication interactions, particularly interactions affecting coagulation. Preoperative consultation should include screening for the use of herbal medicines and the potential interactions with prescription medications. It is recommended that most herbal medications be discontinued at least 2-3 weeks prior to anesthesia or elective surgery.

SUGGESTED READINGS

American Society of Anesthesiologists. What you should know about your patient's use of herbal medicines. Available at http://www.asahq.org. Accessed on April 21, 2013.

Kaye AD, Baluch A, Kaye AJ, Frass M, Hofbauer R. Pharmacology of herbals and their impact in anesthesia. *Curr Opin Anaesthesiol* 2007;20:294-299.

TABLE 47-1   Effects of Commonly Used Herbal Medications

Supplement	Uses	Possible Interactions
Echinacea	Common colds, wounds and burns, UTIs, coughs and URIs, bronchitis	Hepatotoxicity; potentiation of hepatotoxic effects of amiodarone, ketoconazole, methotrexate, anabolic steroids; may decrease effects of corticosteroids and cyclosporine; anaphylaxis
Ephedra	Dietary aid for weight loss, antitussive actions, increased energy	Potential interactions with cardiac glycosides, MAOIs, oxytocin, guanethidine, MI, stroke, hypertension, tachycardia, arrhythmias
Feverfew	Migraines, antipyretic	Inhibit platelet activity, rebound headache
Garlic	Lowering lipids, vasodilatation, antihypertensive, antiplatelet effects, antioxidant, cardiovascular disease prevention	Potentiate effects of warfarin, heparin, aspirin, leading to abnormal bleeding time; risk for perioperative hemorrhage
Ginger	Antiemetic, antivertigo	Potentiate anticoagulant effects of drugs, inhibits thromboxane synthetase
Ginkgo biloba	Antioxidant, circulatory stimulation, vertigo, memory loss, sexual dysfunction, tinnitus, intermittent claudication	Potentiate anticoagulant effects of drugs (ASA, NSAIDs, warfarin, heparin); may decrease effectiveness of anticonvulsant drugs, may lower seizure threshold in patients taking TCAs; spontaneous hyphema and intracranial bleeds
Ginseng	Enhance energy levels, antioxidant, aphrodisiac, promote diuresis, facilitate digestion	Sleepiness, hypertonia, edema, hypoglycemia, tachycardia, hypertension, mania in patients taking MAOIs, inhibition of platelet aggregation, epistaxis, Stevens–Johnson syndrome
Goldenseal	Diuretic, laxative, antiinflammatory	Paralysis, hypertension, electrolyte abnormalities
Kava-kava	Anxiolytic, skin disorders, antiepileptic, antipsychotic	Potentiate effects of barbiturates, benzodiazepines, and ethanol; increased suicide risk, can inhibit norepinephrine, decreased MAC requirements; hepatotoxicity, hallucinations
Licorice	Gastritis, gastric and duodenal ulcers, cough and bronchitis	Hypertension, hypokalemia, edema, renal insufficiency, hypertonia, can worsen chronic liver diseases
Saw palmetto	Antiandrogenic, treatment for benign prostatic hyperplasia	Additive effects with other hormone replacement therapy, headaches, GI discomfort
St. John's wort	Depression, anxiety, sleep-related disorders, vitiligo	Interact with MAOIs, prolonged effects of anesthesia, photosensitivity, possible serotoninergic syndrome with patients taking SSRIs, restlessness, dizziness fatigue, nausea
Valerian	Anxiolytic, sedative	Potentiate effects of barbiturates, benzodiazepine-like withdrawal syndrome, prolonged effects of anesthesia

UTI, urinary tract infections; URI, upper respiratory tract infections

Anesthetic Gases: Principles

Brian A. Kim, MD and Anna Katharine Hindle, MD

CHEMICAL STRUCTURE

The most commonly used volatile anesthetics are desflurane, sevoflurane, and isoflurane. The chemical structures can be classified as substituted halogenated ethers. Additionally, halothane is a substituted halogenated alkane, a derivative of ethane. Isoflurane and enflurane are isomers that are methyl ethyl ethers. Desflurane differs from isoflurane in the substitution of fluorine for a chlorine atom, and sevoflurane is a methyl isopropyl ether.

MECHANISM OF ACTION

The mechanism of action of inhalational anesthetics has not been completely elucidated. Broadly, they are postulated to enhance inhibitory receptors (GABA$_A$ and glycine) while dampening excitatory pathways (nicotinic and glutamate).

Unspecified mechanisms also include suppression of nociceptive motor responses within the spinal cord, as well as supraspinal suppression causing amnesia and hypnotic state.

PHYSICAL CHARACTERISTICS

The end goal of administering inhaled gases is to create an anesthetic state by reaching effective concentrations within the central nervous system (Table 48-1). To arrive at this end point, effective partial pressures must be established within the lung's alveoli, allowing the gases to equilibrate in the pulmonary vasculature and ultimately within the CNS. At equilibrium, the partial pressure of the gases in the alveoli will be equivalent with the partial pressures in the patient's blood and brain. Inhaled anesthetics reach equilibrium due to the following: rapid bidirectional transfer of gases between alveoli, blood,

TABLE 48-1 Physiochemical Properties of Volatile Anesthetics

Property	Sevoflurane	Desflurane	Isoflurane	Enflurane	Halothane	N$_2$O
Boiling point (°C)	59	24	49	57	50	−88
Vapor pressure at 20°C (mm Hg)	157	669	238	172	243	38770
Molecular weight (g)	200	168	184	184	197	44
Oil:gas partition coefficient	47	19	91	97	224	1.4
Blood:gas partition coefficient	0.65	0.42	1.46	1.9	2.50	0.46
Brain:blood solubility	1.7	1.3	1.6	1.4	1.9	1.1
Fat:blood solubility	47.5	27.2	44.9	36	51.1	2.3
Muscle:blood solubility	3.1	2.0	2.9	1.7	3.4	1.2
MAC in O$_2$ 30-60 yr, at 37°C P_B760 (%)	1.8	6.6	1.17	1.63	0.75	104
MAC in 60-70% N$_2$O (%)	0.66	2.38	0.56	0.57	0.29	
MAC, >65 yr (%)	1.45	5.17	1.0	1.55	0.64	—
Preservative	No	No	No	No	Thymol	No
Stable in moist CO$_2$ absorber	No	Yes	Yes	Yes	No	Yes
Flammability (%) (in 70% N$_2$O/30% O$_2$)	10	17	7	5.8	4.8	
Recovered as metabolites (%)	2–5	0.02	0.2	2.4	20	

MAC, minimum alveolar concentration; N$_2$O, nitrous oxide.

(Reproduced with permission from Barash PG, *Clinical Anesthesia*, 7th ed. Philadelphia, PA: Wolters Kluwer Health/Lippincott Williams & Wilkins; 2013.)

and CNS; the low capacity of tissue and plasma to absorb inhaled anesthetics; and the low metabolism, excretion, and redistribution of volatile agents relative to the rate at which they are removed or added to the lungs. Simply put, inhaled agent levels in the brain are heavily dependent on the anesthetic gas concentrations in the alveoli.

$$P_{alveoli} = P_{blood} = P_{brain}$$

MINIMUM ALVEOLAR CONCENTRATION

One minimum alveolar concentration (MAC) of a volatile anesthetic is the alveolar concentration of the gas, at 1 atmosphere, for which 50% of patients will not have a motor response to painful stimulus (ie, surgical incision). A MAC of 1.3 will eliminate motor response in 99% of patients. MAC was developed to compare potencies of inhaled agents, and the potency is inversely proportional to MAC. For example, the MAC of the most common agents, desflurane, sevoflurane, and isoflurane, are roughly 6, 2, and 1, respectively. Isoflurane has the lowest MAC, requiring the lowest alveolar concentration to abolish motor response, and is the most potent agent of the three mentioned. In contrast, desflurane is the least potent and requires the highest concentration to abolish motor response, as it has the largest MAC of the three agents considered.

MAC *increases* (decreases in potency) with the following: hyperthermia, stimulants (cocaine, amphetamines), and chronic alcoholism. The highest MAC values are in infants aged 6-12 months.

MAC *decreases* (increases in potency) with the following: hypothermia, hyponatremia, opioids, barbiturates, alpha-2 blockers, Ca^{2+} channel blockers, acute alcohol intoxication, and pregnancy. Additionally, MAC decreases with prematurity and aging.

MAC is not affected by gender, thyroid function, hyperkalemia, hypocarbia, or hypercarbia.

PARTITION COEFFICIENTS

The partition coefficient represents the distribution of gases at equilibrium between tissues and blood. An increased blood-to-gas partition coefficient means that the volatile anesthetic diffuses more readily into the bloodstream. Therefore, an increased blood-to-gas partition coefficient correlates directly with a higher solubility, as more gas distributes into the vasculature from the alveoli. Furthermore, anesthetic gas diffusion into blood decreases the concentration of the gas within the alveoli. This leads to the prolongation or deceleration of the speed of induction, as the ability of the gas to concentrate in the alveoli is proportional to its rate of induction.

High partition coefficient = High solubility = Slow rate of induction

Rate of induction ∝ Alveolar concentration of gas

For example, the blood-to-gas coefficient for desflurane, sevoflurane, and isoflurane are 0.4, 0.6, and 1.4, respectively. Isoflurane has the highest partition coefficient among the three and, therefore, has the highest solubility and the slowest rate of induction. This is because isoflurane has a disinclination for concentrating within the alveoli, while favoring diffusion into the bloodstream when compared to desflurane and sevoflurane. In contrast, desflurane has the lowest partition coefficient, lowest solubility, and fastest speed of induction.

Speed of Induction	*Slowest*	*Fastest*
	Isoflurane > Sevoflurane > Desflurane	
Solubility	*Highest*	*Lowest*

ANESTHETIC POTENCY

As the speed of induction is dependent on the ability of anesthetic gases to concentrate within the alveoli, factors that accelerate the rate of induction are increasing the delivered concentration, increasing gas flow, and increasing minute ventilation. In contrast, slowing the rate of induction can be achieved by decreasing the concentration and flow of the gas administered. Additionally, increases in cardiac output and high anesthetic lipid solubility both decrease the ability of gases to concentrate in the alveoli and slows the rate of induction.

METABOLISM

The P450 enzymes that metabolize inhaled agents in the process of biotransformation reach saturation before anesthetic doses have been reached. Therefore, metabolism is believed to play a minimal role in the induction phase of inhaled anesthesia but may have more implications postoperatively. Halothane is heavily metabolized by the P450 system, and in hypoxic states, may lead to harmful metabolites that cause hepatic necrosis.

Second, fluoride-associated renal dysfunction can occur with methoxyflurane. Sevoflurane also produces fluoride byproduct, but has not been directly implicated with this particular mechanism of toxicity. Moreover, sevoflurane undergoes base-catalyzed degradation with the soda lime found in CO_2 absorbents, producing a vinyl ether known as compound A. This byproduct may be nephrotoxic. Compound A is most likely to accumulate with higher concentrations of sevoflurane, low-flow, increased-duration cases, and dry absorbents.

Last, carbon dioxide absorbents have been shown to interact with volatile anesthetics, most commonly desflurane, producing carbon monoxide (CO). Expired/desiccated absorbents and absorbents containing more alkaline agents are most likely to interact with desflurane to produce CO. Desiccation of an absorbent may occur with exposure to prolonged high gas flow.

SUGGESTED READING

Campagna JA, Miller KE, Forman SA. Mechanisms of actions of inhaled anesthetics. *N Engl J Med* 2003;348:2110-2124.

Anesthetic Gases: Organ System Effects

Catherine Cleland, MD, and Christopher Jackson, MD

CARDIOVASCULAR EFFECTS

Mean arterial pressure (MAP) decreases with the use of all volatile agents, except halothane, by decreasing systemic vascular resistance (SVR). Halothane decreases cardiac output (CO), and thus MAP, with little to no change in SVR. Nitrous oxide leads to unchanged or increased MAP.

Heart rate (HR) increases with all volatile agents at a minimum alveolar concentration (MAC) of 0.25 for isoflurane, 1 for desflurane, and 1.5 for sevoflurane. Abrupt increases in desflurane concentrations at the initiation of therapy may result in rapidly increasing HR and blood pressure (BP). This may be attenuated with the administration of beta-blockers or opioids.

All volatile anesthetics sensitize the myocardium to epinephrine and depress myocardial contractility.

Sevoflurane should be avoided in patients with a known history of congenital long QT syndrome. Isoflurane has coronary vasodilating properties.

PULMONARY EFFECTS

All inhaled anesthetics decrease tidal volume and increase respiratory rate with little effect on minute ventilation. $Paco_2$ also increases in proportion to anesthetic concentration. All volatile anesthetics blunt the ventilatory stimulation caused by hypoxemia and hypercarbia. Patients also experience increased atelectasis with spontaneous respiration and a decrease in functional residual capacity (FRC). All volatile anesthetics cause bronchodilation. Sevoflurane, halothane, and nitrous oxide are nonpungent, whereas desflurane and isoflurane are pungent and can lead to airway irritation with inhalational inductions and concentrations greater than 1 MAC.

CENTRAL NERVOUS SYSTEM EFFECTS

All inhaled anesthetics increase cerebral blood flow and decrease cerebral metabolic rate for oxygen ($CMRO_2$). Nitrous oxide, however, will increase $CMRO_2$. Nitrous oxide, as well as inhaled anesthetics, causes cerebral vasodilation. However,

if the patient's blood pressure drops, the increase in cerebral blood flow will be attenuated or abolished because volatile anesthetics inhibit autoregulation. Isoflurane causes the least cerebral vasodilation, maintaining autoregulation better than other volatile anesthetics. Isoflurane also has no effect on cerebrospinal fluid (CSF) production and decreases resistance to CSF absorption. Desflurane increases CSF production without significantly effecting CSF reabsorption.

Intracranial pressure (ICP) increases with all volatile anesthetics, but this can be counteracted by hypocapnia. Narcotics, barbiturates, and hypocapnia can blunt the increase in ICP seen with nitrous oxide use.

All volatile anesthetics and nitrous oxide depress the amplitude and increase the latency of somatosensory evoked potentials (SSEPs).

Increasing depth of anesthesia from the awake state leads to initial increased amplitude and synchrony of EEG tracings. As doses increase, the electroencephalogram (EEG) tracing progresses to electrical silence with an isoelectric pattern at 1.5-2 MAC. Sevoflurane may be associated with epileptiform activity on the EEG with higher concentrations.

Volatile anesthetics also produce dose-related skeletal muscle relaxation and work synergistically with neuromuscular blocking agents.

HEPATIC EFFECTS

Immune-mediated liver injury, though rare, can happen following anesthesia with any of the volatile anesthetics, typically requiring prior drug exposure.

Mild liver injury (related to halothane administration) can also occur, presumably due to decreases in hepatic blood flow and reductions in oxygen delivery to the liver in the presence of reductive metabolism of halothane.

RENAL EFFECTS

Transient volatile anesthetic effects on the cardiovascular, endocrine, and sympathetic nervous system affect renal function. They cause a dose-dependent reduction in renal blood flow, glomerular filtration rate, and urine output secondary to decreased blood pressure and CO. Sevoflurane, when used with soda lime CO_2 absorbent, produces compound A, a nephrotoxic metabolite, at low flows.

MUSCULOSKELETAL EFFECTS

All volatile anesthetics can act as triggering agents for malignant hyperthermia in susceptible individuals.

Minimum Alveolar Concentration

50

Vinh Nguyen, DO

The concept of minimum alveolar concentration (MAC) was first introduced by Dr. Edmund Eger in 1965. Prior to this time, there was no accurate way to measure the anesthetic potencies or adequate dosing. Earlier methods focused on the assessment of clinical signs, such as pupil diameter, eyelid reflex, and lacrimation during the different stages of anesthesia. Compared to the limitations associated with these signs, the principle of MAC targets a single clinical end point: immobility in response to surgical stimulus. MAC is defined as the minimum alveolar concentration of inhaled anesthetic at sea level required to suppress movement to a surgical incision in 50% of the patients. It is often referred to as the ED_{50} for immobility, MAC-movement, or median alveolar concentration.

Minimum alveolar concentration values were extrapolated from volatile agents using a pool of healthy human volunteers aged 30-55 years. After equilibration for 15 minutes at a particular end-tidal anesthetic concentration, a standard noxious stimulus was applied to the volunteer and observed for head or limb movement. A dose–response curve was developed based on the increasing or decreasing anesthetic concentration against movement (Figure 50-1). Minimum alveolar concentration or ED_{50} is the point on the curve at which 50% did not move in response to the stimulus. One standard deviation (SD) is about 10% of the MAC value. Therefore, 2 SDs will indicate a MAC value of 1.2 corresponding to the ED_{95}; 95% of the patients will not move with noxious stimulation. MAC is quantitative and can be applied to all inhaled anesthetics. The summation of each volatile agent's MAC value is additive, but the equipotent administration may differ on the physiologic effects, such as respiratory and hemodynamic effects.

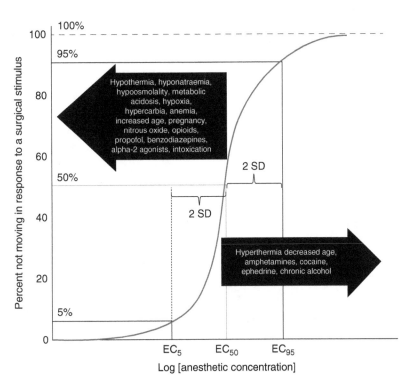

FIGURE 50-1 The anesthetic concentration and the percentage of patients not moving in response to noxious stimulus. (Reproduced from Aranake A et al. Minimum alveolar concentration: ongoing relevance and clinical utility. *Anaesthesia.* 2013; 68(5):512-522.)

COMPONENTS OF MAC

Voluntary Response (MAC-Awake)

The definition of MAC is generally used to measure the potency for immobility. Minimum alveolar concentration can be used to determine the potency for other desirable clinical features, which includes unconsciousness, amnesia, and eye-opening and autonomic response. *MAC-awake* has been used to measure the potency at which voluntary response to verbal command (ie, eye opening). It is defined as the anesthetic concentration needed to suppress the response to verbal command in 50% of the patients when anesthetic concentration is lowered during emergence. In contrast, *MAC-unawake* occurs when 50% of the patients remains responsive to verbal commands during an increase in anesthesia concentration during induction. Therefore, the induction pathway requires higher concentration for immobility and unresponsiveness than the concentration for restored movement. *MAC-awake* is generally one-third of its MAC for the commonly used inhaled agents (desflurane, sevoflurane, isoflurane) except halothane, which is half its MAC (Table 50-1).

Hypnosis and Amnesia (MAC-Amnesia)

MAC-amnesia is the anesthesia concentration required to suppress recollection or explicit memory of a noxious stimulus. The goal of anesthesia is to eliminate any explicit awareness of surgical or procedural events that can lead to post-traumatic stress disorder. In general, MAC-amnesia is much lower than MAC-skin incision. The activity of volatile agents affects the subcortical and cortical region of the brain, which mediate amnesia and unconsciousness. More specifically, the amygdala, hippocampus, and cortex are responsible for the formation of explicit episodic memory (conscious memory of events). Anterograde amnesia is achieved at a lower concentration (0.25 MAC) as compared to unconsciousness (0.5 MAC).

Suppress Autonomic Response (MAC-Blockade of Autonomic Responses [MAC-BAR])

MAC-BAR is the alveolar concentration of volatile anesthetic that blocks sympathetic response to surgical incision in 50% of the patients. These responses would correspond to changes in hemodynamic and pupil dilation. The determination of MAC-BAR is a measurement of catecholamine in venous blood. Its value has been calculated to be approximately 50% more than MAC (MAC 1.5).

Immobility (MAC)

Minimum alveolar concentration measures the immobility of a patient to a noxious stimulus. According to the early studies, the suppression of cortical electrical activity by inhaled anesthetic did not prevent movement. This suggested that another site beside the cortex was involved in immobility. Further studies using goats suggested that the spinal cord is involved. Goats were subjected to the separation of the brain and the spinal cord perfusion. Minimum alveolar concentration values were because of much higher concentration of isoflurane or halothane required for immobility. In additional studies, where a lesion severed the connection between the spinal cord and the brain, there was no alteration in MAC.

FACTORS THAT ALTER MAC (TABLE 50-2)

Numerous physiologic and pharmacological factors can alter the dose–response curve to change the potency of anesthetic by certain factors to the left (increase MAC) or to the right (decrease MAC). In certain situations, higher concentration of anesthetic is required, whereas those factors that decrease MAC may require lower anesthetic concentration to obtain similar clinical outcome. These alterations may not have the same impact on all the other MAC derivatives.

TABLE 50-2   Factors that Increase or Decrease the Value of MAC

Factors Increasing MAC	Factors Decreasing MAC	No Effect on MAC
Drugs	Drugs	Sex
Alcohol	Benzodiazepines	Duration of
(chronic)	(midazolam)	anesthesia
Ephedrine	Barbiturates	Hypocarbia or
Cocaine	Alpha-2 agonists (clonidine,	Hypercarbia
(acute)	dexmedetomidine)	Hypertension
Amphetamine	Opioid analgesia	Isovolemic
(acute)	Local anesthetics	anemia
Others	Ketamine	
Hypernatremia	Etomidate	
Hyperthermia	Amphetamine (chronic)	
Young age	Cocaine (chronic)	
(highest at	Lithium	
2-6 mo)	Verapamil	
Red hair	Alcohol (acute)	
	Others	
	Hyponatremia	
	Hypothermia	
	Elderly patients	
	Pregnancy	
	Anemia (hemoglobin	
	<5 g/dL)	
	Hypoxia	
	CNS injury or pathology	

TABLE 50-1   Commonly Used Volatile Agents: MAC and MAC-Awake Values

Agents	MAC	MAC-Awake	MAC-Awake/ MAC
Halothane	0.76	0.41	0.55
Isoflurane	1.15	0.49	0.38
Sevoflurane	2.0	0.62	0.34
Desflurane	6.0	2.5	0.34

Physiologic Factors

Although gender may not affect the anesthetic potency on MAC, MAC is age dependent. Human studies demonstrated that MAC is highest at 6 months of age, whereas age more than 40 years decreases in a linear relationship. A metaanalysis applied by Mapleson determined the relationship between age and MAC. The relationship suggests that each increasing decade of life after 40 years of age is associated with an approximately 6.0% decrease in MAC.

Temperature and its relationship to MAC have been extensively studied in animal and murine models. Minimum alveolar concentration decreases by 4%-5% per degree centigrade in a linear fashion. This may be due to the temperature effect on cerebral oxygen consumption.

Electrolyte disturbances, especially the sodium level, have similar MAC alteration compared to temperature. Hyponatremia has been determined to decrease MAC, whereas hypernatremia has been associated with an increase in MAC level. This can be due to changes in osmolality by sodium level in the CSF. Lower amount of anesthesia is required in pregnancy due to the increased production of progesterone affecting the CNS. Other causes that decrease MAC include severe anemia and hypoxia.

Pharmacological Factors

Certain pharmacological factors and substances can have a dramatic impact on MAC. Those patients who have an increased catecholamine level in the CNS will require a higher amount of anesthetic. Such drugs as acute usage of amphetamine or cocaine increase MAC, whereas their chronic usage lowers MAC requirements. On the other hand, the chronic usage of alcohol increases MAC, whereas acute usage decreases it. Prior to volatile anesthetic administration, adjuvant drugs such as barbiturates, benzodiazepines, and narcotics can cause a reduction in MAC. This is due to potentiating the activation of gamma-aminobutyric acid (GABA) causing mild sedative–hypnotic effect. In addition, non-GABAergic drugs, alpha-2 agonist or ketamine, have their own sedative property causing a reduction in MAC.

OTHER FACTORS

Those patients with cerebral vascular injury such as stroke, subdural hemorrhage, and traumatic brain injury have a decrease in anesthetic requirements. Degenerative brain disease, such as dementia, or hypoxic brain injury, such as cerebral palsy, will also have a dramatic lowering in MAC requirement. Other causes can include those with increased intracranial pressure such as hydrocephalus, large tumor, or subarachnoid hemorrhage that crowds the cranial vault and exerts pressure on the cortex. In general, any patient with a depressed level of consciousness will not need much anesthesia.

SUGGESTED READINGS

Ararnake A, Mashour G, Avidan M, et al. Minimum alveolar concentration: ongoing relevance and clinical utility. *Anaesthesia* 2013;68:512-522.

Eger E. Age, minimum alveolar anesthetic concentration and minimum alveolar anesthetic concentration-awake. *Anesth Analg* 2001;93:947-953.

Sonner JM, Antognin IE, Dutton RC, et al. Inhaled anesthetics and immobility: mechanism, mysteries, and minimum alveolar anesthetic concentration. *Anesth Analg* 2003;97:718-740.

Opioids

Sami Badri, MD, and Mehul Desai, MD, MPH

PHYSIOLOGY

Opioids are a class of endogenous, naturally occurring, and synthetic compounds that primarily provide analgesia. The effects of opioids are generated at an array of receptors found in peripheral, spinal cord, and brain tissues. Individual opioid receptors may be responsible for analgesia, muscle rigidity, depressed respiratory drive, bradycardia, hypotension, constipation, urinary retention, nausea, and sedation, to name several important clinical effects.

Pain is transmitted via a three-neuron system that originates at the periphery and ends at the cerebral cortex. At periphery tissues, noxious stimuli are mainly received and transmitted by A beta, A delta, and C fiber neurons. These first-order neurons synapse with second-order neurons in the dorsal horn of the spinal cord level. Second-order neurons travel up the spinal cord via the dorsal column and spinothalamic tract and synapse with third-order neurons at the thalamus, which then transmit signals to the cerebral cortex, the site of pain perception. Opioids exert their effects at receptors at all three levels of this system.

SPECIFIC PAIN MEDIATORS

Tissue injury at peripheral tissue causes the release of many different chemical mediators responsible for pain and physical changes at the site of injury. A host of major pain-inducing mediators originate from activated cells at the site of injury.

- **Bradykinin**—Originating from macrophages and plasma kininogen, this mediator activates nociceptors.
- **Serotonin**—Originating from platelets, this mediator activates nociceptors.
- **Histamine**—Originating from platelets and mast cells, this mediator causes vasodilation, edema, and pruritis.
- **Prostaglandin**—Originating from the cyclooxygenase (COX) pathway, this mediator sensitizes nociceptors.
- **Leukotriene**—Originating from the lipoxygenase pathway, this mediator sensitizes nociceptors.
- **H^+ ions**—Originating from tissue injury and ischemia, this mediator causes hyperalgesia associated with inflammation.

- **Cytokines (tumor necrosis factor [TNF], interleukins)**—Originating from macrophages, these mediators sensitize nociceptors.
- **Adenosine**—Originating from tissue injury, this mediator activates nociceptors and causes hyperalgesia.
- **Glutamate**—Originating from injured nerve terminals, this mediator activates nociceptors.
- **Substance P**—Originating from injured nerve terminals, this mediator activates macrophages and mast cells.
- **Nerve growth factor**—originating from macrophages, this mediator stimulates mast cells to release histamine and serotonin.

These pain mediators signal various receptors located throughout the three-neuron pain signal system. The transmitted signal travels to the cerebral cortex and is perceived as pain. Opioid therapy aims to block or attenuate a nociception signal by activating receptors that counter signal transmission. The major receptors activated by opioids are mu, delta, and kappa. These are G-coupled receptors, which carry the mediator-induced signal in conjunction with a second messenger such as cyclic adenosine monophosphate (cAMP). They are located at the periphery, the dorsal horn of the spinal cord, and finally the brainstem, thalamus, and cortex. At these locations, the three major mechanisms of action are:

1. Inhibition of presynaptic Ca^{2+} influx, which depolarizes the cell and inhibits the release of neurotransmitters at the synaptic cleft.
2. Increasing postsynaptic K^+ efflux, which depolarizes and inhibits cellular signal transmission.
3. Activation of the descending inhibitory pain pathway via inhibition of GABAergic receptors found in the brainstem.

By activating brainstem receptors, opioids also inhibit the release of nociceptive and inflammatory mediators such as substance P. In addition, opioids bind with other local and distant receptors that are responsible for the various side effects associated with opioid use. Each opioid compound has its own side effect profile-based receptor activity levels.

Specific Opioid Receptors

Receptor	Analgesia	Respiratory	Gastrointestinal (GI)	Endocrine	Other
mu	Peripheral		⇓GI secretions		Pruritis
			Biliary spasm		Muscle rigidity
					Urinary retention
mu1	Supraspinal		⇓GI transit	Prolactin release	Catalepsy
mu2	Spinal and supraspinal	Respiratory depression	⇓GI transit		Most cardiovascular effects
mu3					⇓Inflammation
kappa	Peripheral			⇓ADH	Sedation
kappa₁	Spinal				Antipruritic
kappa₂					
kappa₃	Supraspinal				
delta	Peripheral	Respiratory depression	⇓GI transit		Urinary retention
delta₁	Spinal				Dopamine turnover
delta₂	Supraspinal				

OPIOID EFFECTS

Analgesia

Opioid analgesia is primarily achieved at the brain, spinal cord, and peripheral tissues via mu1 and mu2 receptors. In the spinal cord, opioids target mu2 receptors. Supraspinal (periaqueductal gray matter, locus coeruleus, and nucleus raphe magnus) effects are achieved at mu1 receptors.

Minimum Alveolar Concentration (MAC) Effects

In animal studies, morphine decreases the MAC of volatile anesthetics in a dose-dependent manner. The maximum effect reduces volatile anesthetic requirements to 0.65 MAC. Morphine (1 mg/kg) in combination with nitrous oxide (60%), known as a "nitrous-narcotic" anesthetic, inhibits the adrenergic response to skin incision in 50% of patients (minimum alveolar concentration-blockade of adrenergic responses [MAC-BAR] effect). Fentanyl can also decrease the MAC requirement of volatile anesthetics. A fentanyl dose of 1.5 μg/kg 5 minutes prior to skin incision can block the adrenergic response to stimuli of isoflurane or desflurane in 60% nitrous oxide by 60%-70%.

Other CNS Effects

Opioids can cause sedation as well as cognitive and fine motor impairment. Additionally, opioids can cause euphoria, dysphoria, and sleep disturbances (decreased REM and slow-wave sleep). Dose-dependent miosis correlates well with opioid-induced ventilatory depression in the absence of other drugs. Hypoxemia from depressed ventilation, however, causes papillary dilation. Normeperidine, the meperidine metabolite, can cause CNS excitation, myoclonus, and seizures. Fentanyl causes a decrease in airway reflexes, especially cough, in a dose-dependent manner.

Endocrine Effects

Morphine decreases anti-diuretic hormone (ADH), adrenocorticotropic hormone (ACTH) beta-endorphin, follicle-stimulating hormone (FSH), and luteinizing hormone release. Opioids can increase prolactin and growth hormone (GH) concentrations. High-dose fentanyl (100 μg/kg) can decrease plasma epinephrine, cortisol, GH, free fatty acid, and glucose levels during surgery by inhibition of the stress response.

Respiratory Depression

Morphine and other mu1 agonists decrease CO_2 responsivity in the medullary respiratory center. There is a right shift and decrease in the slope of the ventilatory response to CO_2 curve.

Muscle Rigidity

High-dose morphine or fentanyl can reduce abdominal muscle and thoracic wall compliance via supraspinal mu receptors. This effect is greatly increased with the addition of nitrous oxide (70%). Myoclonus resembling seizure activity can occur (no EEG changes). Muscle rigidity can increase the difficulty of intubation if the masseter muscle is affected, and rigidity can also interfere with mechanical ventilation. Naloxone or GABA agonists reduce this side effect.

Gastrointestinal Effects

Morphine and other opioids decrease gastrointestinal (GI) motility and propulsion by stimulation of mu, kappa, and delta receptors at the brain, spinal cord, enteric, and smooth muscle tissues. Muscular tone is increased in both the small and large bowel, resulting in constipation. Morphine decreases lower esophageal sphincter tone, causing gastroesophageal reflux. Additionally, morphine increases the tone of the common bile duct and sphincter of Oddi. This is thought to be mediated by histamine release.

Genitourinary Effects

Inhibition of urethral sphincter relaxation causes urinary retention, and can be seen after systemic and neuraxial morphine administration.

Cardiovascular Effects

High-dose morphine administration can cause arteriolar and venous dilation, peripheral vascular tone reduction, and baroreceptor reflex inhibition. Opioids produce a dose-dependent bradycardia via sympatholytic and parasympathomimetic effects. They can be given to prevent tachycardia and myocardial O_2 demand. The action of morphine on mu3 receptors reduces inflammation in patients undergoing cardiopulmonary bypass (CPB). A 40-mg dose of morphine prior to CPB has been shown to improve global ventricular function and prevent postoperative hypothermia. Fentanyl has an excellent cardiovascular side effect profile. At high doses, fentanyl causes unconsciousness. It can be used as a sole agent for anesthesia due to its reliable hemodynamic stability although recall commonly occurs. Unlike morphine and meperidine, which can cause hypotension from histamine release, fentanyl does not significantly induce histamine release and hypotension is uncommon. Combining fentanyl with benzodiazepines, however, can cause marked cardiovascular depression. Fentanyl-induced bradycardia can be seen in anesthetized patients and responds to atropine therapy. Methadone can cause prolonged QT syndrome. Prolongation of the QT interval is used as a surrogate marker for the risk of developing potentially fatal arrhythmias such as torsades de pointes.

Protein Binding and Metabolism

Morphine is 35% protein bound (mostly albumin). It is primarily metabolized by hepatic phase II conjugation (3-glucuronidation) to form morphine-3-glucoronide (40% renal excretion) and morphine-6beta-glucoronide (M6G; 10% renal excretion). Morphine-6beta-glucoronide has high mu receptor affinity and, in chronic morphine therapy, M6G concentrations can be higher than parent compound levels. Since the kidneys excrete M6G, renal failure patients are more sensitive to morphine, necessitating caution. Methadone is 90% protein bound and undergoes N-demethylation in the liver. Fentanyl is extremely lipid soluble and has a rapid onset (<10 seconds) and roughly 60-minute plasma elimination. Fentanyl is 40% bound to red blood cells. Plasma fentanyl is 79%-87% protein bound (alpha-1-glycoprotein and albumin). Fentanyl is metabolized in the liver by N-dealkylation to norfentanyl and only 6% is excreted unchanged by the kidneys.

Other Effects

Meperidine has local anesthetic properties based on its chemical structure; therefore, neuraxial meperidine can cause sensory, motor, and sympatholytic effects not seen with other opioids. Through kappa-opioid receptors, meperidine and butorphanol can reduce shivering.

SPECIAL CONSIDERATIONS

The fentanyl derivatives *sufentanil* and *alfentanil* are very similar to fentanyl in regards to the above effects. An exception, alfentanil has been shown to increase cerebrospinal fluid pressures in patients with intracranial tumors. *Remifentanil* is most notably known for its short context-sensitive half-life: the time to 50% reduction in plasma concentration as a function of infusion duration. It is an ultra-short-acting opioid and is metabolized by blood and tissue esterases. Whereas all opioids and propofol suppress motor evoked potentials (MEPs) in a dose-dependent manner, remifentanil suppresses MEPs to a lesser extent.

The partial agonists and mixed agonist–antagonists *nalbuphine*, *butorphanol*, and *buprenorphine* have clinical effects at mu and kappa receptors. When combined with low doses of a full agonist compound, the effects of the partial agonist are additive up to the maximum, or "ceiling" effect of the partial agonist. With increasing doses of a full agonist, the partial agonist will behave as an antagonist.

Hydromorphone

Hydromorphone has 4-6 times the potency of morphine. The oral bioavailability is 20%-50%; additionally, hydromorphone has excellent subcutaneous bioavailability (78%). Its active metabolites are dihydromorphine and dihydroisomorphine. The inactive metabolite hydromorphone-3-glucuronide can accumulate in renal failure patients and cause neuroexcitation and cognitive impairment. Traditional opioid side effects, such as nausea, vomiting, sedation, cognitive impairment, and pruritis, are much less intense with hydromorphone when compared to morphine. The incidence of pruritis from neuraxial administration of hydromorphone is roughly 5% compared to 11%-77% with neuraxial morphine.

Barbiturates

Michelle Burnett, MD

Barbiturates are derivatives of barbituric acid. The presence of oxygen in the pyrimidine nucleus at carbon 2 position makes the drug an oxybarbiturate (eg, methohexital). In contrast, thiobarbiturates (eg, thiopental) have a sulfur atom at the carbon 2 position. Substitutions at carbon 5 position with either aryl or alkyl groups produce hypnotic and sedative effects. Phenyl groups enable the potent anticonvulsant activity. Thiamylal and thiopental, both thiobarbiturates, have similar pharmacological profiles and are available as racemic mixtures. Methohexital is marketed as a racemic mixture of two alpha isomers. The beta-1 stereoisomer form of methohexital produces excessive motor responses.

All of these barbiturates are available as sodium salts, and are mixed with either sodium chloride or sterile water to produce the solutions used for intravenous injection.

Thiobarbiturates have about 2 weeks' stability in solution, whereas methohexital has 6 weeks. Decreasing the solution's alkalinity by mixing the barbiturate with acidic solutions, lactated Ringer's solution, or water-soluble drugs can cause precipitation and occlusion of an intravenous line.

INDICATIONS

- Alternative induction drug for a patient allergic to propofol.
- Used for cerebral protection during incomplete brain ischemia.
- Facilitates electroconvulsive therapy or during identification of epileptic foci during surgery (methohexital).

CONTRAINDICATIONS

- Porphyrias (induces aminolevulinic synthetase and stimulates the formation of porphyrin).
- Hypovolemia (may cause significant reductions in cardiac output and blood pressure).

MECHANISM OF ACTION

Barbiturates depress nerve synapses in the reticular activating system, the portion of the nervous system responsible for the level of consciousness. Cellular mechanisms include inhibition of excitatory neurotransmission (acetylcholine and N-methyl-D-aspartate [NMDA]) and enhancement of inhibitory neurotransmission mediated by gamma-aminobutyric acid (GABA).

The GABA receptor is a chloride ion channel. When GABA binds to its receptor, chloride ion conductance increases. The cell membrane hyperpolarizes and increases the threshold for excitability. Thus, GABA is an inhibitory neurotransmitter and the principal one in the CNS. The GABA receptor consists of five subunits, each containing specific binding sites for GABA as well as for barbiturates. Barbiturates bind to the GABA receptor, and at lower concentrations, enhance the effects of GABA. The enhancement effect results from decreased GABA dissociation from the receptor with increased duration of activated-ion chloride channel openings. Higher barbiturate concentrations produces anesthesia from agonist binding of the barbiturate to a specific subunit of the GABA receptor. Barbiturates also inhibit excitatory neurotransmission via the NMDA glutaminergic system and suppression of acetylcholine release.

PHARMACOKINETICS

Barbiturates produce rapid (30-45 seconds) onset of unconsciousness following intravenous administration. Most barbiturates exist as a nonionized form and readily pass through the blood–brain barrier, leading to their fast onset of action. The degree of lipid solubility, nonionization state, and degree of protein binding affect the passage of barbiturates across the blood–brain barrier. Higher brain uptake occurs when there is a lowering of serum albumin (decreased protein binding) or plasma pH (increased nonionized fraction). Although thiopental is highly protein bound (80%), its highly nonionized fraction (60%) and great lipid solubility allow maximal brain uptake. Methohexital is 75% nonionized at physiologic pH and has a slightly faster onset than thiopental.

Redistribution is responsible for the awakening from a single induction dose of barbiturate. First, the drug is in the central blood compartment, followed by distribution to brain within 30 seconds. Next, redistribution to the peripheral compartment of lean tissue (muscle) terminates the effect of an induction dose. However, with infusion therapy or larger doses, a compartmental model with consideration of adipose tissue uptake and metabolic clearance explains recovery.

METABOLISM

With the exception of renally cleared phenobarbital, all barbiturates are metabolized by the liver with production of almost all inactive water-soluble metabolites. Desulfuration of higher doses of thiopental can result in an active metabolite pentobarbital. Excretion of metabolites occurs through urine and bile. Methohexital has a higher hepatic clearance than thiopental because of a higher hepatic extraction ratio. Methohexital shows an earlier return to psychomotor recovery than thiopental.

PHARMACODYNAMICS

Central Nervous System

Barbiturates produce a spectrum of effects on the central nervous system (CNS) from sleep, sedation to general anesthesia with loss of consciousness, amnesia, and cardiovascular depression. With low levels, barbiturates may be antianalgesic and decrease the pain threshold. Higher levels of barbiturates, such as with general anesthesia, obtund the response to pain. They do not produce muscle relaxation. Methohexital can provoke involuntary muscle contractions and may also elicit seizure activity. Thiopental in small doses (50-100 mg) can control grand mal seizures.

The multitude of effects of barbiturates on the CNS makes them useful drugs in the management of space-occupying cranial lesions:

- Dose-dependent cerebral vasoconstriction and cerebral metabolic rate.
- Reductions in intracranial pressure (ICP) and cerebral blood flow.
- Preservation of cerebral autoregulation.
- Dose-dependent depression of EEG activity.
- Minimal effects on somatosensory evoked potentials (SSEPs), motor evoked potentials (MEPs).
- Dose-dependent depression of brainsteam auditory evoked potentials (BAEP).
- Provides neuroprotection for focal cerebral ischemia but not for global ischemia.

Cardiovascular

Through peripheral and central mechanisms, barbiturates decrease blood pressure and increase heart rate:

- Depression of medullary vasomotor center vasodilates peripheral capacitance vessels.
- Decreases preload to the right atrium.
- Decrease in contractility from reduction of available calcium in myofibrils.
- Central vagolytic effect with tachycardia.

The effects will vary depending on volume status, autonomic tone, presence of cardiac disease, and concurrent beta-adrenergic receptor blockade.

Respiratory

- Dose-dependent central respiratory depression.
- Diminished minute ventilation.
- Depression of the medullatory ventilatory response to hypercapnia and hypoxia.
- Airway obstruction with sedation.
- Incomplete suppression of noxious airway reflexes with bronchospasm in asthmatics or laryngospasm in lightly anesthetized patients.

Renal and Hepatic

- Reduces renal and hepatic blood flow and glomerular filtration rate in proportion to the fall in blood pressure.
- Induction of hepatic enzymes with increased metabolic rate of some drugs.
- Combination with cytochrome P450 enzyme interferes with biotransformation of others.

SIDE EFFECTS AND TOXICITY

- Garlic or onion taste (thiopental).
- Rare anaphylactic and anaphylactoid allergic reactions.
- Sulfur-containing thiobarbiturates evoke mast cell histamine release *in vitro*.
- Intraarterial injection results in severe vasoconstriction.

Propofol

Chris Potestio, MD, and Brian S. Freeman, MD

Since its introduction in the early 1980s, propofol has been a cornerstone of anesthetic practice. Propofol is an intravenous anesthetic used for the induction and maintenance of general anesthesia and for sedation in and outside of the operating room.

STRUCTURE AND FORMULATION

The structure of propofol is 2, 6-diisopropylphenol (Figure 53-1). As an alkylphenol derivative, propofol exists as an oil at room temperature. Because it is highly lipophilic and insoluble in aqueous solution, propofol is formulated in a rather complicated 1% (10 mg/mL) lipid solution, containing 10% soybean oil, 2.25% glycerol, 1.2% purified egg phosphatide, and 0.0005% sodium edetate (antimicrobial).

The incidence of anaphylactic reactions to propofol is around 1:20 000, but more common in patients with eczema and/or multiple food allergies. Common clinical practice is to avoid administering propofol to patients with soybean, peanut, and egg allergies due to its formulation with similar products. Despite this "clinical wisdom," most egg allergies are to egg protein (whites) rather than the egg phosphatide (yolk) that makes up the propofol solution. Avoiding the use of propofol in those with egg allergy may not be warranted.

PHARMACOKINETICS

Propofol has a very favorable pharmacokinetic profile (Table 53-1). After a single bolus injection, it is quickly redistributed and eliminated. It is rapidly metabolized in the liver

TABLE 53-1 Pharmacokinetic Profile for Propofol

	Time	Implication
Time to peak effect	90-100 seconds	"Vein to brain" time
Initial distribution half-life	2-8 min	Distribution to highly perfused organs (heart, brain, liver)
Slow distribution half-life	30-70 min	Distribution to organs with limited perfusion (muscle, fat)
Context-sensitive half-life	40 min	Time it takes to decrease concentration by half after achieving steady state via infusion—remains the same for the first ~8 h of infusion
Central volume of distribution	20-40 L	
Volume of distribution (steady state)	150-700 L	

by conjugation to glucuronide and sulfate to produce inactive water-soluble compounds that are excreted by the kidneys. Clearance of propofol exceeds liver metabolism, suggesting extra-hepatic metabolism. This fact is confirmed during the anhepatic phase of liver transplant surgery. The kidneys account for roughly 30% of total body clearance. The lungs have also been implicated in propofol metabolism and are responsible for 30% uptake and first-pass metabolism after bolus dose. Propofol exhibits concentration-dependent inhibition of cytochrome P450, specifically CYP 3A4. It may alter metabolism of other drugs that are metabolized by this system, such as opiates and midazolam, which are both often coadministered during induction.

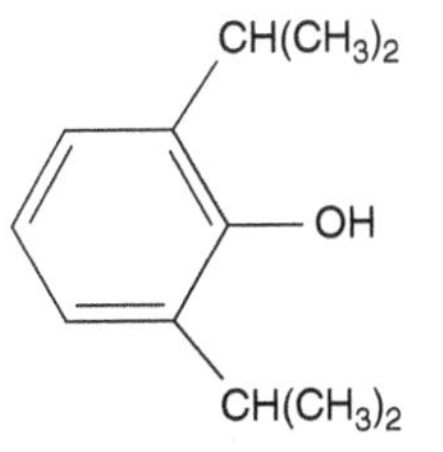

Fospropofol (phosphono-O-methyl 0-2, 6-diisopropylphenol) is a prodrug of propofol with a slightly longer time to peak effect and a prolonged effect. Fospropofol undergoes hydrolysis by endothelial cell surface alkaline phosphates, releasing propofol, along with formaldehyde and an inorganic phosphate group. It is approved for use but not often utilized due

FIGURE 53-1 Structure of propofol.

to its unpredictable pharmacokinetics. The time to maximum concentration of fospropofol is approximately 7 minutes.

EFFECTS ON ORGAN SYSTEMS

Central Nervous System

The hypnotic effects of propofol are achieved by agonism at the beta subunit of GABA-A receptors in the central nervous system (CNS). Stimulation of gamma-aminobutyric acid (GABA-A) receptors produces diffuse CNS inhibition with specific attention to the inhibition of acetylcholine release in the hippocampus and prefrontal cortex. The hypnotic effect may also be due to the inhibition of the N-methyl-D-aspartate (NMDA) subtype of glutamate receptors.

Due to its global potentiation of GABA inhibition, propofol has many advantageous effects in the CNS, namely hypnosis, sedation, and amnesia. Propofol is not an analgesic but lacks the antianalgesic effects of barbiturates. At high induction doses (2.5 mg/kg), propofol will cause rapid hypnosis that will last for 5-10 minutes. Its duration of action is dose dependent and varies with age. Younger patients require a higher induction dose. At lower doses (<2 mg/kg/hour), propofol can cause sedation and amnesia, while not causing hypnosis.

EEG monitoring during propofol infusion gives some insight into its effect on the CNS. When it is administered with a loading dose of 2.5 mg/kg followed by infusion, propofol causes burst suppression and is, therefore, a recommended therapy for refractory status epilepticus. Although there have been reports of seizures after propofol administration, these seizures are likely from withdrawal of propofol's anticonvulsant effect in patients with epilepsy. EEG during propofol administration shows an initial increase in alpha frequency, followed by increased gamma and theta frequencies.

Propofol decreases intracranial pressure (ICP) by 30%-50% by decreasing cerebral metabolic rate of O_2 consumption ($CMRO_2$) and cerebral blood flow (CBF). This decrease in ICP would imply that propofol should cause an increase in cerebral perfusion pressure (CPP); however, administration of propofol has a greater effect on mean arterial pressure (MAP) than it does on ICP. The net effect is a reduction in CBF and CPP, despite a decrease in ICP.

Propofol also acutely decreases intraocular pressure (30%-40%).

Respiratory System

Propofol is a profound respiratory depressant, more so than any other IV anesthetic. Propofol will cause respiratory depression in a dose-dependent manner, with induction dose (2.5 mg/kg) causing apnea in 25%-35% of the patients. Respiratory depression is potentiated by concomitant premedication, such as opiates or benzodiazepines.

In a healthy patient, the medullary respiratory center causes reflexive breathing in response to normal $Paco_2$ levels (~40 mm Hg). Propofol blunts this response, and the $Paco_2$

required for spontaneous ventilation during propofol administration will be much higher than 40 mm Hg. In addition, propofol decreases tidal volume by roughly 15%, even with low-dose infusions (100-200 µg/kg/min).

Cardiovascular System

At induction doses (2.5 mg/kg), propofol produces a 25%-40% decrease in systolic and diastolic blood pressure via effects on preload, afterload, and contractility. It is primarily a vasodilator, leading to decrease in preload. In addition, propofol decreases myocardial contractility, reducing stroke volume and cardiac output. Systemic vascular resistance is also reduced. The effect of propofol on the cardiovascular system can be linked to its attenuation of the sympathetic drive of the heart and vasculature. Blunting of the baroreceptor reflex means that heart rate does not change significantly with propofol induction. Propofol, in combination with fentanyl, increases the incidence of hypotension with induction. An infusion of propofol decreases both myocardial blood flow and myocardial oxygen consumption; hence, the overall supply and demand of myocardial oxygen remains the same. It may have cardioprotective properties.

Other Effects

Propofol causes a sense of euphoria. The drug has been associated with increased dopamine concentrations in the nucleus accumbens, a region which is part of the "pleasure pathway" implicated in many euphoria-inducing drugs.

Propofol has antiemetic properties. When administered as an infusion, it can be more effective than antiemetics like ondansetron in preventing postoperative nausea and vomiting. A bolus dose of 10 mg propofol has also been shown to be effective as an antiemetic. As a result of potentiation of GABA receptor activity, propofol also decreases serotonin levels in the area postrema. This decrease in serotonin is likely the reason for its antiemetic effect.

Propofol decreases pruritis after administration of spinal opioids.

Unlike potent inhalation anesthetics, propofol does not potentiate neuromuscular blockade. Propofol is a useful option during neurosurgery cases where neurologic monitoring is used and neuromuscular activity must be preserved.

SIDE EFFECTS

Although the chief concern when administering an induction dose of propofol is profound hypotension and respiratory depression, other side effects have also been documented:

- Since the lipid formulation is a friendly medium for bacterial growth, there is an increased incidence of bacteremia and sepsis. An opened vial or syringe of propofol should be discarded after 6 hours.

- The lipid formulation may lead to hypertriglyceridemia and the development of pancreatitis.
- Pain on injection is associated with propofol administration. Several strategies have been employed to decrease pain on injection, such as using a large vein and mixing the propofol solution with lidocaine.
- Myoclonus is a less common side effect. It is self-limiting and usually lasts for less than a minute.
- Thrombophlebitis in the injected vein is a rare complication but causes significant morbidity when it does occur.
- Propofol infusion syndrome (PRIS) is a rare but serious side effect of propofol infusion (>4 mg/kg/hour) over long periods (>48 hours). It was first observed in the pediatric ICU setting, but later related to the adult critical care population. Long-term exposure to propofol infusion may lead to acute refractory bradycardia and eventually asystole. There is also concomitant metabolic acidosis, rhabdomyolysis, hyperlipidemia, and enlarged or fatty liver. The proposed mechanisms of PRIS include mitochondrial toxicity, tissue dysoxia, and carbohydrate deficiency. Risk factors include high propofol dose, sepsis, shock, previous cerebral injury. Lipemia, likely related to poor hepatic function secondary to hepatic dysoxia, has been reported as a laboratory abnormality that may signal the early development of PRIS.
- Propofol does not cause malignant hypothermia.

USES

1. **Induction**—Propofol is a widely used agent for induction of general anesthesia (1-2.5 mg/kg). Premedication with opiates and/or benzodiazepines potentiates the effect of propofol and lowers the induction dose. A lower dose is also recommended for patients older than 60 years (1-1.75 mg/kg). Hemodynamic depression is a major concern during anesthetic induction, with older patients. Patients with multiple comorbidities (ASA physical status III or IV) are more likely to experience a sharp drop in blood pressure during induction. Hypotension during induction can be partially prevented by aggressive fluid resuscitation prior to induction, as well as by diluting the propofol solution to 0.5 mg/mL.

2. **Maintenance**—Propofol is also a widely used agent for anesthetic maintenance. It provides rapid recovery from anesthesia comparable to that of older volatile anesthetics. When compared to newer volatile anesthetics (desflurane, sevoflurane), propofol has a slightly slower recovery period but is associated with far less postoperative nausea and vomiting. It can be given as intermittent boluses of 10-40 mg as needed or as an infusion of 50-250 µg/kg/min. It can be combined with opiates, midazolam, clonidine, and ketamine to provide total intravenous anesthesia (TIVA).

3. **Sedation**—Propofol is also used for sedation during minor surgical procedures and in the ICU setting. Again, its rapid rate of recovery after stopping the infusion makes it an ideal drug in this setting. The rapid recovery does not increase with infusion time, making it ideal for long-term sedation in the ICU setting. At 24 and 96 hours, the recovery to consciousness when the infusion is discontinued is about 10 minutes. Also the plasma concentration decreases at a similar rate at either time point. For small procedures, conscious sedation may be the preferred method of anesthesia. Infusions as low as 30 µg/kg/min cause amnesia in most patients.

SUGGESTED READING

Kam PC, Cardone D. Propofol infusion syndrome. *Anaesthesia* 2007;62:690-701.

Etomidate

Elizabeth E. Holtan, MD

First introduced into clinical practice in 1972, etomidate has a long history of use as an intravenous anesthetic and sedative. Like propofol, etomidate has a hypnotic effect but does not provide any analgesia. It is preferred primarily for its stable effect on circulatory hemodynamics in patients with decreased myocardial contractility. Etomidate is also indicated for anesthetic induction in patients with severe neurologic disease, such as elevated intracranial hypertension, who require maintenance of cerebral perfusion pressure. Etomidate may also be particularly useful as an anesthetic for emergency intubation in ICU or trauma patients.

Etomidate has the chemical structure of a carboxylated imidazole (Figure 54-1). Its mechanism of action targets the major inhibitory ion channels in the brain: the gamma-aminobutyric acid (GABA$_A$) receptors. Potentiation, or positive modulation, of GABA$_A$ receptors increases chloride ion conduction, leading to neuronal hyperpolarization and depression of the reticular activating system.

PHARMACOKINETICS AND METABOLISM

The standard induction dose is 0.2-0.3 mg/kg. Because of its high lipid solubility, etomidate has a rapid onset of action. Its elimination half-life is 2-4 minutes with a duration of 3-8 minutes. Every 0.1 mg/kg dose leads to about 100 seconds of unconsciousness. Redistribution is responsible for the recovery and emergence from etomidate. Although the drug has a short context-sensitive half-life, it is rarely given in repeated doses or by infusion due to concern over adrenocortical suppression. More than 75% of the drug will bind to plasma proteins but with decreased protein binding in severe liver disease and uremia. End-stage liver disease leads to increased volume of distribution and decreased clearance of etomidate.

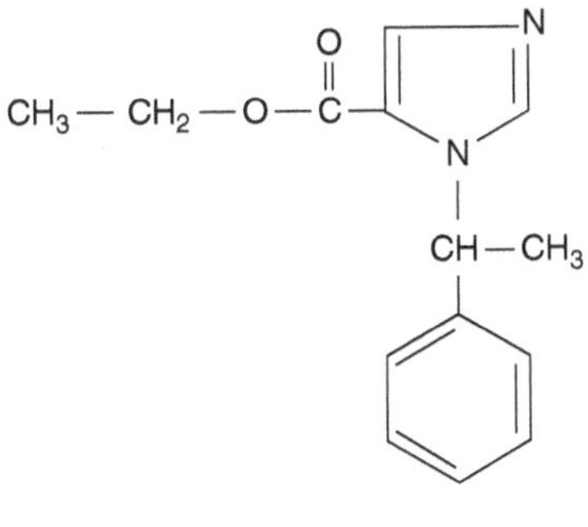

Degradation into inactive metabolites occurs mostly due to ester hydrolysis, primarily in the liver but also in the plasma. Etomidate has a high rate of clearance. Metabolites are excreted in urine (80%) and bile (20%). Less than 3% of etomidate is excreted unchanged in urine.

EFFECT ON ORGAN SYSTEMS

1. **Circulation**—Most anesthetic induction agents are associated with cardiovascular instability. In contrast, etomidate decreases systemic vascular resistance to a much lesser degree. Mean arterial blood pressure usually is maintained or only slightly decreased. Etomidate does not cause significant alterations in heart rate, cardiac output, central venous pressure, pulmonary artery pressure, and pulmonary occlusion pressure. Decreases in myocardial contractility can occur but are negligible with common induction doses. Blood pressure is more likely to decrease in patients with hypovolemia. Of note, etomidate does not blunt the sympathetic responses to laryngoscopy and intubation, so opioids are usually coadministered at induction. Because of these properties, etomidate is the induction agent of choice in patients for whom cardiac stability is of upmost importance.

2. **Respiration**—Etomidate can cause respiratory depression but to a lesser degree than other induction agents. Apnea is more likely to occur when etomidate is combined with opioids and inhalation anesthetics. Due to the lack of histamine release, etomidate is a safe anesthetic for patients with reactive airway disease as it is not associated with histamine release. Hiccups or coughing may occur during its administration.

3. **Endocrine**—Etomidate inhibits 11-beta-hydroxylase, the enzyme that converts cholesterol to cortisol. Decreased synthesis of cortisol and aldosterone can lead to adrenal

FIGURE 54-1   Structure of etomidate.

155

insufficiency. After a single induction dose, the adrenocortical suppression effect may last for up to 8 hours. Due to these concerns, etomidate is contraindicated in a patient at higher risk for the effects of adrenal suppression, such as those receiving chronic steroids. Furthermore, etomidate should not be given in repeated boluses or as a continuous infusion. Continuous infusions of etomidate for sedation in the intensive care unit have been associated with increased mortality.

4. **Central nervous system**—Etomidate reduces cerebral blood flow and intracranial pressure due to cerebral vasoconstriction. Adequate cerebral perfusion pressure is maintained by the stable mean arterial blood pressure. Although etomidate decreases the cerebral metabolic rate of oxygen and causes burst suppression, it has not been shown to be effective in neuroprotection in humans. Etomidate may increase excitatory spikes on EEG and lower the seizure threshold, making the drug useful during electroconvulsive therapy to produce longer seizures. Up to 50% of the patients will have myoclonus when given etomidate, which is often hidden by coadministration of muscle relaxants, opioids, or benzodiazepines. These muscle contractions can be associated with seizure activity on EEG. Unlike most other intravenous anesthetics, etomidate increases the amplitude and minimally decreases the latency of somatosensory evoked potentials. Etomidate can also be associated with decreased intraocular pressure.

5. **Hematologic**—Etomidate may inhibit platelet function and prolong bleeding time.

SIDE EFFECTS AND TOXICITY

Since etomidate is insoluble in water, the drug requires formulation with 35% propylene glycol to achieve stability at normal pH. This solvent can cause burning on injection, vein irritation, and thrombophlebitis. Administration of intravenous lidocaine prior to etomidate may decrease the pain on injection. The propylene glycol solvent may cause hemolysis.

Etomidate has significant emetogenic properties. It is not an ideal choice in patients who are at risk for severe postoperative nausea and vomiting.

Toxicity is unlikely in most patients because the lethal dose is 30 times greater than the effective dose. Therefore, it has a wider margin of safety. Even so, decreased dosing is appropriate for patients with end-stage liver disease.

SUGGESTED READINGS

Cuthbertson BH, Sprung CL, Annane D, et al. The effects of etomidate on adrenal responsiveness and mortality in patients with septic shock. *Intensive Care Med* 2009;35:1868-1876.

Forman SA. Clinical and molecular pharmacology of etomidate. *Anesthesiology*. 2011;114:695-707.

Benzodiazepines

Michelle Burnett, MD

The most common intravenous benzodiazepines administered in the perioperative setting are midazolam, diazepam, and lorazepam. Benzodiazepines produce hypnosis, sedation, anxiolysis, anterograde amnesia, anticonvulsion, and centrally produced muscle relaxation. They do not provide any analgesia. Benzodiazepines are primarily used for premedication and sedation and also for induction of general anesthesia in high doses. Benzodiazepines may be associated with higher risk of postoperative cognitive dysfunction in the elderly.

The chemical structure of this class of drugs consists of a benzene ring with a seven-member diazepine ring. Substitutions at various positions on the rings distinguish the drugs. The imidazole ring of midazolam allows for water solubility at a low pH (3.5) and preparation in an aqueous solution. At physiologic pH, midazolam increases its lipid solubility by an intramolecular rearrangement. Intravenous diazepam and lorazepam solutions contain propylene glycol (associated with venous irritation) due to their water insolubility.

MECHANISM OF ACTION

Benzodiazepines act by enhancing inhibitory neurotransmission through their interaction with the gamma-aminobutyric acid (GABA) receptors. These drugs enhance the efficiency of coupling between the chloride ion channel and the GABA receptor, leading to enhanced inhibition via cellular hyperpolarization. Different GABA receptor subtypes mediate each clinical effect. Alpha-1 receptors modulate sedation, anterograde amnesia, and anticonvulsion. Alpha-2 receptors modulate anxiolysis and muscle relaxation. Central nervous system (CNS) effects depend on each drug's particular stereospecific affinity for a receptor subtype as well as their degree of binding. The order for receptor affinity is lorazepam>midazolam>diazepam. Effects are dose dependent. Receptor saturation can produce a ceiling effect. Flumazenil reverses the effects of benzodiazepines by acting as an antagonist on these same receptors.

PHARMACOKINETICS

Benzodiazepines may be administered orally, intramuscularly (not diazepam), or intravenously. Diazepam and lorazepam are well absorbed from the gastrointestinal tract. Midazolam undergoes first-pass effect, requiring an increase in its oral dosing.

Due to high lipid solubility with intravenous administration, both diazepam and midazolam readily cross the blood–brain barrier with onset of CNS effects within 2-3 minutes. Moderately lipid-soluble lorazepam has a slightly longer onset of action. Effects of a single dose are terminated by redistribution with awakening, which occurs within 3-10 minutes. The elimination phases of these drugs are dependent upon their metabolism.

METABOLISM

Hepatic metabolism via oxidation and glucuronide conjugation transforms benzodiazepines into water-soluble end products which are excreted in the urine. The phase I metabolite of diazepam, desmethyldiazepam, is an active compound with a long half-life. Enterohepatic circulation of diazepam produces a secondary peak in plasma concentration at 6-12 hours with possible resedation. Midazolam results in an active metabolite, hydroxymidazolam, which has mild CNS effects and can accumulate in renal failure.

Hepatic clearance for midazolam is 5 times that of lorazepam and 10 times that of diazepam. Elimination half-lives vary from 2 hours for midazolam, 11 hours for lorazepam, and 20 hours for diazepam. Midazolam has a higher hepatic extraction ratio; most of the drug is removed from the blood as it flows from the liver (perfusion-limited clearance). Elimination of lorazepam and diazepam rely more on enzyme activity and less on hepatic flow (capacity-limited clearance).

Benzodiazepine oxidation may be impaired with liver disease, and inhibited by some hepatic enzyme inhibitors. Cimetidine binds to cytochrome P450 and reduces the metabolism of diazepam. Erythromycin inhibits the metabolism of midazolam with a two- to threefold prolongation of effects. Heparin displaces diazepam from protein binding sites and increases the unbound percentage of drug.

PHARMACODYNAMICS

Cardiovascular

- Minimal cardiovascular depression even with induction doses.
- Slight reduction in arterial blood pressure from a decrease in systemic vascular resistance.
- Heart rate may rise due to preservation of homeostatic reflex mechanism or vagolysis.
- Combination with an opioid will produce greater decreases in systemic blood pressure and reduce sympathetic tone.

Respiratory

- Dose-related central respiratory system depression (more pronounced in patients with chronic obstructive pulmonary disease (COPD) and additive synergistic effect in combination with opioids.
- Depresses ventilatory response to carbon dioxide.
- Depresses swallowing reflex and upper airway reflex activity.

Cerebral

- Dose-related reduction in cerebral metabolic oxygen consumption ($CMRO_2$) and cerebral blood flow (CBF).
- Normal ratio of $CMRO_2$ to CBF.
- Preserves cerebral vasomotor responsiveness to CO_2.
- Potent anticonvulsant, but not neuroprotective.
- Increases the seizure threshold to local anesthetic.
- Does not produce burst suppression isoelectric pattern on electroencephalography (EEG).

FLUMAZENIL

Flumazenil is a competitive antagonist for benzodiazepines at the GABA receptor. Reversal occurs within 2 minutes with a peak effect at 10 minutes. It is short acting and has a 1-hour half-life. Flumazenil is rapidly metabolized by the liver. Recurrence of sedation may occur. Flumazenil should not be given if benzodiazepines are used to treat convulsions.

SIDE EFFECTS AND TOXICITY

- Superficial thrombophlebitis and pain with propylene glycol vehicles in diazepam and lorazepam.
- Crosses the placenta causing neonatal depression.
- Possibility of increased risk of cleft palate with administration during first trimester of pregnancy.

Ketamine

Kumudhini Hendrix, MD

Ketamine is a water-soluble intravenous anesthetic that is structurally related to the psychotropic drug phencyclidine (PCP). It was first synthesized in 1962 and named "C1581" by Parke-Davis Research Laboratory. Clinical evaluation began in 1965 with approval for patient use 5 years later. In the early 1970s, ketamine was widely used as a field anesthetic by the United States during the Vietnam War.

Ketamine has an aryl cyclohexamine chemical structure in which one asymmetric carbon atom results in two optical isomers. The S(+) enantiomer is 3 times more potent and longer acting than the R(–) enantiomer. Unlike other intravenous anesthetics, ketamine produces a unique dissociative anesthetic state in which there is functional and electrophysiologic separation of the thalamocortical and limbic systems. This state is characterized by profound analgesia, amnesia, and catalepsy. The patient is unconscious but appears awake.

PHARMACODYNAMIC PROFILE

Central Nervous System

The primary site of action of ketamine occurs within the thalamus and limbic system where the drug binds to *N*-methyl-D-aspartate (NMDA) receptors. These receptors are thought to play a major role in the relay of sensory information. Noncompetitive antagonism of NMDA receptors by ketamine results in catalepsy and high-amplitude slowing of EEG waves. However, ketamine also interacts with other CNS receptors. Binding of ketamine to the mu-opioid receptor provides its unique analgesic effects at subanesthetic doses. Not surprisingly, ketamine has cross-tolerance with morphine. However, the analgesic effect of ketamine cannot be reversed by naloxone. In addition, ketamine can bind to the sigma opioid (PCP binding site) receptor resulting in dysphoria. Lastly, ketamine interacts with muscarinic and nicotinic cholinergic receptors producing a dose-dependent potentiation of the nondepolarizing muscle relaxants. Physostigmine may reverse some of the effects of ketamine.

Historically, ketamine has been thought to increase intracranial pressure (ICP), making the drug contraindicated in patients with brain injury. An increase in mean arterial pressure (MAP) leads to higher cerebral perfusion pressure, thus raising ICP. Antagonism of the NMDA receptor causes vasodilation of the cerebral vasculature, increasing cerebral blood flow by nearly 80% and contributing to higher ICP. Preadministration of benzodiazepines or thiopental may attenuate this pressure increase. However, recent studies show that ketamine does not always cause an increase in ICP. Ketamine may actually reduce cerebral infarct volume and improve neurologic outcome in rats with brain trauma. Antagonism of the neurotoxic effects of glutamate at the NMDA receptor may serve as the underlying mechanism.

Cardiovascular

Ketamine is a direct myocardial depressant and vascular smooth muscle relaxant. At the same time, however, the drug also increases circulating catecholamines by decreasing neuronal reuptake. These increases in norepinephrine levels are easily blocked by alpha and beta adrenergic receptor and sympathetic ganglion blockade. Benzodiazepines may also attenuate the cardiovascular stimulating effects of ketamine. In the pulmonary vasculature, ketamine increases pulmonary vascular resistance through vasoconstriction. Overall, the cardiovascular stimulating effects of ketamine outperform its myocardial depressant effects. The net result after ketamine induction is an increase in blood pressure, heart rate, cardiac output, and myocardial oxygen consumption. In contrast, ketamine will cause a decrease in blood pressure and cardiac output in critically ill patients who have depleted their catecholamine stores and lack the ability to compensate via the sympathetic nervous system.

Respiratory

Unlike other general anesthetics, ketamine maintains minute ventilation, skeletal muscle tone, and laryngeal reflexes. The minute ventilation–carbon dioxide curve is shifted to the left with the slope unchanged. Apnea only occurs through a rapid bolus or concomitant administration of respiratory depressants like opioids. Patients will develop minimal atelectasis, changes in ventilation or pulmonary perfusion, or depression of functional residual capacity. However, ketamine does not prevent the risk of aspiration. Ketamine is a potent stimulator of salivary and tracheobronchial secretions. It is possible to attenuate the secretions to concomitant administration of anticholinergic drugs (with glycropyrrolate being more effective than atropine). In addition, ketamine is a potent bronchodilator that directly relaxes the smooth muscle of the tracheobronchial tree and stimulates the sympathetic nervous system. Continuous infusion of ketamine has been used to treat refractory asthma attacks.

Maternal–Fetal System

Ketamine is classified as a fetal category C medication (benefits should clearly outweigh the risks). In chick embryos, large doses of ketamine resulted in neural tube defects. Conversely, in rats, up to 120 mg/kg of ketamine to the mother did not result in teratogenesis. No reproductive studies have been performed in humans. Ketamine passes rapidly to placenta and reaches peak levels within 2 minutes of administration. Compared to sodium thiopental (3 mg/kg), an induction dose of ketamine (1 mg/kg) in parturients results in neonates with similar Apgar scores. However, a 2 mg/kg ketamine induction dose produces neonatal depression and increased uterine tone. If ketamine is used for labor analgesia prior to delivery of the baby, it should be administered in incremental doses that do not exceed 1 mg/kg in 30 minutes or 100 mg total.

Other Effects

The addition of S(+) ketamine to caudal bupivacaine results in prolonged analgesia compared to intravenous S(+) ketamine. This effect suggests a possible neuraxial component to the analgesic properties of ketamine. Ketamine is safe for use in patients at high risk for malignant hyperthermia or porphyria. Intravenous infusions of ketamine are now in use for the management of refractory depression. N-methyl-D-aspartate antagonism seems to be the underlying mechanism for this antidepressant effect. The treatment can be effective as quickly as 15 minutes.

PHARMACOKINETIC PROFILE

Ketamine may be administered by intravenous (1-2 mg/kg), intramuscular (5-10 mg/kg), oral (8 mg/kg), and rectal (8 mg/kg) routes without irritation. Peak plasma concentration occurs within 1, 10, 30, and 45 minutes, respectively. In the plasma, ketamine becomes highly lipid soluble and distributed to highly perfused tissues, including the brain, where it quickly achieves a concentration about 4 times the plasma level. Redistribution occurs within 10 minutes, but the elimination half-life is about 2 hours. In the liver, cytochrome P450 enzymes methylate ketamine into its active metabolite norketamine, which has about one-third anesthetic potency. Eventually, norketamine becomes hydroxylated and conjugated to a water-soluble compound for excretion into the urine. Diazepam inhibits cytochrome P450, thereby prolonging the effects of ketamine. Because its hepatic clearance has a high intrinsic extraction ratio (0.9), changes in hepatic blood flow can greatly impact ketamine metabolism. Oral administration of ketamine results in high levels of norketamine due to the first-pass effect, resulting in prolonged anesthesia. This results in prolonged anesthetic effect. Ketamine is finally eliminated in the urine. Only a small percentage of the drug is unchanged in urine. Chronic ketamine administration, such as in burn patients, results in enzyme induction and tolerance. Dependence may also occur.

ADVERSE EFFECTS

- Increased secretions.
- Preserved or increased muscular tone.
- Difficulty assessing depth of anesthesia (due to maintenance of corneal reflexes).
- Prolonged recovery time.
- Dysphoria, unpleasant dreams, hallucinations, and emergence delirium (attenuated with benzodiazepines).

SUGGESTED READINGS

Oye I. Ketamine analgesia: NMDA receptors and the gates of perception. *Acta Anaesthesiol Scand* 1998;42:747-749.

Rabben T, Skjelbred P, Oye I. Prolonged analgesic effect of ketamine, an N-methyl-D-aspartate receptor inhibitor, in patients with chronic pain. *J Pharmacol Exp Ther* 1999;289:1060-1066.

Werther, JR. Ketamine anesthesia. *Anesth Prog* 1985;32(5):185-188.

Local Anesthetics

Brian S. Freeman, MD

Local anesthetics are used to provide intraoperative regional anesthesia and postoperative analgesia. Synthesized from the coca plant in 1860, cocaine was the first local anesthetic adapted for clinical use. Although quite effective, cocaine has significant limitations. It has addictive potential, can irritate nerves, and is still the only local anesthetic capable of blocking norepinephrine reuptake at postganglionic sympathetic nerve terminals. The introduction of lidocaine in 1948 began the modern era of local anesthetics.

GENERAL PROPERTIES

Chemical Structure

All currently available local anesthetics consist of three components:

1. Aromatic benzene ring
2. Tertiary amine
3. Intermediate hydrocarbon linkage
   - Ester (–COO–)
   - Amide (–NH–CO–)

Based on the chemical bond, local anesthetics are classified into two groups: esters and amides (Figure 57-1).

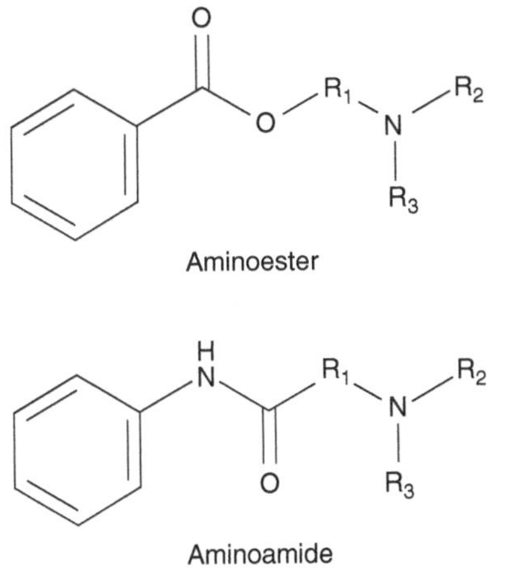

Aminoester

Aminoamide

FIGURE 57-1

Commonly used ester local anesthetics include benzocaine, 2-chloroprocaine, cocaine, procaine, and tetracaine. Since ester links are more easily broken, these drugs are relatively unstable in solution. Commonly used amide local anesthetics include bupivacaine, etidocaine, levobupivacaine, lidocaine, mepivacaine, prilocaine, and ropivacaine. Amide solutions are very stable and can be autoclaved.

Stereoisomerism

Stereoisomerism, or chirality, describes molecules with the same structural formula but are different spatial orientations around the specific chiral center. Enantiomers are stereoisomers that exist as nonsuperimposable mirror images when rotating the plane of polarized light. Local anesthetics exist as either single enantiomers or racemic mixtures (solutions containing equal amounts of the two enantiomers). The two isoforms can possess different clinically important pharmacological properties (potency, adverse effects). For example, bupivacaine, a racemic mixture, has greater potential for cardiac toxicity than the single enantiomers, ropivacaine and levobupivacaine. Differences in chirality perhaps lead to differences in affinity for myocardial sodium channels.

Vasoactivity

Except for cocaine, all local anesthetics exert a biphasic effect on vascular smooth muscle. At low concentrations (not clinically relevant), they produce vasoconstriction. At high concentrations, such as that used for regional anesthesia, they are local vasodilators. Lidocaine and mepivacaine have greater intrinsic vasodilatory effects than bupivacaine and ropivacaine. This vasodilation leads to greater vascular uptake, increased systemic absorption, and decreased local anesthetic duration.

PHARMACOKINETICS

Compared to drugs administered systemically, local anesthetics do not abide closely to classic pharmacokinetics. This is because local anesthetics are deposited directly at the target site, whether in the skin, subcutaneous tissue, muscle, or epidural space. Absorption, distribution, and elimination help to decrease their clinical effects.

Absorption

After a local anesthetic is placed around the intended nerve or plexus, some of the drug becomes absorbed into the circulation. Systemic absorption is determined by a variety of factors, including dose, site of injection (vascularity), local tissue blood flow, use of vasoconstrictor adjuvants, and the physiochemical properties of the drug itself. Vascular uptake is slower for local anesthetics with high lipophilicity and protein binding.

The site of drug injection is a significant factor in determining systemic absorption and potentially toxic plasma blood levels. Highly vascular areas, such as the tracheal mucosa, promote greater absorption compared to poorly perfused areas, such as adipose tissue. Peak plasma drug levels depend upon the specific site of injection. From the highest absorption/vascularity to the lowest:

Intravenous > Tracheal > Intercostal > Paracervical > Caudal > Epidural > Brachial plexus > Sciatic > Subcutaneous

Distribution

The distribution of a local anesthetic is determined by its degree of binding to nervous tissues and plasma proteins. Greater protein binding confers a longer duration of action, since the free drug is slowly made available for metabolism. Distribution is also influenced by the local vascular effects of the particular drug. Lidocaine, a potent local vasodilator, has a shorter clinical effect because increased absorption leads to decreased distribution to the nerve tissue.

Elimination

The metabolism of a local anesthetic depends upon its chemical class. Amides are degraded in the liver by the P450 microsomal enzymes (hydroxylation and *N*-dealkylation). Because of this slow process, amides have a longer half-life and can accumulate with repeated doses. Disease states that reduce hepatic blood flow can decrease amide anesthetic elimination.

In contrast, ester anesthetics are hydrolyzed by pseudocholinesterases found in plasma. (Cocaine, which is primarily metabolized in liver, is an exception.) Inactive metabolites include an alkylamine and para-aminobenzoic acid (PABA). Esters have a short half-life because hydrolysis is rapid. The risk of ester toxicity is increased in neonates and patients with atypical pseudocholinesterase levels.

PHARMACODYNAMICS

Acid–Base Chemistry

Local anesthetics are weak bases. In its tertiary form, the terminal amine is lipid soluble. But it can accept a hydrogen ion to form a conjugated acid (quaternary form), which is positively charged and therefore water soluble. Clinically, drug solutions are formulated as hydrochloride salts to maintain solubility and stability. Therefore, at the time of injection, the drug molecules exist primarily in a quaternary, water-soluble state. But in the body, at physiologic pH (7.4), local anesthetics exist in two conformations in equilibrium, the uncharged base form (lipid soluble) and the cationic charged (water soluble) conjugated acid.

Mechanism of Action

Local anesthetics inhibit electrical conduction through nerves by blocking the voltage-gated sodium channels within the nodes of Ranvier. To reach these targets, local anesthetics must cross the axonal membrane into the cytosol of the neuron by diffusing through the lipid bilayer of the nerve sheath. The lipid-soluble unionized base (B) form penetrates through the axonal membrane much more effectively than the charged form (Figure 57-2).

Once inside the axoplasm, the lower pH promotes reequilibration back to the protonated charged form of the drug. The cationic form (BH$^+$) binds to its receptor site on the inner vestibule of the sodium channel. Blockade of the sodium channel leads to inhibition of the fast inward sodium current underlying the nerve action potentials. As a result, local anesthetics decrease the rate of depolarization in response to excitation thereby preventing achievement of the action potential. They do not alter the resting transmembrane potential (−90 to −60 mV) or the threshold potential.

Differential Blockade

Nerve fibers are classified according to diameter, the presence or absence of myelin, and function (Table 57-1). Larger-diameter nerves have more rapid conduction of action potentials. Myelin, which forces current to flow through the nodes of Ranvier, also increases conduction velocity. The sensitivity to local anesthetic blockade is inversely related to nerve fiber diameter. Local anesthetics preferentially block smaller-diameter fibers first. In addition, myelinated nerves, such as preganglionic B fibers, tend to be blocked before unmyelinated nerves of the same diameter, such as C fibers. The order of

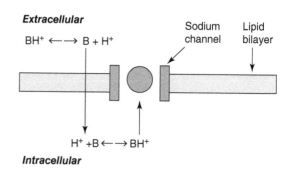

FIGURE 57-2 Local anesthetic site of action.

TABLE 57-1 Classification of Nerve Fibers

Type	Subtype	Fiber Diameter (μm)	Conduction Velocity (m/s)	Function
A (myelinated)	Alpha	12-20	80-120	Proprioception, large motor
	Beta	5-15	35-80	Small motor, touch, pressure
	Gamma	3-8	10-35	Muscle tone
	Delta	2-5	5-25	Pain, temperature, touch
B (myelinated)		3	5-15	Preganglionic autonomic
C (unmyelinated)		0.3-1.5	0.5-2.5	Dull pain, temperature, touch

neural blockade in clinical practice proceeds as loss of sympathetic transmission followed by pain, temperature, touch, proprioception, and then skeletal muscle tone. The dermatomal spread of spinal anesthesia particularly illustrates this order of modality loss.

When local anesthetics are deposited around a peripheral nerve, they diffuse from the outer surface (mantle) toward the center (core) of the nerve along a concentration gradient. As a result, nerve fibers located in the mantle of a mixed nerve are blocked first. Mantle fibers innervate proximal structures while core fibers supply distal structures. This arrangement explains the initial development of proximal anesthesia with later distal involvement as local anesthetic eventually reaches the central core nerve fibers. However, motor blockade may appear before the sensory block if motor fibers are located more peripherally.

Another important factor underlying differential block is a result of the state-dependent, or frequency-dependent, block by local anesthetics. Voltage-gated sodium channels within the nerve membrane move between several different conformational states. Local anesthetics bind to the activated (open) and inactivated (closed) states more readily than the reactivation (resting) state. Therefore, repeated depolarization in rapidly firing axons produces more effective anesthetic binding, and hence progressive enhancement of conduction blockade.

PHYSIOCHEMICAL CHARACTERISTICS (TABLE 57-2)

Potency

The potency of a local anesthetic is determined by and is directly proportional to its lipid solubility. Physicochemical features such as the aromatic ring structure and hydrocarbon chain length determine lipid solubility. Local anesthetics with more carbon atoms in its backbone have higher lipid solubility. Higher concentrations are necessary for less potent anesthetics to achieve neural blockade. For example, bupivacaine is more lipid soluble and, therefore, about 4 times more potent than lidocaine. This is why bupivacaine is formulated in a 0.25% solution, whereas lidocaine is formulated in a 1-2% solution.

Duration

The duration of action of local anesthetics is determined primarily by protein binding. Local anesthetics with a high affinity for protein remain bound to the sodium channel longer. The degree of protein binding depends upon the addition of larger chemical radicals to the amine or aromatic end. For example, bupivacaine (95% protein bound) has a longer duration of action than lidocaine (65% protein binding).

TABLE 57-2 Properties of Local Anesthetics

Agent	Lipid Solubility	Relative Potency	Protein Binding (%)	Duration	pKa
Procaine	<1	1	6	Short	8.9
2-Chloroprocaine	>1	3	—	Short	9.1
Mepivacaine	1	2	77	Medium	7.6
Lidocaine	3	2	65	Medium	7.8
Bupivacaine	28	8	95	Long	8.1
Tetracaine	80	8	76	Long	8.4
Etidocaine	140	8	95	Long	7.9
Ropivacaine	14	8	94	Long	8.1

Duration of action is also influenced by the rate of vascular uptake of local anesthetic from the injection site. Injection of local anesthetics at a highly vascular site such as the intercostal space has a higher rate of vascular uptake leading to a shorter duration of action.

Speed of Onset

The rapidity of onset depends on the pKa (ionization constant) of the local anesthetic. The closer the pKa of the local anesthetic is to tissue pH, the more rapid the onset time. The pKa is defined as the pH at which 50% of the molecules exist in the unionized lipid-soluble tertiary form (B) and 50% in the ionized quaternary, water-soluble form (BH^+). The percentage of local anesthetic present in the unionized form when injected into the tissue (pH 7.4) is *inversely proportional* to its pKa. Local anesthetics with pKa closer to physiologic pH will have a higher concentration of unionized lipid-soluble base. Therefore, more molecules can cross the lipid membrane into the axoplasm, yielding a faster speed of onset.

Since all local anesthetics are weak bases, the Henderson–Hasselbalch equation (pH = pKa + log [B]/[BH^+]) illustrates how the speed of onset differs between local anesthetics.

Lidocaine (pKa 7.8) at tissue pH:

$$7.4 = 7.8 + \log B/BH^+$$

$$-0.4 = \log B/BH^+$$

$$0.4 = \log BH^+/B$$

$BH^+/B = 10^{0.4} = 2.5{:}1 => 70\%$ ionized, 30% unionized

Bupivacaine (pKa 8.1) at tissue pH:

$$7.4 = 8.1 + \log B/BH^+$$

$$-0.7 = \log B/BH^+$$

$$0.7 = \log BH^+/B$$

$BH^+/B = 10^{0.7} = 5{:}1 => 83\%$ ionized, 17% unionized

Lidocaine has a faster speed of onset than bupivacaine because of its nearly 2 times greater percentage of unionized drug when injected into the tissue. The pKa of most local anesthetics ranges from 7.5 to 9.0; therefore, at physiologic pH, the cationic form will make up the greatest percentage.

Local anesthetics have poor penetration and very delayed onset in infected tissue. Inflamed tissues are acidic environments. The low extracellular pH favors production of a greater percentage of quaternary ionized form and reduced fractions of the important neutral form.

Example:

Lidocaine (pKa 7.8) at acidic tissue pH:

$$4.9 = 7.8 + \log B/BH^+$$

$$-2.9 = \log B/BH^+$$

$$2.9 = \log BH^+/B$$

$BH^+/B = 10^{2.9} = 794{:}1 => 99.8\%$ ionized, 0.2% unionized

The onset of action of local anesthetic also depends on the route of administration and the dose or concentration of the drug. For instance, local anesthetics injected into the cerebrospinal fluid reach their targets quickly because of the lack of sheath around the nerve roots. This is why spinal anesthesia has a faster onset than peripheral nerve blockade. Higher local anesthetic concentrations can increase the speed of onset. 2-Chloroprocaine has a pKa of 9.1, which suggests that its onset should be much slower than lidocaine at equal concentrations. Yet, 2-chloroprocaine has the fastest onset of all local anesthetics because clinically it is used in a much higher (3%) concentration solution. Compared to the usual concentrations of other local anesthetics, there are more molecules of 2-chloroprocaine present to reach target sites.

COMMON ADJUNCTS AND ADDITIVES

Epinephrine

Drugs with vasoconstrictive effects (epinephrine, 1:200 000) can be added to local anesthetic solutions to slow the rate of systemic vascular absorption. The result is twofold: (1) increased duration of action due to higher sustained tissue concentrations; and (2) decreased potential for systemic toxicity due to lower peak blood levels. The effect of vasoconstrictors is greater for local anesthetics of intermediate duration and for those with higher intrinsic local vasodilatory action (eg, lidocaine).

Epinephrine will decrease perfusion to the nerve that could potentiate neurotoxicity, especially in patients with diabetes. It may also lead to ischemia in areas that have adequate collateral blood flow (digits, ear, nose, and penis). Systemic absorption of epinephrine may also cause hypertension and dysrhythmias. It should be used with caution in patients with ischemic heart disease, hypertension, and preeclampsia.

Bicarbonate

The addition of sodium bicarbonate to a local anesthetic solution will raise the pH and shifts the equilibrium to increase the effective concentration of the nonionized form. This should hasten the onset time. The effects of alkalinization are greater for lidocaine than for bupivacaine.

Clonidine

Clonidine is an alpha-2-adrenergic agonists that can prolong block duration and decrease local anesthetic requirements. It produces analgesic effects mediated by supraspinal and spinal adrenergic receptors. Side effects include hypotension, bradycardia, and sedation.

Opioids

Opioids are often coadministered with local anesthetics in neuraxial blocks. They do not affect the pharmacokinetics or pharmacodynamics of local anesthetic effect.

Ketamine

Ketamine may prolong postoperative analgesia when coadministered with local anesthetics in peripheral nerve blocks. The analgesic effects are primarily due to N-methyl-D-aspartate (NMDA) receptor antagonism but may also involve opioid receptor agonism.

ADVERSE REACTIONS

Allergy

True allergies to local anesthetics are rare. Since local anesthetic molecules are too small to be antigenic, the protein-bound complex serves as the antigen. Allergic reactions are much more common with ester local anesthetics than with the amides. The suspected antigen is the PABA metabolite. Some amides are formulated with a methylparaben preservative that has a similar structure as PABA and may be responsible for allergic reactions to amides. Most reactions that seem allergic in nature are likely due to either the effects of systemically absorbed coadministered epinephrine, systemic toxicity, or a vasovagal reaction. Since there is no cross-sensitivity between local anesthetic classes, a patient allergic to esters may safely receive an amide local anesthetic (assuming that the antigen was not a common preservative). Patients allergic to ester local anesthetics should receive preservative-free amide local anesthetic.

Methemoglobinemia

Some local anesthetics can overwhelm the oxidative defense mechanisms within erythrocytes and increase the normally low levels of methemoglobin. The most commonly cited drugs are prilocaine and benzocaine, although lidocaine has also been implicated. Prilocaine is metabolized in the liver into o-toluidine, which can oxidize hemoglobin in doses greater than 600 mg. Benzocaine, usually used in the form of a spray, can lead to methemoglobinemia if used in greater than recommended doses.

Direct Neurotoxicity

Local anesthetics have the potential for direct dose-dependent neurotoxicity. The deleterious effects are numerous and include membrane damage, cytoskeletal disruption, disruption of axonal transport, growth cone collapse, and apoptosis.

A. Transient Neurologic Symptoms

Transient neurologic symptoms (TNS) are the result of transient direct neurotoxicity of the lumbosacral nerves by local anesthetics. The classic symptoms are severe pain and dysesthesia in the lower back, buttocks, and lower extremities within 12-24 hours after uneventful spinal anesthesia. There is no sensory loss, motor deficits, or bowel and bladder dysfunction. Known risk factors include the use of lidocaine, higher local anesthetic doses, lithotomy position, and ambulatory

procedures. Symptoms resolve within a week; permanent neurologic damage is rare. Some patients may require hospital readmission for pain control. Nonsteroidal anti-inflammatory drugs are the first-line treatment. The high incidence of TNS has lead to abandonment of lidocaine for spinal anesthesia.

B. Cauda Equina Syndrome

Cauda equina syndrome (CES) is the result of direct neurotoxicity of the sacral nerves. Reports of CES increased in the late 1980s after the introduction of microcatheters for continuous spinal anesthesia. It was thought that pooling of the drug through these catheters exposed the lumbosacral nerves to very high concentrations of local anesthetics. Rare cases in the absence of microcatheters have also been reported. The CES symptoms range from sensory anesthesia to bowel and bladder sphincter dysfunction to paraplegia.

KEY POINTS ABOUT SPECIFIC LOCAL ANESTHETICS

Tetracaine—Tetracaine is primarily used for spinal anesthesia when a long duration is needed. It is available in a 1% solution or in crystal form. Tetracaine is rarely used for epidural anesthesia or peripheral nerve blocks because of its slow onset, profound motor blockade, and potential neurotoxicity when administered at high doses.

Cocaine—As the only naturally occurring local anesthetic used clinically, cocaine is the only local anesthetic that causes intense vasoconstriction. This is why it is most often used as a topical anesthetic. Cocaine inhibits the neuronal reuptake of catecholamines, which can lead to hypertension, tachycardia, and dysrhythmias.

Chloroprocaine—Chloroprocaine produces epidural anesthesia of a relatively short duration. Epidural administration of chloroprocaine is sometimes avoided, because it impairs the action of subsequent epidural bupivacaine and of opioids used concurrently or sequentially. There are reports of back pain associated with epidural chloroprocaine administration.

Mepivacaine—Mepivacaine causes less local vasodilation and has a slightly longer duration of action compared to lidocaine. It is ineffective as a topical anesthetic. Its metabolism is prolonged in the fetus, and hence not used as obstetric anesthesia.

Ropivacaine—Ropivacaine is the S(−) enantiomer of bupivacaine. It produces a less pronounced motor block. Its reduced cardiotoxicity profile may be the result of its greater propensity to produce vasoconstriction.

Levobupivacaine—Levobupivacaine is the S(−) enantiomer of bupivacaine. Compared with racemic bupivacaine, levobupivacaine has less systemic toxicity risk. Its pharmacokinetic profile is similar to that of bupivacaine.

Local Anesthetic Toxicity

Brian S. Freeman, MD

Local anesthetics can have several adverse side effects, including allergic reactions, methemoglobinemia, and direct nerve toxicity. Local anesthetic systemic toxicity (LAST) is perhaps the most devastating complication and can lead to significant morbidity and mortality, particularly cardiovascular and neurologic.

By definition, LAST is characterized by excessive plasma concentrations of local anesthetic that lead to systemic symptoms. Toxic local anesthetic levels occur either due to (1) accidental direct intravascular injection or (2) systemic absorption during and after regional anesthesia. Unintentional intravascular injection of an appropriately dosed nerve block will produce a rapid increase in plasma levels due to the large volumes and/or high concentrations of local anesthetic. Less commonly, the slow vascular absorption of inappropriately dosed local anesthetic at the site of injection can cause LAST. The extent of systemic absorption depends on the specific agent, dose given, presence of epinephrine in the solution, and the vascularity of the tissue injection site (Table 58-1). Whether by direct intravascular injection or systemic vascular absorption, LAST ultimately depends on the quantity of free local anesthetic on the plasma, which is determined by the dose and the rate of injection.

TABLE 58-1　Rate of Local Anesthetic Systemic Absorption Based on Injection Site

Intravenous (highest)
Tracheal
Intercostal
Paracervical
Caudal
Epidural
Brachial plexus
Sciatic
Subcutaneous (lowest)

MANIFESTATIONS

To produce local and regional anesthesia, local anesthetics inhibit voltage-gated sodium channels in the axons of peripheral nerves and decrease action potential conduction velocity. These agents can block potassium and calcium channels as well. The variety of clinical problems due to LAST result from blockade of all of these ion channels in multiple organ systems. In addition, local anesthetics have been shown to inhibit electron transport and uncouple oxidative phosphorylation in mitochondria, thus interrupting ATP synthesis. This effect may be the reason why the brain and heart, two organs highly intolerant of anaerobic metabolism, are most affected by local anesthetic toxicity.

Central Nervous System

The signs of LAST occur on a spectrum that almost always begins with effects on the central nervous system (CNS). Initial signs and symptoms of CNS toxicity may be subtle or nonspecific, such as subjective reports of lightheadedness, dizziness, circumoral paresthesias, and metallic taste. These symptoms are usually followed by visual and auditory disturbances, such as tinnitus, diplopia, and nystagmus. As plasma concentrations rise, local anesthetics then produce greater blockade of sodium channels of GABA-ergic inhibitory cortical interneurons, principally in the temporal lobe. The now-unopposed excitatory neurons have a higher discharge rate that leads to agitation, confusion, muscle twitches (usually of the face and distal extremities), and finally tonic–clonic seizures. Higher plasma levels of local anesthetic are necessary to block the more resistant excitatory neurons. At this later stage, inhibition of excitatory neural circuits lead to a state of generalized CNS depression. EEG activity slows down as patient shows signs of obtundation, loses consciousness, and enters a coma. Respiratory depression may eventually lead to apnea.

Seizures lead to hypoventilation that can add a respiratory component to the underlying metabolic acidosis. Respiratory acidosis can significantly potentiate the risk of CNS toxicity from local anesthetics. In fact, the convulsive threshold of local anesthetics is inversely related to the arterial Pco_2. Acidosis decreases local anesthetic binding to plasma proteins, thereby increasing the amount of unbound drug available for diffusion into the CNS. Hypercapnia also increases cerebral blood flow, thereby delivering local anesthetic more quickly to the brain. In addition, CO_2 will also diffuse into neurons, decrease intracellular pH, and promote conversion of local anesthetics into their charged, cationic form that cannot easily diffuse across the axonal membrane. Toxicity increases as a result of this "ion trapping" phenomenon.

Cardiovascular System

Cardiovascular effects of severe LAST occur when plasma concentrations of local anesthetics are greater than the levels causing CNS toxicity. The cardiovascular manifestations of LAST also follow a similar continuum and pattern as the CNS. The initial signs of toxicity are often hyperdynamic in nature. The patient may develop hypertension, tachycardia, and reentry dysrhythmias such as ventricular tachycardia (including torsades) or fibrillation. The PR intervals and QRS complex will increase on the ECG. Eventually severe hypotension and cardiac depression ensue. The patient may develop decreased contractility, peripheral vasodilation, sinus bradycardia, conduction defects, and asystole. The most common and fatal dysrhythmia in LAST is refractory ventricular fibrillation.

The mechanism of cardiovascular toxicity is multifactorial. The principal direct effect is the binding and inhibition of myocardial sodium channels by local anesthetics. Conduction blockade at the sinoatrial (SA) node creates favorable conditions for reentry dysrhythmias. High levels of local anesthetics also have direct negative inotropic effects by decreasing calcium release from the sarcoplasmic reticulum in the myocyte, which decreases excitation–contraction coupling. By inhibiting the impulses of neurons in the nucleus tractus solitarius, local anesthetics depress the baroreceptor reflex, decrease cardiac output, and promote unopposed sympathetic nervous system activity (which can lead to further dysrhythmias). Local anesthetics also disrupt cellular homeostasis by uncoupling oxidative phosphorylation and decreasing the production of cAMP second messengers.

Each local anesthetic carries a differential potential for the degree of CNS versus cardiac toxicity. There is an inverse relationship between local anesthetic potency and the dose required to elicit CNS toxicity. Based on animal models, the CC/CNS ratio is the dose or plasma level that causes cardiac collapse (CC) divided by the dose or plasma level causing seizures (CNS). Lower CC/CNS ratios indicate a greater degree of selective cardiac toxicity. For instance, bupivacaine (CC/CNS 3) has a lower safety margin than lidocaine (CC/CNS 7), because it can cause dysrhythmias at lower plasma levels. This ratio also explains why cardiac arrest could precede seizures or even occur in the absence of seizures for potent drugs like bupivacaine. The CC/CNS ratios follow the rank order of local anesthetic potency. The newer local anesthetics levobupivacaine and ropivacaine have lower toxicities since higher plasma levels are tolerated before seizures begin. However, once plasma concentrations reach higher levels, all local anesthetics, no matter the potency, can cause severe myocardial depression.

There can be substantial variability in the presentation of LAST. Immediate signs of LAST (<1 minute) suggest direct intravascular injection, whereas delayed presentations (1-5 minutes) suggest intermittent intravascular injection or delayed systemic absorption. In some patients, CNS depression without a preceding excitatory phase is seen. With the more highly protein-bound local anesthetics, the excitement stage of CNS toxicity can be brief and mild. Cardiovascular toxicity can occur without the initial signs of CNS toxicity. The patient may lose consciousness and develop severe bradycardia even without a grand mal seizure. Under general anesthesia, which suppresses the CNS signs, patients typically present with cardiotoxicity as the first evidence of LAST. Because of variability in symptoms and timing, anesthesiologists should maintain high vigilance for atypical presentations when it comes to diagnosing local anesthetic toxicity.

MANAGEMENT

1. **Stop the injection of local anesthetic.**
2. **Call for help.**
3. **Initiate prompt and effective airway management**—The patient should receive 100% oxygen by face mask or endotracheal tube. Since hypoxemia and acidosis will exacerbate CNS toxicity, hyperventilation may be necessary to maintain oxygenation, correct hypercapnia, and increase plasma pH. Airway management equipment should always be available when conducting regional anesthesia.
4. **Seizure suppression**—Benzodiazepines such as midazolam, in small incremental doses, are the preferred treatment for convulsions. If not readily available, sodium thiopental is acceptable. Propofol has anticonvulsant properties but should not be used if there are also signs of concurrent or impending hemodynamic collapse. Large doses of propofol will cause significant myocardial depression. If seizures are refractory to benzodiazepine therapy, neuromuscular blocking drugs such as succinylcholine should be considered to assist ventilation and oxygenation.
5. **Begin advanced cardiac life support for patients in cardiac arrest**—Prompt restoration of cardiac output and oxygen delivery is essential. Depressed myocardial contractility and poor coronary perfusion pressure will potentiate acidosis and prevent washout of local anesthetic from the myocardium.

   Managing cardiac arrest due to LAST involves slight changes to advanced cardiac life support (ACLS) protocols:
   a. Consider using smaller initial doses of epinephrine (<1 μg/kg rather than 1 mg). Animal studies have shown that epinephrine is highly dysrhythmogenic, resulting in poorer outcomes in resuscitation from LAST, and can reduce the effectiveness of lipid therapy.
   b. Consider avoiding the use of vasopressin. Animal studies have shown poorer outcomes that were associated with pulmonary hemorrhage.

c. For treating ventricular dysrhythmias, avoid using calcium channel blockers, beta-blockers, procainamide, or lidocaine. In the past, bretylium, a class III antidysrhythmic drug, was the preferred choice for treating refractory ventricular fibrillation due to local anesthetic toxicity. Since bretylium is no longer manufactured, amiodarone has become the recommended antidysrhythmic drug.

6. **Administer lipid emulsion therapy (Intralipid [Baxter Healthcare])**—In case reports and animal studies, lipids have been shown to increase the success rate of resuscitation from LAST. Intralipid® is a 20% lipid emulsion solution most commonly used as part of total parenteral nutrition. It contains soybean oil, glycerol, and egg phospholipids. It is theorized that these lipids act as a "sink" that bind lipid-soluble local anesthetics within the myocardium and reduces its free fraction. Lipid therapy should be implemented based on the severity and rate of progression of LAST. Early use during prolonged seizures can prevent cardiac toxicity.

The recommended bolus dose is 1.5 mL/kg IV (lean body mass) followed by an infusion of 0.25 mL/kg/min. If cardiovascular instability persists, the bolus may be repeated up to two more times and the infusion rate may be doubled. The infusion should be continued for a minimum of 10 minutes after a perfusing rhythm is restored. Successful use of lipid therapy should be reported at *www. lipidrescue.org* and *www.lipidregistry.org*. Propofol has low lipid content and causes myocardial depression, so it is not a substitute for lipid emulsion.

7. Begin preparations to institute cardiopulmonary bypass for patients unresponsive to pharmacological therapy and ACLS. Alert the closest facility having cardiopulmonary bypass (CPB) capability at the first signs of hemodynamic compromise. This step can be life saving.

8. Monitor patients for at least 12 hours for delayed recurrences of LAST. Redistribution of local anesthetic depots into the circulation can reinitiate cardiovascular toxicity.

PREVENTION

A number of preventive measures can decrease the risk and severity of LAST:

- Use the lowest effective dose (mg) of local anesthetic to achieve the desired block extent and duration. Practitioners should minimize both concentration and volume. For instance, reports of fatal cardiac arrest in obstetric patients due to 0.75% bupivacaine led to its withdrawal for use in labor analgesia.

- Substitution of the less potent enantiomers ropivacaine or levobupivacaine may reduce the potential for systemic toxicity.

- Needles and catheters should be aspirated prior to each injection while observing for blood. There is a 2% false negative rate for intravascular identification.

- Local anesthetic should be injected incrementally in 3-5 mL aliquots. A 15-30 second pause in between injections allows for at least one circulation time to observe for signs and symptoms of LAST. Incremental injections can, however, increase the overall injection time and increase the risk of needle movement. Some may argue that incremental injections are less important for blocks done under ultrasound guidance, in which there are usually more needle passes.

- Test doses with pharmacological markers for intravascular placement are reliable and essential when injecting large volumes of local anesthetic. If injected intravascularly, epinephrine in a 1:200 000 concentration will produce a 15-30 beat increase in heart rate or a 15 mm Hg systolic pressure increase within 30 seconds. Epinephrine test doses are less reliable in patients of advanced age, in active labor, taking beta-blockers, or anesthetized with general or neuraxial anesthesia. Fentanyl (100 μg) is less commonly used marker but can reliably produce sedation or sleepiness if injected intravascularly.

- Ultrasound guidance may reduce the frequency of intravascular injection and LAST. Using ultrasound has been shown to reduce the number of vascular punctures and frequency of seizures compared to peripheral nerve stimulation. Since ultrasound guidance involves more frequent needle movements compared to the fixed needle approach of nerve stimulation, symptomatic intravascular injection can still occur.

- Use standard American Society of Anesthesiologists (ASA) monitors and maintain a high level of vigilance. Frequent communication with the patient regarding toxicity symptoms is essential. The patient should be monitored for at least 30 minutes after completion of injection for delayed LAST.

- Avoid oversedation during block placement. Sedatives such as benzodiazepines are helpful in increasing the seizure threshold. However, sedatives may prevent the patient from reporting systems of LAST. In addition, oversedation may lead to hypoventilation. Local anesthetic toxicity will be exacerbated by the resulting hypoxemia, hypercapnia, and acidosis.

- Choose patients for regional anesthesia carefully. Patients who have slower circulation times have a higher risk of developing local anesthetic toxicity. These conditions include severe cardiac dysfunction, heart failure, ischemia heart disease, and conduction abnormalities. Other factors that can increase plasma local anesthetic levels are renal disease, acidosis, hepatic dysfunction, hypoalbuminemia, and patients at extremes of age (<4 months or >70 years).

SUGGESTED READING

Neal JM, Bernards CM, Butterworth JF, et al. ASRA practice advisory on local anesthetic systemic toxicity. *Reg Anesth Pain Med* 2010;35:152-161.

59

Muscle Relaxants

Choy R.A. Lewis, MD

DEPOLARIZING MUSCLE RELAXANTS

Depolarizing muscle relaxants physically resemble acetylcholine (ACh), and because of this resemblance, they are able to act as competitive agonists by binding to ACh receptors (AChR) and generating action potentials.

Succinylcholine (SCh) is the only depolarizing muscle relaxant in clinical use. It is generally used when there is risk for aspiration of gastric contents or when there is need for rapid paralysis. It is essentially two ACh molecules joined together.

Because of its low lipid solubility and relative overdose, SCh has a very rapid onset of action. Onset of action is approximately 30-90 seconds and its duration of action 5-10 minutes. Succinylcholine is not metabolized by acetylcholinesterase, which is located in the neuromuscular junction (NMJ). Instead, it is metabolized by plasma cholinesterase (pseudocholinesterase), an enzyme present in the blood. Succinylcholine, therefore, has a longer duration of action at the motor end plate. This leads to prolonged depolarization known as a phase I block. Phase I block is often preceded by muscle fasciculation. This is probably the result of the prejunctional action of SCh, stimulating AChR on the motor nerve, causing repetitive firing and release of neurotransmitter. Recovery from phase I block occurs as SCh diffuses away from the NMJ and is metabolized by plasma cholinesterase in plasma.

Repeated boluses or an infusion of SCh may lead to either a desensitization block, or a phase II block. A **desensitization block** occurs when the continued presence of an agonist causes the AChR to become insensitive to the binding of the agonist. This is thought to be a safety mechanism to protect against overexcitation of the NMJ. With a **phase II block** the membrane potential is in a resting state despite an agonist being present and subsequent neurotransmission is blocked throughout. The block takes on the characteristics of a block induced by a nondepolarizing muscle relaxant (Table 59-1). Phase II block may be antagonized by anticholinesterases but the result is hard to predict. For this reason, spontaneous recovery is recommended.

Succinylcholine has numerous side effects:

1. Stimulation of muscarinic receptors may lead to *bradyarrhythmias*, including sinus bradycardia, junctional rhythm, ventricular escape beats, or asystole. Effect is more pronounced in children.
2. Trigger for *malignant hyperthermia*. Fatal, if left untreated.
3. Some patients may have isolated *masseter muscle spasm* when given SCh. This may be isolated and the patient may not be at increased risk for malignant hyperthermia but it has been said that this could be an early sign or mild form of malignant hyperthermia.
4. Prolonged administration of SCh may lead to phase II or desensitization block. One proposed mechanism is desensitization of the prejunctional membrane. Block takes on the characteristic of that of nondepolarizing muscle relaxant. There is variable reversibility by cholinesterase inhibitors and increased sensitivity to depolarizing muscle relaxants. Spontaneous recovery is very slow and attempts at reversal are often inadequate to attain spontaneous ventilation.
5. *Myalgias* thought to be due to fasciculations. A defasciculating dose of a nondepolarizing muscle relaxant may be beneficial.
6. *Increase Increased intracranial pressure (ICP)*. Mechanism not completely understood but defasciculation may help suggesting fasciculation as a contributing factor.
7. *Hyperkalemia may occur* when SCh is used in the presence of immature extrajunctional receptors. Examples include spinal cord or denervation injuries, upper/lower motor neuron damage, burn, neuromuscular disease, and prolonged immobility. On average, SCh increases the potassium by 0.5 mEq/L. Defasciculation does not protect patients from hyperkalemia.
8. *Increased intraocular pressure* proposed to be from fasciculation of extraocular muscles. This may lead to extrusion of the orbit in the situation of an open globe injury. It is still controversial whether or not this is clinically significant. A defasciculating dose of a nondepolarizing muscle relaxant may prevent this.

TABLE 59-1   **Nondepolarizing Muscle Relaxants and Their Properties**

Relaxant	Intubating Dose (mg/kg)	Onset after Intubating Dose (Min)	Duration (min)[a]	Primary Excretion	Metabolism	Histamine Release	Other
Short Acting							
Mivacurium	0.2	1-1.5	15-20	Insignificant	Pseudochol inesterase	Yes	
Intermediate Acting							
Vecuronium	0.15-0.2	1.5	60	75% biliary; 25% renal	Small extent by liver	No	Metabolite has NMB[b] activity
Rocuronium	0.6	2-3	30	>75% liver;	None	No	
	1.2	1	60	<25% renal			
Atracurium	0.75	1-1.15	45-60	<10% biliary + renal	Nonspecific Esterases[c] + Hofmann degradation[d]	Yes	Intermediate (laudanosine) associated with CNS excitation
Cisatracurium	0.2	2	60-90	None	Hofmann	No	
Long Acting							
Pancuronium	0.08-0.12	4-5	90	Limited degree by liver	40% renal;10% bile	No	Metabolite has NMB activity; vagolytic
Pipecuronium	0.07-0.85	3-5	80-90	Minor hepatic	70% renal; 20% biliary	No	
Doxacurium	0.05-0.08	3-5	90-120	Minor plasma cholinesterase	>75% renal; minor hepatobiliary	No	

[a]Duration measured as return of twitch to 25% of control.

[b]NMB, neuromuscular blocking.

[c]Hofmann: spontaneous degradation in plasma at physiologic pH and temperature.

[d]Nonspecific esterases: plasma esterases other than pseudocholinesterase or acetylcholinesterase.

(Modified from Duke J, *Anesthesia Secrets*, 4th ed. Philadelphia, PA: Mosby/Elsevier; 2011.)

Succinylcholine is metabolized by pseudocholinesterase, which is produced in the liver. Quantitative deficiencies may be observed in liver disease, pregnancy, malnutrition, malignancy, and hypothyroidism. This leads to a slightly prolonged duration of action of SCh.

Qualitative deficiencies may be seen in situations where the enzyme function is impaired. Genetic diseases leading to this are either homozygous or heterozygous in nature. This can be assessed by the dibucaine-resistant cholinesterase deficiency study. Dibucaine is a local anesthetic that inhibits pseudocholinesterase by 80% when added to the serum. Atypical pseudocholinesterase is inhibited by only 20%. Normal pseudocholinesterase will have a dibucaine number of 80, whereas someone who is homozygous for atypical pseudocholinesterase will have a dibucaine number of 20. The latter person will have an extremely prolonged block with SCh (40-200 min) with phase II block characteristics. The heterozygous person will have a dibucaine number of 40-60 and will have a moderately prolonged block from SCh.

NONDEPOLARIZING MUSCLE RELAXANTS

Nondepolarizing muscle relaxants are competitive antagonists in that they also bind to the AChR but they are unable to induce the conformational changes needed for depolarization. In doing so, they inhibit activation of the AChR by ACh as well as by the subsequent depolarization and muscle contraction that it generally induces.

Nondepolarizing muscle relaxants are either steroidal compounds (eg, vecuronium, pancuronium, rocuronium) or benzyl isoquinolines (eg, cisatracurium, atracurium, mivacurium). Each has unique characteristics and side effects, which are widely related to its structure. Because of structural similarity, a person may be allergic to all relaxants within a class if there is a history of allergy to one drug within the group.

It is believed that a *priming dose*, 10%-15% of the dose of nondepolarizing muscle relaxant, when given 1-3 minutes prior to administration of the full dose, enhances onset of action.

TABLE 59-2   **Response to Nerve Stimulation**

| Normal Evoked Stimulus | Depolarizing Block | | Nondepolarizing Block |
	Phase I	Phase II	
Train-of-four	Constant but diminished	Fade	Fade
Tetany	Constant but diminished	Fade	Fade
Double-burst stimulation (DBS$_{3,2}$)	Constant but diminished	Fade	Fade
Post-tetanic potentiation	Absent	Present	Present

(Reproduced with permission from Butterworth JF, Mackey DC, Wasnick JD, *Morgan and Mikhail's Clinical Anesthesiology*, 5th ed. McGraw-Hill; 2013.)

Several agents may potentiate the action of muscle relaxants. This includes volatile anesthetics, local anesthetics, calcium channel blockers, beta-blockers, antibiotics (aminoglycosides), magnesium, long-term use of steroids, dantrolene. Respiratory acidosis, metabolic alkalosis, hypothermia, hypokalemia, hypercalcemia, and hypermagnesemia may also prolong duration of action of muscle relaxants. Hepatic and renal failure will prolong block of relaxants with significant renal or hepatic clearance.

It is also believed that the combination of different nondepolarizing muscle relaxants may *potentiate the neuromuscular blockade*; a possible synergistic effect.

Certain disorders may make a patient more susceptible or resistant to groups of muscle relaxants. Patients with *myasthenia gravis* are more susceptible to depolarizing and more resistant to depolarizing muscle relaxants. Patients with Lambert–Eaton myasthenic syndrome are more susceptible to both depolarizing and nondepolarizing muscle relaxants.

Muscle relaxants are capable of inducing paralysis of all skeletal muscles. Core muscles are more susceptible to and peripheral muscles more resistant to the actions of muscle relaxants. As a result, laryngeal muscles, orbicularis oris, and diaphragm respond to and recover from muscle relaxants more easily than muscles of the limb. For surgical purposes, adequate relaxation is generally present when there are one to two twitches by train-of-four measurement (TOF).

Patients who have received depolarizing or nondepolarizing muscle relaxants display characteristic patterns to nerve stimulation (Table 59-2).

Antagonism of Neuromuscular Blockade

Choy R.A. Lewis, MD

Muscle relaxation caused by a muscle relaxant drug can be terminated spontaneously by diffusion, redistribution, metabolism, and excretion or via pharmacological antagonism using specific reversal agents known as cholinesterase inhibitors. Acetylcholinesterase is an enzyme found at the motor end plate. It functions by breaking down and reducing the amount of acetylcholine (ACh) at the nerve terminal. By inhibiting acetylcholinesterase, cholinesterase inhibitors indirectly increase the amount of ACh molecules that are available to compete with the nondepolarizing muscle relaxant for the binding sites of the ACh receptors.

Drugs within the class of cholinesterase inhibitors are neostigmine, pyridostigmine, physostigmine, and edrophonium (Table 60-1). Neostigmine and edrophonium are most commonly used clinically. The use of physostigmine as a reversal agent is limited because it crosses the blood–brain barrier (BBB).

ADVERSE EFFECTS

Cholinesterase inhibitors will increase acetylcholinesterase not just at the neuromuscular junction of skeletal muscles, but at all sites of acetylcholinesterase action. These locations include autonomic ganglia and muscarinic receptors of the cardiovascular, gastrointestinal, genitourinary, and respiratory systems. The use of these reversal agents can, therefore, lead to numerous side effects, including some potentially lethal ones (Table 60-2).

The effect on the cardiac conduction system is particularly concerning. Unopposed muscarinic activity at the sinoatrial node can lead to bradycardia and even asystole. To avoid this (and other) effects, cholinesterase inhibitors are administered simultaneously with muscarinic anticholinergics, such as glycopyrrolate and atropine. The pharmacodynamics and pharmacokinetic profiles of each drug will determine the specific pairings. For example, neostigmine is usually paired with glycopyrrolate, whereas edrophonium is usually paired with atropine.

The dose of acetylcholinesterase inhibitor administered should be altered based on the degree of block. An overdose can lead to too much ACh in the neuromuscular junction. This can lead to an antagonistic effect where it may act to potentiate rather than reverse a block.

TIMING OF ADMINISTRATION

There is no real evidence to suggest that the timing of administration of the reversal agent alters the time to full reversal. Nevertheless, most anesthesiologists advocate waiting to administer the reversal agent until there is at least some evidence of spontaneous reversal. A return of at least 10% of a single twitch suffices. There is a ceiling effect with acetylcholinesterase inhibitors such that increasing reversal agent dosing to overcome profound block is unlikely to provide adequate reversal.

TABLE 60-1 Cholinesterase Inhibitors and Anticholinergics

Cholinesterase Inhibitor	Usual Dose of Cholinesterase Inhibitor	Recommended Anticholinergic	Usual Dose of Anticholinergic per mg of Cholinesterase Inhibitor
Neostigmine	0.04–0.08 mg/kg	Glycopyrrolate	0.2 mg
Pyridostigmine	0.1–0.25 mg/kg	Glycopyrrolate	0.05 mg
Edrophonium	0.5–1 mg/kg	Atropine	0.014 mg
Physostigmine[1]	0.01–0.03 mg/kg	Usually not necessary	NA

[1]Not used to reverse muscle relaxants.

(Reproduced with permission from Butterworth JF, Mackey DC, Wasnick JD, *Morgan and Mikhail's Clinical Anesthesiology*, 5th ed. McGraw-Hill; 2013.)

TABLE 60-2   Side Effects of Acetylcholinesterase Inhibitors

Organ System	Muscarinic Side Effects
Cardiovascular	Decreased heart rate, bradyarrhythmias
Pulmonary	Bronchospasm, bronchial secretions
Cerebral	Diffuse excitation[1]
Gastrointestinal	Intestinal spasm, increased salivation
Genitourinary	Increased bladder tone
Ophthalmological	Pupillary constriction

[1]Applies only to physostigmine.

(Reproduced with permission from Butterworth JF, Mackey DC, Wasnick JD, *Morgan and Mikhail's Clinical Anesthesiology*, 5th ed. McGraw-Hill; 2013.)

INDICATIONS

The body does not need all receptors to be free from neuromuscular blockade to function normally. If adequate strength has been demonstrated, reversal may not be required. Some believe reversal should be given to all patients who received neuromuscular blockade. Evidence suggests that there is increased risk of aspiration with train-of-four (TOF) ratio less than 0.9, so adequate reversal is only achieved after TOF is greater than 0.9. In addition, qualitative assessment (visual or tactile) of response to nerve stimulation is limited, and inter-individual variability in the duration of action and time until recovery to TOF is greater than 0.9 for muscle relaxants is significant. Even with sustained head lift there may still be 30% of receptors blocked.

Neuromuscular Potentiation

A. Sugammadex

Sugammadex is a member of a relatively new class of drugs called muscle relaxant binding agents or steroidal muscle relaxant encapsulators (SMREs). It is a modified cyclodextrin that specifically binds to and inactivates steroidal nondepolarizing muscle relaxants. It can immediately reverse blockade caused by the administration of rocuronium, and to a lesser extent than caused by vecuronium. Once injected into the bloodstream, sugammadex encapsulates the steroidal muscle relaxant in a 1:1 molecular ratio. Binding results in a reduction in the number of free molecules of the muscle relaxant in the blood. A gradient is created that favors diffusion of the muscle relaxant from the neuromuscular junction into the bloodstream where there can be immediate binding and inactivation by sugammadex.

Since the complex is 100% excreted by the kidneys, the drug is not recommended for use in patients with renal failure. It is also not recommended for use in neonates and infants less than 2 years old. The only absolute contraindication to its use is hypersensitivity toward the drug. Potential implications include immediate reversal after rocuronium use where paralysis is not desired, and immediate reversal in a "cannot intubate, cannot ventilate" situation where rocuronium was used for paralysis. Sugammadex is currently being used in Europe but has not been FDA approved for clinical use in the United States.

SUGGESTED READING

Fink H, Hollmann MW. Myths and facts in neuromuscular pharmacology—new developments in reversing neuromuscular blockade. *Minerva Anesthesiolgica*. 2012;78:473-482.

61

ASA Preoperative Testing Guidelines

Victor Leslie, MD, and Lisa Bellil, MD

Practice advisories are not concrete guidelines, but rather a source to assist in clinical decision making. Although supported by scientific evidence, the same rigor is not applied to these advisories as would be to standards or guidelines due to insufficient number of adequately controlled studies.

The definition of preanesthesia evaluation is subjective, but encompasses an anesthesiologist's preparation before various procedures, including but not limited to reviewing the patient's medical records, consulting additional specialties, and performing the preoperative evaluation.

The preanesthesia history and physical examination includes evaluation of pertinent medical records, patient interview, and physical examination. Baseline evaluation should include examination and analysis of airway, heart, lungs, and vital signs. Additional information such as relevant diagnosis with severity, treatments, and prognosis are beneficial to evaluate as well. The purpose of preoperative tests is to elucidate unknown patient pathology, verify and further characterize known patient pathology, and to assist in formulating an individualized clinical plan for the patient. Routine ordering of preoperative tests should be avoided. Rather ordering indicated tests are recommended, especially if aberrant results necessitate a change in anesthetic management for the patient. For highly invasive surgeries, preanesthesia evaluation is recommended before the day of procedure. For minimally invasive surgery, evaluation is recommended before or on the day of procedure.

SPECIFIC RECOMMENDATIONS FROM THE AMERICAN SOCIETY OF ANESTHESIOLOGISTS

Electrocardiogram—May be useful in patients with previously known or newly discovered cardiac risk factors, cardiac pathology, respiratory pathology, and high risk or invasive surgery. Although electrocardiogram abnormalities may increase in older patients, age alone may not be an indication for electrocardiogram.

Cardiac evaluation other than electrocardiogram—It is advisable to consult with relevant specialties, consider cardiac risk factors, understand type and invasiveness of procedure, and compare risks and benefits of additional assessment before ordering tests, including but not limited to echocardiography, cardiac stress test, and cardiac catheterization.

Chest radiography—Consideration of recently resolved respiratory tract infection, stable chronic obstructive pulmonary disease (COPD), stable cardiac disease, smoking, and extremes of age may indicate justification for chest radiography during preanesthesia evaluation; however, the previous risk factors are not definite indications.

Pulmonary evaluation other than chest radiography—Before tests are performed to elucidate extent of pulmonary pathology (including but not limited to pulmonary function tests, pulse oximetry, and arterial blood gas), it is advisable to consult relevant specialties, evaluate pulmonary pathology, pulmonary risk factors, type and invasiveness of procedure, and compare risks and benefits of tests. The date of prior evaluation, asthma, COPD, and scoliosis should also be considered.

Hemoglobin/hematocrit measurement—Consideration of type and invasiveness of procedure, extremes of age, liver pathology, history of anemia, and bleeding diathesis may encourage obtaining hemoglobin and hematocrit levels; however, routine hemoglobin and hematocrit are not indicated.

Coagulation studies—Consideration of liver pathology, renal pathology, bleeding diathesis, and type and invasiveness of procedure may indicate justification for selected coagulation studies. Additional perioperative risks may be associated with anticoagulant medication and alternative therapies. There is lack of sufficient evidence to encourage or discourage coagulation studies before regional anesthesia.

Serum chemistries—Consideration of perioperative treatments, medications, alternative therapies, and pathology within the endocrine, hepatic, and renal systems may indicate justification for serum chemistries (basic metabolic panel, liver function tests, and renal function tests). It is advisable to be cognizant that normal range varies with extremes of age.

Urinalysis—Indications for urinalysis include symptomatic urinary tract infection and specific procedures, including but not limited to urologic procedures and prosthesis implantation.

Pregnancy testing—The literature is inconclusive regarding harmful anesthetic effects on early pregnancy. If the surgical or anesthetic management will need to be adjusted based on potential pregnancy, women of reproductive age may be offered pregnancy testing.

Timing of preoperative testing—The literature is insufficient to provide a conclusion regarding timing of preoperative testing in relation to individual patient factors. Test results obtained 6 months prior to procedure may be generally accepted if there are no significant changes in medical history. If, however, significant changes in medical history have occurred or if test results will affect anesthetic plan, it may be advisable to obtain more recent test results.

FURTHER READING

Practice advisory for preanesthesia evaluation: an updated report by the American Society of Anesthesiologists Task Force on Preanesthesia Evaluation. *Anesthesiology* 2012;116:522-538.

ACC/AHA Guidelines for Perioperative Cardiovascular Evaluation

Todd Stamatakos, MD, and Jason Hoefling, MD

The American College of Cardiology and the American Heart Association have established a set of guidelines, written by a consortium of physicians involved in the perioperative care of patients undergoing noncardiac surgery. These guidelines are a tool to help health-care providers assess risk and administer therapies that will optimize both outcomes and cost. Quality preoperative evaluations take into consideration patient risk factors and preexisting conditions, and order appropriate tests based on peer-reviewed evidence.

STRENGTH OF EVIDENCE

In the development of these guidelines, the authors classified each recommendation on the strength of the underlying studies:

- Class I: There exists evidence or general agreement that treatment or procedure is of useful and/or effective. Procedure/Treatment should be performed.
- Class II: Conditions with conflicting evidence and/or controversy with regard to usefulness/efficacy of a procedure or therapy.
  - Class IIa: The amount of evidence and general opinion demonstrate that benefits likely outweigh risks; however, additional studies with focused objectives are still needed. It is reasonable to perform procedure/administer treatment.
  - Class IIb: Evidence and general opinion suggests a possible benefit with procedure/treatment. Additional studies with larger populations, and broad objectives are needed. A procedure or treatment may be considered.
- Class III: Consensus agreement with respect to procedure or treatment is of no use or ineffective or can cause harm.

FURTHER PREOPERATIVE TESTING TO ASSESS CORONARY RISK

The history, physical examination, and electrocardiogram should focus on identifying preexisting cardiac abnormalities, such as symptomatic arrhythmias, coronary artery disease (CAD), prior myocardial infarction (MI), heart failure (HF), implantable cardiac devises, or a history of orthostatic instability. If abnormalities are identified, problems need to be ranked in order of severity, disability, and treatments.

An algorithm-based approach to preoperative evaluation was developed to assess CAD in a cost-effective manner (Figure 62-1). This algorithm is based on clinical markers, previous coronary evaluations/treatments, functional capacity, and risk stratification commensurate with various types of surgery.

1. **Clinical markers**—Major clinical predictors associated with increased perioperative cardiovascular hazard include: acute coronary syndrome (ACS) such as acute MI (<7 days before procedure), unstable or severe angina, decompensated HF, symptomatic arrhythmias, or severe valvular disease.

   Intermediate clinical predictors of increased cardiac risk include: mild angina, history of MI (>1 month before procedure), compensated HF, preoperative creatinine greater than or equal to 2.0 mg/dL, and diabetes mellitus.

   Minor clinical risk predictors include: advanced age, abnormal ECG, rhythm other than sinus, low functional capacity, history of stroke, and uncontrolled hypertension.

2. **Functional capacity**—Functional capacity is defined via the system of metabolic equivalents (MET) in which activities of daily living are assigned a value based on cardiovascular demand (Table 62-1).

3. **Surgery-specific risk**—Surgical cardiac risk can be assessed by the type of surgery and the cardiovascular stress associated with the procedure. Surgeries can be ranked as high, intermediate, or low risk. High-risk surgeries include major emergency surgeries, vascular surgeries, and long procedures with the potential for large fluid shifts. Intermediate-risk procedures include intrathoracic or peritoneal surgery, carotid endarterectomy, head or neck surgery, orthopedic surgery, and prostate surgery. Low-risk surgeries include endoscopic and superficial surgeries, cataract or breast surgery.

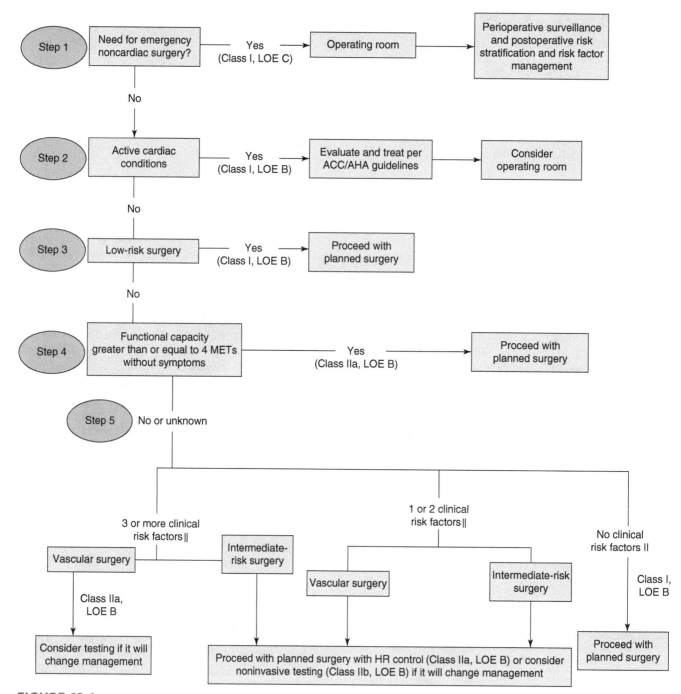

FIGURE 62-1 Cardiac evaluation and care algorithm for noncardiac surgery based on active clinical conditions, known cardiovascular disease, or cardiac risk factors for patients 50 years of age or more. (Reproduced with permission from Fleisher L et al. ACC/AHA 2007 Guidelines on perioperative cardiovascular evaluation and care for noncardiac surgery: executive summary. *Circulation.* 2007;116(17):1971-1996.)

TABLE 62-1 Estimated Functional Capacity Requirements for Various Activities

1 MET	Can you… Take care of yourself? Eat, dress, or use the toilet?	4 METs	Can you… Climb a flight of stairs or walk up a hill? Walk on level ground at 4 mph (6.4 kph)?
	Walk indoors around the house?		Run a short distance?
	Walk a block or 2 on level ground at 2 to 3 mph (3.2 to 4.8 khp)?		Do heavy work around the house like scrubbing floors or lifting or moving heavy furniture?
4 METs	Do light work around the house like dusting or washing dishes?		Participate in moderate recreational activities like golf, bowling, dancing, doubles tennis, or throwing a baseball or football?
		Greater than 10 METs	Participate in strenuous sports like swimming, singles tennis, football, basketball, or skiing?

(Reproduced with permission from Fleisher L., et al. ACC/AHA 2007 Guidelines on perioperative cardiovascular evaluation and care for noncardiac surgery: executive summary. *Circulation.* 2007;23;116(17):1971-1996.)

MANAGEMENT OF SPECIFIC PREOPERATIVE CARDIOVASCULAR CONDITIONS

Hypertension—Blood pressure should optimally be controlled days to weeks before an elective procedure. If the surgery is urgent, beta blockers are of particular use. Patients should continue their hypertension medications perioperatively.

Valvular heart disease—Indications for evaluation and intervention are the same for those not having surgery. Symptomatic stenotic lesions can result in perioperative HF and therefore, often require valvotomy or valve replacement before noncardiac surgery. Regurgitant valve disease symptoms can often be managed with medical therapy and monitoring, and tends to be better tolerated perioperatively.

Myocardial disease—Dilated and hypertrophic cardiomyopathies are associated with worst postoperative outcomes, so emphasis is largely placed on maintaining preoperative hemodynamics and intense postoperative surveillance and medical therapy.

Arrhythmias and conduction abnormalities—Presence of conduction abnormalities or arrhythmia should prompt care and evaluation for metabolic abnormalities, cardiopulmonary disease, and/or drug toxicity. Premature ventricular contractions and nonsustained ventricular tachycardia are not associated with perioperative cardiac morbidity; therefore, treatment in the perioperative setting is usually not required.

Implantable pacemakers or implantable cardioverter-defibrillators (ICDs)—Optimally, the type of device, degree of dependency should be ascertained and ICDs should be turned off before procedure, then immediately turned back on postoperatively.

Supplemental Preoperative Evaluation

1. **Resting left ventricular function**—Determining the resting left ventricular function is not a consistent predictor of perioperative ischemic events. Those who would benefit from noninvasive preoperative left ventricular function include patients with active or poorly controlled heart failure (Class I evidence) and patients with prior heart failure or dyspnea of unknown origin (Class IIa evidence)

2. **12-Lead ECG**—Patients who require preoperative ECG include those with recent episodes of chest pain for intermediate- and high-risk surgical procedures (Class I), patients with diabetes mellitus (regardless of symptoms, Class IIa), patients with prior revascularization of coronaries, prior hospitalizations for causes related to cardiac condition, men over 45 years of age, women over 55 years of age (Class IIb)

3. **Pharmacological or exercise stress testing**—Patients who require this evaluation have an intermediate pretest probability of CAD or an initial evaluation of proven CAD, or require it for the evaluation of medical therapy status post-ACS (Class I). When subjective assessment is not possible, patients should have an exercise capacity evaluation (Class IIa). Patients with ST-depressions less than 1 mm, ECG findings of left ventricular hypertrophy, patients on digitalis therapy, patients with high or low pretest probability of CAD, or patients where concerns rest with restenosis within a month of percutaneous coronary intervention (PCI) (Class IIb)

4. **Coronary angiography**—These recommendations are appropriate for evaluations before and after noncardiac surgery, comprise patients with diagnosed or suspected CAD where there is an elevated risk or poor outcomes based on noninvasive testing, angina in the setting of maximal medical therapy or unstable angina when intermediate- or high-risk noncardiac surgery is planned, or when equivocal noninvasive testing suggests a high cardiac risk for a high-risk surgery (Class I). Patients with several markers of intermediate clinical risks for vascular surgery after first considering noninvasive testing, moderate to extensive ischemia with noninvasive testing in the absence of high-risk features and diminished left ventricular ejection fraction (LVEF), patients with intermediate clinical risk in setting of inconclusive

nondiagnostic test results for planned high-risk surgery, patients recovering from recent MI who require urgent noncardiac surgery (Class IIa), or patients with perioperative MI (Class IIb).

PERIOPERATIVE THERAPY OR PREVIOUS CORONARY REVASCULARIZATION

The indications for coronary artery bypass grafting (CABG) before a noncardiac procedure are the same as the ACC/AHA guidelines for CABG. For patients planning elective noncardiac procedures with high-risk coronary anatomy and who may otherwise benefit from the long-term advantages of CABG should undergo revascularization prior to intermediate or high-risk noncardiac elective procedures.

The indications for PCI in the preoperative setting are similar to the ACC/AHA general guidelines for PCI. For patients who require PCI and may require noncardiac surgery in next 12 months should undergo either angioplasty or get a bare-metal stent with 4-6 months of dual platelet therapy. For those patients who receive a drug eluding stent (DES) within 12 months of nonurgent noncardiac procedures should stop their thienopyridine medications while continuing aspirin therapy in the perioperative period and restart thienopyridine therapy postoperatively.

SUGGESTED READING

Fleisher L, Beckman JA, Brown KA, et al. ACC/AHA 2007 guidelines on perioperative cardiovascular evaluation and care for noncardiac surgery: Executive summary. *Circulation* 2007;116:1971-1996.

Prophylactic Cardiac Risk Reduction

Jason Hoefling, MD

Cardiovascular complications are the most common cause of perioperative morbidity and mortality in patients undergoing noncardiac surgery. For elective surgery, the application of evidence-based strategies can significantly reduce the risk of adverse cardiovascular events in high-risk patients. The following guidelines, developed by the American College of Cardiology (ACC) and the American Heart Association (AHA), are based on an extensive review of the literature. The recommendations are based on the strength of the clinical evidence and are considered the standard for the perioperative management of cardiac patients.

CORONARY REVASCULARIZATION

Preoperative coronary revascularization with coronary artery bypass grafting (CABG) or percutaneous coronary intervention (PCI) can reduce the risk of cardiac morbidity and mortality in patients who meet the following criteria:

1. Stable angina—who have significant left main coronary artery stenosis
2. Stable angina—who have 3-vessel disease
3. 2-vessel disease with significant proximal left anterior descending (LAD) stenosis and either ejection fraction less than 0.50 or demonstrable ischemia on noninvasive testing
4. High-risk unstable angina or non–ST-segment elevation MI
5. Acute ST-elevation MI.

The usefulness of preoperative coronary revascularization is not well established in high-risk ischemic patients with abnormal dobutamine stress echocardiograph and it is not recommended that routine prophylactic coronary revascularization be performed in patients with stable coronary artery disease before noncardiac surgery.

Managing patients with recently placed coronary stents can be broken down into two groups. (a) For patients in whom coronary revascularization with PCI is appropriate for mitigation of cardiac symptoms and who need elective noncardiac surgery in the subsequent 12 months, a strategy of balloon angioplasty or bare-metal stent placement followed by 4-6 weeks of dual-antiplatelet therapy is probably indicated. (b) For patients who received drug-eluting coronary stents and who must undergo urgent surgical procedures that mandate the discontinuation of thienopyridine therapy, it is reasonable to continue aspirin if at all possible and restart thienopyridine as soon as possible.

Medical Management

Medical therapies for cardiac patients include beta blockers, statins, aspirin, calcium channel blockers, and insulin.

A. Beta-Blockers

Class I recommendations:

1. Beta blockers should be continued in patients undergoing surgery, who are currently receiving beta blockers to treat angina, symptomatic arrhythmias, hypertension, or other ACC/AHA Class I guideline indications.
2. Beta blockers should be given to patients undergoing vascular surgery who are at high cardiac risk owing to the finding of ischemia on preoperative testing.

Class IIa recommendations: Beta blockers are recommended for:

1. Patients undergoing vascular surgery in whom the preoperative assessment identifies coronary heart disease (CHD).
2. Patients in whom preoperative assessment for vascular surgery identifies high cardiac risk, as defined by the presence of more than one clinical risk factor.
3. Patients in whom preoperative assessment identifies CHD or high cardiac risk, as defined by the presence of more than one clinical risk factor, who are undergoing intermediate-risk or vascular surgery.

B. Statins

1. Class I—For patients currently taking statins and scheduled for noncardiac surgery, statins should be continued.

2. Class IIa—For patients undergoing vascular surgery with or without clinical risk factors, statin use is reasonable.
3. Class IIb—For patients with at least one clinical risk factor who are undergoing intermediate-risk procedures, statins may be considered.

C. Calcium Channel Blockers

A 2003 metaanalysis of perioperative calcium channel blockers in noncardiac surgery identified 11 studies (1007 patients). The study showed that calcium channel blockers significantly reduced the incidence of myocardial ischemia and supraventricular tachycardia. Calcium channel blockers were associated with reduced death rates and myocardial infarction. Most of these improved outcomes were attributable to the use of diltiazem.

Dihydropyridines and verapamil did not decrease the incidence of myocardial ischemia, although verapamil decreased the incidence of supraventricular tachycardia. To further define the value of these agents, large-scale trials are needed.

SUGGESTED READINGS

Fleisher LA, Beckman JA, Brown KA, Calkins H, Chaikof EL, Fleischmann KE, et al. ACC/AHA 2007 guidelines on perioperative cardiovascular evaluation and care for noncardiac surgery. *Circulation* 2007;116:e418-e500.

Wijeysundera DN, Beattie WS. Calcium channel blockers for reducing cardiac morbidity after noncardiac surgery: a meta-analysis. *Anesth Analg.* 2003;97:634-641.

64

Physical Examination and Airway Evaluation

Taghreed Alshaeri, MD, and Marianne D. David, MD

Preanesthesia assessment is the process of clinical evaluation prior to the delivery of anesthesia in patients undergoing both surgical and nonsurgical procedures. This process includes interviewing the patient, reviewing the patient's medical records, performing a physical examination, including an airway examination, ordering and/or reviewing relevant medical tests, and consulting other medical subspecialists as necessary. The goals of preanesthesia evaluation include familiarizing the provider with the patient's medical conditions, determining the severity of illness, and confirming optimization of all identified issues.

PHYSICAL EXAMINATION

Anesthesia providers should, at a minimum, perform a pulmonary, cardiovascular, and an airway evaluation. The patient's vital signs should also be noted. Evaluation of other organ systems may be necessary depending on the patient's current comorbidities.

General

Evaluate for presence of peripheral venous sites; for regional blocks, examine the extremity or the back for presence of infection or distorted anatomy.

Neurologic

Assess baseline level of consciousness and deficits if the patient has had prior neurologic disease (stroke, neuropathies, etc).

Cardiovascular

Auscultate for heart rate, rhythm, and presence of murmurs; note baseline heart rate and blood pressure.

Pulmonary

Auscultate for rales, rhonchi, and wheezing, especially in patients with known pulmonary disease. Note baseline respiratory rate and O_2 saturation at room air.

Airway Examination

Look for clinical signs that predict difficult airway management. Evaluation of the airway includes, but is not limited to assessing the thyromental distance and cervical spine flexion/extension, examining the oral cavity (Table 64-1) and assigning a Mallampati Classification (Figure 64-1 and Table 64-2). If a difficult airway is anticipated, additional assistance and alternative equipment should be readily available.

SUGGESTED READINGS

Mallampati RS, Gatt SP, Gugino LD et al. A clinical sign to predict difficult tracheal intubation: a prospective study. *Can Anaesth Soc J.* 1985;32:249.

Practice guidelines for management of the difficult airway: an updated report by the American Society of Anesthesiologists Task Force on management of the difficult airway. *Anesthesiology* 2013;118:2.

TABLE 64-1   Elements of Airway Examination

Airway Examination	Non-reassuring Finding
Teeth	Edentulous
Length of upper incisors	Relatively long
Relation of maxillary and mandibular incisors during normal jaw closure	Prominent overbite, inability to demonstrate underbite
Relation of maxillary and mandibular incisors during voluntary protrusion of mandible	Patient cannot bring mandibular incisors anterior to maxillary incisors
Interincisor distance	< 3 cm
Visibility of uvula	Not visible with tongue protruded and with patient sitting up
Shape of the palate	Highly arched or very narrow
Compliance of mandibular space	Stiff, indurated, occupied by mass
Thyromental distance	Less than three finger breadths
Thickness of neck	Thick neck
Length of neck	Short neck
Range of motion of head and neck	Patient cannot touch tip of chin to chest or limited neck extension

(Reproduced with permission from Apfelbaum JL, Hagberg CA, Caplan RA et al. Practice guidelines for management of the difficult airway: an updated report by the American Society of Anesthesiologists Task Force on Management of the Difficult Airway, *Anesthesiology*. 2013;118(2):251-270.)

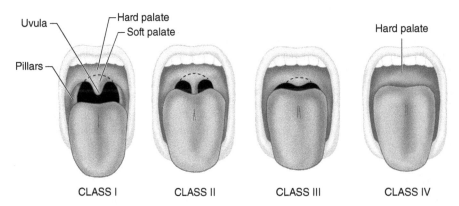

FIGURE 64-1 Mallampati Classification. (Reproduced with permission from Butterworth JF, Mackey DC, Wasnick JD, *Morgan and Mikhail's Clinical Anesthesiology*, 5th ed. McGraw-Hill; 2013.)

TABLE 64-2   Mallampati Classification

Grade View	Visible Structure	Laryngoscope View
I	Tonsillar pillars, soft palate, entire uvula	Entire glottis
II	Soft palate, uvula	Posterior commissure
III	Soft palate, base of uvula	Tips of epiglottis
IV	Hard palate only	No glottal structure

"Full Stomach" Status

Elizabeth E. Holtan, MD

Pulmonary aspiration can cause significant morbidity and mortality to affected patients. It is the anesthesiologist's responsibility to assess a patient's risk for aspiration and determine the best anesthetic plan for the patient to minimize the occurrence and severity of pulmonary aspiration. The anesthesiologist should control gastric contents by minimizing intake of the patient and observing the *nil per os* (NPO) guidelines. When indicated, enhancing gastric emptying and decreasing volume, and increasing pH of gastric contents should also be incorporated into the anesthetic plan. In addition, rapid sequence induction and intubation should also be considered in the anesthetic plan for those with a full stomach status.

NPO GUIDELINES

Before administering any anesthetic, the anesthesiologist should determine the NPO status. One key method to control gastric contents is to minimize intake by following the American Society of Anesthesiologists' (ASA) preoperative fasting practice guidelines (Table 65-1).

Clear Liquids

It is acceptable to ingest clear liquids at least 2 hours before an elective procedure under monitored anesthesia care, regional anesthesia, or general anesthesia. Examples of clear liquids are water, carbonated beverages, juices without pulp, clear tea, and black coffee. Alcohol is not included as an acceptable clear liquid. The amount of liquid consumed is not as significant as the type of liquid consumed.

TABLE 65-1 NPO Guidelines

Clear liquids	2 h
Breast milk	4 h
Infant formula	6 h
Nonhuman milk	6 h
Light meal	6 h
Full meal	8 h

Breast Milk

It is acceptable to ingest breast milk at least 4 hours before an elective procedure under monitored anesthesia care, regional anesthesia, or general anesthesia.

Infant Formula

It is acceptable to ingest infant formula at least 6 hours before elective procedures under monitored anesthesia care, regional anesthesia, or general anesthesia.

Solids and Nonhuman Milk

It is acceptable to ingest nonhuman milk or a light meal 6 hours before elective surgery under monitored anesthesia care, regional anesthesia, or general anesthesia. Consuming meat or foods high in fat content can delay gastric emptying. Extra fasting time, typically 8 hours or more, may be necessary. The total amount and kind of food consumed must be taken into account when deciding an acceptable fasting period. Because nonhuman milk is comparable to solids in gastric emptying time, one must consider the amount ingested to decide on an appropriate fasting period.

Other Methods to Control Gastric Contents

In certain situations, following NPO guidelines may not be feasible. In emergency cases, such as trauma, surgery cannot be delayed by the recommended time to allow for full gastric emptying. Or even if guidelines are followed, the patient may still be at increased risk for aspiration due to a full stomach or an incompetent lower esophageal sphincter. Certain patients carry a higher increased aspiration risk due to medical conditions (Table 65-2). In these cases, the anesthetic plan must be optimized to prevent aspiration and morbidity and mortality if aspiration does occur. Additional steps must be taken to decrease volume and increase pH of gastric contents, as well as enhancing gastric emptying. The anesthesiologist must also consider if, including rapid sequence induction and insertion of an endotracheal tube are part of the appropriate anesthetic plan to protect against pulmonary aspiration.

TABLE 65-2   Factors Increasing Aspiration Risk

Emergency surgery (trauma)
ICU patients
Diabetes mellitus or those with gastroparesis
Poorly controlled gastroesophageal reflux
Hiatal hernia
Gastrointestinal obstruction/abdominal distension
Pregnancy
Morbid obesity
Upper gastrointestinal hemorrhage
Intracranial hypertension
Patient taking opioids
Upper abdominal or laparoscopic surgery
Positioning (lithotomy or Trendelenburg)
Light anesthesia
Insufflation of stomach with bag mask ventilation or LMA

Methods to Decrease Risk of Aspiration

In addition to restrictions on oral intake, increasing gastric emptying and decreasing volume and increasing pH of gastric contents may also help lessen the severity of aspiration, if it occurs. The most significant factor to determine aspiration severity is the pH of aspiration. A pH less than 2.5 usually correlates with worse outcomes. Volume is also a factor; 0.4 mL/kg of aspirate correlates with worse outcomes.

A. Increasing Gastric Emptying/Prokinetics

Metoclopramide is a dopamine antagonist that enhances lower esophageal sphincter tone, increases gastric emptying, and thereby decreases gastric volume. A dose of 10 mg has an onset of 30-60 minutes oral and 2 minutes intravenously. It is contraindicated in patients with Parkinson disease, pheochromocytoma, gastrointestinal obstruction, or in patients taking medications that may interact and cause extrapyramidal side effects. The regular use of prokinetics to decrease the risk of pulmonary aspiration in patients who have no known risk for pulmonary aspiration is not supported by the ASA.

B. Increasing pH and Decreasing Volume of Gastric Contents

- H2-receptor antagonists and proton pump inhibitors—Acidity of gastric contents can be decreased by H2-receptor antagonists and proton pump inhibitors, which can also decrease gastric volume. Famotidine decreases volume and acidity when given a few hours before surgery. Proton pump inhibitors, including omeprazole and lansoprazole, are most effective when given in two repeated doses, the night before and morning of surgery. The regular use of drugs that decrease gastric acidity to prevent the risks of pulmonary aspiration in patients who have no known risk for pulmonary aspiration is not supported by the ASA.

- Nonparticulate antacid—Sodium citrate is a nonparticulate antacid that can be given orally within an hour preoperatively to increase gastric pH above 2.5. Its effect on increasing pH is more rapid than H2-receptor antagonists and proton pump inhibitors, which may be more useful in an emergency case. The regular use of antacids to increase gastric pH to prevent pulmonary aspiration in patients who have no known risk for pulmonary aspiration is not supported by the ASA.

- NG tube—Lastly, a nasogastric (NG) tube can decrease gastric volume in an emergency situation, as well as in cases when there is an increased risk of pulmonary aspiration. An NG tube does not ensure an empty stomach, and it can decrease the upper and lower esophageal sphincter's tone. In high-risk patients, rapid sequence induction and endotracheal intubation may still be indicated.

AIRWAY MANAGEMENT

Airway Protection

Cuffed endotracheal tube by intubation is the method of choice to prevent any regurgitated gastric contents from entering the trachea and lungs. Currently, most commonly used endotracheal tubes have high volume, low pressure cuffs. They do not guarantee prevention of aspiration of gastric contents, but they are still indicated for patients at high risk for aspiration.

Rapid Sequence Induction and Cricoid Pressure

Rapid sequence induction is indicated to secure a patient's airway in the shortest time once consciousness and protective airway reflexes have been lost. First, the patient is well preoxygenated. Then the intravenous anesthetic is given and quickly followed by a rapid onset neuromuscular blocking agent. Once muscle relaxation is established, laryngoscopy and intubation are completed. Cricoid pressure is performed by an assistant from the beginning of induction until the endotracheal tube placement is confirmed.

Cricoid pressure is downward movement of the cricoid cartilage onto the vertebral bodies. The index finger applies downward pressure, while the thumb and middle finger prevent lateral displacement of the cricoid cartilage. The purpose is to close the esophageal lumen while keeping the tracheal lumen patent since it is a circular ring, unlike the other semicircular tracheal rings. The purpose is to prevent passive regurgitation of gastric fluids. Cricoid pressure is contraindicated in patients with cervical spine fracture and in patients with active emesis. Cricoid pressure is controversial as many argue it moves the esophagus laterally and may not truly be efficacious.

As mentioned, the patient should be well preoxygenated prior to induction. Bag mask ventilation should not be used during induction due to concerns of insufflating air in the stomach and increasing risk for aspiration. In the situation where intubation is difficult and oxygen saturation decreases, mild positive pressure ventilation (<25 cm H_2O) is appropriate while maintaining cricoid pressure. If cricoid pressure interferes with essential ventilation, then the pressure may be released.

SUGGESTED READING

American Society of Anesthesiologists Committee on Standards and Practice Parameters: Practice guidelines for preoperative fasting and the use of pharmacologic agents to reduce the risk of pulmonary aspiration: application to healthy patients undergoing elective procedures. *Anesthesiology* 2011;114:495-511.

ASA Physical Status Classification

Kuntal Jivan, MD, FAAP

With an aging and increasingly obese population, patients with significant comorbidities present for surgery. Although age *per se* is not a factor in determining candidacy for ambulatory procedures, each patient must be considered in the context of his or her comorbidities, the type of surgery to be performed, and the expected response to anesthesia. First developed in 1963, the American Society of Anesthesiologists' (ASA) physical status classification system (Table 66-1) summarizes the physiologic fitness of each patient prior to surgery. It serves as a means of communication between health-care providers and is used for record-keeping.

In general, ambulatory surgeries should be of a complexity and duration such that one could reasonably assume that the patient will make an expeditious recovery. Assessment of the patient's ASA physical status and completion of a thorough history and physical examination are crucial in the screening of patients selected for ambulatory or office-based surgery. ASA 4 and 5 patients normally would not be candidates for

TABLE 66-1   ASA's Physical Status Classification of Patients[1]

Class	Definition
1	Normal healthy patient with no organic, physiologic, biochemical, or psychiatric disturbances
2	Patient with mild-to-moderate systemic diseases that have no functional limitations and may not be related to the reason for surgery
3	Patient with severe systemic diseases with some functional limitations that may or may not be related to the reason for surgery
4	Patient with severe systemic disturbances that have incapacitated functions and are a constant threat to life (functionality incapacitated) with or without surgery
5	Moribund patient who has little chance of survival but undergoes surgery as a last resort (resuscitative effort)
6	Brain-dead patient whose organs are removed for donor purposes
E	For an emergency operation, the physical status is followed by "E" (eg, "2E")

[1]Data from Committee on Standards and Practice Parameters.

TABLE 66-2   ASA's Physical Status and Mortality

PS	Mortality (%)
I	0.1
II	0.2
III	1.8
IV	7.8
V	9.4

(Reproduced with permission from Aitkenhead AR, Rowbotham D, Smith G (eds): *Textbook of Anesthesia*. 4th ed. England: Churchill Livingstone; 2001, p. 288.)

ambulatory surgery, whereas ASA 1 and 2 patients would be prime candidates for such surgery. ASA 3 patients with diabetes, hypertension, and stable coronary artery disease would not be precluded from an ambulatory procedure, provided their diseases are well controlled. Ultimately, the surgeon and anesthesiologist must identify patients for whom an ambulatory or office-based setting is likely to provide benefits (eg, convenience, reduced costs, and charges) that outweigh risks (eg, the lack of immediate availability of all hospital services, such as a cardiac catheterization laboratory, emergency cardiovascular stents, assistance with airway rescue, and rapid consultation).

Criticism of the ASA physical status scale is primarily due to its exclusion of age and difficulty of intubation. A study of 1095 patients undergoing total hip replacement, prostatectomy, or cholecystectomy found that both age and ASA physical status accurately predicts postoperative morbidity and mortality. Although it does not predict operative risk, the ASA physical status scale remains a useful application for all patients during the preoperative visit (Table 66-2).

SUGGESTED READINGS

Apfelbaum JL, Connis RT, Nickinovich DG, et al. Practice advisory for preanesthesia evaluation: an updated report by the American Society of Anesthesiologists Task Force on Preanesthesia Evaluation. *Anesthesiology* 2012;116:522.

Cullen DJ, Apolone G, Greenfield S, et al. ASA physical status and age predict morbidity after three surgical procedures. *Ann Surg.* 1994;220:3.

Prophylactic Antibiotics

Sonia John and Jeffrey S. Berger, MD, MBA

Choosing an antibiotic depends on the properties of the antibiotic and the nature of the pathogen. The following considerations are important in selecting the proper course of antimicrobial treatment:

1. Identification of the pathogen determined with testing
2. Susceptibility of the organism to a variety of antibiotics
3. Seriously ill or immunocompromised patients should receive bactericidal rather than bacteriostatic drug
4. Site of infection (ie, does the blood–brain barrier need to be crossed?)
5. Patient limitations such as allergy, immunosuppression, hepatic failure, or renal dysfunction
6. Use of multiple antimicrobials in combination
7. Route of administration
8. Duration of treatment
9. Risk of development of resistant strains
10. Cost

In general, narrow-spectrum antibiotics should be chosen before broad spectrum drugs to avoid disruption of the patient's normal flora of bacteria. Normal bacterial flora are important as they can compete with pathogens for nutrients, produce antibacterial substances, and combat nosocomial-resistant organisms. The recommended dosing of antibiotics should be strictly followed. Morbidly obese patients may require increased dosing to achieve adequate tissue levels of antibiotics, while patients with hepatic or renal dysfunction may require decreased dosing. A listing of commonly used perioperative antibiotics can be found in Table 67-1.

INDICATIONS FOR PROPHYLACTIC ANTIBIOTICS

Prophylactic antibiotics are indicated for surgeries that are contaminated or clean-contaminated. Prophylaxis is also warranted for clean procedures that involve implants, immunocompromised patients, or patients at risk for endocarditis.

Procedures for which antibiotic prophylaxis is generally NOT indicated include: cardiac catheterization, varicose vein surgery, most dermatologic surgeries, arterial punctures, thoracocentesis, paracentesis, repair of simple lacerations, outpatient burn treatment, dental extractions, root canal therapy, plastic surgery (cefazolin may be helpful for operations lasting more than 3 hours).

SURGICAL CARE IMPROVEMENT PROJECT

Antibiotic prophylaxis is one of the core measures of surgical care improvement project (SCIP). Perioperative standardization with SCIP has several evidence-based facets. One element of SCIP is an outcome improvement intervention for choosing and delivering an antibiotic prior to surgical incision. Surgical care improvement project requires practitioners to give appropriate antibiotic prophylaxis for specific procedures in specific body areas. Administration must occur within 1 hour of skin incision, except for vancomycin and fluoroquinolones, which must be given within 2 hours. When a tourniquet is to be used, antibiotics must be delivered prior to inflation. With prolonged surgeries, antibiotic redosing should occur after two half-lives of the antibiotic. Antibiotic prophylaxis must be stopped within 24 hours of surgery (48 hours after cardiac surgery). This project aims to decrease surgical site infections as well as reduce the frequency of antibiotic-resistant infections.

TABLE 67-1   Common Perioperative Antibiotics

Antibiotic	Class and Mechanism	Surgery	Microbe Coverage	IV Adult Dose (D), Redose (R)	Route of Elimination	Notes
Ampicillin	Penicillinase-susceptible; inhibits bacterial cell wall synthesis	Colorectal, appendectomy	Gram-negative bacilli such as *Escherichia coli, Proteus,* and *Streptococcus*	D: 1–2 g R: 4–6 h	Hepatic metabolism; renal excretion	SE: allergic reaction (1–10%)
Cefazolin	First generation Cephalosporin; inhibits mucopeptide layer of bacterial cell wall synthesis	All at-risk surgery	Gram-positive cocci: *Staphylococci* and Nonenterococcal *streptococci*	D: 1 g (if > 80 kg, 2 g) R: 2–6 h (Postop R: 8 h)	Renal excretion	SE: allergic reactions (1–10%)
1. Cefoxitin, 2. Cefotetan, 3. Cefuroxime	Second generation Cephalosporin	1,2: Colorectal; 3: cardiac, thoracic, vascular	Resistant to cephalosporinases, extended gram-negative activity. 3: *H. flu,* meningitis	D: 1–2 g R: 1: 6–8 h; 2:12 h; 3: 8 h	Renal excretion	SE: allergic reactions, prolonged thrombin time, neutropenia
Ceftriaxone	Third generation Cephalosporin	Neurosurgery, epiglottitis	Resistant to beta-lactamase hydrolysis of gram-negative bacilli, including: *E. coli, Klebsiella, Proteus, and H. influenza.* Can cross blood–brain barrier for meningitis	D: 1–2 g R: 24 h	Renal excretion	SE: allergic reactions, prolonged thrombin time, neutropenia
Ciprofloxacin	Fluoroquinolones; broad spectrum; bactericidal; inhibits DNA gyrase in bacteria	Respiratory tract, bone and joints, colorectal, GI, GU	*M. tuberculosis, Salmonella,* enteric gram-negative bacilli, osteomyelitis, otitis	D: 400 mg R: 8–12 h	Hepatic metabolism (active metabolite); renal excretion	SE: allergic reactions, long QT, tendinitis, photosensitivity, teratogenicity; GI irritation
Clindamycin	Lincomycin (similar to Macrolide); acts on bacterial ribosome to inhibit protein synthesis	Cardiothoracic, GI, colorectal, neurosurgery, ENT, and with gentamycin for GU	Most gram-positive bacteria: *Streptococcus pneumoniae, S. aureus, Moraxella catarrhalis, H. flu, Mycoplasma, Chlamydia, Corynebacterium diphtheriae.* Also, anaerobes	D: 600–900 mg over 60 min R: 6–8 h	Biliary excretion	SE: skin rash (10%), pseudo-membranous colitis, NMJ effects resistant to calcium or anticholinesterase drugs, neuromuscular blockade, alcohol intolerance, neuropathy

Drug	Class/Mechanism	Indications	Dosing	Elimination	Notes
Gentamycin	Aminoglycoside; bactericidal; poor lipid solubility; acts on bacterial ribosome to inhibit protein synthesis	Penetrates pleural, ascitic and synovial fluid, GI, colorectal, ENT, and with clindamycin for GU	Gram-negative bacilli, *Pseudomonas aeruginosa*	D: 1–2.5 mg/kg over 60 min R: 8–12 h	Renal excretion	Check for toxicity (<9 μg/mL) to avoid SE: ototoxicity, nephrotoxicity, skeletal muscle weakness and potentiation of NMB drugs
Metronidazole	Antiprotozoal; bactericidal by forming toxic metabolites in the bacterium	Colorectal, neurosurgical (distributes to CNS), orthopedic (bone and joint), abdominal sepsis, and endocarditis	Anaerobic, gram-negative bacilli, *Clostridium*, and pseudomembranous colitis	D: 500 mg over 60 min R: 6–8 h	Hepatic metabolism and renal excretion	SE: antabuse reaction, GI irritation, dry mouth, seizures, neuropathy teratogenicity, and pancreatitis
Piperacillin/ Tazobactam	Antipseudomonal penicillin, beta-lactamase inhibitor; broad spectrum	Sepsis, skin/soft tissue infections	*Pseudomonas aeruginosa*	D: 3.375 g R: 6–8 h	Hepatic metabolism and renal excretion	Does not cover MRSA, VRE, or atypicals SE: neutropenia
Vancomycin	Glycopeptide derivative; bactericidal; impairs cell wall synthesis	Cardiothoracic, orthopedic, vascular, and neurosurgery. Add gentamycin when treating enterococcal endocarditis	Gram-positive bacteria (staphylococcal or streptococcal), MRSA, *Staphylococcus epidermitis* (on prosthetic valves)	D: 1 g (>70 kg); 500–700 mg (<70 kg) or 10–15 mg/kg over 60 min R: 6–12 h	Renal excretion	SE: histamine release causing hypotension ("red-man syndrome") Alternative for PCN-allergic patients for prosthetics, shunts, and valves as prophylaxis

SE, side effect; GI, gastrointestinal; GU, genitourinary; ENT, ear, nose, and throat; NMJ, neuromuscular junction; NMB, neuromuscular blocking; MRSA, Methicillin-resistant *Staphylococcal aureus*; CNS, central nervous system.

68

Premedication

Douglas Sharp, MD

Premedication refers to the administration of medication before the induction of anesthesia. These medications are neither part of the surgical patient's usual medical regimen nor are they part of the anesthetic. They are given to reduce anxiety, control pain, decrease the risk of aspiration pneumonitis, and lower the incidence of postoperative nausea and vomiting. Perioperative beta-blockade and glucocorticoid supplementation are also considered premedication. Antimicrobial therapy for prevention of bacterial endocarditis is briefly reviewed. There are certainly other types of medication that can be given preoperatively, such as erythropoietin for anemia, but these are either not common or not considered the standard of practice.

ANXIOLYTICS

Anxiety levels are typically high for patients presenting for surgery. Anxiety not only interferes with patient comfort, but also increases stress hormone production, gastric secretions, initial anesthetic requirements, and preoperative procedure difficulty (ie, intravenous placement). Children, in particular, may have high anxiety levels that can lead to lack of cooperation. Many centers withhold anxiety premedication out of concerns for reducing throughput, prolonging recovery room stay, and over sedation. None of these concerns have been validated with judicious administration of anxiolytics.

The classes of medications used for anxiolysis premedication include benzodiazepines and, less commonly, alpha-2 adrenergic agonists. Melatonin and ketamine are occasionally chosen for particularly uncooperative pediatric patients.

Less respiratory depression and hemodynamic effects occur with benzodiazepines compared to other sedative-hypnotic agents. Additionally, the amnestic effects are desirable in the preoperative setting. The three commonly used intravenous benzodiazepines are midazolam, Ativan, and diazepam. Midazolam has the fastest onset of action, has an inactive metabolite, and is well tolerated during parenteral administration. It has, therefore, become the predominant preoperative anxiolytic. In adults, a dose of 1-2 mg is typically sufficient for premedication.

Oral benzodiazepines have found a role in pediatric anesthesia, with liquid midazolam at a dose of 0.5 mg/kg typically producing sedation within 10 minutes. Oral diazepam in tablet form has a long history of use in adults. Consideration of an oral benzodiazepine prescription the night before or the morning of surgery is useful for the particularly anxious adult before they enter a surgical facility.

Clonidine and dexmedetomidine may have a role in reducing anxiety preoperatively and also have some anesthesia sparing effects. The hemodynamic side effects and longer duration of action of these drugs limit their clinical utility.

Ketamine as a premedication is reserved for children who need a deeper level of sedation than oral benzodiazepines may provide. Oral ketamine in a dose of 4-6 mg/kg is usually given in conjunction with oral midazolam and an anti-sialagogue. If this approach is considered too slow or if a child does not cooperate with oral medications, then ketamine 2-4 mg/kg may be given intramuscularly, although this may be painful and risks formation of aseptic abscesses.

Melatonin has recently seen more consideration as a preoperative sedative. Melatonin produces anxiolysis without psychomotor skills impairment. Premedication with oral 0.2 mg/kg melatonin provides sedation and anesthetic sparing properties. Other novel anxiolytic premedicants include gabapentin and pregabalin.

ANALGESICS

Opioids are not generally given as premedication unless the patient requires analgesia or is on a preexisting opioid regimen. In these cases, fentanyl or one of its analogs may be given. Withholding opioids in the immediate preoperative period for a narcotic-dependent patient will have significant physiologic and psychological effects on that patient, potentially complicating induction of anesthesia. Care should be taken while administering opioid medications as respiratory depression can occur in a preoperative patient without close monitoring. Other analgesics given preoperatively include NSAIDs. Celecoxib 400 mg PO in adults provides analgesia without increasing the risk of surgical bleeding.

ANTIEMETICS

Premedication for the prevention of postoperative nausea and vomiting is limited as most are preferentially given intraoperatively. Agents with a long duration of action or a delayed onset of action are appropriately given as a premedication. Transdermal scopolamine has been shown to be as efficacious as ondansetron for the prevention of postoperative emesis. Effective plasma levels are generally obtained within 4 hours. Side effects include dry mouth, dizziness, mydriasis. Patients with open angle glaucoma should not be given this medication. Aprepitant, a neurokinin-1 antagonist, has a longer duration of action than ondansetron and, therefore, may have more use as a premedication in the high-risk patient.

ASPIRATION PROPHYLAXIS

The use of agents to reduce the risk of pulmonary aspiration is not routinely warranted in the fasted patient. Non-fasted patients, patients with bowel obstruction, autonomic neuropathy, advanced pregnancy, gastroesophageal reflux disease, scleroderma, and several other conditions should be considered for the administration of agents to decrease both gastric pH and residual gastric volumes. H_2-receptor blocking drugs (ie, ranitidine 50 mg IV in adults) are effective in reducing gastric pH if given 2-3 hours prior to anesthetic induction. Gastric stimulants, such as metoclopramide and proton pump inhibitors, such as pantoprazole can also be helpful but have not been shown to have additional benefit to the H_2-receptor antagonists. Nonparticulate antacids such as sodium citrate and magnesium trisilicate can quickly increase gastric pH and can be considered in patients at risk for aspiration.

BETA-BLOCKADE

The addition of perioperative beta-blockade is recommended for a small preoperative population, specifically the high-risk cardiac patient undergoing high-risk vascular surgery. Ideally, this therapy should be started at least a week before the surgery and titrated to a heart rate of less than 60 if there is no concomitant hypotension. The POISE trial indicated a possible increased mortality risk if instituted in a broader patient population. Beta-blockade has other benefits, however, in addition to the reduction of cardiac morbidity, including decreased analgesic requirements and the control of hypertensive responses during surgery.

STEROIDS

Supplementation of glucocorticoid therapy should be considered in the patient at high risk for suppression of the hypothalamic—pituitary—adrenal axis. Those at risk for such suppression include patients taking more than the equivalent of 20 mg of prednisone daily for more than a 3-week period prior to the scheduled surgery. Hydrocortisone or its equivalent should be dosed depending on the type of surgery. Minimally invasive procedures do not require any supplementation of the patient's regular glucocorticoid dose. A dose of 50 mg IV hydrocortisone with continuation for 1-2 days is appropriate for most surgeries. High-risk surgeries may require 100 mg IV doses, with continuation for 2-3 days postoperatively.

ANTIBIOTICS

In regards to antibiotic prophylaxis for the prevention of bacterial endocarditis, the guidelines published by the American Heart Association underwent a major revision in 2007. Currently, it is recommended that only the highest risk patients should get prophylaxis and that it should be given only for specific procedures involving gums or roots of teeth, the respiratory tract (bronchoscopy only if incision of respiratory mucosa), and infected tissues. The highest risk patients include those with artificial heart valves, prosthetic material in the heart, certain congenital heart defects that have been incompletely or not treated, a previous history of endocarditis, and in heart transplant patient with acquired valvular disease.

SUGGESTED READING

Devereaux PJ, Yang H, Yusuf S, et al. Effects of extended-release metoprolol succinate in patients undergoing non-cardiac surgery (POISE trial): a randomised controlled trial. *Lancet* 2008;371:1839-1847.

Management of Chronic Medical Therapy

69

Douglas Sharp, MD

With a few exceptions, chronic medical therapy should not be adjusted prior to presentation for surgery. It is prudent to maintain adequate treatment of medical conditions, including administration of oral medications with small sips of water on the day of surgery. Surgery presents problems such as bleeding, fasting, and physiologic stresses that require anticipation prior to surgery. Additionally, preoperative examination and testing may dictate the need for the initiation or adjustment of medications.

Chronic medical therapy must be reviewed in a timely fashion before surgery. This review can take place in a variety of settings, including the surgeon's office, a primary medical provider or specialist's office, or in a preanesthesia testing unit. A phone discussion may be appropriate in many circumstances. Particular attention should be focused on anticoagulation treatment, including herbal remedies, diabetes mellitus therapy, and antihypertensive treatment.

ANTICOAGULATION

The surgical patient on anticoagulation therapy needs special attention, especially with the proliferation of novel anticoagulants and new management guidelines. Surgical bleeding risk must be weighed against thrombosis risk. Abruptly stopping anticoagulants may induce a hypercoagulable state. This adds to the prothrombotic nature of the surgical period itself.

- Example 1—A patient on aspirin therapy for primary prevention of stroke or cardiovascular disease scheduled for a procedure with a high risk of bleeding. Aspirin therapy should be withheld for seven days, or less for lower-dose aspirin regimens.
- Example 2—A patient on dual antiplatelet therapy for recent coronary intervention with unclear surgical bleeding risk. The clinical decision making is less clear; institutional guidelines should inform decisions.

Warfarin therapy is stopped 5 days prior to surgery unless the risk of surgical bleeding is very low. If the starting INR is greater than 2.5, then more than 5 days may be necessary to normalize the INR ratio, and laboratory findings should guide surgical preparedness. For emergency surgery, vitamin K, fresh frozen plasma, or a combination of the two may expedite anticoagulation reversal. Bridging therapy with heparin, fractionated or unfractionated, should be considered. Temporal relation of the initial thrombotic event can dictate the need for bridging therapy; a recent thrombotic event suggests the need for bridging therapy. For atrial fibrillation and mechanical heart valves, recent trends in perioperative care favor bridging therapy for high-risk patients only.

Newer, oral, direct thrombin inhibitors, such as dabigatran do not require bridging therapy because of rapid onset and offset. Patients with normal renal function can stop dabigatran 2 days prior to surgery. If creatinine clearance is decreased, longer stoppage time may be necessary. Thrombin clotting time can be used to assess residual anticoagulant effects. These agents can be started 24–72 hours after surgery depending on bleeding risk.

Patients on aspirin therapy for secondary stroke prevention or cardiovascular events should continue the therapy intraoperatively. However, bleeding risk may be unacceptably high during certain procedures such as spine surgery, plastic surgery, neurosurgery, and some urologic surgeries and aspirin therapy may be stopped in these cases. Patients with coronary stents should not have any elective procedure within certain time frames of stenting.

Preoperative history should uncover use of herbal medications and vitamin therapy associated with bleeding. Specifically, gingko, garlic, ginseng, feverfew, and vitamin E have been associated with increased bleeding. These supplements should be stopped for at least a week prior to surgery. Also, NSAIDs can be stopped within several days of a procedure if alternate pain management options are provided.

DIABETIC THERAPY

Ideally, presurgical fasting should adhere to the 8 hour minimum for solid food and 2-hour period for clear liquids. A slight modification of medication regimen may be needed for adequate perioperative control; if fasting is to be continued postoperatively, then intravenous regimens including both insulin and substrate (ie, dextrose) should be implemented.

Fasting patients with glucose levels greater than 250 mg/dL or HgA1c greater than 8.5% should be referred for medical optimization prior to elective surgery.

Goal of perioperative glucose levels are 70-150 mg/dL. Perioperative level checks commence preoperatively and continue hourly intraoperatively. Postoperative glucose levels should also be monitored closely.

Oral hypoglycemic agents are held on the day of surgery with some exceptions. Metformin should not be stopped for a prolonged period before surgery since the risk of fasting hypoglycemia is low and its abrupt withdrawal may lead to difficulty controlling glucose levels. Renal dysfunction and IV contrast exposure risk development of lactic acidosis on metformin. Therefore, metformin should be withheld for 48 hours prior to surgery in those patients.

Insulin preparations are typically adjusted preoperatively. Long-acting agents, including insulin glargine (Lantus) are continued, reflecting basal insulin replacement and minimal fasting hypoglycemia. Intermediate-acting insulin preparations are curtailed to half the usual neutral protamine Hagedorn (NPH) or Humulin lente dosages on the evening before and the morning of surgery. Short-acting insulin preparations are withheld during the fasting period.

ANTIHYPERTENSIVES

Induction of anesthesia typically results in hypotension and vasodilation. Although most antihypertensive therapy should be continued on the day of surgery, many centers instruct patients not to take angiotensin-converting enzyme inhibitors and angiotensin-receptor blockers on the day of surgery to minimize hypotensive episodes and the risk of vasoplegic syndrome.

PSYCHIATRIC MEDICATIONS

Most psychiatric medications including antidepressants, anxiolytics, and antipsychotic medications should be continued on the day of surgery to avoid withdrawal. The exception is monoamine oxidase inhibitors (MAOIs), such as phenelzine, which are associated with several severe perioperative risks. Hypertensive crisis may result if a patient is also given indirect acting sympathomimetics (ie, ephedrine). Additionally, MAOIs given with meperidine may initiate serotonin syndrome. MAOIs should be stopped 3 weeks preoperatively in conjunction with the patient's psychiatrist.

SUGGESTED READINGS

Baron TH, Kamath PS, McBane RD. Current concepts: management of antithrombotic therapy in patients undergoing invasive procedures. *New Engl J Med.* 2013;368.

Mercado DL, Petty BG. Perioperative medication management. *Med Clin N Am.* 2003;87:41-57.

Rivera RA. Preoperative medical consultation: maximizing its benefits. *Am J Surg.* 2012;204:787-797.

Spinal Anesthesia

Jonah Lopatin, MD, and Kuntal Jivan, MD

ANATOMY

The epidural space lies between the walls of the vertebral canal and the meninges. The meninges are composed of three distinct layers (dura, arachnoid, and pia mater) that are continuous cephalad with the cranial meninges. Dura mater, the outermost layer, extends from the foramen magnum to S2 in adults where it fuses with the filum terminale. The innermost layer of dura mater is highly vascular and serves as the principal route for elimination of drugs in the epidural and subarachnoid space. The arachnoid mater lies deep in the dura and serves as a tight barrier, separating the spinal cord from the epidural space. A potential space exists between the dura and arachnoid mater. The pia mater is the deepest layer of the spinal meninges and adheres to the spinal cord. The subarachnoid space lies between the arachnoid and pia mater, and contains the cerebrospinal fluid (CSF).

The CSF is produced by the choroid plexus and cerebral and spinal capillaries at a rate of 25 mL/h. In an adult, the CSF volume is approximately 100–150 mL. The entire volume of CSF is replaced every 4–6 h as it is removed through the spinal nerve roots and in the sagittal sinus.

TECHNIQUE

Access to the subarachnoid space is accomplished using the spinal needles. The outside diameter of the needle determines the gauge of the needle. Smaller gauge needles lower the risk of postdural puncture headaches but can be difficult to introduce and are often deflected by the interspinous ligaments. Insertion of spinal needles smaller than 22 gauges is often accomplished with the use of an introducer to pass through the supraspinous ligament. Inner stylets prevent plugging of the needle with skin or epidural fat, and subsequent introduction of these substances into the subarachnoid space.

Patient position is critical for successful spinal anesthesia. For obese patients or patients with otherwise difficult anatomy, the sitting position is useful in identifying the midline landmarks of spinous processes. This position can also be useful in restricting spinal anesthesia to more caudal dermatomes when using a hyperbaric local anesthetic. Similarly,

the lateral decubitus position can be used to localize a spinal block to one side when bilateral anesthesia is not required for an operation or procedure, limiting the side effects of spinal anesthesia. The spinal canal narrows above L2, so insertion of a spinal needle above L2-L3 is generally avoided to decrease the risk of spinal cord injury.

The midline approach for access to the subarachnoid space starts with identification of the desired level. Once local anesthesia has been accomplished, the introducer needle is inserted at the top of the vertebral body that forms the lower border of the intended interspace. The introducer should be angled slightly cephalad to avoid the spinous process of the superior vertebra. As the spinal needle is introduced, it will cross the skin, subcutaneous tissue, supraspinous ligament, interspinous ligament, ligamentum flavum, epidural space, dura mater, and arachnoid mater into the subarachnoid space. Dural penetration is accompanied by a characteristic "pop." Once the spinal needle is in the subarachnoid space, the stylet is withdrawn to allow the return of CSF to be observed.

The paramedian approach may be useful in cases of calcification of the supraspinous or interspinous ligaments, or in patients where flexion may be difficult. Local anesthesia is achieved cutaneously 1 cm lateral to midline and following the intended track of the spinal needle. The paramedian approach requires a more cephalad orientation of the introducer and spinal needle as well as a slight medial orientation. The first change in resistance encountered from this angle will be the ligamentum flavum, as the supraspinous and interspinous ligaments do not run lateral to the midline. From this approach, the ligamentum flavum will not be as thick in comparison to the midline approach.

Block Level

The level of the desired block is dictated by the intended surgical procedure. Since spinal needle access is not generally attempted above the level of L2-L3, patient position (gravity) and baricity of the local anesthetic in relation to CSF are important in obtaining appropriate block height. Baricity is the ratio of the local anesthetic density to that of the CSF. Baricity plays a more important role than dose, volume, or concentration of local anesthetic in determining block level. Most local anesthetics are delivered as a hyperbaric solution, which is accomplished through the addition of dextrose (between 1.25% and 8.25%) to the local anesthetic. Block laterality can be achieved by using a hyperbaric solution and by maintaining the patient in a lateral decubitus position with the operative side down. Blocks above the level of needle insertion can be achieved by placing the patient in a Trendelenburg position until the desired level of block is observed.

The initial onset of spinal anesthesia is rapid (in minutes) and is similar for all local anesthetics. Generally, lidocaine and mepivacaine reach peak block effect prior to tetracaine and mepivacaine. Epinephrine, phenylephrine, or clonidine can be added to local anesthetics to extend the duration of action of local anesthetics for spinal anesthesia.

	Dose (mg)	Duration (min)
Procaine	75	45
Bupivacaine	4–10	90–120
Tetracaine	4–8	90–120
Lidocaine	25–50	60–75
Ropivacaine	8–12	90–120

SENSORY, MOTOR, AND AUTONOMIC EFFECTS

Local anesthetics provide the desired sensory blockade through interruption of afferent transmission of painful stimuli from the level of the block. This sensory blockade will block somatic as well as visceral stimuli through blockade of nociceptive A-delta and C fibers. Differential blockade of additional afferent and efferent fibers is dependent on the diameter and myelination of those fibers as well as the decreasing concentration of local anesthetic with distance from level of injection, and will result in additional effects of neuraxial anesthesia, including motor and autonomic blockade.

Sympathetic blockade can be tested through temperature perception and generally extends 1-2 levels cephalad of the sensory block, which is measured by fine touch perception. The most caudal of the nerves impacted through spinal anesthesia are the efferent fibers, responsible for a motor blockade that is observed 1-2 levels caudal to the sensory blockade. Both the A-alpha motor fibers and A-beta mechanoreceptors are more heavily myelinated than the nociceptive fibers, leading to limited persisting motor control and pressure sensation in the setting of appropriate pain control with spinal anesthesia.

SIDE EFFECTS

Cardiovascular side effects are the most common changes observed with spinal anesthesia and are due to blockade of sympathetic control of the anesthetized region, resulting in hypotension and bradycardia. In healthy individuals, lumbar spinal anesthesia can be expected to produce a 15%-20% decrease in mean arterial pressure as well as a decrease in peripheral vascular resistance. The severity of these changes is proportional to block height and, when allowed, can be decreased with lateralization of spinal blockade. Hypotension results from venous and arterial dilation, which in turn leads to decreased preload and afterload, and decreased cardiac output. These changes are offset through the renin–angiotensin-aldosterone system, and accordingly are more pronounced in patients taking angiotensin-converting enzyme inhibitors or angiotensin-receptor blocking drugs.

Administration of fluid boluses to patients prior to spinal anesthesia and ensuring normovolemia can decrease the incidence of hypotension. Epinephrine may increase peripheral vascular resistance, and unlike fluid restoration, will also result in increased cardiac output. Prolonged treatment with epinephrine may lead to increase in heart rate, so dopamine is favored for long-term blood pressure maintenance, if needed.

Nausea is a common side effect of spinal anesthesia. The likely mechanism involves chemical sympathectomy that enables unopposed parasympathetic tone, as well as hypotension leading to decreased splanchnic blood flow. Unopposed parasympathetic input will also lead to increased peristalsis and relaxation of intestinal sphincters; this increased motility may contribute to nausea. Treatment of hypotension will often relieve feelings of nausea.

Interruption of autonomic control of the kidneys will result in decreased glomerular filtration rate through a decrease in renal blood flow. Similar changes are observed with hepatic blood flow in high spinal blocks. These changes are proportional to changes in arterial pressure.

Blocks that cover the thoracic area, including intercostal and abdominal muscles, may influence respiratory function, especially in patients with chronic lung disease. In healthy patients, decreased sensation of chest and abdominal movement with normal breathing may lead to a sensation of dyspnea. As long as the patient is speaking and oxygenating comfortably, reassurance is often the only necessary treatment.

COMPLICATIONS

The most common complication associated with spinal anesthesia is back pain at the site of needle insertion following the procedure. This pain is caused by ligament strain, local anesthetic irritation, and trauma from the spinal needle and introducer. Back pain is generally self-limited and requires only supportive care.

There is a risk of postdural puncture headache whenever meningeal puncture occurs, which is a prerequisite for spinal anesthesia. It has characteristic symptoms, including frontal and occipital pain that is worse when the patient is upright and relieved or absent when the patient is supine, and may be accompanied by nausea and vomiting. The incidence of these headaches increases with increasing needle diameter and decreases with age. These headaches are usually self-limiting and will resolve over the course of a week. If a patient is unable to tolerate spontaneous resolution, an epidural blood patch may be employed, in which 10-20 mL of autologous blood is injected into the epidural space at the site of needle insertion to cover the meningeal puncture site.

Perhaps the most potential severe complication of spinal anesthesia is direct damage to the spinal cord or nerve roots, resulting in permanent neurologic deficits. Direct trauma to spinal nerves may occur when the spinal needle is introduced. If paresthesia is reported by the patient, needle advancement should be stopped and the stylet removed. If the needle is in the epidural space, no CSF will be observed and the needle has likely contacted a spinal nerve root, which is likely if the paresthesia occurs in the dermatome of the level of needle insertion. If CSF return is observed, the needle has likely contacted a nerve root in the cauda equina, indicating the needle is appropriately situated in the subarachnoid space, which is also occupied by the cauda equina nerve roots. Diffuse injury to these roots may result in cauda equina syndrome.

Although a rare outcome, the knowledge of this potential complication can cause extreme anxiety in patients if they experience more common side effects such as transient neurologic symptoms (TNS). Patients with this syndrome have lower extremity pain that occurs following full muscular and sensory recovery of spinal anesthesia in the immediate postoperative period. It is most commonly seen following spinal anesthesia with lidocaine and is thought to be due to the transient neurotoxicity of concentrated local anesthetics. TNS is self-resolving, usually within 5 days.

Spinal hematoma, although rare, occurs when blood pools around the spinal cord. Because the vertebral canal is fixed, pooled blood within the canal may lead to ischemia of the spinal cord, resulting in permanent neurologic deficits. Definitive treatment is surgical decompression and the diagnosis is made by MRI, but any patient complaining of numbness or lower extremity weakness extending beyond the anticipated duration of the block should raise concern for the presence of a spinal hematoma. The greatest risk factor is impaired coagulation, either secondary to an inherent bleeding disorder or pharmacological anticoagulation.

Epidural Anesthesia

Victor Leslie, MD, and Brian S. Freeman, MD

ANATOMIC BOUNDARIES

Epidural anesthesia is typically implemented in the clinical realms of surgery, obstetrics, and in the subspecialty of pain management. The epidural space is considered a potential space, which is filled with nerve roots, blood vessels, lymphatic vessels, and fat. The anatomic boundaries of the epidural space are:

- foramen magnum (rostrally)
- sacrococcygeal ligament (caudally)
- posterior longitudinal ligament (anteriorly)
- ligamentum flavum and vertebral lamina (posteriorly)
- vertebral pedicles (laterally)

The epidural space varies in width from the cervical to lumbar region and is 2-3 mm wide at C3-C6, 3-5 mm wide in the thoracic spine, and widest (5-6 mm) in the lumbar spine.

MECHANISM OF ACTION

In the epidural space, the primary site of action for local anesthetics is the spinal nerve roots. Sodium channel blockade occurs in the dural sleeve, the region where nerves travel through the intervertebral foramen. Secondary and minimal influence occurs from diffusion of local anesthetic from the epidural space into the subarachnoid space, which invariably affects the nerve roots and spinal cord tracts.

With implementation of a successful epidural anesthetic, several physiologic changes occur in the order of sympathectomy first, then sensory blockade, and finally motor blockade. Sympathectomy is induced by epidural anesthesia, which may lead to profound hypotension in individuals predisposed to reduced preload. A reduction in afterload also contributes to hypotension. In response to decreased systemic vascular resistance, tachycardia has been well documented. Upper thoracic sympathectomy (T1-T4) inhibits cardioaccelerator fibers, thus causing decreased cardiac contractility and heart rate. Sympathectomy at T8 and above may inhibit sympathetic afferent neurons to the adrenal medulla leading to a decreased stress response. With phrenic nerve paralysis (C3-C5), ventilation and airway protection may be compromised. However, cranial nerves are unaffected because the foramen magnum serves as the rostral boundary of the epidural space. It is important to differentiate between high epidural blockade and a total spinal anesthetic. With the latter, oculomotor nerve function is compromised as pupillary dilation is present accompanied by an absent light reflex.

Other manifestations of sympathectomy include increased bowel motility and contraction, urinary retention, and increased propensity for decreased core body temperature secondary to peripheral vasodilation if external warming measures are ignored. Advantages of sympathectomy include decreased probability of ileus from unopposed parasympathetic tone and decreased blood loss during procedure from hypotension. Disadvantages include increased risk for decreased perfusion, resulting in ischemia to vital organs (brain—stroke, spinal cord—myelopathy, heart—myocardial infarction).

CONTRAINDICATIONS

Absolute contraindications to epidural anesthetics are patient refusal, sepsis with hemodynamic instability, hypovolemia, and coagulopathy. Once a patient has been properly informed about regional anesthesia and subsequently expresses disapproval, avoid further attempts to convince. Sepsis with hemodynamic instability presents a vasodilated patient at baseline predisposed to further reductions in systemic vascular resistance and afterload with administration of local anesthetics. Epidural anesthesia may contribute to hemodynamic instability; sepsis increases the possibility of catheter infection and epidural abscess. Hypovolemia contributes significantly to hypotension and decreased venous return. A patient's intravascular volume status must be replenished before receiving epidural anesthesia to help counteract sympathectomy. Vasopressor effects are also suboptimal in an intravascularly depleted patient. Coagulopathy and bleeding diathesis predispose the patient to epidural hematoma and potential neurologic deficits.

Relative contraindications are prior back injury with neurologic deficit, progressive neurologic disease, chronic back pain, localized infection at injection site, various forms of stenosis, and elevated intracranial pressure. Prior back injury with neurologic deficit and progressive neurologic diseases, such as multiple sclerosis, may mask important symptoms used in determining successful placement of epidural anesthesia and symptoms of local anesthetic toxicity. Chronic back is associated with influencing psychological factors. Some patients may associate further pain with epidural placement even if the epidural did not contribute to increased pain. Infection at the site of epidural injection may facilitate bacteremia in a patient. Patients with mitral stenosis, aortic stenosis, and idiopathic hypertrophic subaortic stenosis are intolerant of acute decreases in systemic vascular resistance. Elevated intracranial pressure is recognized as a contraindication because epidural anesthesia increases intracranial pressure, thus potentially decreasing cerebral perfusion pressure and brain perfusion.

ADVANTAGES/DISADVANTAGES

When formulating an anesthetic plan, it is important to be cognizant of the advantages and disadvantages of epidural anesthesia compared with spinal and general anesthesia. Advantages of epidural anesthesia over general anesthesia include:

- patient being awake for procedure;
- no airway intervention;
- reduced body stress response;
- decreased pulmonary complications;
- decreased probability of ileus;
- decreased thromboembolic events;
- reduced postoperative nausea and sedation;
- superior postoperative pain management.

Advantages of epidural anesthesia over spinal anesthesia include:

- providing focused segmental block only at the site of procedure;
- increased onset time of local anesthetic that provides additional time to manage potential hypotensive episodes;
- continuous infusion through epidural catheter that increases duration of blockade;
- ability to manipulate local anesthetic concentration to affect density of block;
- reduced potential for postdural puncture headache.

Disadvantages of epidural anesthesia compared with spinal anesthesia include:

- less reliability;
- subjective end point for determining location of epidural space;
- slower onset of anesthetic block;
- less intense sensory and motor blockade;
- propensity for unintentional patchy, segmental, and unilateral blockade.

TECHNIQUE

Common landmarks to be cognizant of when evaluating the surface anatomy of the back include the vertebra prominens (C7), root of scapular spine (T3), inferior angle of the scapula (T7), iliac crest (L4), and the posterior superior iliac spine (S2), which is also the caudal boundary of the dural sac. Unlike spinal anesthesia, thoracic kyphosis and lumbar lordosis are of minimal significance in regards to epidural anesthesia.

The median or paramedian approach may be implemented. Median approach is most often associated with lumbar epidurals. Advantages include a more direct approach as the needle traverses skin, subcutaneous fat, supraspinous ligament, interspinous ligament, and ligamentum flavum to enter the epidural space (latissimus dorsi and trapezius muscles are avoided). Second, there is a decreased possibility of injuring spinal nerves. The paramedian approach is usually associated with thoracic epidurals due to steep angulation of thoracic spinous processes. Patients with inability to adequately flex the back, hypertrophied bone spurs, or additional spinal abnormalities often benefit from this technique.

Begin procedure ensuring availability of oxygen, devices to secure an airway, emergency drugs, and administration of intravenous fluids if patient is considered hypovolemic. Patient may be placed in sitting or lateral decubitus position, flexing back, with vertebrae aligned vertically or horizontally. Appreciate surface landmarks, in particular the iliac crest which approximates the L4 vertebrae. Palpate intervertebral spaces above and below L4, and subsequently sterilely prep the desired placement of epidural. Make skin wheal with local anesthetic and insert epidural needle into wheal. After needle is inserted several millimeters, remove stylet and connect syringe filled with fluid or air. Apply continuous or intermittent pressure to syringe, aspirating every couple of millimeters during insertion. Since recognizing the endpoint of reaching the epidural space is subjective, appreciating the tactile sensation of skin, fascia, and ligaments is of utmost importance. Ligamentum flavum, the final layer before the epidural space, may be described as having a gritty, sandy tactile sensation. Once loss of resistance is achieved, remove syringe and thread epidural catheter approximately 5 cm. Remove needle over catheter, aspirate, and administer 3 mL test dose of local anesthetic with epinephrine. If test dose is negative, secure catheter and titrate local anesthetic to desired effect.

PHARMACOLOGY

Choice of Anesthetic

The choice of anesthetic for epidural anesthesia depends on patient characteristics, procedure, and quality of local anesthetic. The most significant factors affecting spread of epidural anesthesia are dose (concentration × volume) and site of injection. The baricity of local anesthetic agents does not affect spread of epidural anesthesia. The duration of anesthesia is influenced by choice of local anesthetic and addition of vaso-constrictor, most commonly epinephrine.

Adjuvants

Epinephrine assists in extending the duration of action of local anesthetic, enhances blockade, decreases local anesthetic peak blood levels, and serves as a marker of intravascular injection (tachycardia). Opioids, characterized as lipophilic or hydrophilic, may assist with analgesia and improve quality of blockade. Lipophilic agents such as fentanyl have a faster onset, shorter duration of action, and less side effects (most important of which is respiratory depression). Hydrophilic agents have longer onset, longer duration of action, and more side effects. The addition of sodium bicarbonate decreases local anesthetic onset time by facilitating a predominance of the nonionized form. However, with bupivacaine, alkalinization promotes precipitation.

COMPLICATIONS

- *Hypotension* occurs from the chemical sympathectomy. The extent of hypotension is proportional to degree of sympathectomy and patient's volume status. Hypotension may be augmented by patient positioning and administration of intravenous fluids before procedure.

- *Subarachnoid injection* of epidural local anesthetic dose may result in total spinal blockade. Goals of treatment are supporting respiration with positive pressure ventilation and maintaining hemodynamic stability with vasopressors. Intrathecal normal saline may prevent significant neurologic damage.

- *Postdural puncture headache* occurs when the dura is accidentally traversed by the epidural needle. Initial treatment involves positioning the patient supine and expectant management. If conservative treatment fails, administration of blood patch is warranted. Caffeine and analgesics may also be implemented.

- *Epidural hematoma and abscess* may be induced or spontaneous and commonly present as acute radicular back pain. When epidural hematoma is suspected, emergent imaging (MRI or CT scan) and decompression within 6-8 hours is warranted to prevent neurologic sequelae.

- *Intravascular injection* may result in local anesthetic toxicity. Aspirating before injection and test dose with epinephrine reduces probability, but catheter may migrate intravascularly. If this occurs, administer induction agents or anticonvulsant to stop convulsions, intubate if indicated and counteract hemodynamic instability with vasopressors, inotropes, and ACLS protocol. Additional symptoms of local anesthetic toxicity are slurred speech, restlessness, and tinnitus. Bupivacaine has well-documented cardiotoxic effects.

Combined Spinal–Epidural Anesthesia

Victor Leslie, MD, and Brian S. Freeman, MD

First documented in 1937, combined spinal–epidural anesthesia (CSE) is a technique in which both spinal and epidural anesthesia are administered simultaneously. The combination of the two approaches can present complications that are absent from each individual procedure.

INDICATIONS AND CONTRAINDICATIONS

Indications include patients in need of rapid anesthesia and analgesia with subsequent extended postprocedure analgesia. Labor analgesia, including emergent and elective cesarean sections, utilize CSE anesthesia because it offers timely, reliable anesthesia with adequate muscle relaxation and minimal drug toxicity to both mother and fetus. The CSE technique has been documented to be superior to sole individual and epidural anesthesia for abdominal procedures such as hysterectomies. Thoracic procedures have been performed with CSE anesthesia. However, the inhibition of cardioaccelerator fibers and respiratory depression may necessitate use of cardioactive drugs and general anesthesia with a secure airway. For certain lower extremity orthopedic procedures (eg, total hip arthroplasty, femur fractures, and total knee arthroplasty), implementation of CSE anesthesia provides benefits of decreased blood loss and decreased incidence of postoperative deep vein thrombosis.

Absolute contraindications include patient refusal, sepsis, hypovolemia, coagulopathy or therapeutic anticoagulation, elevated intracranial pressure, and infection at procedure site. Relative contraindications include current neurologic pathology, severe psychiatric disease, dementia, aortic stenosis, left ventricular outflow tract obstruction, and alteration of vertebral column secondary to prior surgery.

ADVANTAGES AND DISADVANTAGES

Ideally, CSE anesthesia incorporates the advantages of each procedure while avoiding the disadvantages. The spinal portion allows rapid onset of blockade and more reliable blockade, while the epidural portion provides ability for extended analgesia through redosing or continuous infusion of local anesthetic. Intensity of blockade may be altered by manipulating local anesthetic concentration. Although there is increased preparation time for surgery compared with general anesthesia, the technique of CSE anesthesia decreases recovery time in the postanesthesia care unit, time to postoperative patient fluid intake, narcotic requirements, and episodes of emesis.

Disadvantages potentially avoided include the single administration of local anesthetic and unpredictable level of blockade with spinal anesthesia and patchy blockade, poor sacral spread, and possible local anesthetic toxicity associated with epidural anesthesia.

COMBINED SPINAL–EPIDURAL TECHNIQUES

Single pass—First performed in 1980 (Vitenbeck), using the same needle, local anesthetic is first injected into the epidural space, and then further inserted into the subarachnoid space for intrathecal local anesthetic administration.

Needle-through-needle—First described in 1982, this most commonly used technique involves locating the epidural space with a needle and subsequently inserting a small diameter spinal needle through the epidural needle lumen to administer local anesthetic intrathecally. Once the spinal needle is removed, the epidural catheter may be inserted into the lumen of the epidural needle and placed in the desired position. The epidural catheter may be placed before the spinal needle is introduced, but this may increase the risk of damage to the spinal needle and the catheter or increased difficulty of correctly positioning the spinal needle.

Eldor needle technique—This technique may be viewed as a variation of the needle-through-needle technique. However, it enables placement of the epidural catheter before spinal anesthesia, allowing administration of an epidural test dose. Before placement of the epidural needle, the spinal needle is inserted in a small channel within the lumen of the epidural needle. When the epidural space is successfully identified, the catheter is threaded through the epidural needle lumen without contacting the spinal needle due to the intraluminal spinal channel. An epidural test is administered. Subsequently, the spinal needle is inserted into the subarachnoid space to inject local anesthetic. Lastly, both spinal and epidural needles are removed, leaving the epidural catheter in proper position.

Huber needle technique—This technique incorporates a small hole in the greater curvature of the Tuohy needle, also referred to as a "back-eye." The back-eye assists in positioning the dural puncture away from the epidural catheter. The technique begins with identification of the epidural space with the Tuohy needle. Insertion of spinal needle within lumen of Tuohy needle, exiting through the "back-eye," transverses dura and injects local anesthetic in the subarachnoid space. Once spinal needle is withdrawn, an epidural catheter is appropriately placed.

Separate needles—Separate epidural and spinal needles used to facilitate each portion of the block may be administered in the same interspace or in separate interspaces. Single interspace technique involves making separate passes with the spinal and epidural needles in a single interspace. Separate interspaces allow for administration and verification of epidural catheter placement before spinal anesthetic. Potential risk of spinal needle damaging catheter is present if second injection site is less distance away from first puncture site than length of inserted epidural catheter.

Dual catheter techniques—This technique involves placement of both epidural and spinal catheters in either the same or separate intervertebral spaces. Advantages include epidural catheter administration before spinal anesthesia and titration of spinal anesthetic dosing. Be cautious of epidural and spinal catheter entanglement and unintentional placement of epidural catheter into subarachnoid space.

FACTORS AFFECTING COMBINED SPINAL–EPIDURAL ANESTHESIA

Patient Positioning and Drug Baricity

The literature provides conflicting views; therefore, no consensus has been obtained regarding an optimal approach. Procedure may be completed quicker with patient in sitting position, however, with hyperbaric solutions prolongation of procedure may result in insufficient anesthetic blockade. Hyperbaric solutions provide more reliable blockade, decreased probability of cephalad spread, less hypotension, and nausea. Isobaric solutions are less dependent on positioning, therefore, if hypotension ensues, tilting patient's head downward may facilitate venous return without promoting cephalad spread of anesthetic blockade.

Midline vs Paramedian Approach

The epidural–dural distance is reduced with midline approach, improving the success of spinal component. Paramedian approach may be advantageous for epidural placement for the following reasons: decreased unintentional dural puncture, decreased probability of postdural puncture headache with oblique approach to dural fibers and increased probability of cephalad catheter placement.

COMPLICATIONS

Failed CSE anesthesia may be due to the inability to obtain cerebrospinal fluid due to nerve root obstruction of spinal needle and inappropriate positioning of spinal needle. The distance the spinal needle must extend past the epidural needle to traverse the dura ranges from 0.3 to 1.05 cm, and the spinal needle may simply be too short. Also, angulation error upon entering epidural space may result in excessive lateral placement and inability to locate subarachnoid space. Unilateral spinal blockade has been documented due to lateral patient positioning, necessary for placement of epidurals in particular patients.

Complications with administration of epidural anesthetic before spinal blockade include damage to either epidural catheter or spinal needle due to friction occurring during same interspace spinal needle insertion. This friction may result in metallic microparticles being introduced into the epidural and subarachnoid space.

Complications with administration of spinal anesthetic before epidural blockade include an inability to recognize paresthesia during epidural placement. Inability to accurately evaluate epidural test dose may result in incorrect placement of epidural catheter, with subsequent total spinal blockade, seizures, or cardiorespiratory arrest from opioid overdose. Cephalad extension of spinal blockade may occur due to expanding volume of epidural space as well as transfer of epidurally placed local anesthetic into subarachnoid space via site of dural puncture. Catheter migration may occur from epidural to subarachnoid space through dural puncture site or secondary to rupture of a subdural bleb. In addition, rupture of the membrane separating lateral epidural space from anterior venous confluence may allow catheter migration and intravascular delivery of anesthetic.

Patients may also experience complications associated with individual spinal and epidural procedures including hypotension, bradycardia, cardiorespiratory arrest, subarachnoid injection of epidural-dosed local anesthetic resulting in total spinal, postdural puncture headache (rotation of epidural needle may contribute to dural tear), epidural—spinal hematoma and abscess, meningitis, intravascular injection, and nerve injury.

Caudal Anesthesia

Jamie Barrie, MD, and Kuntal Jivan, MD

ANATOMIC CONSIDERATIONS

1. In neonates and infants, the conus medullaris is located at L3, which is more caudal than in adults (L1). Because of the difference in the rates of growth between the spinal cord and the bony vertebral column, the conus medullaris reaches L1 at approximately 1 year of age. Thus, lumbar puncture for subarachnoid block in neonates and infants should be performed at L4-L5 or L5-S1 so as not to injure the spinal cord. The midline approach is preferred over paramedian because the vertebral laminae are poorly calcified in neonates and infants.

2. The sacrum is narrower and flatter in neonates. This difference affects the approach to the subarachnoid space from the caudal canal. It is much more direct in neonates than in adults. The needle must not be advanced deeply in neonates because dural puncture is much more likely.

3. The distance from the skin to the subarachnoid space in neonates is approximately 1.4 cm, progressively increasing with age. The ligamentum flavum is much thinner and less dense in children than adults, which makes it more difficult to detect engagement of the epidural needle and results in unintended dural puncture.

4. Cerebrospinal fluid (CSF) volume per percentage of body weight is greater in infants than in adults. This may account for the comparatively larger doses of local anesthetics required for surgical anesthesia with subarachnoid block.

5. A caudal block may be contraindicated in the presence of a deep sacral dimple because this may indicate the presence of spina bifida occulta, thus greatly increasing the probability of dural puncture.

PHYSIOLOGIC CONSIDERATIONS

1. **Cardiovascular system**—Subarachnoid and epidural blockade in children is characterized by hemodynamic stability even if the block reaches the level of the upper thoracic dermatomes. The heart rate is preserved because of parasympathetic activity and modulating the heart rate appears to be attenuated in infants. The attenuated vagal tone allows the heart rate to compensate for alterations in peripheral vascular tone.

2. **Respiratory system**—Central neuraxial blockade can affect the respiratory mechanics of the chest wall and diaphragm by diminished activity of the intercostal muscles. In infants and young children, the chest walls are very compliant due to limited ossification of the ribs. They rely on the diaphragm for the maintenance of tidal volume more than adults. Studies of infants have demonstrated that during rapid eye movement and deep sleep, paradoxical inward chest wall motion occurs commonly and increases as the force of diaphragmatic excursion increases. When high thoracic levels of motor blockade is achieved during spinal anesthesia in infants, outward motion of the lower rib cage decreases and paradoxical motion of the lower rib cage occurs. The diaphragmatic contribution to respiration is increased. This suggests a shift in respiratory workload from the rib cage to the diaphragm in compensation for the loss of the intercostal muscle contribution to breathing. The ability of the diaphragm to compensate for the loss of contribution of the rib cage to breathing is adequate in the vast majority of infants.

INDICATION

Caudal epidural anesthesia is used as an alternative to general anesthesia to reduce the incidence of perioperative apnea. Data suggest that regional anesthesia is the preferable anesthetic technique in former preterm infants. However, the most common indication is for the augmentation of general anesthesia and postoperative pain management.

TECHNIQUE

The child is placed in either lateral decubitus or prone position with a small roll beneath the anterior iliac crest. The cornua of the sacral hiatus are best palpated as two bony ridges, about 0.5-1 cm apart. When the sacral cornua cannot be easily appreciated, the space can also be found by palpating the L4-L5 intervertebral space in the midline and then palpating in the caudal direction until the sacral hiatus is reached. However, the space between the sacrum and coccyx may be mistaken for the sacral hiatus. Thus, more caution is needed when using this technique. The proper location is often located just at the beginning of the crease of the buttocks.

A short-bevel 22-gauge stiletted needle should be used because a long-bevel needle may increase the risk of intravascular injection. The needle is initially directed cephalad at a 45-75-degree angle to the skin until it "pops" through the sacrococcygeal ligament into the caudal canal which is contiguous with the epidural space. If a bone is encountered before the sacrococcygeal ligament, the needle should be withdrawn several millimeters, then the angle with the skin decreased to approximately 30 degrees. Subsequently, the needle is again advanced in the cephalad direction until the sacrococcygeal ligament is pierced. As the needle is advanced slightly farther, bone (the anterior table of the sacrum) is encountered, and the needle should be leveled in orientation before further advancement so that it is nearly parallel to the plane of the child's back.

Once the caudal–epidural space has been entered, the needle is advanced several millimeters. Caution should be used because in infants the dural sac lies relatively caudad and it is easy to enter the subarachnoid space. Confirm the placement of needle by aspirating and ensure that no blood or CSF is seen.

Caudal Epidural Test Dose

Caudal epidural analgesia requires a test dose of local anesthetic. Studies suggested new pediatric criteria for positive intravascular placement: an increase of heart rate greater than or equal to 10 bpm or systolic blood pressure greater than or equal to 15 mm Hg. Hemodynamic changes do not always occur early, with some patients developing heart rate (HR) or blood pressure changes 60-90 s after injection. During halothane or isoflurane anesthesia, but not during sevoflurane anesthesia, the sensitivity of the hemodynamic criteria is increased with the administration of atropine or the use of a larger dose of epinephrine (0.5 vs 0.75 μg/kg). Although larger doses of epinephrine may increase the sensitivity of the test dose, there is also a concern that these larger doses may be associated with ventricular arrhythmias. Atropine premedication with sevoflurane anesthesia prolongs the duration of the tachycardia or the hypertension with the test dose.

Observation of not only the HR and systolic blood pressure, but also the T-wave amplitude should increase the sensitivity of the test dose and aid in the recognition of inadvertent systemic injection. T-wave changes occur first, followed by HR changes, and then by blood pressure changes. However, T-wave changes do not occur with isoproterenol, suggesting that the mechanism is a beta-adrenergic receptor effect. The mechanisms responsible for these ECG changes have not been clearly delineated. T-wave changes have been described when only epinephrine is given, when only the local anesthetic is given, and when both agents are administered together.

If neither hemodynamic nor ECG changes are seen, then for "single shot epidural" the remainder of the local anesthetic may be given. The local anesthetic should be administered slowly and in an incremental fashion over several minutes. It is also possible to mistakenly inject into the intramedullary cavity of the sacrum, which would result in rapid uptake (similar to direct intravascular injection), resulting in circulatory collapse.

DRUG SELECTION

The drug dose required for epidural blockade to a given dermatomal level depends on the volume of the local anesthetic and the volume of the epidural space. A common approach is to administer 1 mL/kg (up to 20 mL) of 0.125% bupivacaine with 1:200 000 epinephrine. This provides a sensory block with minimal motor blockade up to about T6-T4. The concentration of local anesthetic is based on the desired density of the block and on the risk of toxicity. For continuous infusions, a maximum of 0.4 mg/kg/h of bupivacaine after the initial block is established. A reduced dose by 30% is needed for infants younger than 6 months of age.

COMPLICATIONS

1. Intravascular or intraosseous injection
2. Hematoma
3. Neural injury
4. Infection
5. Perforation of bowel or pelvic organs

SUGGESTED READINGS

Fortuna A. Caudal analgesia: a simple and safe technique in paediatric surgery. *Br J Anaesth.* 1967;39:165-170.

Tobius J. Caudal epidural block: a review of test dosing and recognition of systemic injection in children. *Anesth Analg.* 2001;93:1156-1161.

Epidural Test Dose

Brian S. Freeman, MD

A catheter positioned properly in the epidural space can provide excellent surgical anesthesia, postoperative analgesia, and labor analgesia. Inadvertent placement of the catheter into the cerebrospinal fluid (CSF) (intrathecal) or an epidural vein (intravascular) could lead to catastrophic complications. Positive aspiration of blood or CSF from the catheter confirms catheter misplacement. However, the absence of an aspirate cannot rule out whether or not the catheter is actually in the epidural space. The incidence of false negative aspiration is lower for multiorifice epidural catheters (<1%) compared to single-hole catheters (2%). Aspiration of fluid may fail due to low epidural venous pressure, air locking within a filter, mechanical obstruction due to tissue or blood, or simply incorrect identification of the aspirate. For these reasons, a "test dose" should be administered subsequent to epidural catheter placement and prior to incremental dosing of small volumes of local anesthetic.

THE "IDEAL" TEST DOSE

An epidural test dose involves injecting local anesthetic to determine accidental intravenous or intrathecal catheter placement. The most popular and effective test dose is 3 mL of lidocaine 1.5% with epinephrine 1:200 000. From a practical standpoint, an ideal test dose should be a single solution that produces objective evidence of intravascular or intrathecal injection within several minutes of administration. A test dose should be safe for a parturient and her fetus, and should not increase the risk of complications for all patients. It should not significantly delay the onset of epidural anesthesia.

The ideal epidural test dose would have both high sensitivity and specificity. As sensitivity increases, more intravascular catheters would be detected. A high false-positive rate (low specificity) would lead to unnecessary manipulations or replacements of correctly positioned epidural catheters. In general, the epidural test dose has high (>90%) sensitivity but poor specificity (around 50%). Therefore, a negative test dose does not guarantee—it only decreases the probability—that the catheter is not in the intravascular or intrathecal space. A negative test dose also does not ensure proper placement in the epidural space.

The epidural test dose should always be injected rapidly. Slow administration may cause the drugs (both epinephrine and local anesthetic) to undergo redistribution and metabolism before a sufficient mass could bind to its receptors. Furthermore, most anesthesiologists use closed-tip multiorifice epidural catheters. Any number of the three orifices could be positioned in blood or CSF while the other is in the proper space. Slow administration may mean that the epidural test dose exits the proximal orifice and does not reach the most distal orifice. As a result, part of the catheter may remain undetected within the intravascular or intrathecal space.

Testing for Intrathecal Placement

The test dose for accidental intrathecal catheter placement should produce relatively rapid sensory changes to allow for easy identification. The intrathecal component of the test dose should not cause cardiovascular compromise, high or total spinal anesthesia, or neurotoxicity. For these purposes, 3 mL of lidocaine 1.5% is the ideal local anesthetic. Lidocaine allows for reliable detection of intrathecal injection within a short period of time. If the catheter is placed in the CSF, 45 mg lidocaine produces detectable sensory block (leg warmth and sensory loss to pinprick) within 1-2 minutes and a motor block (leg weakness and impaired straight-leg raise) within 3-4 minutes. This onset time contrasts to the 20 minutes required when properly injected into the epidural space.

In contrast, using 7.5 mg bupivacaine (3 mL of 0.25%) or 15 mg ropivacaine requires a longer waiting period (at least 5-6 minutes) to produce sensory and motor changes when injected into the CSF. In addition, isobaric bupivacaine has greater variability of dermatomal level achieved and onset time compared to isobaric lidocaine.

It is important to keep in mind that most lidocaine solutions used for test dosing are slightly hypobaric compared to CSF. Patients may develop high spinal anesthesia and rapid hypotension due to sitting in an upright position. Furthermore, a positive intrathecal test dose with lidocaine does not necessarily mean that the patient will develop the transient neurologic syndrome (TNS) associated with this drug. In fact, it is possible that pregnancy actually decreases the incidence of TNS in patients who receive intrathecal lidocaine.

Testing for Intravascular Placement

The epidural veins of a parturient are larger during pregnancy due to higher intraabdominal pressures. The incidence of accidental intravascular catheter placement is about 6% in parturients and 5% in children. Failure to recognize intravenous epidural catheter placement could lead to local anesthetic systemic toxicity (seizures, cardiac arrest). Using both local anesthetic and epinephrine in a test dose solution provide different pieces of data to help rule out intravascular catheter placement.

A. Local Anesthetic

Accidental intravascular injection of a subconvulsant dose of local anesthetic (eg, 45 mg lidocaine) generally causes subjective signs and symptoms of subclinical central nervous system (CNS) toxicity: dizziness, tinnitus, circumoral paresthesia, metallic taste, or blurred vision. These responses may be unreliable in an anxious parturient or a sedated patient. It is unlikely that this small dose could achieve plasma levels leading to full CNS local anesthetic toxicity (seizures, unconsciousness, or apnea) or cardiovascular local anesthetic toxicity (cardiac arrest, dysrhythmias).

B. Epinephrine

The typical test dose contains 3 mL of a 1:200 000 solution of epinephrine (concurrently mixed with a local anesthetic). Compared to the local anesthetic component, a positive test dose from 15 µg epinephrine results in objective signs: sudden tachycardia (>10 bpm within 45-60 seconds) and hypertension (increase in systolic blood pressure by 20 mm Hg). The amplitude of the epinephrine response is attenuated by a number of factors, including concomitant use of beta-adrenergic blocking drugs, benzodiazepines, opioids, and inhalation anesthetics. Furthermore, the pregnant patient may respond less reliably to catecholamines, leading to a depressed chronotropic response.

Since maternal heart rate is quite variable during labor, it is important that the test dose be administered between uterine contractions when heart rate is stable. The inability to easily distinguish tachycardia from uterine contraction pain versus IV epinephrine reduces test specificity. However, in laboring patients, epinephrine-induced tachycardia is usually different from contraction-associated tachycardia. Within a minute after epinephrine injection, the heart rate increases but is then followed by a rapid return to baseline with delayed hypertension. Some patients may report subjective symptoms like palpitations and lightheadedness. If the response is equivocal, test doses should be repeated. Only rapid, sudden increases in heart rate are considered positive.

Using epinephrine could potentially have adverse effects. Epinephrine may cause a transient decrease in uterine blood flow due to uterine artery vasoconstriction. Parturients have altered sensitivity to vasopressors and chronotropes which may lead to an exaggerated response. Contraindications to the use of epinephrine in a test dose include patients with pregnancy-induced hypertension, uteroplacental insufficiency, stenotic valvular disease, and coronary artery disease (CAD). A patient with preeclampsia may respond to 15 µg epinephrine IV with malignant hypertension. Patients with stenotic valvular lesions and CAD may develop myocardial ischemia as a result of the tachycardia-induced increase in myocardial oxygen consumption. A non-reassuring fetal HR tracing is not a contraindication to using epinephrine in a test dose.

C. Air

It is possible to use air to rule out intravascular catheter placement. Like epinephrine, air serves as an objective marker. Intravenous injection of 1-2 mL of air through an open-tipped catheter causes changes in heart sounds. It is necessary to listen with a Doppler device, such as the external fetal heart monitor, placed over the maternal precordium. False negative results can occur in multiorifice catheters.

D. Fentanyl

Administration of fentanyl 100 µg can be a highly sensitive and specific test to rule out intravascular catheter placement. Reported symptoms include feelings of dizziness, sedation, euphoria, and analgesia. Reliability of this test depends heavily on the subjective reporting of symptoms.

Epidural Test Dose and General Anesthesia

The test dose is typically given just prior to administering the total volume of local anesthetic desired to produce epidural analgesia or anesthesia. Most patients, such as parturients or patients scheduled for lower extremity operations are fully conscious or lightly sedated. However, epidural catheters are also sometimes dosed in patients who are fully unconscious under general anesthesia, such as children or adults undergoing intrathoracic or intraabdominal procedures. For instance, children may receive lumbar or caudal epidurals while under general anesthesia due to lack of cooperation. The simultaneous administration of a potent volatile inhalation anesthetic may blunt the cardiovascular response to the epinephrine test dose. During accidental intravascular injection, a positive response to epinephrine includes an increase in hear rate by greater than 10 beats per minute, increase in systolic blood pressure by greater than 15 mm Hg, and an increase in T-wave amplitude by greater than 25% on lead II.

The Test Dose Controversy

Because of its debatable sensitivity and specificity, some anesthesiologists still question the value of the epidural test dose. Arguments against routine use of an epidural test dose that includes epinephrine are:

- The test dose with epinephrine has a low positive predictive value. High false negative rates may lead to the conclusion that the catheter is not placed in an epidural vein despite the possibility.

- Significant side effects, such as decreased uterine blood flow, are possible.
- The incidence of undetected intravascular misplacement with the use of multiorifice catheters is extremely low (<1%).
- Intravascular placement can be considered if small incremental doses of local anesthetic fail to provide sensory block or analgesia.
- Epinephrine should preferentially be used in a test dose only when large volumes of local anesthetic are planned for surgical anesthesia; it is not necessary for small doses required for analgesia

The epidural test dose is simply another means to verify proper placement of an epidural catheter and prevent adverse outcomes. The American Society of Anesthesiologists' closed claims study showed that some cases of local anesthetic toxicity may have been prevented if a test dose with epinephrine had been included. The test dose should always be combined with clinical judgment, aspiration, and slow incremental injection followed by careful observation of the patient. Since a positive epidural test dose has the most diagnostic value, each step is equally important.

SUGGESTED READING

Gaiser R. The epidural test dose in obstetric anesthesia: it is not obsolete. *J Clin Anesth*. 2003;15:474-477.

Complications of Neuraxial Anesthesia

Joseph Myers, MD

Awareness of potential problems is one of the best ways to avoid complications during the administration of neuraxial anesthesia. Anticipating problems and preparing for their treatment also improves safety. For example, recognizing the risk of infection improves one's focus on sterile technique and realizing the potential for a sudden drop in blood pressure implores one to have an IV and medications available to treat hypotension. "Know thy enemy..." is a good advice for avoiding complications.

Complications specific to the placement of a spinal, epidural, combined spinal–epidural, or a caudal block are best organized into three groups: (1) exaggerated responses to their placement; (2) problems related to the placement of the needle or catheter; and (3) drug toxicity issues.

ADVERSE OR EXAGGERATED PHYSIOLOGIC RESPONSES

A method for looking at problems associated with exaggerated physiologic responses to neuraxial anesthesia is to describe the stepwise onset of an inadvertent spinal anesthetic while attempting to place an epidural block. Local anesthetics are approximately 10 times as potent in the spinal space versus the epidural space. In addition, the dose volume is usually much greater for epidural administration. Therefore, an exaggerated response is nearly unavoidable. The complete sequence of events would proceed as follows. First, there would be a sudden and profound drop in blood pressure. This occurs because sympathetic nerve fibers are extremely sensitive to the effects of local anesthetics and the subsequent vasodilation leads to hypotension. The hypotension may be accompanied by nausea and vomiting. As the block spreads higher, the accessory muscles of respiration (sternocleidomastoid, scalene, and abdominal muscles) are affected and tidal volumes reduced. At thoracic levels T1 through T4, the function of the cardiac accelerator fibers is impaired and the heart rate falls. Combined with already profound hypotension, cardiac arrest is possible. If the block spreads higher, sensory and motor function to the upper extremities and hands become impaired (C5-T1). The patient starts to panic and becomes dyspneic.

When they are no longer able to talk, the diaphragm (C3-C5) becomes paralyzed and breathing stops. If the brain is bathed in local anesthetic, unconsciousness is assured.

Besides the development of a "high spinal" from an overdose of local anesthetic, a similar situation could develop from a spinal block if hyperbaric local anesthetic is used and the patient is immediately placed in the Trendelenburg position. Although this same sequence is possible with an epidural or caudal block, it is rare. The local anesthetic dose would have to be excessive and/or the patient would have to be particularly sensitive (eg, short stature, pregnant, or elderly) for it to occur.

Now consider what would happen if there was an inadvertent intravascular injection of local anesthetic. This complication could result from either a large bolus or a prolonged intravascular infusion. First, the signs of mild systemic local anesthetic toxicity would occur, including tinnitus and circumoral numbness. If epinephrine has been included in the local anesthetic, a sudden and significant increase in heart rate will ensue. This rise in heart rate will be transient, lasting only several minutes. Next, the patient would start to slur their speech and become restless or start twitching. A tonic–clonic seizure would follow. Cardiac toxicity then occurs and brings profound consequences. Blockade of cardiac sodium channels reduces automaticity and impairs conduction. The ECG shows prolongation of the PR interval and widening of the QRS complex. Hypotension and arrhythmias may follow. Finally, there is direct cardiac toxicity with cardiovascular collapse, in particular with the use of bupivacaine. There may be variability in the stepwise pattern described above but central nervous system (CNS) effects reliably precede cardiovascular effects.

PROBLEMS RELATED TO THE PLACEMENT OF THE NEEDLE OR CATHETER

Puncture of the skin with an epidural or spinal needle introduces the potential risks of bleeding and infection. The bleeding we are concerned about is that which would lead to an epidural hematoma. As blood accumulates in the epidural space, pressure could be applied to the spinal cord or nerve roots resulting in ischemia, and eventually, irreversible nerve damage. The risk is increased following difficult placement, multiple attempts, low platelet count, or the use of antithrombotic agents by the patient. In particular, aspirin, enoxaparin, clopidogrel, and other anticoagulants can increase the risk of hematoma. They should be discontinued for an appropriate time period before the procedure and not restarted until at least 2 hours after the epidural catheter is removed. The signs and symptoms of an epidural hematoma include pain at the site, epidural effect not wearing off in an appropriate amount of time, or a rising level of muscle weakness. Treatment, which consists of surgical evacuation of the hematoma, cannot be delayed since neurologic function will not return if the ischemia persists.

Infection can be a minor superficial skin infection, a life-threatening epidural abscess, or meningitis. Warmth and redness at the needle entry site with a discharge, along with pain, fever, and an elevated white blood cell count are indications of infection. Headache, neurologic symptoms, seizures, and death may follow. Aggressive treatment is necessary with antibiotics; and possibly, incision and drainage of the epidural abscess.

Neurologic injury can result from neuraxial anesthesia for reasons besides epidural hematoma or abscess. While transient neurologic symptoms are most common, a permanent deficit is possible. Fortunately, a permanent neurologic injury is extremely rare with an incidence of 0.08%-0.16%. Needles and catheters can damage nerves not only when anatomic landmarks are misidentified, but also when a paresthesia is disregarded during placement of a neuraxial block. The appropriate reaction to paresthesia should be to redirect the needle or catheter until the paresthesia is alleviated. It should also be noted that the analgesia provided by neuraxial anesthesia presents a risk in itself. Pain can be protective. A patient who has sciatica or is delivering a baby may be positioned such that a paresthesia would develop but the pain impulses are not detected because of the anesthetic. A prolonged or permanent deficit could be the consequence.

Postdural puncture headache can occur following a neuraxial anesthetic. When the dura mater is punctured, a cerebrospinal fluid (CSF) leak is created. This is commonly referred to as a "wet tap." The leak may be sufficient to reduce the buoying effect of CSF on the brain, causing traction and stretching of the meninges as the patient assumes the upright position. A headache will likely develop. It will be relieved by lying down. A small hole from a spinal needle rarely causes a dural puncture headache. But a larger hole, such as that created inadvertently during epidural placement, is very likely to cause one. The differential diagnosis for headache includes meningitis. An association with fever and an increased WBC count, along with the lack of a postural component to the headache, differentiates it from a postdural puncture headache. A dural puncture headache can be treated with increased fluid intake, NSAIDs, caffeine, narcotics, and/or an epidural blood patch. It could take 2 weeks for relief of the headache without treatment.

Finally, needles and catheters can break and be left in the patient. And, although rare, the tip of a catheter can be sheared off if pulled back through the opening of a needle. Epidural catheters are occasionally difficult to remove and will break if enough tension is applied. Often, by placing the patient into the same position that they were in for the placement of the epidural, the catheter can be removed easily. The sheared-off tip of an epidural catheter should probably not be searched for surgically unless there are symptoms. The catheter is placed sterilely and is made of a nonreactive material, such as polyamide.

PROBLEMS ASSOCIATED WITH DRUG TOXICITY

Arachnoiditis is a rare but devastating complication of neuraxial anesthesia. Injection of inappropriate drugs can lead to inflammation with resulting adhesions and a variety of neurologic deficits (eg, paraplegia, quadriplegia, hydrocephalus, and syringomyelia). In the past, lack of cleaning or the cleaning solutions themselves were known causes when epidural trays were reused. There is always the potential for arachnoiditis since an inadvertent injection of a caustic solution is as easy as a syringe swap or lack of vigilance toward contamination of solutions. If noticed, it is possible to treat the inadvertent injection by "washing it out" with saline, a technique described by Tartiere.

Cauda equina syndrome is a variable group of neurologic deficits originating from the nerves L1-S5 which come together below the conus medullaris. From an anesthesia perspective, the cause is typically due to an injection of a contaminant into the CSF at the lumbar level. The resultant severe inflammation of these nerves can cause the syndrome.

Local anesthetics can be directly neurotoxic at high concentrations. Preservatives and additives which cause extremes in the pH levels of local anesthetics can also be neurotoxic.

Failure of a neuraxial block is not usually considered a risk until a backup plan such as, endotracheal intubation in a less than ideal candidate, is initiated. And failure of block does not have to be a complete failure. Even a small "window" of unanesthetized abdomen will prevent surgery from continuing. The reasons for failure are multiple. Precisely placing the tip of a needle into the several-millimeters-wide epidural space is always a challenge. Epidural catheters can migrate to one side or pass through the paravertebral foramina causing a one-sided block. Pulling the catheter back several centimeters will often, but not always, take care of the problem. And finally, anatomic variability, including septa and scar tissue, may prevent the spread of local anesthetic. Until a way is found to more precisely place a needle or catheter, neuraxial blocks will never be as reliable as general anesthesia.

SUGGESTED READINGS

Murphy TM, O'Keefe D. Complications of spinal, epidural, and caudal anesthesia. In:Benumof JL, Saidman LJ (Eds.). *Anesthesia and Perioperative Complications*. Chicago: Mosby Year Book, 1992;38-51.

Tartiere J, Gerard JL, Peny J et al. Acute treatment after accidental intrathecal injection of hypertonic contrast media. *Anesthesiology* 1989;71:169 [letter].

Weinberg GL. Resuscitation for local anesthetic and other drug overdose. *Anesthesiology* 2012;117:180-187.

American Society of Regional Anesthesia and Pain Medicine (ASRA) Guidelines: Neuraxial Anesthesia and Anticoagulation

Lisa Bellil, MD

Venous thromboembolism is an important health-care problem and the source of significant morbidity and mortality. Nearly all hospitalized patients have at least one risk factor for thromboembolism, with 40% having three or more risk factors. Therefore, many hospitalized patients are candidates for thromboembolism and receive thromboprophylaxis.

The estimated incidence of neurologic dysfunction resulting from bleeding complications associated with neuraxial blockade has been reported as less than 1/150 000 for epidurals and less than 1/220 000 for spinal anesthetics. However, some studies show that the incidence may be as high as 1/3000 in some patient populations. The risk of clinically significant bleeding increases with age, existing problems with the spinal cord or vertebral column, underlying coagulopathy, difficulty with needle placement, and sustained anticoagulation with indwelling epidural catheter.

Bleeding is the major complication of anticoagulant and thrombolytic therapy, and is classified as major if it is intracranial, intraspinal, intraocular, mediastinal, retroperitoneal, or results in hospitalization or death. The most dreaded complication for patients with indwelling epidural catheter is a spinal hematoma. The term spinal hematoma is defined as bleeding within the spinal neuraxis and it most commonly occurs in the epidural space because of the prominent epidural venous plexus. Neurologic compromise presents as progression of sensory or motor block or bowel/bladder dysfunction and not as severe radicular back pain. Spinal cord ischemia tends to be reversible if patients undergo laminectomy within 8 hours of onset of neurologic dysfunction, with 38% of patients having partial or complete neurologic recovery in one study.

UNFRACTIONATED HEPARIN (UFH)

The mechanism of action of heparin is to bind to antithrombin with high affinity and subsequently inactivate thrombin (IIa), factor Xa, and factor IXa. IV injection of heparin results in immediate anticoagulant activity compared to subcutaneous injection which results in a delay of effect for 1-2 hours. Administration of small dose (5000 U) of subcutaneous heparin does not prolong activated partial thromboplastin time (aPTT), however, it can result in unpredictable blood concentrations in some patients 2 hours after administration. Heparin is rapidly revered by protamine and each milligram of protamine can neutralize 100 U of heparin.

Intravenous Unfractionated Heparin

Intraoperative heparin doses range from 5000 to 10 000 U IV, especially during vascular surgery to prevent coagulation during cross clamping. The use of neuraxial procedures after administration of IV heparin may be associated with an increased risk of epidural hematoma. As a result, performance of neuraxial procedures should take place at least 1 hour before the administration of heparin and removal of the epidural catheter should take place 2-4 hours after the last heparin dose. Careful assessment of the patient's neurologic status in the lower extremities should take place for at least 12 hours after catheter removal.

Subcutaneous Unfractionated Heparin

The administration of 5000 U subcutaneous unfractionated heparin (SCUFH) every 12 hours is used extensively as prophylaxis against deep vein thrombosis (DVT). There is often no significant change in the aPTT, but approximately 15% of patients may develop a prolongation of the aPTT to 1.5 times normal. With therapy longer than 5 days, a small subset of patients will develop a drop in platelet count.

Based on the 2008 ACCP conference guidelines, more patients are being treated with SCUFH three times per day rather than two times per day. Three times a day dosing of UFH may be associated with an increase in aPTT. The use of three times a day heparin dosing may lead to an increase of surgical-related bleeding; it is unclear whether there is an increased risk of spinal hematoma. It is advised that patients not receive three times a day SCUFH while epidural analgesia is maintained. These patients should be treated with twice daily dosing and compression devices because there is no apparent difference between twice daily dosing of SCUFH with the use of compression devises and thrice daily dosing.

The risk of spinal hematoma in patients receiving SCUFH is very low. There are only four published cases of neuraxial hematomas in patients receiving UFH. Performing neuraxial block in patients before the injection of subcutaneous heparin is preferable and waiting 2 hours after injection of heparin may coincide with peak effect, so delaying needle placement may not be justified. Patients can have epidurals placed before the next dose of UFH and have the catheter removed ideally one hour before the next scheduled dose.

Heparinization during Cardiopulmonary Bypass

There has been only one case report to date of a case of spinal hematoma after heparinization for cardiopulmonary bypass. The patient was treated with other anticoagulants and thrombolytics on the second postoperative day. Therefore, the ASRA practice advisory panel advises that the following precautions be taken to minimize the risk of spinal hematoma:

1. Neuraxial blocks should be avoided in a patient with known coagulopathy from any cause.
2. Surgery should be delayed 24 hours in the event of a traumatic tap.
3. Time from instrumentation to systemic heparinization should exceed 60 minutes.
4. Heparin effect and reversal should be tightly controlled (smallest amount of heparin for the shortest duration compatible with therapeutic objectives).
5. Epidural catheters should be removed when normal coagulation is restored, and patients should be closely monitored postoperatively for signs and symptoms of hematoma formation.

The committee also states that in addition to the above recommendations, epidural catheters should be placed 24 hours in advance of surgery.

A. Anesthetic Management of Patient Receiving UFH

- Dosing regimens of 5000 U twice daily—there is no contraindication to the use of neuraxial techniques (Grade 1C).
- Dosing regimens of UFH greater than 10 000 U/day—unclear if increased risk of spinal hematoma. Risks/benefits are evaluated on an individual basis (Grade 2C).
- Epidural catheter in place for more than 4 days—check platelet count prior to placing or removing catheter due to increased risk of heparin-induced thrombocytopenia (HIT) (Grade 1C).

- Currently, there is insufficient data to determine the risk of full anticoagulation during cardiac surgery. Postoperative monitoring of neurologic function is recommended (Grade 2C).
- Intraoperative heparin use:
  ○ Ensure there is no preexisting coagulopathy
  ○ Delay heparin 1 hour after needle placement
  ○ Remove catheter 2-4 hours after last heparin dose; wait 1 hour to restart heparin
  ○ Monitor postoperatively and use minimal amount of local anesthetic to increase early detection of spinal hematoma
  ○ There is no data to support mandatory case cancellation if bloody or difficult needle placement occurs. Direct communication with the surgeon is recommended

Low Molecular Weight Heparin

Several pharmacological and biochemical properties of low molecular weight heparin (LMWH) differ from those of UFH. Most important is the lack of monitoring of the anticoagulant response from LMWH and its irreversibility with protamine. Anti-Xa levels peak 3-4 hours after administration and significant activity of LMWH is still present 12 hours after injection. The plasma half-life of LMWH increases in patients with renal failure.

There are several risk factors for spinal hematoma in patients receiving LMWH, including: female sex, advancing age, renal insufficiency, spinal stenosis/ankylosing spondylitis, traumatic placement, indwelling epidural catheter, epidural–spinal, immediate preoperative (or intraoperative) drug administration, twice daily drug dosing, concurrent antiplatelet, or anticoagulation medications.

A. Anesthetic Management of Patients Receiving LMWH

- Because the anti-Xa level is not predictive of the risk of bleeding, no routine use of monitoring the anti-Xa level (Grade 1A).
- Antiplatelet and oral anticoagulants used in combination with LMWH increase risk of spinal hematoma. However, concurrent use is not recommended (Grade 1A).
- Traumatic or bloody placement of epidural needle and catheter does not require delay of surgery. First dose of LMWH should be delayed 24 hours (Grade 2C).
- Preoperative LMWH:
  ○ Prophylactic dose—Wait 10-12 hours before needle placement (Grade 1C).
  ○ High dose (1.5 mg/kg q 12 hours or 1.5 mg/kg daily)—Wait 24 hours before needle placement (Grade 1C).
  ○ In patients who received LMWH 2 hours preoperatively, recommend against neuraxial technique (Grade 1A).

- Postoperative LMWH:
  - Twice daily dose—First dose should be given 24 hours postoperatively. Indwelling catheters should be removed 2 hours prior to first dose (Grade 1C)
  - Once daily dosing—First dose should be administered 6-8 hours postoperatively, subsequent dose 24 hours after first dose. Indwelling catheters are okay but should be removed 10-12 hours after last dose and redosing should not occur for 2 hours after catheter removal (Grade 1C).

ORAL ANTICOAGULANTS

Warfarin

Warfarin exerts its effect by interfering with the synthesis of Vitamin K-dependent clotting factors (II, VII, IX, X). Clinically, Warfarin therapy is monitored with the prothrombin time (PT) though international normalized ratio (INR) allows for standardization and comparison of PT values between laboratories. The INR is less reliable in the early course of treatment of Warfarin. The initial rise in PT and INR after Warfarin therapy is due to reduction of factor VII due to a short half-life of only 6 hours. Factor VII is also the first to recover after discontinuation of Warfarin therapy. Factors II and X have longer half-lives (50-80 and 25-60, respectively) and is responsible for PT prolongation as therapy continues.

A. Anesthetic Management of Patients Receiving Warfarin

- In the first 3 days after discontinuation of Warfarin therapy, factor II and X levels may not be adequate for hemostasis despite an increased INR. Recommendation is that Warfarin be stopped 4-5 days before planned procedure. The INR should be normalized before neuraxial block (Grade 1B).
- Concurrent use of aspirin, clopidogrel, ticlodipine, UFH, LMWH, and NSAIDs is not recommended (Grade 1A).
- If patients have received a first dose of Warfarin 24 hours before surgery, INR should be checked prior to neuraxial block or if a second dose of oral anticoagulant has been administered (Grade 2C)
- In patients on low-dose Warfarin therapy with indwelling epidural catheter:
  - Monitor INR daily (Grade 2C)
  - Routine neurologic assessment of sensory and motor functions (Grade 1C)
  - Choose local anesthetic to minimize degree of sensory or motor block (Grade 1C)
- When Warfarin therapy is being initiated, neuraxial catheters should be removed while the INR is less than 1.5. Neurologic assessment should be performed for 24 hours (Grade 2C).
- In patients with INR between 1.5 and 3, removal of indwelling catheter should be done with caution and the

record should be reviewed to ensure no concomitant use of other medications that may affect hemostasis (Grade 2C). Neurologic status should be assessed before catheter removal and until INR has normalized (Grade 1C).
- In patients with INR greater than 3 and indwelling neuraxial catheters, Warfarin dose should be held or reduced (Grade 1A). No definitive recommendation for catheter removal.

Antiplatelet Medication

Drugs which inhibit function of platelets include cyclooxygenase inhibitors (aspirin, NSAIDs), adenosine diphosphate inhibitors (clopidogrel, ticlodipine), and glycoprotein IIb/IIIa inhibitors (abciximab, eptifibatide, tirofiban). NSAIDs do not present a significant risk for the development of spinal hematoma. Several studies have shown the relative safety of antiplatelet therapy with neuraxial anesthesia.

A. Anesthetic Management of Patients Receiving Antiplatelet Medication

- NSAIDs do not pose specific concerns for the performance of single shot or catheter techniques, or removal of neuraxial catheters (Grade 1A).
- In patients receiving NSAIDs and concurrent oral anticoagulants, UFH and LMWH, performance of neuraxial techniques should be avoided (Grade 2C).
- The suggested time interval between discontinuation of ticlodipine therapy and neuraxial blockade is 14 days (Grade 1C).
- The suggested time interval between discontinuation of clopidogrel therapy and neuraxial blockade is 7 days (Grade 1C).
- Platelet GP IIb/IIIa inhibitors exert a profound effect on platelet function. Normal platelet aggregation is 24-48 hours for abciximab and 4-8 hours for eptifibatide and tirofiban. Neuraxial techniques should be postponed until platelet function has recovered (Grade 1C).

HERBAL MEDICATIONS

Garlic and ginkgo affect platelet function by inhibiting platelet aggregation, whereas Ginseng potentially increases PT and aPTT. However, the herbal drugs, by themselves, represent no added significant risk for the development of spinal hematoma. ASRA does not recommend mandatory discontinuation of these medications prior to neuraxial block.

NEW ANTICOAGULANTS

Direct Thrombin Inhibitors

Recombinant hirudin derivatives include desirudin, lepirudin, and bivalirudin. These drugs inhibit both free and clot bound thrombin. Argatroban has a similar mechanism of action. These drugs are often used in patients with heparin-induced thrombocytopenia or during angioplasties. The pharmacological effects of thrombin inhibitors cannot be reversed, and prolonged PPT is present for up to 3 hours.

There are no large series examining the use of neuraxial techniques on patients receiving direct thrombin inhibitors. There are case reports of spontaneous intracranial bleeds in these patients. Given the lack of data, ASRA recommends against the use of neuraxial blocks in patients receiving direct thrombin inhibitors.

Fondaparinux

Fondaparinux works by inhibiting factor Xa. Its long half-life (21 hours) allows for once daily dosing. A series of 3600 patients with neuraxial block and fondaparinux reported no additional spinal hematomas. However, performance of the neuraxial block was strictly controlled. Patients were only included if the needle placement was atraumatic and achieved on the first attempt, and no indwelling catheters were placed.

Given these studies, the ASRA consensus statement suggests that performance of neuraxial techniques on patients receiving fondaparinux should only be attempted in clinical scenarios similar to study conditions (atraumatic needle placement on the first attempt; NO indwelling catheters).

Antithrombotic Therapy in Pregnancy

It is established that the risk of thrombosis increases during pregnancy, ranging from 5 to 50 times higher in pregnant women. In most women, the risk of DVT prophylaxis outweighs maternal and fetal benefits. However, the use of thromboprophylaxis is becoming more common in patients with acquired or hereditary thrombophilia. There is limited data regarding the risk of neuraxial anesthesia in these patients.

The frequency of spinal hematoma in obstetric patients is unknown, but there have been several case reports of spontaneous hematomas in healthy patients. In published case reports about obstetric patients with spinal hematoma, a significant number displayed abnormal coagulation at the time of needle placement or catheter removal.

Because there are no large series of neuraxial techniques in pregnant patients on thromboprophylaxis or VTE treatment, the ASRA guidelines for surgical patients should be applied to parturients (Grade 2C). In addition, the authors also offer the following recommendations:

- At no later than 36 weeks oral, anticoagulants should be switched to LMWH or UFH.
- At least 36 hours prior to delivery, LMWH should be discontinued and the patient converted to IV or SubQ UFH, if indicated.
- IV UFH should be stopped 4-6 hours prior to delivery.
- Resumption of prophylaxis should be held until at least 12 hours after vaginal delivery or epidural removal (whichever occurs later).
- Thromboprophylaxis should be held at least 24 hours after cesarean section.
- If higher doses are required, prophylaxis should be held at least 24 hours, regardless of vaginal or surgical delivery.

Plexus and Peripheral Blockade in the Anticoagulated Patient

There are few studies examining the frequency or severity of bleeding complications after peripheral or plexus blocks in anticoagulated patients. The largest study involved 670 patients with continuous lumbar plexus catheters who were receiving Warfarin. Roughly, one-third of the patients had their catheter removed on postoperation day 2 with an INR greater than 1.4 without adverse events. There is insufficient data to make recommendations; however, trends suggest that significant blood loss rather than neural deficits may be the most serious complication of regional anesthesia in anticoagulated patients. Additionally, hemorrhagic complications in these patients tend to cause major morbidity. Based on the available data, the ASRA recommendation for patients undergoing plexus or peripheral block is to follow the recommendations regarding neuraxial techniques (Grade 1C).

SUGGESTED READING

Horlocker TT, Wedel DJ, Rowlingson JC et al. Regional anesthesia in the patient receiving antithrombotic or thrombolytic therapy: American Society of Regional Anesthesia and Pain Medicine evidence-based guidelines (third edition). *Reg Anesth Pain Med.* 2010;35:64-101.

77

ASA Monitoring Standards

Elizabeth E. Holtan, MD

PRINCIPLES OF MONITORING

Because of the possibility of frequent alterations of patient vital signs and physiology due to the administration of anesthesia, the anesthesiologist must monitor the patient to assess for problems and allow for ample time to intervene. One must apply monitors, observe, and interpret the data, as well as begin appropriate treatment when necessary. The purpose of monitoring is to promote optimal care of the patient and notice trends and abnormalities before they become irreversible. Even so, following these guidelines does not ensure any particular outcome for patients.

The American Society of Anesthesiologists (ASA) has developed Standards for Basic Anesthetic Monitoring, which was last updated in 2011. According to this document, an authorized anesthesia provider must remain with a patient throughout the duration of any general, regional, or monitored anesthesia care, to administer anesthesia and monitor the patient. In some instances, short lapses in monitoring may occur and are sometimes inevitable. For certain patients, particular monitoring techniques may be unfeasible. In the rare situation where there is an exposure or danger to the anesthesia care provider, distant discontinuous monitoring may be necessary. If there is an emergency that would require the anesthesia provider to temporarily leave the patient, the anesthesiologist must determine the importance of the emergency and its effect on the patient. The anesthesiologist must also decide who will continue to deliver the anesthetic and monitor the patient until the anesthesia care provider is able to return.

These standards apply to patients receiving monitored anesthesia care, general anesthesia, as well as regional anesthesia. These standards do not necessarily apply to obstetrical patients or pain management patients. It is also the anesthesiologist's responsibility to determine if additional monitoring is required beyond the basic monitors.

The ASA Standards for Basic Anesthetic Monitoring emphasizes the assessment of a patient's circulation, oxygenation, ventilation, and body temperature:

Circulation

It is important to monitor the patient's circulation while under anesthesia. Every patient must have a blood pressure and heart rate assessed at least every 5 minutes. Patients must also have an electrocardiogram continually assessed from the start of the anesthetic until the patient leaves the operating or procedure room. Lastly, patients under general anesthesia are also required to have assessment of circulation continuously by an additional method. The possible methods are pulse oximetry, intraarterial blood pressure monitor, auscultation of patient's heart, feeling of patient's pulse, or peripheral pulse assessment with ultrasound.

Oxygenation

The anesthesia provider must assess that the patient has sufficient oxygen concentration in inspired gas and blood. During any general anesthetic that utilizes an anesthesia machine, an oxygen analyzer must be used to evaluate the concentration of oxygen in the breathing circuit. The machine must have a working low oxygen concentration limit alarm.

During any type of anesthesia, blood oxygenation must be measured by certain means, such as a pulse oximeter. The anesthesia provider must be able to hear the variable pitch tone, and the alarm must be set if the saturation falls below the set level. The patient should also be exposed enough to be able to evaluate color.

Ventilation

It is imperative that any patient under anesthesia be continually assessed to have satisfactory ventilation. Clinical signs such as visualizing chest rise and auscultating breath sounds are helpful in assessing ventilation in all types of anesthesia. During local anesthesia or regional anesthesia without sedation, these clinical signs must be observed. During moderate or deep sedation or general anesthesia, clinical signs are important, as well as continually assessing end-tidal carbon dioxide. When using a mechanical ventilator, tidal volumes should be observed.

After insertion of a laryngeal mask airway or an endotracheal tube, the proper placement must be confirmed by clinical signs, as well as by end-tidal carbon dioxide in the expired gas. Capnography to evaluate end-tidal carbon dioxide must be monitored from time of insertion of the endotracheal tube or laryngeal mask airway until removal of the device. The end-tidal CO_2 alarm must be audible when $P_{ET}CO_2$ is above or below preset levels. The anesthesia breathing machine must also have an audible alarm to identify a circuit disconnect.

Body Temperature

It is important to maintain a patient's body temperature while under anesthesia. When considerable alterations in body temperature are expected, probable, or planned, body temperature should be monitored.

SUGGESTED READINGS

Eichhorn JH. Review article: practical current issues in perioperative patient safety. *Can J Anaesth*. 2013;60:111-118.

Merry AF, Cooper JB, Soyannwo O, Wilson IH, Eichhorn JH. International Standards for a Safe Practice of Anesthesia 2010. *Can J Anaesth*. 2010;57:1027-1034.

Stages and Signs of General Anesthesia

Brian S. Freeman, MD

WHAT IS GENERAL ANESTHESIA?

The American Society of Anesthesiologists has specific criteria for the definition of general anesthesia. General anesthesia is the induction of a loss of unconsciousness by pharmacological means. In this state, the patient will be unarousable to verbal, tactile, and painful stimuli. Because of upper airway obstruction, some form of intervention, usually insertion of a laryngeal mask airway or endotracheal tube, is typically required to maintain airway patency. Spontaneous ventilation is frequently inadequate, necessitating the use of partial or full mechanical support with positive pressure ventilation. Cardiovascular function may be impaired, often leading to hypotension and dysrhythmias.

The primary goals of general anesthesia are to achieve:

- Amnesia
- Sedation/hypnosis
- Analgesia
- Areflexia (motionlessness)
- Attenuation of autonomic (sympathetic) nervous system responses.

HISTORICAL PERSPECTIVE

In 1846, Dr. William Morton gave the first public demonstration of general anesthesia by ether. At the time, physical examination of the patient provided the only clues to the depth of anesthesia. Inexperienced anesthetists could easily overdose the patient. It was not until World War I that the anesthesia community had the first true systematic approach to monitoring. Dr. Arthur Guedel, better known for his widely used oropharyngeal airway, was responsible for this system. As the medical officer responsible for supervising anesthesia services for the U.S. Army, he was concerned about the safe administration of ether by the nonmedical personnel. Guedel created one of the first safety systems in anesthesiology with his chart that explained the signs of ether anesthesia with increasing depth. He published this classification system as an article in 1920 and later in a textbook in 1937.

The Guedel classification for the stages of general anesthesia is based on the administration of a sole volatile anesthetic: diethyl ether. Although patients were commonly premedicated with atropine and morphine, ether was the only induction agent available at the time. It provided amnesia, analgesia, and muscle relaxation. Ether has not been used in the United States since the early 1980s. Today, "balanced anesthesia" uses multiple classes of drugs (intravenous anesthetics, opioids, neuromuscular blocking agents, and benzodiazepines) for induction that can easily mask the classical clinical signs of each Guedel stage of anesthesia. These drugs also have a greater safety profile compared to diethyl ether. In addition, modern monitors of respiration, circulation, and consciousness add to the clinical information provided by physical examination of the patient. Some anesthesiologists, therefore, may consider Guedel's work to be obsolete. Others still use his classification when it comes to describing emergence from anesthesia and inhalation inductions in children.

STAGES AND SIGNS OF GENERAL ANESTHESIA

Stage 1 (Disorientation)

The first stage of anesthesia, sometimes known as the induction stage, begins with the initial administration of anesthesia and ends with loss of consciousness. The patient experiences sedation, analgesia (but can still feel pain), and eventually amnesia. However, the patient should still be able to maintain a conversation during this stage. Respiration is slow but regular. The eyelid reflex is intact.

Stage 2 (Excitement)

The second stage of anesthesia is the period immediately following loss of consciousness until regular spontaneous ventilation resumes. The characteristic features are disinhibition, delirium, and uncontrolled spastic movements. Examination of the eyes reveals loss of lash reflex, divergent gaze, and reflex pupillary dilatation. The airway is irritable and has more secretions. As a result, there is an increased risk of eliciting intact reflexes like coughing, vomiting, laryngospasm, and bronchospasm. Respirations are irregular with periods of breath holding. Hypertension and tachycardia are common.

Because of the risk of clinically significant airway compromise, contemporary anesthetic techniques use rapidly acting intravenous hypnotics such as propofol to minimize time spent in Stage 2. However, all patients emerging from an inhalation anesthetic, and children who receive an inhalation induction, will show evidence of progressing through this stage. External stimulation, particularly of the airway, should be kept to a minimum. Endotracheal intubation and extubation should never occur during Stage 2.

Stage 3 (Surgical Anesthesia)

The third stage of anesthesia begins when the patient resumes spontaneous respiration and ends with respiratory paralysis. Stage 3 is the period when the target level of surgical anesthesia has been reached. It is also the stage in which it is appropriately safe to intubate the patient without neuromuscular blocking agents. Characteristic features include cessation of eye movement, skeletal muscle relaxation, and respiratory depression. Stage 3 is divided into four planes:

Plane 1—The patient has regular spontaneous breathing. A number of reflexes (eyelid, conjunctival, swallowing) disappear. Ocular muscles become less active. The patient has constricted pupils and central gaze.

Plane 2—The patient's spontaneous respirations have slight pauses between inhalation and exhalation. Additional reflexes are lost (corneal, laryngeal) while tear secretion increases. Eyeball movements cease completely. The patient no longer responds to skin stimulation with movement or deep breathing. Intercostal muscles begin to weaken.

Plane 3—Intercostal and abdominal muscles are completely relaxed, so ventilation is solely controlled by the diaphragm. The light reflex is lost. Surgical anesthesia has now been achieved.

Plane 4—Respirations become irregular and shallow with paradoxical rib cage movement as a result of complete intercostal muscle paralysis. Eventually, apnea results from full paralysis of the diaphragm.

Stage 4 (Overdose)

This stage of anesthesia begins from the cessation of respiration and ends at death. An overdose of anesthetic, relative to the degree of surgical stimulation, results in severe medullar depression leading to death unless support is provided. Otherwise, respiratory arrest and cardiovascular collapse result. Pupils are fixed and widely dilated. Skeletal muscles are flaccid.

SUGGESTED READING

Urban BW, Bleckwenn M. Concepts and correlations relevant to general anaesthesia. *Br J Anaesth.* 2002;89:3-16.

Awareness Under General Anesthesia

79

Hiep Dao, MD

INCIDENCE

The advent of movies and media reports have brought the fear of awareness under anesthesia into the forefront of patients' anxiety going into surgery. Intraoperative awareness under general anesthesia rarely occurs, with a reported incidence of 0.1%-0.2%. While rare, significant psychological consequences may occur after such an occurrence and the patient may be affected for some time. Oftentimes intraoperative awareness may be unavoidable in hemodynamically unstable patients, such as patients in trauma or cardiac surgery.

DEFINITION

Intraoperative awareness occurs when a patient becomes conscious during a procedure performed under general anesthesia, and subsequently has recall of these events. Recall can take the form of explicit memory (assessed by patient's ability to recall specific events that took place during general anesthesia) and implicit memory (assessed by changes in performance or behavior without the ability to recall specific events that took place during general anesthesia that led to those changes).

RISK FACTORS

Studies have suggested that certain procedures such as cesarean delivery, cardiac surgery, emergency surgery, trauma surgery as well as anesthetic techniques (rapid sequence inductions, reduced anesthetic doses with or without paralysis, difficult intubations, total intravenous anesthesia, use of nitrous oxide-opioid anesthetic technique) may be associated with an increased risk of intraoperative awareness. Furthermore, certain patient characteristics may place a patient at risk for intraoperative awareness including substance abuse (eg, opioids, benzodiazepines, cocaine), American Society of Anesthesiologists (ASA) physical status of IV or V, limited hemodynamic reserve, and history of awareness.

PREINDUCTION PREVENTION

Preventive measures in the preinduction phase of anesthesia management may minimize the occurrence of intraoperative awareness. Such measures include checking the functioning of the anesthesia machine and the prophylactic administration of benzodiazepines. There have been reported cases of intraoperative awareness resulting from low inspired volatile anesthetic concentration or drug errors.

Double-blind randomized clinical trials have shown a lower frequency of intraoperative awareness, with the prophylactic administration of midazolam as an anesthetic adjuvant. Consultants from ASA agree that benzodiazepines or scopolamine should be used in patients requiring smaller dosages of anesthetics, cardiac surgery patients, and patients undergoing trauma surgery. Caution should be taken with benzodiazepines due to delayed emergence.

INTRAOPERATIVE MONITORING

Intraoperative awareness cannot be measured during the intraoperative phase of general anesthesia because the recall component of awareness can only be determined postoperatively by speaking to the patient. Clinical techniques used to assess intraoperative consciousness include checking for patient movement, response to voice commands, eye opening, eyelash reflex, papillary response, perspiration, and tearing. Furthermore, conventional monitoring systems such as ECG, blood pressure, heart rate, end-tidal anesthetic analyzer, capnography are also valuable and help assess intraoperative depth of anesthesia.

There are a multitude of devices designed to monitor brain electrical activity for the purpose of assessing anesthetic effect. They record electroencephalographic activity from electrodes placed on the forehead. Several systems process spontaneous electroencephalographic and electromyographic activities, and others acquire evoked responses to auditory stimuli (auditory evoked potentials [AEP]). Various signal processing algorithms are applied to the frequency, amplitude, and latency relationship derived from the raw electroencephalography (EEG) or AEP to generate an "index" number, typically scaled from 0 to 100 indicating the progression of states of consciousness from awake to deep anesthesia (100 associated with awake state and 0 occurring with an isoelectric EEG and deep sedation).

Bispectral Index

The bispectral index (BIS) is a proprietary algorithm that converts a single channel of frontal electroencephalograph into an index of hypnotic level. BIS values are scaled from 0 to 100, with specific ranges (40-60) indicative of a low probability of consciousness under general anesthesia. In some randomized controlled trials, the BIS monitor has decreased the incidence of explicit recall, times to awakening, first response, or eye opening and consumption of anesthetic drugs. Other studies have shown no decreased incidence of intraoperative awareness with its use. Thus, the current data and recommendations on its use are mixed. Intraoperative events unrelated to titration of anesthetic agents can produce rapid changes in BIS values (cerebral hypoperfusion, gas embolism, and hemorrhage). Other routine intraoperative events (use of depolarizing muscle relaxants, activation of electromagnetic equipment, patient warming, or hypothermia) may interfere with BIS functioning.

Auditory-Evoked Potential Monitor

Auditory-evoked potentials (AEP) are the electrical responses of the brainstem, auditory radiation, and auditory cortex to auditory sound stimuli (clicks) delivered via headphones. The typical AEP response to increasing anesthetic concentrations is increased latency and decreased amplitude of the various waveform components. From analysis of the AEP waveform, the monitor generates an "AEP index" that correlates anesthetic concentration to a level of consciousness (low probability of consciousness with values < 25).

The ASA states that a brain electrical activity monitor should be used in patients on a case-by-case basis with conditions that may place them at risk and patients requiring smaller doses of anesthetics (trauma surgery, cesarean delivery, and total intravenous anesthesia). There is insufficient evidence that such a monitor truly reduces the risk of intraoperative awareness for all patients undergoing general anesthesia. Furthermore, maintaining low brain function monitor values in an attempt to prevent intraoperative awareness may conflict with other important anesthetic goals (hemodynamic stability).

INTRAOPERATIVE AND POSTOPERATIVE INTERVENTIONS

1. Intraoperative administration of benzodiazepines to patients who may become conscious.
2. Providing a postoperative interview to patients to define the episode of awareness.
3. Providing a postoperative questionnaire to patients with intraoperative awareness.
4. Offering postoperative counseling or psychological support.

SUGGESTED READINGS

Bergman IJ, Kluger MT, Short TG. Awareness during general anaesthesia: a review of 81 cases from the Anaesthetic Incident Monitoring Study. *Anaesthesia* 2002;57:549-556.

Domino KB, Posner KL, Caplan RA, Cheney FW. Awareness during anesthesia: a closed claims analysis. *Anesthesiology* 1999;90:1053-1061.

Sandin RH, Enlund G, Samuelsson P, Lennmarken C. Awareness during anaesthesia: a prospective case study. *Lancet* 2000;355:707-711.

Sebel PS, Bowdle TA, Ghoneim MM, et al. The incidence of awareness during anesthesia: a multicenter United States study. *Anesth Analg.* 2004;99:833-839.

Techniques of General Anesthesia

80

Brian S. Freeman, MD

General anesthesia is a state of unconsciousness in which pharmacological agents produce hypnosis, amnesia, and analgesia. Other endpoints met during most general anesthetics include muscle relaxation, immobility, and attenuation of sympathetic and somatic reflexes. The induction of general anesthesia is achieved by either intravenous or inhalation routes. The "maintenance" phase begins when the amnestic patient is not only unconscious, but also unable to produce movements in response to surgery. At this point, there are several techniques available for the anesthesiologist to maintain general anesthesia during a given operation or procedure.

TOTAL INHALATION ANESTHESIA

This technique involves the sole administration of potent volatile agents such as sevoflurane to maintain general anesthesia. Advantages of this approach include the ability to maintain spontaneous ventilation and satisfactory blunting of sympathetic responses to noxious stimulation. Modern inhalation agents are easier to titrate to the patient's blood pressure, pulse, minute ventilation, and movements. The major disadvantage of this technique is significant dose-dependent cardiovascular depression. In addition, volatile anesthetics do not provide any degree of analgesia. This approach is most amenable for short procedures for which intraoperative and postoperative pain is expected to be minimal, such as myringotomy, cystoscopy, and examinations under anesthesia.

TOTAL INTRAVENOUS ANESTHESIA

The technique of "total intravenous anesthesia" (TIVA) can be used for the complete maintenance of general anesthesia or for the administration of deep sedation. TIVA utilizes continuous infusions or repeated doses of a short-acting sedative-hypnotic drug. Opioids, either in bolus form or through an infusion, are often added for these procedures that may produce more than minimal stimulation.

There are several advantages to TIVA:

- Decreased incidence of postoperative nausea and vomiting.

- Rapid induction and easy titration.
- Rapid emergence even after long infusions due to favorable context-sensitive half-times.
- No risk of malignant hyperthermia.
- Minimal suppression of neurophysiologic-evoked potentials.
- Avoidance of occupational exposure or environmental pollution by volatile agents.
- No need for gas delivery or scavenging systems.
- No expansion of gas cavities.
- May reduce intracranial pressure (propofol).

TIVA is used quite extensively for deep sedation and maintenance in ambulatory surgery. It is a simple technique that leads to rapid and clear emergence with minimal postoperative nausea and vomiting. TIVA is especially useful for maintaining general anesthesia in patients for whom delivery of inhalation anesthetics may be compromised or difficult. For example, pulmonary diseases that impair ventilation and perfusion to the lung can lead to inconsistent drug uptake. TIVA allows for a much more rapid onset of action that does not depend on the adequacy of alveolar ventilation. TIVA is also suitable for operations in which ventilation is interrupted, such as laser airway surgery or bronchoscopy.

There are several disadvantages to TIVA for maintenance or deep sedation:

- Need for multiple infusion pumps (compared to just one agent vaporizer).
- More expensive: is the cost worth the benefit?
- Variability in patient dose requirements and pharmacokinetics.
- Inability to measure blood concentration of intravenous anesthetics.
- Greater incidence of patient movement.

Many different drugs can be chosen to provide total intravenous anesthesia. The most popular combination is a sedative-hypnotic plus opioid. Propofol (75-150 µg/kg/min) has become the mainstay of TIVA infusions. It provides amnesia, hypnosis, and even antiemetic properties—all with a short duration of action. Adding a concurrent opioid infusion, usually remifentanil, allows for short-acting analgesia.

Titration of drug dosages can take place against measurement of the bispectral index (BIS), for propofol, and hemodynamic changes to surgical stimulation, for opioids. Other options for TIVA include infusion of dexmedetomidine, a central acting alpha-2 adrenergic agonist and low-dose ketamine, an NMDA receptor antagonist.

BALANCED ANESTHESIA

General anesthesia using a single drug may require doses that produce excessive cardiovascular compromise. Providing "balanced" anesthesia is probably the most common approach to maintenance of general anesthesia. The concept of balanced anesthesia is based on combining multiple classes of drugs to achieve the desired endpoints of general anesthesia. Targeting different receptors enables lower dosages and fewer side effects for each type of medication. A balanced anesthetic will often produce less hypotension and cardiovascular depression than a pure inhalation or intravenous technique. This concept is not a new one. As new drugs were synthesized over the past century, they quickly became part of the administration of anesthesia. For instance, meperidine was often used as an adjunct to the administration of nitrous oxide anesthesia starting back in the 1940s.

A typical balanced anesthetic includes:

- a potent inhalation agent such as sevoflurane (amnesia, unconsciousness, immobility, autonomic attenuation);
- a benzodiazepine such as midazolam (amnesia);
- an opioid such as fentanyl (analgesia);
- a muscle relaxant such as rocuronium (immobility);
- an intravenous sedative-hypnotic such as propofol (unconsciousness).

Opioids are one of the key components of a balanced anesthetic. Their primary function is reduction of pain. Opioids also decrease requirements for both intravenous and inhalation anesthetics, attenuate autonomic responses to airway and surgical stimulation, and help to maintain hemodynamic stability. These drugs should be given prior to the onset of the noxious stimulus. For instance, if fentanyl is not given at least 5 minutes before surgical incision, it is much less effective in suppressing hemodynamic surges now that catecholamines have been released. Sufficient time is necessary for opioids to be truly effective. The most rapidly titratable opioids are remifentanil and alfentanil (1-2 minutes before onset of peak effect). With more favorable kinetics and better hemodynamic stability, fentanyl and its derivatives are generally found to be superior to morphine, meperidine, and hydromorphone in the administration of balanced anesthesia.

NITROUS OXIDE–OPIOID–RELAXANT TECHNIQUE

Because of their low solubility, volatile agents such as desflurane and sevoflurane are key agents used today during inhalation anesthesia. Back in the days when more soluble drugs such as enflurane and halothane were the only options, nitrous oxide was the most commonly administered inhalation anesthetic. Nitrous oxide has a very low potency (MAC 104%) but extremely favorable pharmacokinetics due to its low solubility. One technique of general anesthesia less commonly used today is the administration of high dose nitrous oxide along with intravenous opioids and muscle relaxants. The patient receives an inspired gas mixture of about 70% nitrous oxide with 30% oxygen. Opioids are administered in response to changes in the pulse and blood pressure due to surgical stimulation. It is important to dose opioids regularly throughout the case to prevent delayed emergence. Muscle relaxants are necessary to prevent patient movement. Controlled mechanical ventilation is necessary to prevent hypercapnia.

Using this technique, emergence from general anesthesia is usually quite smooth (due to the opioids) and rapid (due to the nitrous oxide). In addition, patients tend to have less anesthetic-induced vasodilation and hypotension during the case. However, the potential for intraoperative awareness is an important concern when using this "light" anesthesia technique (especially when combined with muscle relaxants). Benzodiazepines should be considered.

COMBINED GENERAL–REGIONAL ANESTHESIA

General anesthesia may be combined with regional anesthesia to maximize the advantages of both techniques while minimizing the potential complications. The most common approach involves the administration of an epidural anesthetic or peripheral nerve block followed by the induction of general anesthesia (or deep sedation). Epidural catheters should be placed at the appropriate level depending on the type of surgery (T5-T6 for thoracic surgery, T7-T8 for upper abdominal surgery, T9-T10 for lower abdominal surgery). For epidural catheters, this technique assumes that local anesthetics will be administered during the procedure.

Advantages to a combined general–regional technique for maintenance include:

- Avoidance of opioids;
- Less postoperative nausea and vomiting;
- Higher quality of postoperative analgesia;

- Preemptive analgesia;
- Maintaining a secure airway with an endotracheal tube or laryngeal mask airway (LMA) device;
- Less patient movement;
- Improved suppression of endocrine stress response to surgery;
- Faster return of bowel function;
- Lower incidence of postoperative pulmonary complications.

This approach may yield several disadvantages, such as:

- Greater degree of hypotension due to the sympathectomy (neuraxial technique only);
- Nerve injury;
- Epidural hematoma;
- Higher risk of local anesthetic systemic toxicity;
- Time consuming placement.

Assessment and Identification of the Difficult Airway

Raymond A. Pla, Jr. MD

The American Society of Anesthesiologist's (ASA) Closed Claims Project reports that difficult intubation leading to death or brain injury account for 9% of all claims. Some were classified as preventable. Preoperative evaluation with medical, surgical, and anesthetic history as well as physical examination and radiographic study evaluation minimizes the chances of unrecognized difficult intubation. No single factor reliably predicts difficult airway management. The more the predictors of difficulty in a given patient, the greater the likelihood of difficult airway. Once difficult intubation is recognized, practitioners may prepare additional equipment, modify induction agents, and secure backup support as necessary.

DEFINITIONS

- Difficult mask ventilation is an inability to face mask ventilate the patient.
- Difficult laryngoscopy is an inability to visualize the vocal cords after multiple laryngoscopy attempts.
- Difficult intubation is encountered when multiple attempts are required to intubate the trachea.
- Failed intubation is the inability to place an endotracheal tube despite multiple attempts.

These definitions presume best operator and optimized positioning (ie, sniff position).

PREDICTION CRITERIA

Although no single criterion envisages difficulty, a history of difficult airway is the single best predictor of future difficulty. Consequently, a thorough anesthetic history should include previous airway concerns. Interval change in the patient's medical history or condition, such as new oral or pharyngeal pathology, significant weight or height gain (ie, previous surgery as a child), cervical spine injury, or pregnancy discounts previous airway success.

1. **Mallampati/Samsoon–Young Scoring**—The Mallampati/ Samsoon–Young scale classifies airways according to the base of tongue to overall open mouth ratio. The underlying premise is that during direct laryngoscopy, the base of the tongue obscures the view of the larynx. Thus, a higher ratio would suggest a greater likelihood of difficult laryngoscopy. This test is performed with the patient's head in the neutral position without phonation. A class I view includes the entire uvula, hard, and soft palates; class II—only a partial uvula view in addition to the hard and soft palates; class III—hard and soft palates with base of uvula visible; and class IV—hard palate only is visualized. Classes III and IV are associated with a higher incidence of difficulty with intubation (see Chapter 64).

2. **Macroglossia**—Macroglossia predicts difficult intubation as a large tongue is difficult to be completely displaced by a rigid laryngoscope into the submandibular space.

3. **Thyromental distance**—Thyromental distance is the distance between the thyroid cartilage and the mentum of the mandible. It is normally greater than 6.5 cm; thyromental distance predicts difficulty with intubation when less than 6 cm. This measurement suggests that the mandibular size is measured with the head extended at the atlanto-occipital joint.

4. **Mandibulohyoid distance**—The mandibular–hyoid distance predicts a large, hypopharyngeal tongue blocking visualization of the glottic opening; hence, direct laryngoscopy and intubation difficulty is increased. This distance should be greater than 4 cm.

5. **Neck circumference**—A short, thick neck with a circumference greater than 44 cm predicts difficulty with ventilation and intubation.

6. **Cervical spine range of motion**—Decreased cervical spine mobility predicts difficult intubation on the basis of an inability to extend the atlanto-occipital joint and achieve an optimal "sniff position." This condition makes bringing the visual axes of the mouth, pharynx, and the larynx into alignment difficult or impossible. Sitting upright with the head in a neutral position, the neck is maximally extended and the examiner estimates the angle traversed by the occlusal surface of the maxillary incisors. This angle is normally greater than 35 degrees. Extension deficit may be graded: grade I greater than 35 degrees; grade II 22-34 degrees; grade III 12-21 degrees; and grade IV less than 12 degrees.

7. **Temporo-mandibular joint (TMJ) translation**—TMJ translation is necessary for mouth opening and laryngoscopy. Inability to extend the mandibular incisors anterior to the maxillary incisors suggests difficult intubation.

8. **Dentition**—The state of dentition can predict difficulty. Several dental conditions warrant particular concern: (1) loose or broken teeth, especially maxillary or mandibular incisors; (2) interincisor distance less than 3 cm; and (3) maxillary incisors that override mandibular incisors, commonly referred to as an overbite. Edentulous patients carry higher risk for difficult ventilation and intubation as well.

MEDICAL HISTORY

A number of disease states, syndromes, and conditions predict difficulty. The following conditions are often associated with difficult airway management:

1. **Obesity**—Obesity is defined as a body mass index (BMI) greater than 30. The BMI is calculated as weight in kg/height in meters^2. Obese patients have adipose deposits in the pharynx, which protrude and narrow the airway. Additionally, obesity is associated with macroglossia and a short, large neck. Ventilation and intubation may be difficult in obese patients. They quickly desaturate O_2 following induction of anesthesia due to lower functional residual capacity (FRC); consequently, difficult airway management decisions are time-sensitive in this population.

2. **Pregnancy**—Airway difficulties pose a particular risk in the parturient, resulting in pulmonary aspiration of gastric contents, hypoxia, cardiac arrest, and even death. Parturients suffer from edematous and friable airways. Large, pendulous breasts make placing the laryngoscope difficult as the long handle contacts the chest wall. The parturient risks rapid arterial desaturation with apnea due to reduced FRC. Further, delayed gastric emptying and inadequate esophageal sphincter tone predispose parturients to aspiration.

3. **Burns, thermal injury, and smoke inhalation**—These injuries are often associated with airway edema.

4. **Cervical spine injury**—Instability of the c-spine decreases the degree of safe neck extension. This makes alignment of the three principal axes (oral, pharyngeal, and laryngeal) difficult. Intubation requires in-line stabilization to prevent neck extension.

5. **Acromegaly**—Acromegaly is caused by excessive growth hormone production. It is associated with macroglossia and prognathism.

6. **Epiglottitis**—Epiglottitis is a life-threatening infection of the epiglottis and periepiglottic structures that causes upper airway edema and potentially complete airway obstruction. Airway instrumentation can completely obstruct the airway and is contraindicated in the awake patient. If emergent intubation is required, they should be performed in a setting with emergency tracheostomy immediately available.

7. **Submandibular cellulitis (Ludwig angina)**—The infection and resulting swelling of the submandibular space forces the tongue in a cranial and caudad direction blocking the airway. The infection causes pharyngeal and tongue swelling. Like epiglottitis, this disease can cause life-threatening airway compromise and requires emergent intubation, preferably in the operating room.

8. **Rheumatoid arthritis**—Limitations in cervical range of motion and TMJ mobility may compromise mouth opening. Cervical spine arthritis limits the neck's degree of extension, preventing axis alignment and laryngeal view. Additionally, atlanto-axial (C1-C2) subluxation and separation of the odontoid process can occur. The free-floating odontoid process can impinge upon the spinal cord or vertebral arteries during induction and intubation. This diagnosis can be made with lateral, flexion–extension radiographs of the neck.

9. **Diabetes**—Patients with long-term, insulin-dependent diabetes present with diabetic stiff joint syndrome. This occurs as a result of glycosylation of collagen and its deposition in joints. Consequently, achieving optimal intubating sniff position is difficult.

10. **Beards**—Facial hair can make mask ventilation difficult.

Approaches to Difficult Airway Management

Raymond A. Pla, Jr., MD

Analysis of the American Society of Anesthesiologist's (ASA) Closed Claims database (1985-1992) focusing on management of difficult airway, in part, led to development of the ASA Difficult Airway Algorithm in 1993. Subsequently, death and brain damage claims resulting from difficult airway management on induction of anesthesia decreased. In contrast, claims associated with the other phases of anesthesia (maintenance, emergence, and recovery) did not change. Over the years, many techniques have been developed to manage a difficult airway. Each technique has been proven valuable. However, anatomy and disease state of an individual patient and the clinical judgment and experience of the operator influence the technique applied to each patient.

Managing a patient with a known or suspected difficult airway has, as its central goal, to avoid major complications, including, but not limited to: injury to airway structures, hypoxic brain injury, cardiopulmonary arrest, unnecessary tracheostomy, or death. To this end, securing the airway while the patient is awake and breathing spontaneously may be indicated or necessary.

INDUCTION

Airway Avoidance

This technique involves the exclusive use of regional or neuraxial anesthesia, avoiding the use of apnea-inducing sedatives or protective airway reflex compromise. While this technique poses the risks of incomplete block, local anesthetic systemic toxicity, and patient anxiety, it effectively achieves the goal of anesthesia while maintaining a patent airway. Before attempting, practitioners should consider: regional anesthetic contraindications, patient anxiety level, duration, and anatomic extent of the surgery relative to the duration and anatomic distribution of the block and intraoperative airway access.

Laryngeal Mask Airway

Laryngeal mask airway (LMA) is an inflatable, supraglottic device that overlies the laryngeal inlet and seals the hypopharynx, allowing for delivery of positive pressure (up to 20 cm H_2O). Since it overlies the larynx, an LMA serves as a conduit through which an endotracheal tube (ETT) can be passed (either blindly or fiberoptically) into the trachea. As there is no subglottic cuff, LMAs do not provide definitive airway protection from aspiration.

Flexible Fiberoptic Intubation

This technique uses a fiberoptic bronchoscope (FOB) as a visually guided stylet over which an ETT is directed into the trachea. This technique can be administered nasally or orally, when the patient is asleep or awake. Supplemental oxygen, either via a nasal cannula or through the bronchoscope itself, maintains oxygenation during intubation. If performed with anesthetized patient, jaw-thrust or gentle anterior traction on the tongue opens the pharynx, raises the epiglottis, and aids in glottic opening visualization.

If attempted in an awake patient, psychological and anesthetic (topically and/or airway nerve blocks) preparation is necessary. Psychological preparation of the patient begins with an explanation of what is to occur and why. While physical preparation includes the judicious use of anxiolytics (while maintaining airway protective reflexes and spontaneous ventilation). Anti-sialagogue pretreatment is critical to the success of the procedure as oral secretions prevent mucosal contact of topically applied local anesthetic. Further, saliva obscures visualization of the larynx. Anticholinergics such as glycopyrrolate are effective in this regard, as is suction capability via the FOB.

If the nose is chosen, topical anesthetic to the nasal mucosa, innervated by the greater and lesser palatine nerves and the anterior ethmoid nerve, all branches of the trigeminal nerve, must be applied. Further, local anesthetic may be supplemented by a vasoconstrictor to shrink the nasal mucosa. This facilitates passage of the ETT and reduces the risk of traumatic epistaxis. Phenylephrine or oxymetazoline effectively induces vasoconstriction. Due to bleeding risk, the nasal approach is not advised in pregnancy (engorged-friable mucosa) and in those with coagulopathy or receiving anticoagulant therapy.

Orally inhaled nebulized or atomized local anesthetic should be administered to the posterior oropharynx to inhibit the gag reflex and allow FOB passage through the pharynx and larynx. Finally, the larynx and trachea should be anesthetized using a transtracheal injection of local anesthetic through the cricothyroid membrane, thereby minimizing the cough response to FOB and ETT advancement. These topical techniques can be accomplished using lidocaine 1%, 2%, or 4% or cocaine, paying close attention to the toxic dose of local anesthetic as there can be fairly rapid and significant absorption into systemic circulation from airway mucosa. Airway nerve blocks, specifically the superior laryngeal nerve block and the glossopharyngeal nerve block can supplement airway anesthesia for sensitive patients.

Video Laryngoscopy

Video laryngoscopy is a form of indirect laryngoscopy, in which the clinician views the larynx with a fiberoptic or digital rigid laryngoscope. Video laryngoscopy has recently provided a viable alternative to oral FOB. Indirect view of the glottic opening may be obtained with video laryngoscopy in cases where direct laryngoscopy visualization is difficult or impossible. Specially designed stylets allow for anterior, acute-angle ETT placement.

Lighted Stylet and Gum Elastic Bougie

Lighted stylets such as light wands provide trans-illumination of the anterior neck, demonstrating ETT position. These can be used blindly or in conjunction with direct or video laryngoscopy. The tip of a gum elastic bougie or Eschmann catheter can be manipulated to an angle that allows for anterior manipulation in the larynx. Bougie stylets are used in conjunction with laryngoscopy and allow for ETT placement over the stylet as a guide.

Retrograde Technique

Retrograde wire intubation involves percutaneous passage of a guide wire into the trachea through the cricothyroid membrane, in a retrograde direction, emerging from the mouth or nose. An ETT is then placed over the wire and passed in an anterograde direction, over the wire and into the trachea. This technique can be performed electively or emergently. It can be particularly helpful when blood or copious secretions in the airway would make fiberoptic intubation very difficult or impossible. Though safe, complications such as pneumothorax, bleeding, and coughing (a sign of distal passage of the wire toward the carina) exist.

Cricothyrotomy

Cricothyrotomy involves either: (1) percutaneous, Seldinger technique placement of a catheter through the cricothyroid membrane; or (2) surgical placement of a catheter using a vertical incision through the aforementioned location. This technique is useful when unable to ventilate or intubate.

Transtracheal Jet Ventilation

Transtracheal jet ventilation is a form of cricothyrotomy in which a catheter is introduced into the cricothyroid membrane as described previously and attached to a high-pressure oxygen source (25-50 psi). The patient's lungs are ventilated at a rate of 12-16 times per minute, leaving adequate time for gas exhalation. Exhalation must be ensured passively so as to prevent barotrauma. This technique can be life-sustaining until a more definitive airway is established.

EXTUBATION

The patient who presented difficulty with intubation at induction must be considered a difficult extubation. Difficult extubation refers to the risk of premature or inadvertent extubation that may result in hypoxic brain injury or death. Clinical situations include, but are not limited to: (1) recurrent laryngeal nerve damage, tracheomalacia or hematoma from thyroidectomy; (2) hematoma from carotid endarterectomy; (3) hematoma or subglottic edema from cervical vertebral decompression; (4) airway edema from prone position, anaphylaxis, or thermal injury; and (5) bleeding, laryngospasm or edema from laryngeal biopsy or tonsillectomy.

Options to consider in managing potential difficult extubation include ensuring routine extubation criteria have been met, such as: (1) following commands, including sustained head lift for 5 seconds to verbal command; (2) intact gag reflex; (3) adequate pain control; (4) airway clear of secretions and blood; (5) adequate ventilatory mechanics—tidal volume greater than 5 mL/kg, vital capacity greater than 10 mL/kg; (6) controlled respiratory and cardiac rate and rhythm; (7) hemodynamic stability; and (8) normothermia. Negative inspiratory force measurements, arterial blood gas values, and ETT cuff leaks are additional considerations for extubation management of difficult airway patients. Once extubation conditions have been satisfied, location should be considered: operating room, postanesthesia care unit or intensive care unit. Equipment and personnel availability should aid the decision regarding location of extubation.

Finally, a stylet can be placed in the ETT and left in place to assist with reintubation if the need arises after extubation. Extubation stylets called exchange catheters provide the advantage of serving as a conduit for O_2 administration. The gum elastic bougie, or Eschmann catheter can be used as a stylet, but oxygen cannot be administered with this type of stylet. Equipment for immediate reintubation should be available and close monitoring should be maintained in the hours immediately following extubation.

The ASA Difficult Airway Algorithm

C H A P T E R
83

Christopher Edwards, MD

The difficult airway algorithm was designed to help practitioners deal with both anticipated and unanticipated difficult airway management. Before delivering any anesthetic care, a thorough history and physical examination should be performed to help predict any difficulty with airway management. While there is typically no single finding that predicts a difficult airway, the summation of history and physical data may suggest potential difficulty during airway management.

PLANNING

The difficult airway algorithm (Figure 83-1) is organized to help practitioners navigate various complications that arise during airway management. The first step in the difficult airway algorithm is assessing basic management options such as patient cooperation with various airway plans (ie, an awake intubation), ability to mask ventilate, potential effectiveness of a supraglottic airway device, ease of laryngoscopy, ease of intubation, and surgical airway feasibility. Evaluation should occur before attempting airway manipulation. In addition, there should be a plan to administer supplemental oxygen throughout the airway management process. One such example would be performing an awake intubation with supplemental oxygen via nasal cannula until the airway is secured. The last approach should include a plan to ease various airway management techniques. What is the feasibility of performing an awake versus sleep intubation? Is an awake surgical airway an option? Is video-assisted laryngoscopy warranted? Should preservation of spontaneous ventilation be maintained? These are questions that need to be answered before engaging in airway management as answers to these questions may change the plan. By approaching each of these questions and concerns prior to airway manipulation, the practitioner is prepared to deal with difficulties as they arise.

UNANTICIPATED DIFFICULT AIRWAY

Despite a myriad of recommendations, there will undoubtedly be unanticipated difficulty with airway management. When navigating the difficult airway algorithm, decision points hinge on whether or not oxygenation and ventilation are adequate. The two arms of the flow chart start with either induction of general anesthesia or performing an awake intubation. Most difficulty in common anesthesia practice occurs after the induction of anesthesia has taken place and will initially focus on this arm of the flow chart. Once general anesthesia has been induced by a trained anesthesia provider and intubation has been unsuccessful, the patient is classified as having a difficult airway and swift decisions need to take place. The **most** important consideration is whether or not **mask ventilation is adequate**. All ventilation should be confirmed with exhaled CO_2, in addition to other means of assessing ventilation. Once mask ventilation has been established, the urgency is removed, allowing for nonemergent techniques to establish oxygenation and ventilation. These techniques can include anything from alternate methods of noninvasive airway access, to invasive airway access, to awakening the patient, and choosing an alternate plan. If **mask ventilation is not adequate and awakening the patient is not an option,** alternate means to establish ventilation are needed. Consider placing a **supraglottic airway device,** such as an Laryngeal mask airway (LMA) to aid with ventilation and call for help. If ventilation is still inadequate with the supraglottic airway device, then **invasive access is necessary.** Supplemental oxygen should be delivered while other modalities of securing the airway are in process. Methods of invasive airway access include a surgical airway such as tracheostomy, percutaneous cricothyrotomy, percutaneous jet ventilation, and retrograde wire intubation.

SPECIAL CONSIDERATIONS

In addition to the ASA difficult airway algorithm, there are other considerations during special circumstances. One of those circumstances is the **obstetric patient presenting for emergent cesarean section** (Figure 83-2). The obstetric patient carries another level of complexity in that the wellbeing of the fetus needs consideration along with the mother when deciding how to address difficult airway management. During an emergent cesarean section in which a general anesthetic is required, while the mother is of prime importance

The ASA Difficult Airway Algorithm

American Society of

Anesthesiologists®

DIFFICULT AIRWAY ALGORITHM

1. Assess the likelihood and clinical impact of basic management problems:
    • Difficulty with patient cooperation or consent
    • Difficult mask ventilation
    • Difficult supraglottic airway placement
    • Difficult laryngoscopy
    • Difficult intubation
    • Difficult surgical airway access

2. Actively pursue opportunities to deliver supplemental oxygen throughout the process of difficult airway management.

3. Consider the relative merits and feasibility of basic management choices:

    • Awake intubation vs intubation after induction of general anesthesia
    • Noninvasive technique vs invasive techniques for the initial approach to intubation
    • Video-assisted laryngoscopy as an initial approach to intubation
    • Preservation vs ablation of spontaneous ventilation

4. Develop primary and alternative strategies:

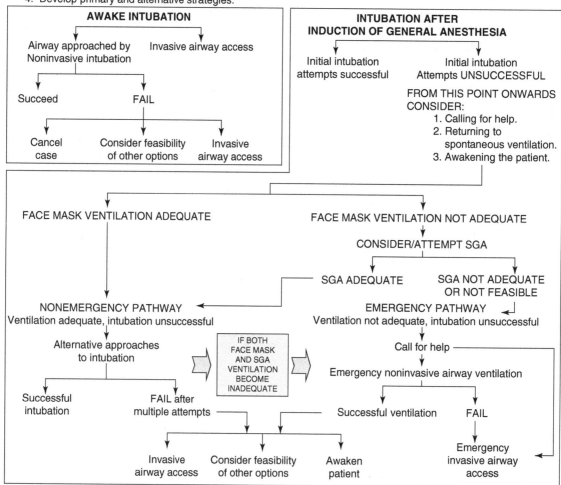

FIGURE 83-1 The difficult airway algorithm. (Reproduced with permission from Apfelbaum JL, Hagberg CA, Caplan RA, et al. Practice guidelines for management of the difficult airway: an updated report by the American Society of Anesthesiologists Task Force on management of the difficult airway, *Anesthesiology.* 2013;118(2):251-270.)

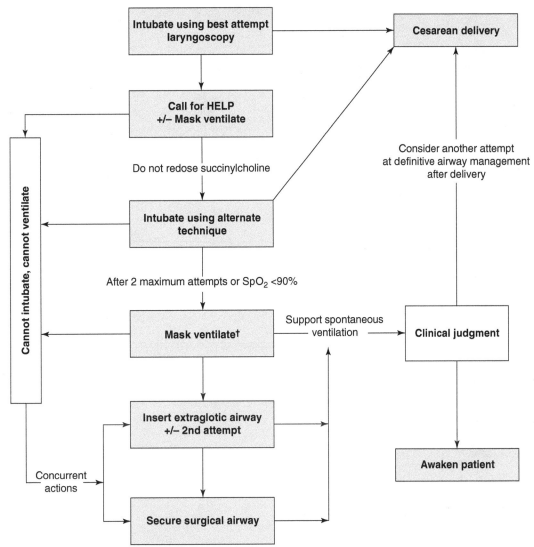

FIGURE 83-2 Difficult airway algorithm for cesarean delivery in a patient with fetal distress. (Reproduced with permission from Mhyre JM, Healy D. The unanticipated difficult intubation in obstetrics. *Anesth Analg.* 2011;112(3):648-652.)

to the anesthesiologist, if unable to intubate but ventilation is adequate, despite the patient being a full stomach, it is reasonable to continue the procedure while ventilating with cricoid pressure if there are nonreassuring fetal tones. If the fetal heart tone is adequate, it would be prudent to awaken the mother and choose another plan.

SUGGESTED READINGS

American Society of Anesthesiologist: practice guidelines for the management of the difficult airway: an updated report. *Anesthesiology* 2013;118.

Mhyre JM, Healy D. The unanticipated difficult intubation in obstetrics. *Anesth Analg.* 2011;112:648-652.

Intubation Devices

84

Sandy Christiansen, MD, and Sudha Ved, MD

Intubation devices are a critical component of administering general anesthesia. By facilitating endotracheal intubation, these devices secure the patient's airway, thereby protecting the patient from aspiration, laryngospasm, and anatomic obstruction.

RIGID LARYNGOSCOPES

The rigid laryngoscope is essentially a retractor-type device. This laryngoscope elevates the tongue and other soft tissues within the pharynx to create a straight line of vision, or "line of sight," between the operator's eye and the larynx. Multiple devices are available that differ in the location of the light source, dimension of the hinges, and shapes of the blades and handles.

1. The **Miller blade** is inserted posterior to the epiglottis and is ideal for children or adults with a large epiglottis that obstructs the view of the vocal cords. Proper placement of the Miller blade will stimulate the vagus nerve (CN X). It is available in sizes 00, 0, 1, 1.5, 2, 3, and 4.
2. The **Macintosh blade** is the most common blade used in adults in the United States. It is inserted into the vallecula from the right side of the oropharynx and advanced midline manipulating the tongue to the left. Once in position, the handle is lifted up and outward to elevate the larynx and expose the vocal cords. Proper placement of the Macintosh blade will stimulate the glossopharyngeal nerve (CN IX). It is available in sizes 0, 1, 2, 3, 3.5, and 4.
3. A **left-handed Macintosh blade** is available. It is a mirror image of the standard Macintosh blade, containing a right-sided groove for directing the tongue rightward as it is advanced midline. It is intended for use by left-handed practitioners or for use on patients with atypical anatomy on the right side of their face. The blade is only available in size 3.
4. The **McCoy blade** is similar to the Macintosh blade but includes an additional hinge with handle to maneuver an adjustable tip at the distal portion of the blade. It is designed to elevate the vallecula and epiglottis when the adjustable tip is flexed.

5. The **Soper blade** is a straight blade with a left-sided groove and is used predominantly for intubating neonates and infants. The flat portion of the blade is used to restrict tongue motion.
6. The **Wisconsin blade** is a straight blade with a semicircular groove to allow passage of the endotracheal tube through the circular portion after establishing a view of the larynx.
7. The **Robertshaw blade** is a curved blade that is rounded at the distal third portion. Similar to the Macintosh blade, it is designed to lift the epiglottis. The benefit of this blade is greatest when facilitating nasotracheal intubation because it provides a superior view of the pharynx compared to the Macintosh blade, particularly after the Magill forceps have been introduced.
8. The **Seward blade** is a straight blade with a curved distal tip. It is predominantly used for assisting nasotracheal intubation in children younger than 5 years of age due to its ability to maintain a view of the pharynx after introducing Magill forceps.
9. The **Oxford blade** is a U-shaped straight blade with a curved tip. The blade becomes gradually narrower as it progresses distally. The blade is most useful in children with cleft palate due to its unique shape.

RIGID FIBEROPTIC LARYNGOSCOPES

There are two subcategories of fiberoptic laryngoscopes, rigid and flexible, both of which depend on fiberoptic technology to generate a view of the larynx. Both types utilize a fiberoptic conductor that transmits the view of the larynx from the end of the scope to an eyepiece or camera, allowing an indirect view of the larynx. In the rigid fiberoptic laryngoscope, the fiberoptic conductor is encased in a solid material that is able to retract tissues as well as project an image on the eyepiece or camera. Some have anti-fogging lenses and most have wide high resolution cameras, which can capture video images.

The **Bullard, WuScope,** and **Upsher** laryngoscopes all have a broadly curved blade with a proximal eyepiece. Owing to their unique design, they are able to elevate the jaw without neck extension. This quality is particularly advantageous in patients with limited mouth opening or trauma patients. The difference between the Bullard and the Upsher laryngoscopes lies in the manner of endotracheal tube passage. The Bullard has a fixed stylet on which to mount the endotracheal tube, whereas the Upsher and WuScope have a semicircular channel for passing the endotracheal tube into the field of view.

Video laryngoscopes, including the **Glidescope, Storz C-MAC,** and **McGrath**, utilize blades that are similar in structure to the Macintosh and Miller blades but with different angles. They contain high resolution cameras, which provide fiberoptic imaging onto a video screen to improve intubating conditions. The Glidescope blade has a 60 degree angle and an anti-fogging mechanism to prevent clouding of the lens. The portable "Ranger" version is rugged and designed for field (ie., emergency medical technician and military) use. The C-MAC Dorges D-Blade has an 80 degree angle for anterior airways. The blades can be autoclaved for sterilization and repeat usage.

The **Airtraq laryngoscope** is a disposable laryngoscope with a reusable video screen, which provides a panoramic view of the larynx without an external video monitor. **Airtraq SP** allows a snap-on camera that can be connected to an external monitor for viewing. This laryngoscope contains two ports: an optical port and an endotracheal tube guiding port. The Airtraq fits endotracheal tubes ranging from size 2.5 to 8.5 mm and is able to support nasotracheal, oral, and double lumen intubations. A unique advantage of the Airtraq is its utility in facilitating tracheal intubation in virtually any position, making it particularly valuable for patients with cervical spine fractures, trauma, and jaw immobility.

FLEXIBLE FIBEROPTIC LARYNGOSCOPES

The flexible fiberoptic laryngoscope is composed of a coherent bundle consisting of thousands of fine glass fibers that cause total internal reflection of an image that is transmitted to the opposite end of the bundle. The fiberoptic bundle is enclosed in a flexible sheath allowing it to bend around anatomic structures. The scope also contains a "working channel" through which instruments can be inserted to perform various functions, such as biopsying tissues, injecting medications, and providing suction. Two angulation wires enable the endoscopist to make fine movements with the tip of the scope. Images can be projected onto the eyepiece of the scope or a video monitor.

Flexible fiberoptic intubation that allows for assessment of even distal airways, can be used orally or nasally, and is a very reliable method for use in difficult intubation. Advanced technologies include improved optics, a video chip camera at the tip of the scope allowing for projection of a wide image of high resolution, increased angulation capabilities, and a completely disposable system. Insufflation of oxygen or jet

ventilation through the suction channel allows additional time for endoscopy and intubation.

The operator can perform fiberoptic laryngoscopy via the oral or nasal route on an awake or asleep patient. Jaw thrust and tongue retraction assist in creating room for the path of the scope. An endotracheal tube is thread over the fiberoptic scope prior to insertion into the patient's mouth. A special bite block, Ovassapain or Bermann, is placed in the patient's mouth to prevent any damage to the scope. Once the fiberoptic scope is advanced beyond the vocal cords, the endotracheal tube is then passed to secure the airway; it is held in place while the scope is removed.

SURGICAL AIRWAY DEVICES

The devices used to place an artificial airway via an invasive approach employ the Seldinger technique through the cricothyroid membrane.

1. **Retrograde intubation** is primarily used for securing a difficult airway, particularly in trauma patients or those with restricted neck mobility. The retrograde intubation set contains a needle with a soft cannula loaded on a syringe designed for piercing the cricothyroid membrane, a "J-tipped" guide wire that is advanced through the soft cannula into the trachea until it exits the oral or nasal opening, and a long and rigid cannula that is then placed over the guide wire and advanced from the oral or nasal orifice into the larynx. Once the rigid catheter is in place, the endotracheal tube may be passed over it in an anterograde fashion thereby securing the airway.

2. As with other surgical airway techniques, **cricothyrotomy devices** are used in difficult airway situations where the anesthesiologist cannot intubate or ventilate the patient. These kits contain kink-resistance catheters for a percutaneous cricothyrotomy or a No. 20 scalpel for a surgical cricothyrotomy, as well as a cuffed tracheal tube with a 6 or 7 mm internal diameter and sometimes equipment for maintaining the sterility of the procedure, including face mask, sterile gloves, and sterilization solution.

3. Surgeons and occasionally anesthesiologists are called upon to perform emergency tracheostomy. The **tracheostomy kits** are similar to the cricothyrotomy kits as they include a needle loaded with a flexible catheter and syringe, guide wire, scalpel, dilator, and usually a cuffed tracheostomy tube. Tracheostomy establishes percutaneous access to the trachea below the level of the cricoid cartilage. Translaryngeal tracheostomy is a newer technique and is considered safe, particularly in coagulopathic patients. Tracheostomy tubes are available in several sizes, most commonly 4, 5, 6, 7, 8, 9, and 10, in both cuffed and uncuffed variations.

4. The **transtracheal jet ventilator** is primarily used in two scenarios: (a) providing oxygenation and ventilation

during rigid bronchoscopy; (b) emergency airway management after placement of a cricothyrotomy catheter. There are several commercially available manual jet ventilation devices. The **Enk Oxygen Flow Modulator** is a device recommended when a jet ventilator is not available. The jet ventilator pressure is carefully titrated starting at 5 psi and increasing by increments of 5 psi until chest rise and fall is observed in the patient. Once the transtracheal jet ventilator is in communication with the patient's airway, the operator manually controls the flow of oxygen to the patient in bursts that create chest excursion. The system itself is composed of high pressure withstanding tubing, a pressure gauge, pressure regulator, and handle or valve for turning the flow on or off.

Alternative Airway Devices and Adjuncts

Sandy Christiansen, MD, and Sudha Ved, MD

SUPRAGLOTTIC AIRWAY DEVICES

Compared to an endotracheal tube (ETT), supraglottic airway devices are considered less secure due to the lack of an inflated cuff protecting the larynx, trachea, and distal airways. Although the supraglottic airways are useful for gas exchange, use of these devices can place the patient at risk for laryngospasm and aspiration of gastric contents. Despite these disadvantages, supraglottic airway devices have an important role in the difficult airway algorithm. When ventilation by face mask proves difficult or impossible, use of a supraglottic airway for rescue ventilation can be life-saving.

For the last three decades, supraglottic airway devices have been gaining popularity worldwide in both the hospital and prehospital settings. While there are several models available, all possess the same essential design components: (1) a seal formed in the pharynx, isolating the respiratory tract from the gastrointestinal tract; (2) an external tube for connection to an oxygen supply and a ventilation device; and (3) a blind insertion technique that requires confirmation of adequate ventilation. There are two main categories of supraglottic airways: periglottic devices that form a seal around the larynx and esophageal obturator devices that block the esophagus and divert gas flow to the respiratory tract.

1. The **Laryngeal Mask Airway (LMA)** is a periglottic airway device with a curved tube connected to a diamond tear-drop (oval) shaped cuff. The device is available in rubber autoclave-safe and disposable models. Both types are designed to sit in the posterior pharynx over the larynx (glottic vestibule) and a fenestrated epiglottic bar in the bowl prevents epiglottic obstruction. The LMA is typically recommended for shorter duration operations, less than 2 hours; however, it is commonly used for longer cases. Standard ETT insertion is possible with all LMAs, except for flexible ones, either blind or with fiberoptic guidance.

Given the increased risk of gastric content aspiration, airway pressures should be kept below 20 cm H_2O to prevent gastric distention. Cuff inflation pressure should be kept below 60 cm H_2O. Similarly, patients with "full stomach" status (such as those with poorly controlled GERD,

hiatal hernia, gastric neuropathy, pregnancy) or pharyngeal obstruction are not candidates for an LMA. Due to related concerns, using the LMA in patients in prone position is controversial since it is not considered a secure airway.

a. The **LMA Classic** is popularly stocked in most operating rooms in the United States. It is available in sizes 1, 1.5, 2, 2.5, 3, 4, 5, and 6. This LMA is designed for single use. It is now listed in the ASA Difficult Airway Algorithm as an airway ventilatory device or a conduit to endotracheal intubation. A distinct disadvantage with Classic LMAs is that only small ETTs can be inserted, which if needed should be changed to a larger ETT with the help of tube exchangers.

b. The **Flexible LMA** has a small diameter tube that is wire reinforced, enabling it to be positioned out of midline and is available in sizes 2-6. This feature is particularly useful during head and neck surgery.

c. The **Proseal LMA** contains a built-in bite block and an esophageal drain. Along with a tighter cuff seal, this drain gives this LMA the unique advantage of higher airway pressure delivery (up to 40 cm H_2O). Gastric distention and stomach contents can be emptied through the esophageal drain. The esophageal drain can also be used to confirm proper placement. The Proseal LMA is available in sizes 1-5.

d. The **Fastrach LMA** available in sizes 3-5 (ETT sizes 6-8), is primarily used for guiding blind ETT intubations in patients with difficult airways, including trauma patients who require manual in-line neck stabilization. The barrel aperture has a single movable elevation bar aligned to the glottic vestibule. The silicone ETT provided in the Fastrach kit is reinforced with stainless steel to prevent kinking. Standard ETTs guided by fiberoptic scope may also be used with the Fastrach LMA but only up to a size 8. Between intubation attempts, the Fastrach LMA can be used for oxygenation and ventilation.

e. The **LMA Supreme**, available in sizes 1-5, contains aspects of both the Proseal LMA and Fastrach LMA. Similar to the Proseal LMA, it has an esophageal drain port and a cuff seal able to withstand high airway pressures. The LMA Supreme also has an integral bite block and a fixed curve shaft for smooth insertion. As in all LMAs, it has molded fins in the bowl of the mask to protect the airway from epiglottic obstruction.

f. The **LMA C-Trach** contains a fiberoptic camera within the cuff that assists in laryngoscopy and tracheal intubation in patients with difficult airways. It is available in sizes 3, 4, and 5.

2. The **Intersurgical i-gel**, available in sizes 1-5, is a noninflatable periglottic airway device with an integral bite-block created from medical-grade thermoplastic elastomer. As in the Proseal, it contains a port for gastric drainage. Preliminary studies have demonstrated faster insertion than the LMA Classic. It is being further studied for its potential role in the prehospital setting.

3. The **Air-Q Blocker**, available in sizes 2.5-4.5, is a disposable periglottic airway device with a gastric port and an ETT access port for patients who are difficult to intubate. The gastric port is able to support an 18 French orogastric tube and the airway port can accommodate ETT sizes 6.5, 7.5, and 8.5, depending on the size of the air-Q Blocker. On its own, the air-Q Blocker can also facilitate gas exchange similar to an LMA.

4. The **Pharyngeal Airway Xpress** is another single-use supraglottic airway device. The design concept is similar to the LMA but differs in that it has a distal gilled tip and proximal laryngeal cuff with an opening located in between. It was designed to provide an improved seal for ventilation compared to the LMA.

5. The **Glottic Aperture Seal (GAS) Airway** is a periglottic device similar in shape to the LMA Classic, except it contains a spongy foam piece on the posterior surface of the mask creating a tight seal for improved ventilation.

6. The **Combitube** is a disposable esophageal obturator device that has a double-lumen tube with two cuffs. It is commonly carried by Emergency Medical Service personnel for establishing urgent airway access in patients in the out-of-hospital arena. The device is inserted blindly and usually leads to an esophageal intubation; however, occasionally blind placement in the trachea occurs. The tube contains two distinct holes distal to each cuff that connect to a separate lumen of the Combitube. This design enables the provider to ventilate from the distal port if the tube is in the trachea and from the proximal port if the tube is in the esophagus. In most instances, ventilation is accomplished through the proximal port while the distal port is used for gastric decompression. The greatest concern with the Combitube is gastric distention that increases the risk of aspiration or esophageal rupture from increased transluminal pressure.

7. The **Laryngeal Tube**, available in sizes 0-5, commonly known as the **King Airway LT and LT-D**, is another example of an esophageal obturator device. It is a single-lumen tube with two cuffs that are inflated within the oropharynx and the esophagus. The distal esophageal cuff seals off the esophagus, thereby preventing gastric insufflation. Similar to the Combitube, there is a hole between the two cuffs that enables gas exchange with the patient's airway. Unlike the Combitube, however, it is unlikely that the laryngeal tube would be successfully placed in the trachea, as the device is much shorter in length. This device can also facilitate the nasal approach to tracheal intubation by introducing a flexible fiberoptic scope into the laryngeal tube that can help guide the user to manipulate the ETT into its correct position. The **Laryngeal Tube Sonda** and **King LTS-D** are similar in design to the King Airway but also include a gastric drainage tube.

8. The **Cobra Perilaryngeal** Airway, available in sizes 1/2-6, has a wide distal striated tip and a proximal oropharyngeal cuff that serve to isolate the upper airway. The Cobra Airway is particularly useful in pediatric patients as it retracts both the soft tissues and epiglottis away from the airway opening.

ENDOTRACHEAL TUBE GUIDES

The **intubating stylet** is a malleable wire that is inserted into the ETT lumen to give the tube more rigidity during laryngoscopy. Once the operator has verified that the ETT is correctly positioned, the stylet is removed and the tube connected to the ventilator. There are several designs of the stylet available, including the commonly used disposable stylet, as well as the reusable rigid stylet that is specially conformed to follow the 60 degree angle of the Glidescope blade.

The **bougie**, also known as the **gum-elastic bougie (GEB)**, is used when complete visualization of the larynx is not possible with standard intubation devices. The curved tip of the bougie enables it to be passed into the trachea, which is confirmed by the notched feeling of the tracheal rings upon advancement of the device. Once in the trachea, the ETT is passed over the bougie and then the bougie is withdrawn. It is available in both single-use and repeat-use autoclave safe versions.

Airway exchange catheters, available in various sizes and lengths, are another form of ETT guides that serve as a physical guide for reintubation. The **Cook Airway Exchange Catheter (CAEC)** and **Aintree Intubation Catheter (AIC)** are two examples of exchange catheters available in the market. The AIC has a larger internal diameter compared to the CAEC, enabling it to be loaded onto a flexible fiberoptic bronchoscope.

LIGHTED AND OPTICAL STYLETS

A lighted stylet is used to facilitate endotracheal intubation by illuminating neck structures to aid in the placement of the ETT. They can be used alone or in conjunction with direct laryngoscopy.

The most basic style of the lighted stylet is the **Lightwand**. The Lightwand is shaped similar to the standard stylet. It is placed within the ETT during advancement under direct laryngoscopy. In addition to providing structural support to the ETT, it also has a light at the distal tip for illuminating anatomic structures.

The **Trachlight** is based on a similar concept as the Lightwand; however, it is intended for use without direct laryngoscopy. The stylet is more rigid and the ETT is attached to the Trachlight handle. The Trachlight is then placed in oropharynx and rotated until the thyroid cartilage is illuminated midline. Once in the trachea, the ETT is detached and the Trachlight removed.

The **Optical Stylets** incorporate a fiberoptic system into the design that enable the provider to view the patient's laryngeal anatomy either through an eyepiece or on a monitor. Examples include the Bonfils, the Shikani Optical Stylet, the Karl Storz, and the Levitan FPS. The **Bonfils Fiberscope** is often referred to as an "intubating fiberoptic stylet." The stylet has a subtle curve at the distal portion to facilitate passage into the larynx.

SPECIAL AIRWAY DEVICES: FACEMASK VENTILATION

The **Continuous Positive Airway Pressure (CPAP) device** is a method of noninvasive positive pressure ventilation and is regularly used for oxygenation and ventilation of patients who are hypoventilating from obstructive sleep apnea, undergoing ventilator weaning, decompensating from acute respiratory failure (thus temporizing intubation), recovering from general anesthesia, and suffering from other respiratory emergencies, like a COPD exacerbation or pulmonary edema. The mask is connected to a machine that administers positive pressure to the patient during exhalation, thereby decreasing atelectasis and increasing the patient's functional residual capacity. The pressure can be titrated, between 2.5 and 20 cm H_2O, to meet the patient's ventilation needs. Various mask sizes are available, including the face mask, nasal mask, and head helmet.

Some CPAP machines also provide a **Bilevel Positive Airway Pressure** mode, which provides positive airway pressure on both inhalation and exhalation. This mode supports patient's inhalation efforts by providing pressure to increase tidal volume and then provides pressure on exhalation, as does the CPAP mode, to prevent alveolar collapse.

Transcutaneous and Surgical Airways

Alex Pitts-Kiefer, MD, and Lorenzo De Marchi, MD

A transcutaneous or surgical airway is indicated following unsuccessful orotracheal or nasotracheal intubation attempts in the context of an inability to mask ventilate and the presence of an immediate need for definitive airway management. The placement of a surgical or transcutaneous airway is the final endpoint for the "unsuccessful arm" of the emergency pathway for the American Society of Anesthesiologists (ASA) Difficult Airway algorithm. Once the presence of a "can't intubate, can't ventilate" situation is clear, a surgical or transcutaneous airway should be immediately considered. A delay can increase the patient's risk of hypoxic brain injury and death. A surgical or transcutaneous emergent airway can be achieved using different methods, including a surgical cricothyrotomy, needle cricothyrotomy with jet oxygenation, and percutaneous cricothyrotomy using the Seldinger technique.

SURGICAL CRICOTHYROTOMY

Cricothyrotomy is the creation of a surgical opening in the airway through the cricothyroid membrane (CTM) with the subsequent placement of a tube for ventilation. In an emergency situation, the speed, lower complication rate, and relative ease of performance make a cricothyrotomy preferable to a tracheostomy.

All difficult airway carts should contain the necessary instruments for the cricothyrotomy, which include a scalpel and a 5.0-7.0 cuffed endotracheal tube (ETT). Forceps and hemostats are optional. Briefly, the skin is prepared with standard antiseptic technique, the CTM is identified just superior to the cricoid cartilage, the trachea and larynx is stabilized with the nondominant hand, and a generous vertical incision is made over the membrane. The pretracheal tissue and fascia is rapidly divided, a horizontal incision is made through the CTM, the incision is dilated using an instrument or finger, and an ETT is inserted with the aid of a stylet to a depth of approximately 5 cm.

This procedure can be conducted in less than 30 seconds and provides a stable airway for up to 72 hours. Acute complications include procedure failure, hemorrhage, pneumothorax, pneumomediastinum, subcutaneous emphysema, and misplaced ETT. Tracheal stenosis and infection are the most common late complications. The only absolute contraindication is age less than 12 years. Traditionally, a needle cricothyrotomy is recommended for children younger than 12 years of age.

Percutaneous Cricothyrotomy

Because anesthesiologists are often hesitant to perform unfamiliar surgical procedures, other methods of establishing airway access are commercially available. These kits contain components that are based on the insertion of a needle and wire, followed by insertion of a cannula using a modified Seldinger technique. Although this procedure is considered simpler by nonsurgeons, it requires the execution of more steps than a surgical cricothyrotomy and is limited by the relatively small lumen of the cannula. This technique is preferred in children younger than 12 years as incision of the CTM can produce irreparable damage in this population.

Needle Cricothyrotomy with Jet Ventilation

This method of establishing a surgical airway involves the combined use of a needle or cannula inserted through the cricothyroid membrane and high-pressure ventilation (often referred to as "jet ventilation").

Briefly, a needle with cannula (often a 12- or 14-gauge angiocath with Luer-Lok connection) is inserted through the CTM; the tracheal position is confirmed by the aspiration of air with a 20 mL syringe, the cannula is connected to the high pressure ventilation system, and ventilation is begun cautiously. The inflation and deflation of the lungs should be confirmed by monitoring chest rise and exhalation should be noted through the upper airway, which should remain open during ventilation. Chin lift, jaw thrust, or LMA placement may be required to ensure sufficient exhalation. If an obstruction to exhalation is present, a second cannula may be placed to relieve built-up pressure. If ventilation of the patient fails, a surgical cricothyrotomy should be performed immediately.

Barotrauma, secondary to high initial inflation pressure, is a serious complication, the risk of which can be reduced by using caution when initiating ventilation. This procedure does not provide a definitive airway and is best used as a bridge until a stable airway can be placed. The build-up of CO_2 and subsequent respiratory acidosis limit the duration of this technique's efficacy.

TRACHEOSTOMY

A tracheostomy differs from a cricothyrotomy in the location of entry into the airway. The cricothyrotomy enters the airway at the larynx through the CTM, whereas a tracheostomy enters inferiorly into the larynx through the trachea. A tracheostomy is an elective surgical procedure and should not be attempted in an emergency setting, secondary to the increased length and anatomic complexity of the procedure.

Endobronchial Intubation

Lorenzo De Marchi, MD

Endobronchial intubation is the placement of the endotracheal tube (ETT) in either the left or right mainstem bronchus. Unintentional endobronchial, or "mainstem," intubation can lead to high peak inspiratory pressures during mechanical ventilation, hypoventilation, and hypoxemia. However, the ETT may also be placed into the mainstem bronchus intentionally for surgery. In addition, endobronchial intubation may be useful in managing patients with unilateral lung pathology and is essential in certain emergency situations.

Absolute indications for endobronchial intubation and subsequent one-lung ventilation (OLV) include:

- Massive bleeding in one lung;
- Infection with pus in one lung;
- Bronchopleural/bronchocutaneous fistulas;
- Lung bullae with/without pneumothorax;
- Alveolar lavage (alveolar proteinosis or cystic fibrosis);
- Minimally invasive cardiothoracic surgery.

On the other hand, *relative* indications for endobronchial intubation and subsequent OLV include:

- Pneumonectomy;
- Lobectomy (upper>middle or lower);
- Esophagectomy;
- Thoracic aortic aneurysm repair.

The most frequent applications of OLV are for relative indications. Successful endobronchial intubation and ventilation depend primarily on the patient's underlying pathology and the preferences and skill of the thoracic surgeon.

METHODS OF ENDOBRONCHIAL INTUBATION

Double-Lumen Endotracheal Tubes

The most widely adopted devices for achieving OLV by endobronchial intubation are the double-lumen ETTs. These tubes possess a fixed conformation that differentiates the left and right versions. Initially manufactured in red rubber, disposable double-lumen tubes (DLTs) are now produced using polyvinyl chloride with a blue cuff on the bronchial lumen for better fiberoptic identification. Sizes range from 35 to 42 French for adults. Smaller sizes of 28 and 32 French are also available for small-sized adults or pediatric population.

Placement of a DLT involves a number of steps. After the larynx is visualized with regular direct laryngoscopy, the DLT is introduced into the trachea, rotated 90 degrees toward the tracheal side (short lumen), then the stylet is removed, the tube rotated back 90 degrees, and advanced until resistance is felt. Since these tubes are preformed, they should allow correct endobronchial positioning in the vast majority of the cases (Figure 87-1).

After inflation of the high volume, low pressure tracheal cuff, tracheal breath sounds should be checked immediately in both lung fields. The bronchial cuff should then be inflated gradually to avoid excessive pressure that can damage the bronchial mucosa. Since the bronchial cuff is not a high volume, low pressure cuff, generally no more than 2 mL of air is required. The chest should be auscultated again for bilateral breath sounds to rule out herniation over the tracheal carina of the bronchial cuff. Herniation of this cuff can compromise the ventilation of the contralateral lung.

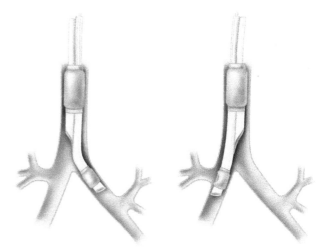

FIGURE 87-1 Correct position of a left- and right-sided DLT. (Reproduced with permission from Butterworth JF, Mackey DC, Wasnick JD, *Morgan and Mikhail's Clinical Anesthesiology*, 5th ed. McGraw-Hill; 2013.)

It is mandatory to make sure the bronchial lumen is perfectly placed in the correct main bronchus. A clamp should be applied to one of the lumens at the level of the collector, and the patient should be ventilated through the contralateral port. Inspection and auscultation should reveal absence of movement and murmur of the hemithorax ipsilateral to the clamp. The same operation should be repeated by clamping the contralateral lumen.

Even when DLTs are considered perfectly positioned with inspection and auscultation, fiberoptic bronchoscopy demonstrates a much higher incidence of malposition. If a *left*-sided DLT is chosen, the bronchial lumen may be accidently advanced too deeply within the left main bronchus. This error can lead to obstruction of the left upper lung lobe. Bronchoscopy through the bronchial lumen must identify the left upper bronchus take off from the left main bronchus.

If a *right*-sided DLT is placed, proper ventilation of the **right upper lobe** (RUL) should be confirmed with auscultation. Incorrect placement of a right-sided DLT into the right main bronchus may block the ventilation of the RUL. This can happen due to the short distance between the origin of the right upper bronchus and the carina (average of 1.5 cm). A fiberoptic bronchoscope can more accurately confirm positioning of the Murphy eye in front of the branching point to the right upper bronchus. Management and positioning of a right-sided DLT can become complex, especially after the patient is placed in lateral decubitus. An advanced level of expertise is required to properly conduct OLV through these endobronchial tubes. There are several other problems associated with proper endobronchial placement of DLTs:

- Left DLT may erroneously be introduced into the right main bronchus. In this case, ventilation of RUL will be absent.

- Bronchial cuff herniation above the tracheal carina.
- Tracheal and bronchial lacerations are possible due to the conformation of preformed tubes. A higher incidence of tracheal damage has been found when the stylet is not extracted before rotation and due to the advancement of the DLT in the trachea.

Bronchial Blockers

A bronchial blocker is a long, thin, semi-rigid, hollow catheter that carries an inflatable balloon/cuff at its tip. This device is introduced in the patient's airway through or aside a regular single lumen ETT. It is then advanced into the main bronchus of the lung that is meant to be excluded from ventilation. Once the placement is confirmed with a fiberoptic bronchoscope, the cuff is inflated and lung deflation is allowed throughout the blocker's hollow core.

Bronchial blockers are an ideal way to achieve OLV in cases of difficult intubation. If the only secure airway is a single lumen tube, it is best to place a bronchial blocker in the desired mainstem bronchus rather than exchange to a DLT. In addition, using bronchial blockers allows the possibility to continue the postoperative ventilation with the same ETT. Most intensive care units are ill-prepared to handle a patient with a double-lumen endobronchial tube.

Bronchial blockers are more susceptible to displacement compared to DLTs, and lung deflation might not be always optimal. They can be difficult to place from a technical standpoint and more prone to frequent dislocations due to surgical maneuvers. Endobronchial placement of a bronchial blocker often leads to longer lung collapse times. In addition, suctioning of secretions is very difficult.

Intubation and Tube Exchange Adjuncts

Alex Pitts-Kiefer, MD, and Lorenzo De Marchi, MD

Several devices have been developed that are commercially available to assist with endotracheal intubation and/or tube exchanges.

INTUBATING STYLET

Made of malleable metal wire, this frequently used adjunct is inserted into an endotracheal tube (ETT) prior to intubation and manually shaped to allow the ETT to conform to the upper airway anatomy of the patient. Many anesthesiologists use this stylet to form an ETT into a "hockey stick" shape that allows easier intubation of an anteriorly placed larynx. A variation of this stylet is the Verathon Stylet or "Glidescope Stylet," which is rigid and designed to conform an ETT to the 60 degree angle of an Indirect Video Laryngoscope (Glidescope) blade.

ESCHMANN TRACHEAL TUBE INTRODUCER

This device is commonly referred to as a "gum elastic bougie" and is a 60 cm long, 15 French diameter flexible stylet with an angulated tip that can be used to facilitate a blind endotracheal intubation when the larynx cannot be visualized with direct laryngoscopy. After a direct laryngoscope is inserted into the mouth in the usual manner, the anesthesiologist keeps the laryngoscope midline and estimates the likely location of the larynx behind the epiglottis. The introducer is then passed blindly behind the epiglottis, between the vocal cords, and into the trachea. A tactile sensation of "clicking" as the introducer passes over the cartilaginous tracheal rings is often detected during a successful placement. While keeping the laryngoscope in place, an ETT is then threaded over the introducer and is guided through the larynx by the introducer. A 90° counterclockwise rotation of the ETT may assist during passage through the vocal cords.

This technique cannot be used when the epiglottis cannot be elevated away from the posterior wall of the pharynx with the direct laryngoscope. Despite its wide availability, many experts have questioned the role of this blind technique in modern anesthesia practice due to its potential to cause obstruction of the airway if the initial cause of the difficult intubation was a friable lesion that can be dislodged

unintentionally. Widely available instruments such as Glidescopes and flexible fiberoptic laryngoscopes allow for indirect visualization of the larynx while minimizing these risks.

TRACHEAL TUBE EXCHANGER

These flexible catheters are similar to other introducers and are used when an ETT needs to be replaced in an intubated patient. Length ranges from 56 to 81 cm. The exchanger is inserted through the ETT and held stable as the patient is extubated. Another ETT is then threaded over the exchanger and passed through the larynx. A version of a tracheal tube exchanger called a Cook Airway Exchange Catheter (CAEC) has a central lumen that can be used to administer oxygen to the patient during an ETT exchange ensuring good oxygenation.

OPTICAL STYLET

This stylet incorporates a lens into its distal end and allows indirect visualization of the larynx through an optical system. These devices vary based on manufacturer and can be flexible or rigid, and have distal tips capable of extension or flexion. The stylet is inserted into an ETT and the tube is advanced through the larynx. As the stylet is stabilized, the ETT is advanced further into the trachea.

LIGHTED STYLET

A bright light on the distal tip of this stylet, sometimes called a "lightwand," facilitates light-guided intubation. The quality of the light transmitted through the skin of the neck can be interpreted by the anesthesiologist to indicate the anatomic location of the distal tip of the ETT. The operating room is darkened and the patient's head is maintained in a neutral position. The nondominant hand lifts the jaw forward, which elevates the tongue and epiglottis and allows the ETT to be passed through the pharynx. The dominant hand inserts the ETT/light stylet assembly into the mouth midline. The assembly is advanced until the pretracheal glow (a red, downward streaking glow also known as the jack-o-lantern effect) is visualized. As the

ETT passes further into the airway, a localized glow indicates a tracheal intubation while a diffuse glow indicates an esophageal intubation. The stylet is removed and tracheal intubation is confirmed in the usual manner.

Many anesthesiologists note that this procedure has a high learning curve, but it has been shown to be a successful technique during difficult airway intubations. Conditions that reduce the ability to visualize the glow of the light transcutaneously, such as obesity or diseases of skin pigmentation, are relative contraindications to its use. Because it is a blind technique, other contraindications include airway tumors, infection, trauma, and foreign bodies.

Types of Endotracheal Tubes

Alex Pitts-Kiefer, MD, and Lorenzo De Marchi, MD

Endotracheal tubes (ETT) are an essential and familiar element of anesthesiology practice. The presence of an ETT maintains airway patency, permits oxygenation and ventilation, allows for suctioning of secretions, lowers the risk of aspiration of gastric contents or oropharyngeal secretions, and facilitates the use of inhalation anesthetics.

MATERIAL

The most commonly used ETT material in the United States is polyvinyl chloride (PVC), a transparent plastic that allows the visualization of exhalational condensation ("breath fogging"), secretions, and other foreign materials within the tube. PVC is a semi-rigid material at room temperature, but relatively more pliable as it warms following placement in the trachea, which permits easy manipulation of the tube tip during intubation while reducing the risk of mucosal ischemia following placement. Although not used as commonly, ETTs made of other materials, including nylon, silicone, and Teflon, are also available in the United States.

SIZES

The size of an ETT signifies the inner diameter of its lumen in millimeters. Available sizes range from 2.0 to 12.0 mm in 0.5 mm increments. For oral intubations, a 7.0-7.5 ETT is generally appropriate for an average woman and a 7.5-8.5 ETT for an average man. However, the appropriate tube size is a multifactorial clinical decision based on patient height and weight, type of procedure or surgery, and the presence of pulmonary or airway disease. For nasal intubations, a reduction in size of 0.5-1.0 mm is appropriate. Length is directly proportional to the ETT size. Nasotracheal tubes are approximately 2 cm shorter than orotracheal tubes. Because anatomic variations of tracheas can be difficult to predict, several sizes of ETT should be readily available prior to intubation.

The appropriate pediatric tube size can be calculated using the formula *ID = age in years/4) + 4.* For example, a size of 6.0 ETT would generally be appropriate for an 8-year-old patient.

ANATOMY

The patient end, also known as the distal or tracheal end, is placed into the trachea and commonly has an inflatable cuff, which provides a seal that prevents the aspiration of gastric contents and reduces air leakage during positive pressure ventilation. A cuff is inflated through its pilot balloon, which is located at the machine end (or proximal end) of the ETT. The pilot balloon is connected to the cuff by a pilot tube that runs the length of the ETT and contains a one-way valve that maintains the inflation of the cuff once the inflating syringe is removed. Generally, cuffed tubes are used in patients older than 6 years of age.

Endotracheal tubes can be beveled or nonbeveled. A bevel allows better visualization of the glottis ahead of the ETT tip while permitting it to more easily pass through the vocal folds. In orotracheal tubes, the bevel faces left and is at a 45 degree angle. In nasotracheal tubes, the bevel angle is 30 degrees and the orientation of the bevel is based on whether it is to be passed through the left or right nares. A nasotracheal tube to be inserted into the left nare should have a right-facing bevel and that to be inserted into the right nare should have a left-facing bevel to avoid trauma to the turbinates.

Murphy or Murphy-like ETTs have a Murphy eye, which is a hole on the wall of the distal end of the tube designed to maintain the ability to ventilate the patient if the distal end becomes occluded. ETTs without a Murphy eye are called Magill or Magill-type tubes.

Markings on ETTs state the type of the tube, outer diameter (OD), size or inner diameter (ID), manufacturer, whether the tube is for oral, nasal, or oral/nasal use, and mark centimeters to allow the visual determination of depth of placement. A radiopaque line is often included in the wall of the tube to allow for radiographic confirmation of the position of the distal tip relative to the carina. Pediatric tubes often have a solid marking at the distal end to designate the part of the tube that should be passed distally to the vocal folds.

ENDOTRACHEAL TUBE CUFFS

Endotracheal tubes can have high-volume low-pressure cuffs or low-volume high-pressure cuffs. High-volume cuffs have a larger surface area in contact with the tracheal wall, which minimizes the risk of mucosal ischemia and necrosis. High-volume cuffs may develop wrinkles that may result in an air leak or aspiration of gastric contents or oropharyngeal secretions. Low-volume cuffs, on the contrary, result in a more effective high-pressure seal; but can result in mucosal ischemia and necrosis if used over an extended period of time.

ETTs are also designed without cuffs. Generally, uncuffed tubes are used in children younger than 6 years old. In children younger than 5 years, the narrowest section of the airway is the cricoid cartilage, which allows for a sufficient seal without the use of a cuff. It should be noted that recent studies have shown no difference in the rates of complications with the use of cuffed tubes in children; their use in young children has increased and is generally widely accepted. Cuffed tubes offer children the same advantages as they offer adults, including a reduction in the risk of aspiration of gastric contents and the ability to provide higher airway pressures during ventilation. When using a cuffed tube in a child, a smaller tube size should be chosen and the cuff should not be overinflated so as to avoid mucosal ischemia, secondary to extended pressure on the tracheal wall.

SPECIAL ENDOTRACHEAL TUBES

1. **Preformed**—ETTs for orotracheal intubation have a radius of curvature of 14 cm ± 10% and ETTs for nasotracheal intubation have a radius of curvature of 20 cm ± 10%, which allows the tube to be more easily manipulated through the larynx. Other tubes are manufactured with a more dramatic bend. The most commonly used preformed tube is the "RAE" tube, which is named after its inventors Ring, Adair, and Elwin. The RAE tubes have a 180 degree curvature that allows the proximal end to be directed away from the surgical site and is often utilized in ENT surgeries to provide better surgical access. The RAE tubes are available in cuffed and uncuffed versions as well as orotracheal and nasotracheal designs.

2. **Reinforced**—Some ETTs are reinforced with wire that is spiraled or otherwise integrated into the wall of the tube, which increases the strength of the tube and reduces the risk of kinking. Such tubes are occasionally used during surgeries that require unusual patient positioning or a shared airway with surgeons that can result in an increased risk of tube compression. These reinforced tubes are referred to as anode, armored, reinforced, flexometallic, wire-reinforced, metal spiral, or woven tubes. It should be noted that a bite-block should be used to prevent reinforced tubes from breaking or kinking if bitten by the patient.

3. **Endotrol**—These tubes are similar in anatomy to standard ETTs but are designed to allow the real-time manipulation of the distal end of the tube to facilitate intubation of an anterior airway. A pull ring at the proximal end of the tube is connected to a cord that is integrated into a channel that connects to the distal end of the tube, which allows the clinician to bend the tube tip.

4. **Laser**—When lasers are used during a surgery conducted in close proximity to a standard PVC ETT, there is an increased risk of airway fire. Because of this, special ETTs are manufactured using a metal impregnated silicone or metal foil that is designed to reduce the risk of an airway fire caused by a CO_2, potassium-titanyl-phosphate (KTP), or Nd-YAG laser. The cuffs are filled with saline rather than air to reduce the risk of combustion, to serve as a heat sink for the ETT, and to aid in extinguishing an ETT fire. Methylene blue dye can be injected with the saline so cuff rupture can be readily visualized.

5. **Tubes designed for the intubating LMA**—A specially designed ETT can be utilized when inserting an ETT through an intubating LMA. These tubes contain both a bevel and a Murphy eye, are reinforced with a spiral wire, and can be autoclaved and reused. As with other tubes reinforced with wire, they may kink or break if bitten.

6. **Microlaryngeal**—These ETTs have small inner and outer diameters of a pediatric-sized ETT but with an adult-sized cuff. They can be used during laryngeal surgeries when a standard adult-size tube does not allow sufficient access to the surgical site.

Monitored Anesthesia Care and Sedation

Brian S. Freeman, MD

Monitored anesthesia care (MAC) is an anesthetic technique that achieves many of the similar goals as general anesthesia: sedation, amnesia, anxiolysis, and analgesia. Monitored anesthesia care carries the advantage of invoking less physiologic disturbance and allowing for a more rapid recovery and discharge rate than general anesthesia. While requiring patient acceptance and cooperation, it often leads to greater patient satisfaction. By using drugs with favorable pharmacokinetic profiles, many outpatient operations and satellite procedures are now performed under a MAC technique.

THE SEDATION CONTINUUM

Minimal Sedation

Also referred to as anxiolysis, the lowest level of the continuum is a drug-induced state of impaired cognition. Patients respond normally to verbal commands. The respiratory and cardiovascular systems are unaffected. Airway patency and reflexes are maintained. Typical drugs used include oral benzodiazepines. The Centers for Medicare and Medicaid Services (CMS) do not define minimal sedation as anesthesia.

Moderate Sedation/Analgesia

Previously known by the imprecise term "conscious sedation," this level of sedation involves a slightly deeper depression of consciousness. Patients should still respond purposefully to verbal commands with or without light tactile stimulation. The respiratory and cardiovascular systems are unaffected. Airway patency and reflexes are maintained. Typical drugs used include intravenous benzodiazepines and opioids. CMS also does not define moderate sedation/analgesia as anesthesia.

Deep Sedation/Analgesia

In this deeper level of sedation, significant central nervous system depression occurs. Patients have lost consciousness and are not easily aroused. They should respond purposefully to painful stimulation. Respiratory depression and impairment of spontaneous ventilation occurs. Cardiovascular function may be depressed. Airway patency decreases, often necessitating assistance by hand (chin lift jaw thrust) or with a mechanical appliance (oral or nasal airway). Typical drugs used include

benzodiazepines, opioids, propofol, ketamine, etomidate, and dexmedetomidine.

General Anesthesia

The final step in the continuum involves a complete loss of consciousness and lack of arousability to painful stimulation. Significant respiratory and cardiovascular depression occurs. Airway patency is lost, usually requiring insertion of a laryngeal mask airway or endotracheal tube. Positive pressure ventilation is often necessary due to hypoventilation and drug-induced depression of neuromuscular function. Typical drugs used include any of the intravenous or inhalation anesthetics.

These definitions utilize the term "purposeful response." The reflex withdrawal from a painful stimulus is not considered such a response. Purposeful responses are movements of an extremity specifically to remove the source of pain. Non-purposeful responses include movements of the extremities that are clearly not related to the avoidance of pain.

It is important to note that sedation falls on a continuum. When receiving MAC, each patient may respond differently. As such, every practitioner must be able to rescue a patient from the next level of sedation in the event of an exaggerated and unintended response. A patient can quickly and easily transition from deep sedation/analgesia to general anesthesia, requiring immediate assistance.

DEFINING MONITORED ANESTHESIA CARE: AMERICAN SOCIETY OF ANESTHESIOLOGISTS

The relationship between the term MAC and the sedation continuum is complex. MAC does not refer to any particular level of sedation. Instead, according to the American Society of Anesthesiologists (ASA), MAC is defined as a specific type of anesthesia service requested of the anesthesiologist for the care of a patient undergoing a procedure. MAC requires flexibility to match sedation levels to patient needs and procedural requirements. MAC usually involves the administration of drugs with anxiolytic, hypnotic, analgesic, and amnestic properties, either alone or as a supplement to a local or regional technique. Whether or not the procedure is diagnostic or therapeutic in nature, nearly all MAC cases should involve some form of local anesthesia. In some MAC cases, however, no anesthesia is provided.

Monitored anesthesia care involves various levels of sedation (usually deep), often with multiple transitions during the same case. According to the ASA, there are two significant differences between MAC and moderate sedation/analgesia:

1. Based on the sedation continuum, MAC implies deep sedation/analgesia. MAC should involve some degree of verbal communication with the patient. Administration of MAC may lead to conversion to general anesthesia at any time. By definition, the complete loss of consciousness and lack of purposeful movements to pain indicate a state of general anesthesia. Therefore, MAC should always be administered by a physician capable of rescuing the patient from general anesthesia.

2. An essential feature of MAC is the assessment and management of a patient's medical comorbidities or physiologic disturbances during and after a diagnostic or therapeutic procedure. It is a physician service due to the expectations and qualifications of the provider who must utilize all anesthesia resources available for patient comfort, safety, and physiologic homeostasis. Postprocedure responsibilities go beyond that of moderate sedation. Monitored anesthesia care providers must assure return to full consciousness, pain relief, and management of adverse effects from medications administered during the procedure.

Monitored anesthesia care services must include the following:

- Request by procedure physician;
- Consent and acceptance by patient;
- Performance of a preanesthetic evaluation
- Administration of anesthetic care and nonanesthetic pharmacological therapy as may be deemed necessary in the judgment of the anesthesiologist;
- Personal participation in, or medical direction of, the entire care plan;
- Continuous physical presence of the attending anesthesiologist, resident anesthesiologist, or nurse anesthetist;
- Continuous availability of the attending anesthesiologist for diagnosis and treatment of emergencies;
- Adherence to all institutional regulations regarding anesthesia services;
- Usual noninvasive cardiopulmonary monitoring;
- Oxygen administration when indicated.

DEFINING MONITORED ANESTHESIA CARE: CENTERS FOR MEDICARE AND MEDICAID SERVICES

According to the Centers for Medicare and Medicaid Services (CMS), MAC includes all the necessary components of anesthesia care: preprocedure evaluation, intraprocedure care,

and postprocedure management. This requirement contrasts significantly with that of minimal or moderate sedation/analgesia. Deep sedation/analgesia is included in the definition of MAC.

When administering MAC, the anesthesiologist will provide or medically direct a number of specific services, such as:

- Diagnosis and treatment of clinical problems that occur during the procedure;
- Support of vital functions;
- Administration of sedatives, analgesics, hypnotics, anesthetic agents, or other medications as necessary for patient safety;
- Psychological support and physical comfort;
- Provision of other medical services as needed to complete the procedure safely.

For billing purposes, CMS considers MAC to be a physician service provided to an individual patient. Monitored anesthesia care cases receive the same level of payment as general or regional anesthesia. The same base procedural units, time units, and modifier units used for general anesthesia also apply to MAC.

PROVIDING MONITORED ANESTHESIA CARE

Preoperative Assessment

The preprocedure assessment and evaluation is an essential requirement of MAC. It should be as comprehensive as that performed prior to any general or regional anesthetic. For MAC, patients should also be evaluated on their ability to remain motionless or to cooperate actively during the procedure. The inability to remain still can be hazardous for certain MAC procedures. Both psychological (eg, claustrophobia) and physical (persistent cough, orthopnea) issues could serve as barriers to successful MAC. Patients should also have intact cognition. Continuous verbal communication between patient and anesthesiologist during MAC is necessary for reassurance, patient safety, and monitoring the level of sedation.

Monitoring

The same level of patient monitoring is required during MAC cases. Vigilance is absolutely essential since patients can easily slip from a level of moderate or deep sedation into general anesthesia, placing them at risk for airway obstruction, aspiration, and hypoxia.

Monitoring should include:

- Communication and observation:
  - response to verbal stimulation,
  - observation of rate, depth, and pattern of respiration,
  - palpation of pulse,

- ○ assessment of peripheral perfusion by extremity temperature and capillary refill,
- ○ observation of diaphoresis, pallor, shivering, cyanosis, and acute changes in neurologic status.
- Auscultation by precordial stethoscope;
- Pulse oximetry;
- Capnography;
- ECG;
- Noninvasive blood pressure measurement (minimum every 5 minutes);
- Temperature;
- Bispectral index (not mandatory);
- Preparedness to recognize and treat local anesthetic toxicity.

Techniques

During MAC, the actual "anesthesia," or loss of sensation, is typically provided by local anesthesia instilled by the surgeon or proceduralist. The other goals of MAC include the provision of sedation, amnesia, anxiolysis, and analgesia. Many different sedative–hypnotic drugs can be used during MAC, such as barbiturates, benzodiazepines, propofol, etomidate, ketamine, and dexmedetomidine. There are several ways to deliver these agents: intermittent boluses, variable-rate infusions, target-controlled infusions, and patient-controlled sedation. To avoid excessive levels of sedation, drugs should be titrated in small increments or by adjustable infusions in response to the magnitude of the noxious stimulus. A continuous propofol infusion (50-100 μg/kg/min) is the most commonly used, and perhaps most easily titratable, technique today. The context-sensitive half-time of propofol, which is the time required for the plasma drug concentration to decline by 50% after terminating an infusion of a particular duration, demonstrates a minimal increase as the duration of the infusion increases.

Provision of quality MAC should lead to rapid recovery without side effects. Since there is not a single drug that provides all the requirements of successful MAC, patient comfort is usually maintained with multiple agents. By taking advantage of synergism, lower doses of each individual drugs can be used. For example, using opioid analgesics in addition to propofol hypnosis during MAC can decrease the propofol dosage required to blunt the response to skin incision. Unfortunately, synergism also applies to adverse physiologic effects. Respiratory function can quickly and easily be compromised during MAC due to the effects of sedatives and opioids on respiratory drive, upper airway patency, and protective airway reflexes. For this reason, effective analgesic doses of opioids are usually limited during MAC.

Complications

According to the ASA Closed Claims database, the risk of injury during MAC is similar to the risk incurred during general or regional anesthesia. Both MAC and general anesthesia claims had similar incidences of permanent brain damage and death. Inadequate oxygenation and ventilation, usually due to heavy sedation with propofol, fentanyl, and midazolam, was the most common respiratory complication in MAC claims. Nearly half of these claims involved operations on the head and neck, which restrict access to the patient's airway. Other complications during MAC cases include eye injury secondary to movement during ophthalmologic surgery, fires and burns, and local anesthetic cardiovascular toxicity. There is also the possibility of awareness and recall. Any MAC case may require conversion to general anesthesia. Factors which may contribute to complications during MAC include lack of attention to monitors, disabled monitor alarms, delayed recognition of cardiopulmonary events, and improper resuscitation.

SUGGESTED READING

Bhananker SM, Posner KL, Cheney FW, Caplan RA, Lee LA, Domino KB. Injury and liability associated with monitored anesthesia care: a closed claims analysis. *Anesthesiology* 2006;104:228-234.

ASA Sedation Guidelines for Non-Anesthesiologists

Alan Kim, MD, and Sudha Ved, MD

Sedation and analgesia comprise a wide range of states; from anxiolysis to general anesthesia. The American Society of Anesthesiologists (ASA) has defined four levels of sedation: minimal, moderate, deep, and general. These levels are defined by four physiologic responses: responsiveness, airway, spontaneous ventilation, and cardiovascular function (see Chapter 90). Given the wide range of environments and settings that anesthesia can be delivered, the ASA developed guidelines to guide the practice of sedation and analgesia by non-anesthesia providers.

PREPROCEDURAL ASSESSMENT

A thorough preprocedural and major organ diseases assessment of a patient is one of the best tools to anticipate and minimize potential morbidity and mortality in the delivery of an anesthetic. Providers need to be aware of previous sedation-related adverse events of the patient's medical history, including current drug regimen, allergies, *Nil per os* (NPO) status, and pregnancy status. A thorough physical examination includes the patient's weight, vital signs, pain level, oxygen saturation, airway assessment, general neurologic status, and level of consciousness; in particular, factors such as sleep apnea history, receding chin, obesity, small mouth opening, and limited neck extension which can be associated with difficult airway management. Preoperative studies are guided to more thoroughly assess preexisting medical conditions and their impact on sedation/analgesia. The evaluation needs to be updated immediately before sedation is started.

Patient Selection Criteria

The goal of the preprocedural assessment is to identify "at risk" patients for whom the delivery of moderate sedation by non-anesthesia personnel may or may not be appropriate. A helpful tool in this assessment is the ASA classification system. Patients classified as ASA Class III-V and patients with special needs may not be candidates for sedation by non-anesthesiologists. These patients require further consultation with appropriate subspecialists and/or anesthesiologists to ensure safe and effective sedation. If a difficult airway is anticipated, providers should refer to an anesthesiologist.

Patient Preparation

Patients should have the anesthesia plan thoroughly explained to them, with all risks, benefits, and alternatives to sedation and analgesia. They should be informed of the preoperative guidelines to fasting and their importance in reducing the risk of pulmonary aspiration of gastric contents. Pros and cons of sedation should be weighed in patients with recent oral intake and with other risk factors for regurgitation (such as emergency procedure, trauma, and decreased level of consciousness, obesity, and intestinal obstruction); particularly determining target levels of sedation, delay of procedure, or protection of trachea by intubation.

Monitoring

The key to avoiding complications is early recognition of adverse effects of sedative medications. These include respiratory or cardiovascular impairment or cerebral hypoxia. For moderate and deep sedation, the patient's level of consciousness, ventilation, oxygenation, and hemodynamic measures should be recorded at a minimum during the following five components of the case: (1) preprocedural; (2) during administration of sedative-analgesic medications; (3) every 5 minutes throughout the procedure; (4) during recovery; and (5) prior to discharge.

A. Level of Consciousness

The patient's ability to respond is an accurate measure of their level of consciousness. Verbal responses indicate spontaneous ventilation. In moderate sedation, verbal or physical responses should be monitored when practical to assess level of consciousness.

B. Oxygenation

Oximetry accurately detects oxygen desaturation and hypoxemia. Early detection of desaturation allows appropriate interventions before significant adverse effects can occur. All patients undergoing any form of sedation/analgesia should be monitored by pulse oximetry. An alarm option should be present. Oxygenation is not the same as ventilation; therefore, oximetry should not be used to assess ventilation.

C. Pulmonary Ventilation

In the sedation setting, key concerns are respiratory depression and airway obstruction impairing ventilation. For moderate sedation, monitor ventilation by auscultation and observation. Use of capnography is equivocal in moderate sedation. *However, one should consider capnography if the sedation provider is physically separated from the patient.* For deep sedation, capnography monitoring may reduce risks of adverse outcomes by means of early intervention and should be considered for all patients receiving deep sedation.

The new updated 2011 standards of ASA monitoring require monitoring for the presence of exhaled carbon dioxide unless during moderate or deep sedation, unless precluded or invalidated by the nature of the patient, procedure, or equipment. It remains to be seen whether capnography monitoring will be included for all patients undergoing moderate sedation by non-anesthesiologists in the revised updated version of ASA sedation guidelines. However, the CMS definition of "anesthesia services" excludes topical and local anesthesia, minimal sedation, moderate sedation/analgesia (conscious sedation), and labor epidural analgesia.

D. Hemodynamics

Hemodynamic stability can be affected by either light or excessive anesthesia. Regular monitoring of vital signs, including heart rate and blood pressure can reduce the risk of adverse events in both moderate and deep sedation. However, it should be considered strongly but not necessarily employed in situations where the stimulation of the cuff may affect the procedure. ECG monitoring can be useful and must be used in deep sedation, but not in moderate sedation in normal patients. However, those with a significant prior medical history of cardiovascular instability may benefit from ECG monitoring. Vital signs, blood pressure, heart rate, respiratory rate, and oxygen saturation should be monitored in 5 minute intervals.

Personnel

A. Availability of an Individual Responsible for Patient Monitoring

For moderate sedation, a separate provider who is primarily responsible for administering the medication and monitoring the patient is needed, but this provider can also perform additional roles that involves engaging in minor interruptible tasks. For deep sedation, a separate provider needs to operate in a singular capacity to monitor and intervene in a patient's care.

B. Non-Anesthesia Provider Requirements

Providers need to have proper credentials; should have undergone standardized training and meet competency requirements, demonstrate basic life support skills, including resuscitation and emergency airway management. The provider performing the procedure must be a separate entity from the provider performing the sedation. However the procedural provider may supervise the person providing the sedation.

C. Training of Personnel

Individuals providing sedation/analgesia should have a basic understanding of the medications that they are administering, including available antagonists. They need to understand, recognize, and treat the potential airway and cardiopulmonary complications that may result from medication use. An individual with advanced life support skills should be available within 5 minutes of the patient.

Emergency Services

Hospital facilities must establish and maintain access to back-up emergency services and a code team certified in ACLS available within 5 minutes of the anesthesia site. For non-hospital facilities, ambulance service and activation of EMS system must be available. Emergency carts must be available within the immediate vicinity of the sedation. Each cart must contain supplies required to establish IV access, emergency medications, and resuscitate an apneic or unconscious patient.

Pharmacological antagonists to sedative medications, suction, advanced airway equipment, and resuscitation medications should be immediately available for use. A defibrillator should be available if the patient has a history of mild or severe cardiovascular disease during moderate sedation and during deep sedation.

Sedation Technique

Use of Supplemental Oxygen—For moderate sedation, supplemental oxygen should be available and used if hypoxia occurs. For deep sedation, supplemental oxygen should be used, unless it is specifically contraindicated.

Intravenous Access—For patients who already have IV access, the access should be maintained until a reasonable amount of time after the procedure is finished. In situations when non-IV medications are used, the need for IV access should be considered. However, an individual capable of establishing IV access should be immediately available.

Sedative–Analgesic Agents

Combinations of Sedative–Analgesic Agents—The combination of sedative and analgesic medications can cause respiratory depression and airway obstruction. Set ratios of sedative and analgesic agents are not recommended. Instead tailoring each component to the necessary effects based on patient response are recommended.

Titration of IV Sedative–Analgesic Medications—Benzodiazepines and/or opioids are the most commonly used medications for moderate sedation. Medications should be given in small doses titrated to effect. Medications given in non-IV routes should be allowed time to take effect.

Anesthetic Induction Agents Used for Sedation/ Analgesia—This category includes propofol, barbiturates (methohexital, thiopental, pentobarbital, and phenobarbital), dexmedetomidine, and ketamine. Because of their narrow therapeutic indices, side effect profiles, and lack of pharmacological antagonists, the aforementioned medications should only be given by providers credentialed to perform deep sedation and general anesthesia.

Reversal Agents—Although antagonists, naloxone and flumazenil should be available; there are severe risks of acute reversal of opioids, including severe pain, hypertension, tachycardia, and pulmonary edema. The doses should be tailored to restore respiratory drive in a controlled fashion after more conservative measures are exhausted. These measures include: (1) encouragement of breathing, (2) supplemental oxygen administration, (3) positive pressure ventilation. The use of routine reversal of sedative/ analgesic agents is discouraged.

RECOVERY CARE

Patients remain at significant risk of complications after a procedure. Oxygenation needs to be monitored until restoration of spontaneous ventilation without risk of further hypoxemia. Ventilation and circulation should be measured at regular intervals until the patient is discharged. Appropriate discharge criteria are used to minimize risk of cardiorespiratory depression after discharge.

SPECIAL SITUATIONS

In patients with significant underlying medical conditions with increased risk of developing periprocedural complications, the appropriate specialists should be consulted to optimize the patient for the procedure. Furthermore, in situations with severely compromised or medically unstable patients or in case of a completely unresponsive patient, consult an anesthesiologist to provide anesthesia.

Rescue Therapy

Sedation lies on a continuum that extends from fully awake to general anesthesia. This continuum is associated with a variety of adverse effects. From a pulmonary standpoint, oxygen desaturation, hypoventilation, apnea, upper airway obstruction, bronchospasm, laryngospasm, and aspiration are all potential concerns. From a cardiovascular standpoint, hypotension from NPO-related hypovolemia, hypertension from anxiety, pain, hypoxia, hypercarbia, bladder distension, or cardiac dysrhythmias, and cardiopulmonary impairment are concerns. Prediction of a patient's response to medications is limited due to interindividual variability.

Given this variability, individuals who provide sedation must be able to provide rescue therapy further down the sedation spectrum than their intended range; that is, when administering moderate sedation/analgesia, one should be able to rescue patients who enter a state of deep sedation/ analgesia, and those providing deep sedation/analgesia should be able to rescue patients who may slip into a general anesthesia state. Mastery of a variety of techniques is needed to keep patients safe. Adequate resources for rescue are a prerequisite for moderate sedation.

SUGGESTED READING

American Association of Anesthesiologists: Practice guidelines for sedation and analgesia by non-anesthesiologists. *Anesthesiology* 2002;96:1004-1017.

Intravenous Fluid Therapy

Eric Pan, MD, and Darin Zimmerman, MD

Anesthesiologists must be able to evaluate and optimize volume status and electrolyte balance in the perioperative period. The primary goals of intravenous fluid therapy are the preservation of intravascular volume and the maintenance of left ventricular filling pressure and cardiac output to ensure adequate oxygen delivery to tissues.

FLUID COMPARTMENTS

The average adult man is approximately 60% water by weight, whereas the average woman is approximately 50%. This is referred to as total body water, and it is divided into two major fluid compartments: intracellular fluid (ICF = 40% total body weight) and extracellular fluid (ECF = 20% total body weight). ECF is further subdivided into the interstitial (15% total body weight) and intravascular components (5% total body weight).

Blood plasma is the major component of intravascular fluid volume contained in the vascular endothelium. Electrolytes are freely exchanged between the intravascular space and the interstitium, maintaining near-equilibrium state between the two compartments. Plasma proteins such as albumin do not cross the endothelium freely and therefore provide osmotic forces.

PREOPERATIVE EVALUATION OF INTRAVASCULAR FLUID VOLUME

Determining the fluid volume status of a patient can be challenging. Detailed patient history, physical examination, and laboratory data aid in accurately gauging volume status.

Nil per os (NPO) status, nausea and vomiting, diarrhea, bowel preparation, hemorrhage, burns, history of weight change, and high urine output are all common causes of preoperative hypovolemia. Hyperventilation, fever, and diaphoresis are often overlooked causes of hypovolemia. Tachycardia, orthostatic hypotension, and low urine output with concentrated urine are nonspecific signs of dehydration. Physical examination findings, suggestive of hypovolemia, include dry mucous membranes, flat neck veins, orthostatic

hypotension, concentrated urine, and poor skin turgor. In babies, sunken fontanelles indicate hypovolemia.

Hematocrit is often elevated with dehydration. Hypovolemic shock can cause tissue hypoperfusion leading to metabolic acidosis and elevated lactate production. If renal function is normal during dehydration, sodium is retained, leading to low urine sodium and high urinary specific gravity (>1.025 in adults), and an elevated blood urea nitrogen: creatinine ratio (BUN/creatinine ratio >20).

PERIOPERATIVE FLUID THERAPY

Perioperative fluid therapy entails the replacement of preexisting fluid deficits, administration of maintenance fluids, and replacement of surgical losses.

Compensatory intravascular volume expansion (CVE) counteracts venodilation and cardiac depression from anesthesia as well as the hemodynamic effects of positive-pressure ventilation. CVE with 5-7 mL/kg of a balanced salt solution should occur prior to, or simultaneously with induction of general anesthesia provided there are no patient comorbidities prohibiting fluid administration.

Hourly maintenance of fluid requirements can be estimated using the "4-2-1 rule" (Table 92-1). This hourly rate can also be calculated for any person weighing more than 20 kg as [weight (in kg) + 40]. Maintenance fluid requirements take into account ongoing losses secondary to continued urine production, gastrointestinal secretions, sweat, and other insensible losses through the integumentary and respiratory systems.

A preexisting fluid deficit exists in patients arriving for surgery after an overnight fast. This deficit is directly

TABLE 92-1 Estimating Hourly Maintenance IV Fluid Requirements

Weight	Rate
First 0-10 kg	4 cc/kg/h
Second 11-20 kg	2 cc/kg/h
Every kg >20	1 cc/kg/h

proportional to the length of time since the last *per os* (PO) intake and can be estimated by multiplying the maintenance rate by the number of NPO hours. For example, a 75 kg patient who has been on NPO for 8 hours will present with approximately 1 L fluid deficit (115 mL/h × 8 h = 920 mL). Bleeding, vomiting, diarrhea, and diuresis can worsen preoperative fluid deficits. Every attempt should be made to replace preoperative fluid deficits prior to surgery.

Intraoperative blood losses can be difficult to quantify due to occult blood loss into the surgical field, collection of blood in between surgical drapes, use of surgical sponges, and irrigating fluid in the suction canister. A fully soaked, 4 × 4 gauze sponge can hold approximately 10 mL of blood, whereas a laparotomy pad can hold 100 mL. Scrub technicians and circulating nurses record the number of laparotomy pads and gauze sponges, as well as the amount of irrigating fluid used. Communication with all members of the surgical team contributes to accurate intraoperative blood loss estimation.

Physiologically inactive body fluid is commonly referred to as being within the "third space." Evaporative losses and third spacing contribute to ongoing surgical fluid losses. In cases with large, exposed surface such as open bowel surgery, third space losses can be significant (Table 92-2). Ongoing

TABLE 92-2 **Correcting for Evaporative Fluid Losses**

Severity of Tissue Trauma	Additional IV Fluid Requirements
Minimal (laparoscopic cholecystectomy)	0-2 mL/kg
Moderate (open cholecystectomy)	2-4 mL/kg
Severe (open bowel resection)	4-8 mL/kg

losses come at the expense of the functional extracellular and intracellular compartments, and must be replaced to preserve adequate intravascular volume.

The total rate of fluid administration is determined by adding together the CVE, fluid deficit replacement, maintenance fluids, ongoing losses replacement, and third space losses.

Total rate of fluid requirement = CVE + deficit + maintenance rate + losses + third space loss.

INTRAOPERATIVE ASSESSMENT OF FLUID STATUS

Intraoperative assessment of fluid status relies heavily on nonspecific indicators such as changes in heart rate, blood pressure, and urine output. Sinus tachycardia has many intraoperative causes, including hypovolemia, hypoxemia, hypercarbia, pain, sympathetic stimulation, desflurane, anaphylaxis, and pneumothorax. Rate reduction following a fluid challenge suggests hypovolemia as the cause of tachycardia.

Invasive arterial blood pressure monitoring can provide useful information regarding fluid status. High variation in arterial line systolic blood pressure tracings in patients with sinus rhythm, during positive pressure ventilation, suggests hypovolemia. Cardiac output monitors can also be used intraoperatively in patients with arterial lines.

Foley catheters are inserted perioperatively for a variety of reasons, including urologic surgery, prolonged surgical procedures, anticipated administration of large fluid volumes, and continuous urine output monitoring. Surgical stress and positive pressure ventilation stimulate the release of antidiuretic hormone leading to decreased urine output. Urine output should be maintained at greater than or equal to 0.5 cc/kg/h.

93

Crystalloids versus Colloids

Jeffrey Plotkin, MD

Prior to discussing the controversial topic of whether crystalloids or colloids are superior, one must first understand the distribution of body fluid compartments as well as the control of fluid distribution between these compartments. The first concept is *total body water* (TBW), which is described and broken down as follows:

- 600 cc/kg—varies with age, gender, and adiposity
- 60% body weight in average adult man
- 50% body weight in average adult woman
- 80% body weight in neonate
- 65% body weight in 12-month-old infant.

Total body water is distributed into multiple compartments within the body as follows:

- Intracellular fluid (ICF) = 400-450 cc/kg
- Extracellular fluid (ECF) = 150-200 cc/kg (20%-30% TBW)
  - Interstitial compartment
  - Transcellular compartment
  - Intravascular fluid compartment
- Intravascular blood volume = 65-70 cc/kg in adults, 90 cc/kg in a full term newborn, 100 cc/kg in a premature newborn, and 75-80 cc/kg in an infant.

CONTROL OF FLUID DISTRIBUTION

Cell membranes exist between the intracellular and extracellular fluid compartments, while capillary membranes divide the extracellular fluid compartment into the interstitial and intravascular compartments. These membranes are semipermeable and contain Na/K ATPase pumps which work to create concentration gradients, extruding Na^+ out of the cell and keeping K^+ in. Water passes freely down the concentration gradient, but larger molecules cannot. During ischemia or trauma, these membranes become leaky allowing water and large molecules to pass freely between compartments.

The Starling equation describes the passage of fluids between the capillaries and the tissues, and is given as: $J_v = K_f [(P_{mv} - P_t) - r(COP_{mv} - COP_t)]$. The variables are defined as follows:

- J_v = transcapillary fluid filtration rate
- K_f = filtration coefficient determined by capillary surface area and permeability
- P_{mv} = capillary pressure
- P_t = tissue pressure
- r = reflection coefficient (1.0, no molecular passage; 0, free molecular passage)
- COP_{mv} = colloid oncotic pressure of capillary
- COP_t = tissue colloid oncotic pressure

Osmolality is defined as the number of osmoles per liter solution. It can be calculated using the equation *1.86(Na+) + glucose/18 + BUN/2.8*. *Osmolarity* is defined as the number of osmoles per 100 g solvent. This value is equivalent to osmolality in dilute solutions (human body) and normally ranges from 285 to 295 mOsm/L (approximately $2 \times Na^+$).

Fluid Therapy

The goals of fluid replacement therapy are to replace preoperative deficits, maintenance fluids, insensible fluid losses, electrolyte losses, and blood loss. Insensible losses come from evaporation of H_2O from respiratory tract, sweat, feces, and urinary excretion. Maintenance fluid, therefore, is about 2 mL/kg/h, usually in the form of a crystalloid solution. Preoperative deficits are determined by multiplying the number of hours NPO × maintenance fluid requirements and are replaced as 1/2 in first hour, and a 1/4 in each of the subsequent 2 hours. Third space losses vary with the extent of surgical trauma and are categorized as mild (hernia) 3-4 cc/kg/h, moderate (cholecystectomy) 5-6 cc/kg/h, and severe (AAA) 8 cc/kg/h. These are usually replaced as crystalloid as well.

Replacing blood loss is a bit more complicated, requiring 3 cc of crystalloid solution for every 1 cc of blood lost or 1 cc of colloid solution or blood for every 1 cc of blood lost. Typically, these are the losses where colloids are considered.

Table 93-1 shows the normal values of electrolytes and properties of the extracellular fluid compared to some standard crystalloid solutions.

TABLE 93-1   Crystalloid Solutions

	Dextrose	Na	Cl	K	Mg	Ca	Lactate	pH	mOsm/L
ECF	90-110	140	108	4.5	2.0	5.0	5.0	7.4	290
D5W	50							5.0	253
D5 1/2NS	50	77	77					4.2	407
D5 NS	50	154	154					4.2	561
NS		154	154					5.7	308
LR		130	109	4.0		3.0	28	6.7	273
D5 LR	50	130	109	4.0		3.0	28	5.3	527
PlasmaLyte		140	98	5	3		27*	7.4	294

*Acetate, gluconate.

Colloids

Colloids are fluids that contain protein or large molecules. These synthetic products are able to replace blood loss in a 1:1 ratio. Since they are heat-treated, colloids have no chance of transmitting infections, such as hepatitis or HIV.

1. **Albumin** is the major oncotically active protein produced by the liver and has a half-life of 16 hours in circulation and 2-3 hours in pathologic conditions. Five percent albumin has a colloid pressure of 20 mm Hg, similar to COP_{mv}, while 25% albumin (salt poor) has the potential to draw in 5× the volume infused. Side effects are minimal but include a 0.5%-1.5% incidence of allergic reactions and ionized hypocalcemia if large amounts are given quickly. Further, it is significantly more expensive than crystalloid.
2. **Hydroxyethyl starch**, also known as Hetastarch and Hespan, is a synthetic colloid that resembles glycogen. It has a half-life of 17 days. Despite this, plasma volume will increase by 9% after 500 mL is given, but will return to baseline by 48 hours. Its side effect profile is more extensive than that of albumin and includes coagulopathy due to decreased fibrinogen, platelets, and platelet aggregation, as well as increased PT/PTT. This is rarely seen, however, in doses less than 20 cc/kg. In addition, anaphylactoid reactions can occur in 0.085% and it may increase the serum amylase; this, however, does not lead to pancreatitis. It costs 50% less than albumin, but is still more expensive than crystalloid.
3. **Dextran** is a synthetic colloid originally isolated from sugar beets and comes in molecular weights of 40 and 70. Within 12 hours, 60% of Dextran 40 and 40% of Dextran 70 is renally cleared, while 17% remains intravascular after 24 hours. Its side effect profile includes decreased platelet adhesiveness, decreased platelet factor 3, alteration of the fibrin clot structure, surface coating of RBCs leading to interference with the ability to type and cross, anaphylaxis in 0.01% for 40 and in 0.025% for 70, osmotic diuresis and falsely elevated blood glucose levels.

Crystalloids versus Colloids: The Controversy

For more than 100 years, controversy has existed regarding the use of colloids versus crystalloids in fluid resuscitation. The following are considerations used in making these arguments:

- Colloids will cause less interstitial edema than crystalloid due to the need for less overall volume.
- Colloids will leak into the interstitium when capillaries are leaky, thereby making the interstitial edema worse.
- Colloids have side effects, while crystalloids do not.
- Crystalloid costs less.
- Anesthesiologists can achieve faster resuscitation using colloids.

The bottom line is that no study exists that clearly documents the benefit of one over the other! In practice, the best principles to guide management are as follows:

- Guide fluid management based on the above principles.
- Know your patient.
- Use vital signs and central monitoring, when needed, to help guide resuscitation.

Ultimately, if total fluid requirements are low, crystalloids will suffice. If fluid requirements are high, most anesthesiologists use a combination of colloid, crystalloid, and blood products (when necessary).

Epistaxis

Karen Slocum, MD, MPH, and Marian Sherman, MD

ANATOMY OF NASAL BLOOD SUPPLY

Blood supply to the nose arises from the internal and external carotid artery systems. The external carotid provides arterial flow by way of the facial and internal maxillary arteries. The facial artery forms the superior labial artery, supplying the septum and nasal alae. The internal maxillary artery terminates in five branches, three of which supply the nasal cavity: the sphenopalatine, pharyngeal, and greater palatine branches. The internal carotid artery supplies the nose via terminal branches of the ophthalmic artery and the anterior and posterior ethmoid arteries.

Two anastomotic regions within the nose are particularly common for epistaxis—the Woodruff area and the Kiesselbach plexus. The Kiesselbach plexus is located in the anteroinferior nasal septum and is the source of the majority of nosebleeds. The posterior location of the Woodruff area makes it a common source for severe, nontraumatic bleeds.

ETIOLOGIES OF EPISTAXIS

Epistaxis can be categorized into local and systemic etiologies. Local etiologies include trauma, anatomic deformities, inflammatory reactions, and intranasal tumors. In children, the most common cause of epistaxis is digital trauma to the Kiesselbach plexus causing anterior septal nosebleeds. The improper use of topical nasal sprays, trauma from a foreign body, and nasal cannula can also cause epistaxis due to local irritation. In the operating room, insertion of nasal trumpets and nasal endotracheal tubes can cause trauma leading to nosebleeds. Anatomic deformities may disturb airflow, and the turbulent flow desiccates nasal mucosa, leading to epistaxis. Inflammatory or granulomatous disease such as allergic rhinitis, nasal polyposis, Wegner granulomatosis, and tuberculosis can also cause bleeding. Recurrent, unilateral bleeds without a clear etiology should raise suspicion of intranasal neoplasms or vascular malformations.

Systemic causes of epistaxis include hypertension, coagulopathy, and vascular disease. Hypertension is the most commonly associated finding in the case of severe or refractory bleeding. Anticoagulation medications and liver dysfunction are also common systemic factors affecting epistaxis. Aspirin, clopidogrel, NSAIDs, warfarin and heparin are medications that can singly, or in combination, increase the risk for epistaxis. The most common inherited bleeding disorders associated with epistaxis are hemophilia A, hemophilia B, and von Willebrand disease. Finally, vascular and cardiovascular diseases such as congestive heart failure, arteriosclerosis, and collagen abnormalities can contribute to epistaxis. Specifically Osler–Rendu–Weber disease leads to fragile, injury-prone vessels with deficiencies in elastic tissue and smooth muscle.

MANAGEMENT OF EPISTAXIS

Initial management includes assessment of airway, breathing, and circulation as well as resuscitation, and should be immediately followed by direct therapy, tamponade, and vascular intervention. While epistaxis is typically not an immediate threat to the airway, patients should be placed in a sitting position and encouraged to lean forward to clear clots from the pharynx. Venous access should be established. One of the first priorities is to identify the site of bleeding.

In anterior nasal bleeding, anterior nasal compression for 10-60 minutes, in conjunction with topical vasoconstrictors, should be implemented. Recommended topical vasoconstrictors include epinephrine, phenylephrine, cocaine, or oxymetazoline solution. Direct therapy includes silver nitrate cautery, electrocautery, and electrocoagulation to stop bleeding. If local therapy fails, nasal packing should be employed to achieve tamponade. Once inserted, a pack should be left in place for 24 hours and the patient should be monitored in an appropriate setting. Postnasal packs are often uncomfortable and can cause significant hypoxia. Other complications associated with nasal packing include displacement with airway obstruction, pressure necrosis, sinus infection, and toxic shock syndrome.

In cases of refractory bleeding, surgical ligation or embolization should be attempted. The most common arteries that are ligated are the sphenopalatine artery, anterior ethmoid artery, and external carotid artery. If surgical ligation fails, selective embolization of the internal maxillary artery or facial arteries should be considered.

SUGGESTED READINGS

Barnes ML, Speilmann PM, White PS. Epistaxis: a contemporary evidence based approach. *Otolaryngologic Clin North Am.* 2012;45:1005-1017.

Fatakia A, Winters R, Amedee RG. Epistaxis: a common problem. *Ochsner J.* 2010;10:176-178.

Corneal Abrasions

Joseph Mueller, MD

CORNEA ANATOMY

The cornea makes up the anterior most portion of the sclera. The sclera is a fibrous outer layer that provides both protection and rigidity to maintain the shape of the eye. The cornea is a transparent structure that permits light to pass into the internal ocular structures before forming a retinal image.

The cornea is densely innervated by the ophthalmic division (V1) of the trigeminal nerve (CN V) via the long and short ciliary nerves. Research suggests that the cornea's dense sensory innveration is 300-600 times that of the skin, making injury to the cornea excruciatingly painful (Table 95-1).

CORNEAL ABRASION

Corneal abrasion is the most common ocular complication of general anesthesia. Symptoms include foreign body sensation, pain, tearing, and photophobia. The pain is exacerbated by blinking and ocular movement. Iatrogenic mechanisms of injury include damage caused by anesthetic masks, surgical drapes, intravenous line tubing, stethoscopes, hospital identification cards, and watch bands. Ocular injury may also occur due to loss of pain sensation or decreased tear production. Chemical

TABLE 95-1 Corneal Pathology and Systemic Disease

Metabolic Disease	Connective Tissue Disease
Carbohydrate metabolism disorders	Ankylosing spondylosis
Chronic renal failure	Scleroderma
Cystinosis	Sjögren syndrome
Gout	Wegener granulomatosis
Graves' disease	**Inflammatory Disease**
Wilson disease	Behçet syndrome
Skin Disorders	Reiter syndrome
Erythema multiforme	Rheumatoid arthritis
Pemphigus	Sarcoidosis

injury from antiseptic solutions has also been implicated in corneal abrasion due to de-epithelialization (Table 95-2).

Incidence

The incidence of abrasion varies between 0.03% and 0.17%, depending on the method of reporting. Prolonged surgery, lateral or prone positioning during surgery and operations on the head and neck are the main risk factors. They are most commonly caused by exposure keratopathy, chemical injury, and direct trauma.

General anesthesia reduces the tonic contraction of the orbicularis oculi muscle, which causes lagophthalmos (the inability to close eyelids completely) in a majority of patients. If the eyes are not fully closed, exposure keratopathy may occur in 27%-44% of patients. Anesthesia also inhibits the protective mechanism afforded by Bell's phenomenon (in which the eyeball turns upward during sleep, hence protecting the cornea). This combination of effects may lead to corneal epithelial drying and loss of protection.

Management and Treatment

Common practice for injury prevention involves taping the eyelids closed after induction and during mask ventilation and laryngoscopy. Some providers apply protective goggles and/or instill lubricant to the conjuctiva. Several disadvantages of ointments include possible allergy, inflammation, and blurry vision postoperatively. The blurring and foreign body sensation may actually increase the incidence of abrasion if

TABLE 95-2 Corneal Abrasions Due to Antiseptic Solutions

Cetrimide
Chlorhexidine
Phenols
Alcohols
Povidone-iodine containing alcohols

it triggers excessive eye rubbing during emergence. Special attention should be given to patients in the prone position intraoperatively.

Anesthesia providers should pursue an immediate ophthalmologist consultation for patients suffering from a corneal abrasion. Treatment consists of prophylactic application of antibiotic ointment and patching the injured eye shut. Healing usually occurs within 24 hours but permanent injury is possible.

SUGGESTED READING

White E, David DB. Care of the eye during anaesthesia and intensive care. *Anaesth Intens Care Med.* 2010;11:418-422.

CHAPTER

96

Postoperative Visual Loss

Lisa Bellil, MD

Visual loss after anesthesia and surgery is a rare and devastating complication, with the most frequent cases occurring after spinal fusion and cardiac surgery. It should be considered in any patient who complains of visual loss during the first week after surgery. The most frequently reported cause of postoperative visual loss (POVL) is ischemic optic neuropathy. Ischemic optic neuropathy has also been reported in patients undergoing radical neck operations and robotic-assisted prostatectomy in steep Trendelenburg positioning. Other less common cases of POVL include retinal artery occlusion, cortical blindness, and ophthalmic vein obstruction.

ISCHEMIC OPTIC NEUROPATHY

The optic nerve can be divided into an anterior and posterior segment depending on blood supply. The central retinal artery and small branches of the ciliary artery supply the anterior portion of the optic nerve, while the small branches of the ophthalmic and central retinal arteries supply the posterior portion of the optic nerve. Blood flow to the posterior segment of the optic nerve is less than that of the anterior segment and as such, ischemic events to the segments have different risk factors and physical findings.

Anterior Ischemic Optic Neuropathy

The visual loss due to anterior ischemic optic neuropathy (AION) is due to infarction of the watershed perfusion zones between the small branches of the short posterior ciliary arteries. Visual loss is usually painless and ranges from monocular visual deficits to complete blindness. Optic disc swelling and hemorrhage may be early signs of pathology.

Anterior ION is attributed to decreased oxygen delivery to the optic disk associated with hypotension and/or anemia. This type of visual loss has been associated with cardiac surgery, hemorrhagic hypotension, anemia, head and neck surgery, cardiac arrest, and hemodialysis. There have been reports of AION occurring spontaneously. Another form of AION, arteritic anterior ION, occurs due to inflammation and thrombosis of the short posterior ciliary arteries. The diagnosis is

confirmed by temporal artery biopsy showing giant cell arteritis. Treatment includes high dose steroids.

Posterior Ischemic Optic Neuropathy

Posterior ischemic optic neuropathy (PION) is the more commonly reported cause of ischemic optic neuropathy (ION) in the perioperative period and is most commonly associated with prone posterior spinal fusion, with an estimated incidence of 0.017%-0.1%. Posterior ION has also been reported to occur after robotic procedures where the patient is in steep head down position for prolonged periods of time. Posterior ION presents with acute loss of vision and visual field defects similar to AION. It is caused by decreased oxygen delivery to the posterior portion of the optic nerve between the optic nerve and the point of entry of the central retinal artery. Initial ophthalmologic examination may not reveal any findings, but mild disc edema may be present after a few days.

Literature reviews demonstrate that most ION patients, after prone spine surgery, are relatively healthy (ASA 1-2) and PION has been reported in patients as young as 10-13 years of age. Previously stated risk factors for developing ION are summarized in Table 96-1. However, recent studies suggest that the etiology of ION may be more strongly influenced by intraoperative physiologic conditions than by any preexisting conditions.

TABLE 96-1 Risk Factors for Developing Ischemic Optic Neuropathy

Anemia
Hypotension
Blood loss
Fluid shifts
Venous congestion of the orbits
Coexisting disease: atherosclerosis, diabetes, obesity, hypertension

275

Conditions identified by The Postoperative Visual Loss Study Group as having a significantly increased risk of ION include male sex, obesity, diabetes, use of the Wilson frame, blood loss >2 L, and anesthesia duration ≥4-6 hours. Blood pressure, more than 40% below baseline values for greater than or equal to 30 minutes, was also identified as being a significant risk factor for the development of ION.

Patients who are obese and in the prone position have increased intraabdominal and central venous pressure that leads to increased venous pressure in the head. This causes a reduction in venous return and cardiac output, and leads to decreased end organ perfusion. The use of the Wilson frame also predisposes patients to increased venous congestion in the head due to the positioning of the head in relation to the body while on the frame. Prolonged elevation in venous pressure in the orbit may lead to edema formation and potential decreased perfusion of the optic nerve.

Increased duration in the prone position and increased estimated blood loss (EBL) also contribute to periods of reduced cardiac output and decreased end organ flow. Large EBL increases fluid shifts, capillary leak, and interstitial edema, which may compromise blood flow to the optic nerve. Prolonged duration of surgery allows for increased blood loss and subsequent increased fluid administration, again leading to the potential for venous congestion in the orbit.

CORTICAL BLINDNESS

Cortical blindness has been observed after profound hypotension or circulatory arrest. It results from hypoperfusion and infarction of watershed areas in the parietal or occipital lobes of the brain. Cortical blindness has been observed following surgical procedures such as cardiac surgery, craniotomy, laryngectomy, and cesarean section. It may also result from air or particulate emboli during cardiopulmonary bypass. Cortical blindness is characterized by loss of vision, but retention of pupillary reactions to light. Funduscopic examination is usually normal. Patients may not be aware of focal vision loss, which usually improves with time. CT or MRI abnormalities in the parietal or occipital lobes confirm the diagnosis.

RETINAL ARTERY OCCLUSION

Central retinal artery occlusion presents as painless monocular blindness as a result of occlusion of a branch of the retinal artery. The resulting deficit is limited visual field defects or blurred vision. Visual field defects can be severe initially but improve with time, unlike ION. Ophthalmoscopic examination reveals a pale edematous retina. Unlike ION, central retinal artery occlusion may be caused by emboli from an ulcerated atherosclerotic plaque of the ipsilateral carotid artery, vasospasm, or thrombosis. It can also occur following intranasal injection of α-adrenergic agonists. Stellate ganglion block usually improves vision in these patients.

OPHTHALMIC VENOUS OBSTRUCTION

Obstruction of venous drainage from the eyes may occur intraoperatively as a result of external pressure on the orbits during patient positioning. The prone position and use of headrests during procedures require careful attention to ensure that the patient's orbits are free from external compression. Ophthalmoscopic examination reveals engorgement of the veins and edema of the macula.

SUGGESTED READINGS

Lee LA. ASA Postoperative Visual Loss Registry. www.apsf.org/newsletters/html/2001/winter/09povl.htm.

Apfelbaum JL, Roth S, Connis RT, Domino KB, et al. Practice advisory for perioperative visual loss associated with spine surgery: an updated report by the American Society of Anesthesiologist Task Force on perioperative visual loss. *Anesthesiology* 2012;116:274-285.

Lorri LA, Roth S, Todd MM, et al. The Postoperative Visual Loss Study group. Risk factors associated with ischemia optic neuropathy after spinal fusion surgery. *Anesthesiology* 2012;116:15-24.

Roth S. Perioperative visual loss: what do we know, what can we do? *Br J Anesth*. 2009;103:i31-i40.

Air Embolism

Hiep Dao, MD

The first cases of vascular air embolism (VAE) in both pediatric and adult patients were first reported as early as the nineteenth century. Vascular air embolism is the entrainment of air (or delivered gas) from the operative field or environment into the venous or arterial vasculature, producing systemic effects. Many cases are subclinical and go unreported. Historically, VAE is most often associated with sitting position craniotomies (posterior fossa) but we should also be suspicious of VAE during procedures where gas may be entrained under pressure, both within the peritoneal cavity or vascular access.

PATHOPHYSIOLOGY

The two factors determining the ultimate morbidity and mortality associated with VAE are directly related to the volume of air entrainment and rate of accumulation. Many case reports of accidental intravascular delivery of air in adults show that a lethal volume has been described as between 200 and 300 mL (3-5 mL/kg). Many believe that the closer the vein of entrainment is to the right heart, the smaller the required lethal volume.

The rate of air entrainment is also important because the pulmonary circulation and alveolar interface allow for dissipation of intravascular gas. If entrainment is slow, the heart may be able to withstand large quantities of air despite entrainment over a prolonged time.

Not only negative pressure gradients but also positive pressure insufflations of gas may present a VAE hazard. Injection of gas into the uterine cavity for separation of placental membranes for a variety of laparoscopic procedures can increase the risk of a VAE.

Early animal experiments indicate that VAE increases microvascular permeability and release of platelet activation inhibitor, thus, precipitating systemic inflammatory response syndrome. These changes can lead to pulmonary edema and also cause toxic free radical damage to lung parenchyma. If the embolism is large (5 mL/kg), a gas air-lock can immediately occur, causing complete right ventricular outflow obstruction and cardiovascular collapse. Even with lesser volumes of emboli, the patient may have decreased cardiac output, hypotension, myocardial and cerebral ischemia, and even death. Air in the pulmonary circulation may lead to pulmonary vasoconstriction, bronchoconstriction, and an increase in ventilation/perfusion mismatch.

CLINICAL PRESENTATION

Vascular air embolism may have cardiovascular, pulmonary, and neurologic consequences. Cardiovascularly, tachyarrhythmias are common and the ECG frequently shows ST-T wave changes. Blood pressure may decrease as cardiac output drops. Pulmonary artery pressures may increase as a result of increased filling pressures and reduction in cardiac output. The central venous pressure may increase as a consequence of right heart failure, resulting in jugular venous distention.

Pulmonary symptoms in awake patients include dyspnea, coughing, lightheadedness, and chest pain. As the patient gasps for air resulting from dyspnea, there can be a further reduction in intrathoracic pressure and hence more air entrainment. Pulmonary signs include rales, wheezing, and tachypnea. During anesthesia, decreases in $ETCO_2$, SaO_2, and Pao_2 along with hypercapnia may be observed.

The CNS may be affected by two mechanisms. The reduction in cardiac output can lead to cardiovascular collapse and cerebral hypoperfusion. Secondly, direct cerebral air embolism may occur with the presence of a patent foramen ovale, a defect present in 20% of the general adult population.

Clinical Etiology

Neurosurgical cases remain the highest risk for VAE for a multitude of reasons. The elevated positioning of the wound relative to the heart predisposes to greater risk of air entrainment along with the numerous large, non-compressed, open venous channels. Such factors can also occur in other surgeries with positional changes (thoracotomy) or high degree of vascularity (tumors) or open vessels (trauma). For cesarean deliveries, the period of greatest risk is when the uterus is exteriorized. Patient positioning in reverse Trendelenburg does not appear to attenuate the risk. During laparoscopic surgery, the inadvertent opening of vascular channels through surgical manipulation increases the risk for VAE rather than a complication of insufflation.

DETECTION OF VASCULAR AIR EMBOLISM

The monitors used to detect VAE should ideally be sensitive, easy to use, and noninvasive (Figure 97-1). The detection of an ongoing incident of VAE is a clinical diagnosis that takes into consideration the circumstances under which the clinical changes occur. VAE should be suspected whenever there is any unexplained hypotension or decrease in end-tidal carbon dioxide ($ETCO_2$) intraoperatively, in cases performed in reverse Trendelenburg position or in cases where there may be exposure to venous vasculature to atmospheric pressure. Suspicion should also be raised in case of a patient undergoing insertion or removal of a central venous catheter who reports shortness of breath during or shortly after the procedure. Finally, a high index of suspicion is warranted in any patient undergoing cesarean section who has sustained hypotension and/or hypoxia not explained by hypovolemia alone.

Transesophageal Echocardiography (TEE)

This is the most sensitive monitor for a VAE, detecting as little as 0.02 mL/kg of air. It can detect both venous emboli and also paradoxical arterial embolization that may result in ischemic cerebral complications. The major deterrent to the use of TEE is that it is invasive, expensive, and requires expertise beyond the scope of care of noncardiac anesthesiologists.

Precordial Doppler Ultrasound

The precordial Doppler is the most sensitive of the noninvasive monitors, detecting as little as 0.25 mL of air (0.05 mL/kg). The Doppler is placed on either the right or left sterna border at the second to fourth intercostal spaces. The probe ideally is placed along the right heart border to pick up changes in

signals from the right ventricular outflow tract. The first sign of a VAE is a change in character and intensity of sound. The "washing machine" turbulent sound of normal blood going through the right cardiac chamber is abruptly changed to an erratic high-pitched swishing sound. With greater air entrainment, a "mill wheel" murmur can develop. Major drawbacks of the Doppler include sound artifacts during use of electrocautery, prone and lateral positioning, and morbid obesity.

Transcranial Doppler Ultrasound

Contrast-enhanced transcranial Doppler has been shown to be highly sensitive in detection of air embolism, in the setting of a patent foramen ovale for patients undergoing high-risk procedures.

Pulmonary Artery (PA) Catheter

A PA catheter is a relatively insensitive monitor of air emboli (0.25 mL/kg). The catheter has a limited ability to withdraw air from its small caliber lumen. The use of such catheters are thus limited to those patients who have comorbidities that may benefit from its use as a monitoring device of cardiac output and mixed venous oxygen saturation rather than for VAE detection.

End-Tidal Nitrogen

This monitor is not routinely available on all anesthesia machines. ETN2 is the most sensitive gas-sensing VAE detection method, measuring increases as low as 0.04%. Changes in ETN2 occur 30-90 seconds earlier than changes in $ETCO_2$. The monitor is not useful if nitrous oxide is used as an anesthetic gas or if the patient has moderate hypotension.

End-Tidal Carbon Dioxide ($ETCO_2$)

The $ETCO_2$ monitor is the most convenient and practical monitor used in the operating room. A change of 2 mm Hg $ETCO_2$ can be indicative of a VAE. Unfortunately, the monitor is not very specific and its reliability in the event of hypotension is difficult to assess.

Pulse Oximetry

A change in oxygen saturation is a late and nonspecific finding in cases of VAE.

Esophageal Stethoscope

The sensitivity of this device has been shown to be very low in detecting mill wheel murmurs.

Electrocardiographic Changes

This monitor ranks low in sensitivity for VAE detection. Changes are seen early only with rapid entrainment of air

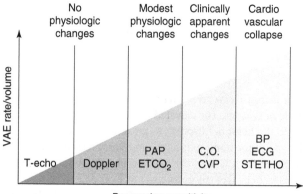

FIGURE 97-1 The relative sensitivity of various monitoring techniques to the occurrence of venous air embolism. (Reproduced with permission from Miller RD, *Miller's Anesthesia*, 7th ed. Philadelphia, PA: Churchill Livingstone/Elsevier; 2010.)

and generally reflect an already compromised cardiac status. Changes in ST-T waves are first noted, followed by supraventricular and ventricular tachydysrhythmias.

Vigilance of the Anesthesiologists

The anesthesiologist should always have timely anticipation of VAE during critical portions of high-risk procedures. Such vigilance is perhaps more important than any aforementioned monitoring devices.

PREVENTION

Central Venous Access Catheter Insertion/Removal

Central venous catheters are most often placed or removed in the Trendelenburg position. Even with an optimal positioning, an air embolism can still occur with an incidence of 0.13%. Conditions that lead to increased risk of VAE include detachment of catheter connections, failing to occlude the needle hub or catheter during insertion or removal, presence of a persistent catheter tract following removal, deep inspiration during insertion or removal, hypovolemia, and upright positioning of the patient. Removal of the catheter should always be in the Trendelenburg position and synchronized with active exhalation if the patient is cooperative and breathing spontaneously. The Valsalva maneuver has proved superior to breath holding for increasing central venous pressure and reducing the incidence of air entrainment in awake patients. Careful attention to occlusion of the entry site is also an important preventive measure.

Surgical Positioning

Surgery in the head-up position places the patient at greatest risk for VAE, occurring most often during craniotomy or spine procedures but also with some incidence in shoulder surgeries and other procedures of the head and neck. To attenuate the negative gradient between the open vein sites and the right atrium, many have advocated increasing right atrial pressure via leg elevation.

Cesarean Delivery

The usual left lateral tilt during cesarean deliveries creates a pressure gradient between the right heart and uterus, thus encouraging air embolism. Some studies have advocated a slight reverse Trendelenburg position which would decrease the risk of VAE.

Hydration

There is an increased incidence of VAE in patients with low central venous pressures, which enhances the negative pressure gradient at the wound site compared to the right atrium. Hence, a well hydrated patient reduces VAE risk (proposed right atrial pressure between 10 and 15 cm H_2O, depending on the degree of head elevation).

Positive End-Expiratory Pressure (PEEP)

Use of PEEP to prevent VAE is controversial. Several studies have shown some benefit for prevention of VAE but others have suggested an actual increase in risk of paradoxical air embolism. PEEP should be used with caution and used to improve oxygenation rather than as a means to minimize VAE.

Avoidance of Nitrous Oxide

Inhaled nitrous oxide allows lower volumes of delivered venous gas to more rapidly exacerbate the hemodynamic effects of the embolism. Nitrous oxide can drastically increase the size of the entrained volume of air due to the fact that it is 34 times more soluble in blood than nitrogen. The anesthesiologist is strongly discouraged to use nitrous oxide in any high-risk case.

MANAGEMENT

Prevention of Further Air Entrainment

The surgeon should be immediately informed if there is a suspected VAE so as to immediately flood the field with saline or saline-soaked dressings. The surgeon should then attempt to close or eliminate any potential entry sites. If the patient is in cranial surgery, air entrainment can be minimized by jugular venous compression. Nitrous oxide should be discontinued and the patient placed on 100% oxygen. It may be possible to relieve the air-lock in the right side of the heart, either by placing the patient in a left lateral decubitus position or by placing the patient in the Trendelenburg position if the patient is hemodynamically unstable. For massive VAE, there may be a need for immediate cardiopulmonary resuscitation with defibrillation and chest compression. Chest compressions may force air out of the pulmonary outflow tract into the smaller pulmonary vessels, thus improving the forward blood flow.

Aspiration of Air from the Right Atrium

Multilumen catheters have been shown to be ineffective in aspirating air, with success rates around 6%. Currently there is no data to support emergent catheter insertion for air aspiration during an acute setting of VAE-induced hemodynamic compromise.

Hemodynamic Support

A large VAE increases the right ventricular afterload, resulting in acute right ventricular failure and subsequent decrease in cardiac output. The goal for hemodynamic support includes optimizing myocardial perfusion, relieving entrained air as much as possible, and providing inotropic support for the right ventricle. Vasopressor or inotropic support has been successfully achieved with dobutamine, epinephrine, ephedrine, and norepinephrine.

Hyperbaric Oxygen Therapy

The proposed mechanisms of benefits of hyperbaric oxygen are believed to be due to a reduction in the size of the air bubbles, secondary to accelerated nitrogen resorption and increased oxygen content of the blood.

SUGGESTED READINGS

Balki M, Manninen PH, McGuire GP, El-Behereiry H, Bernstein M. Venous air embolism during awake craniotomy in a supine patient. *Can J Anesthesiol.* 2003;50:835-838.

Bithal PK, Pandia MP, Dash HH, Chouhan RS, Mohanty B, Padhy N. Comparative incidence of venous air embolism and associated hypotension in adults and children operated for neurosurgery in the sitting position. *Eur J Anaesthesiol.* 2004;21:517-522.

Mirski MA, Lele AV, Fitzsimmons L, Toung TJ. Diagnosis and treatment of vascular air embolism. *Anesthesiology* 2007;106:164-177.

Intraarterial Injections

Rachel Slabach, MD

Inadvertent arterial injections of medications can be a source of great morbidity to patients. Accidental arterial injections can lead to cyanosis of the limb, gangrene, and possible loss of the extremity. Anesthetic medications, specifically benzodiazepines and barbiturates, have been a main source of damage in the past; however, there is an increasing number of medications with poor sequelae if injected arterially. An intraarterial injection can be given at any time in any patient; however, obese patients, patients with darkly pigmented skin, and those with thoracic outlet syndrome are at increased risk. Additionally, patients with arterial catheters in place for blood pressure monitoring are also at increased risk of accidental injection of medication.

SIGNS AND SYMPTOMS OF ARTERIAL INJECTION

Signs suggestive of an intravenous catheter placed in an artery include: bright red blood in the IV tubing, pulsatile movement of blood within the catheter, palpation of a pulse proximal to the catheter, signs of ischemia distal to the catheter, and pain on injection of medications which is worse than expected. More specific signs of unintentional arterial catheterization are a pulsatile waveform on transduction (may be absent in hypotension), or arterial blood gas drawn from catheter site consistent with an arterial blood sample (inaccurate if arterio-venous fistula is present).

Symptoms suggestive of arterial cannulation include: skin pallor, hyperemia, cyanosis, hyperesthesia, profound edema, muscle weakness, paralysis, and gangrene with tissue necrosis proximal and distal to the injection site. These symptoms may not be present immediately, but often develop in a short period of time depending on the medication that is infused into the artery.

TREATMENT

There is no standard treatment for intraarterial injections because there is no one clear cause of damage. However, several therapeutic interventions have become the standard treatment based on proposed mechanism of trauma and successful treatment in case studies. If arterial injection is suspected, treatment should be started immediately and tailored to the medication injected. Treatment endpoints include: cessation of arterial spasm and restoration of blood flow to affected area, treating sequelae from any vascular injury, and symptomatic relief. Although the first response may be to remove the intraarterial catheter, it should be left in place. This allows confirmation of arterial injection either through transduction or blood gas analysis as well as direct treatment to the site of injury. It is recommended to start a slow infusion of isotonic fluid to keep the catheter patent.

Anticoagulation with heparin is the accepted first step in treatment, if the clinical situation allows. An initial bolus should be instituted followed by a heparin drip with the goal of aPTT 1.5-2.3 times higher than normal. The duration of treatment is guided by resolution of symptoms or need of surgical intervention.

Additional specific interventions may also be undertaken. Elevation of the extremity and massage may help to decrease the local edema and provide symptomatic relief to the affected area. Injection of local anesthetic to prevent reflex vasospasm can be given in the affected area, but this is limited by local anesthetic toxicity levels. Sympatholysis of the extremity via a stellate ganglion block prevents prolonged vasoconstriction and reflex vasospasm. However, practical constraints, such as body habitus, may prevent this from being a first line treatment. Additional neuraxial blocks have been described, such as a caudal block and axillary plexus block but each carries its own inherent risks, including the increased risk of these patients being anticoagulated. Calcium channel blockers have been used with varying response. Papaverine, an opium alkaloid that causes smooth muscle relaxation, has also been injected into affected arteries with varying success. Selective intraarterial injection of thrombolytics, hyperbaric oxygen therapy, and corticosteroids have all been used, again with varying degrees of benefit.

Unfortunately, even with prompt recognition and treatment, inadvertent arterial injections often lead to multiple surgical debridements, loss of limb, and severe impairment for patients.

Pressure Injuries

Catherine Cleland, MD, and Christopher Jackson, MD

Both surgeon and anesthesiologist share responsibility in positioning the patient appropriately for surgery. It is important that both parties are involved in the positioning so that each is aware of the potential for pressure injuries. Risk–benefit analysis should consider patient comfort, injury-risk, surgical exposure needs, and padding options.

The basic positions used in most surgeries are supine, prone, lateral, Trendelenburg, and reverse Trendelenburg with numerous variations. Additional positions include lithotomy, jackknife, lateral decubitus, beach chair, and sitting. The most common complication in any position is peripheral nerve injury. Other injuries include tape burns, blisters, skin breakdown, abrasions, and alopecia. Older patients should not be over flexed at the hips, especially in lithotomy. This can cause a sciatic nerve injury. In the prone patient, avoid eye pressure to prevent ischemic optic neuropathy, which can cause permanent blindness. Other injuries that are common in the prone position include stretch or compression injuries to the brachial plexus, ulnar nerve, and lateral femoral cutaneous nerve injury. To avoid lateral femoral cutaneous nerve injury, the anterior iliac crest should be padded. Care also needs to be taken to make sure toes are not supporting the full weight of the legs in the prone position; pillows can be used to relieve pressure.

Brachial Plexus Neuropathy

Brachial plexus neuropathy occurs with median sternotomy or prone position surgeries. Median sternotomy can place pressure on the brachial plexus during rib retraction. Minimizing rib retraction for surgical exposure prevents this injury. In the prone position, injury occurs with arms rotated cranially above the head. Positioning arms tucked at the patient's side decreases intravenous accessibility and brachial plexus injury risk.

Symptoms associated with brachial plexus injury include paresthesia or anesthesia to the arm or hand, decreased reflexes, weakness and lack of arm, hand or wrist control. Weakness patterns depend on brachial plexus injury location and can involve the entire arm or merely a portion. With musculocutaneous nerve injury, elbow flexion and supination weakness occurs. Median nerve injury causes proximal forearm pain.

Ulnar Neuropathy

Ulnar neuropathy can be caused by external nerve compression or stretch. It is associated with the male gender, a BMI greater than 38, and prolonged bed rest. People who develop ulnar neuropathy attributed to surgical positioning may also have contralateral ulnar nerve dysfunction, suggesting preoperative dysfunction. This injury occurs with elbow flexion greater than 110 degrees. Excessive elbow flexion tightens the cubital tunnel retinaculum, which compresses the ulnar nerve. In addition, forearm pronation puts pressure on the postcondylar groove, which can also compress the nerve. Neutral or supinated arm position is recommended.

Ulnar nerve injury symptoms typically present more than 48 hours after surgery. Symptoms associated with ulnar nerve neuropathy include sensory changes to the 4th and 5th digits, and a weak grip.

Radial Nerve Neuropathy

The radial nerve arises from C 6-8 and T1, and courses dorsolaterally around the middle and lower parts of the humerus in the musculospiral groove. It can be compressed most easily on the lateral part of the humerus, 3 fingerbreadths proximal to the lateral epicondyle. This injury can occur with excessive blood pressure cuff cycling or arterial line placement. Symptoms of radial nerve injury include wrist drop, numbness of the back of the hand and wrist, and an inability to straighten fingers.

Sciatic Neuropathy

Sciatic neuropathy is caused by hip hyperflexion and knee extension. This position stretches the nerve, leading to damage if prolonged. Lithotomy positioning is a risk for sciatic neuropathy; it can occur during positioning or intraoperatively. Gentle, coordinated positioning is essential. Sciatic injury results in foot drop.

Femoral Neuropathy

Abdominal wall retractors, causing direct nerve compression, typically account for femoral nerve injury. Improperly placed retractors can place pressure on the iliopsoas muscle. Retractors can also occlude the external iliac artery, causing ischemic neuropathy of the femoral nerve. Symptoms of femoral nerve damage include sensation changes to the thigh, knee or leg, and weakness, which can make stair climbing difficult.

Obturator Neuropathy

The obturator nerve runs through the pelvis and medial thigh, and can be stretched or compressed by retractors or by excessive abduction of the thigh at the hip. This happens most commonly in lithotomy position. The symptoms include transient, medial thigh sensory loss, and also weakness in the quadriceps muscle, making ambulation difficult.

Lateral Femoral Cutaneous Neuropathy

Hip hyperflexion causes lateral femoral cutaneous neuropathy. Hyperflexion exerts pressure on the inguinal ligament, where nerve branches run through. This nerve is purely sensory and when it is damaged, it causes lateral thigh numbness and tingling.

INJURY PREVENTION

Peripheral nerve and pressure injury prevention requires the anesthesiologist to be involved in patient positioning with the surgeon. Cloth, foam, and gel pads can be used to avoid direct compression of the nerves. Padding distributes the compressive forces over a larger area, dissipating pressure on the nerves. A patient should not stay in the same position for prolonged periods (ie, intraoperative repositioning or exercising) to mitigate positioning risks.

100

Iatrogenic Burns

Eric Wise, MD, and Shawn T. Beaman, MD

Iatrogenic burns in the operating room (OR) are relatively rare events, but the consequences can be dramatic and devastating. Nearly all are preventable. Although the use of modern nonflammable inhalation anesthetic gases has lowered the severity of fire occurrence, many anesthesiologists today are less aware of how to properly prevent and manage OR fires. Any fire that occurs on/in the proximity of patients undergoing surgery is considered an OR fire. Surgical fires occur directly on/in a patient, while airway fires specifically occur in the patient's airway. Sources of iatrogenic burns are primarily thermal in nature and include warming devices, OR lights, high-powered light cables, electrocautery devices, lasers, heated probes, and hot retractors.

INCIDENCE AND ADVERSE OUTCOMES

Although impossible to estimate with complete accuracy, approximately 600 surgical fires are thought to occur each year (a comparable incidence to that of wrong-site surgery). In a recent closed claims analysis, 103 OR fire claims were identified, with electrocautery serving as the ignition source in 90% of the claims. Electrocautery-induced fires are increasing, growing from less than 1% of all surgical claims between 1985 and 1994 to 4.4% between 2000and 2009. Oxygen was identified as the oxidizer source in 95% of electrocautery-induced fires. The majority of electrocautery-induced fires occurred during monitored anesthesia care (MAC), with an especially high incidence during plastic surgery on the face. A much smaller percentage of fires occurred during general anesthesia cases, particularly during high-risk cases like tonsillectomy and tracheostomy. Lasers are a growing source of OR fires.

Several patient deaths occur each year due to OR fires. However, the severity of injury is on average less than other surgical claims. Payments are more often made in fire claims than other surgical claims, but the payments are on average lower for fire claims (median $120 166). Other adverse outcomes include minor and major burns, inhalation injuries, psychological trauma, increased hospitalization costs, and liability.

A 1994 closed claims analysis of burns from warming devices found 28 cases. Warmed IV solution bags or plastic bottles accounted for 64% of claims and electrically powered warming devices (particularly, circulating water blankets) made up 29% of claims. Of the other identifiable thermal burn claims, electrocautery devices and hot retractors were largely responsible. More recently, there are case reports of burns from forced-air warming devices, fires originating from anesthesia machines, OR lights, providone-iodine, and isopropyl alcohol pooling on heating pads, and residual disinfectant on a TEE probe. Constant assessment of the patient and potential malfunctioning equipment is the cornerstone for preventing and minimizing severity of these types of burns.

COMPONENTS OF AN OPERATING ROOM FIRE

Three components within a "fire triad" are necessary for an OR fire: (1) an oxidizer, (2) an ignition source, and (3) fuel. All three components must be present in sufficient proportions for a fire to occur. Oxidizers lower the temperature at which a fire will ignite and increase both the likelihood and severity of fire. By far the most common oxidizer in the OR is oxygen, but nitrous oxide also works as an oxidizer. In an oxidizer-enriched atmosphere, the oxygen concentration is greater than that of room air (21%) or contains any amount of nitrous oxide. Oxygen-enriched atmospheres can be found in closed or semiclosed breathing systems including the airway, or locally around open oxygen sources such as nasal cannula or face masks. They can also develop when drapes promote trapping of runoff from open oxygen sources. Electrocautery devices are the most common ignition sources (Table 100-1).

TABLE 100-1   Fuel Sources

Drapes, towels, dressings, surgical sponges
Prepping agents (chlorhexidine, alcohol)
Foam (eg, crate mattresses and pillows)
Patient's hair
Surgical gowns, hoods, and masks
Petroleum jelly ointments

TABLE 100-2   Ignition Sources

Electrocautery
Lasers
Defibrillators
Drill sparks
Fiberoptic light sources

Fuel sources found in the OR include alcohol-containing prepping solutions, drapes, dressings and gauze, tracheal tubes, patient hair, and bowel gases (Table 100-2). Some of these fuels will only burn in an oxidizer-enriched atmosphere.

Preventing fires relies on each member of the OR team understanding the components of the "fire triad," minimizing the risk associated with each component, and recognizing and preparing for high-risk situations. High-risk procedures include those in which the surgical site is located on the head, neck, upper chest, or in the airway. These procedures often create an environment where an ignition source may come in close proximity with an oxidizer-enriched atmosphere.

PREPARING FOR OPERATING ROOM FIRES

Proper OR fire safety education can help teach anesthesiologists about fire prevention and management. Anesthesiologists are responsible for the patient's airway and for controlling anesthetic gases and oxygenation. A recent practice advisory from the American Society of Anesthesiologists recommends that all anesthesiologists have fire safety education with an emphasis on identifying and reducing risk surrounding oxidizer-enriched atmospheres. Although everyone is responsible for prevention measures, anesthesiologists typically have more control over oxidizers, surgeons over ignition sources, and nurses over fuel. Virtually every institution has an OR fire protocol in place. Each member of the team should know this protocol and his/her role in case of a fire. This OR fire prevention and management protocol should be displayed in every OR. Fire drills, including the entire operating team, have been shown to improve staff response time to fire and should be undertaken periodically. Like many other situations in medicine, communication between the entire team is key to preventing, preparing for, and managing OR fires. In addition, every OR should have fire equipment readily available, including containers of sterile saline, a carbon dioxide fire extinguisher, rigid laryngoscope blades, and replacement airway breathing circuits and lines.

PREVENTING OPERATING ROOM FIRES

Operating room fire prevention should target all three components of the "fire triad" simultaneously. To reduce the oxidizer-enriched atmosphere, position the surgical drapes in an open fashion which prevents oxidizer trapping and flow under the drapes onto the surgical site. The anesthesiologist and surgeon should communicate throughout the procedure to minimize the presence of an ignition source near an oxidizer-enriched atmosphere. Supplemental oxygen administered through an open system, such as a face mask, should be avoided when possible in the OR. If an ignition source is necessary around an open oxygen delivery device, the anesthesiologist should stop or reduce as much as possible the delivered oxygen concentration and wait a few minutes before allowing activation of the ignition source. Administration of oxygen concentrations above that of room air should be done with a sealed delivery device such as a laryngeal mask airway. As always, check anesthesia circuits and airway equipment, such as endotracheal tube cuffs, to ensure they are leak free. Avoid nitrous oxide for high-risk procedures.

Reducing ignition source risk focuses on decreasing their ignition power and ensuring adequate distance from oxidizer-enriched atmospheres. According to the Emergency Care Research Institute, no case report exists of a fire when using a bipolar electrosurgical unit. Bipolar devices should be used whenever possible, with the lowest possible setting and always with an audible alarm tone. Safety holsters are essential, and only the person using the device should activate it. Light sources should be turned off when not in use and kept away from flammable items. Do not place the cables on the patient, drapes, or other flammable sources.

Alcohol-containing skin prepping solutions are a common fuel for OR fires. All skin solutions must be thoroughly dried before draping the patient. Gauze and sponges should be moistened if used near an ignition source. It may be necessary to clip the patient's hair if in the vicinity of the surgical field.

MANAGING OPERATING ROOM FIRES

Please refer to Figure 100-1 for the ASA airway fire algorithm. Recognition is the first step in managing an OR fire. Early signs may include a flame or flash, unusual smells or sounds, smoke, heat, and unexpected movement of drapes or the patient. If one of these signs is noted, the surgeon should stop the procedure, and the anesthesiologist should initiate a thorough evaluation for a fire. If a fire is present, the entire OR team should be notified, followed by initiation of the OR fire protocol. Each member should perform his/her task without delay and subsequently assist others. For fires outside the breathing circuit or airway, the flow of airway gases should be stopped, and all drapes and flammable materials removed from the patient. All burning materials must be extinguished with saline, water, or by smothering. A carbon dioxide fire extinguisher may be necessary if the fire is refractory to these measures. If the fire still persists, activate the fire alarm and evacuate the patient and OR team from the room. Ensure that the OR door is closed and the medical gas supply has been turned off. After extinguishing the fire, assess the patient's respiratory status and potential for smoke inhalation injury.

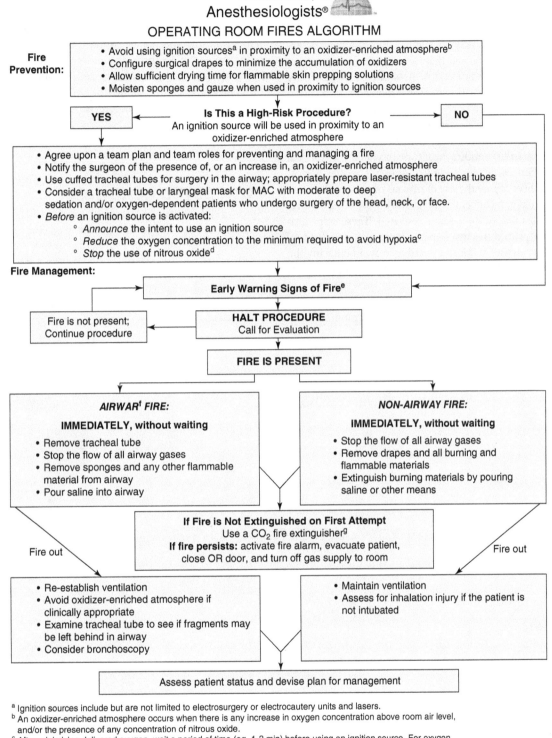

American Society of
Anesthesiologists®
OPERATING ROOM FIRES ALGORITHM

Fire Prevention:
- Avoid using ignition sources[a] in proximity to an oxidizer-enriched atmosphere[b]
- Configure surgical drapes to minimize the accumulation of oxidizers
- Allow sufficient drying time for flammable skin prepping solutions
- Moisten sponges and gauze when used in proximity to ignition sources

Is This a High-Risk Procedure?
An ignition source will be used in proximity to an oxidizer-enriched atmosphere

YES / NO

- Agree upon a team plan and team roles for preventing and managing a fire
- Notify the surgeon of the presence of, or an increase in, an oxidizer-enriched atmosphere
- Use cuffed tracheal tubes for surgery in the airway; appropriately prepare laser-resistant tracheal tubes
- Consider a tracheal tube or laryngeal mask for MAC with moderate to deep sedation and/or oxygen-dependent patients who undergo surgery of the head, neck, or face.
- *Before* an ignition source is activated:
  ○ *Announce* the intent to use an ignition source
  ○ *Reduce* the oxygen concentration to the minimum required to avoid hypoxia[c]
  ○ *Stop* the use of nitrous oxide[d]

Fire Management:

Early Warning Signs of Fire[e]

HALT PROCEDURE
Call for Evaluation

Fire is not present; Continue procedure

FIRE IS PRESENT

AIRWAR[f] FIRE:

IMMEDIATELY, without waiting
- Remove tracheal tube
- Stop the flow of all airway gases
- Remove sponges and any other flammable material from airway
- Pour saline into airway

NON-AIRWAY FIRE:

IMMEDIATELY, without waiting
- Stop the flow of all airway gases
- Remove drapes and all burning and flammable materials
- Extinguish burning materials by pouring saline or other means

If Fire is Not Extinguished on First Attempt
Use a CO_2 fire extinguisher[g]
If fire persists: activate fire alarm, evacuate patient, close OR door, and turn off gas supply to room

Fire out

Fire out

- Re-establish ventilation
- Avoid oxidizer-enriched atmosphere if clinically appropriate
- Examine tracheal tube to see if fragments may be left behind in airway
- Consider bronchoscopy

- Maintain ventilation
- Assess for inhalation injury if the patient is not intubated

Assess patient status and devise plan for management

[a] Ignition sources include but are not limited to electrosurgery or electrocautery units and lasers.
[b] An oxidizer-enriched atmosphere occurs when there is any increase in oxygen concentration above room air level, and/or the presence of any concentration of nitrous oxide.
[c] After minimizing delivered oxygen, wait a period of time (eg, 1-3 min) before using an ignition source. For oxygen dependent patients, *reduce* supplemental oxygen delivery to the minimum required to avoid hypoxia. Monitor oxygenation with pulse oximetry, and if feasible, inspired, exhaled, and/or delivered oxygen concentration.
[d] After stopping the delivery of nitrous oxide, wait a period of time (eg, 1-3 min) before using an ignition source.
[e] Unexpected flash, flame, smoke or heat, unusual sounds (eg, a "POP," snap or "foomp") or odors, unexpected movement of drapes, discoloration of drapes or breathing circuit, unexpected patient movement or complaint.
[f] In this algorithm, airway fire refers to a fire in the airway or breathing circuit.
[g] A CO_2 fire extinguisher may be used on the patient if necessary.

FIGURE 100-1 Operating room fire algorithm. (Reproduced with permission from Apfelbaum JL, Caplan R, Barker S, et al. Practice advisory for the prevention and management of operating room fires: an updated report by the American Society of Anesthesiologists Task Force on Operating Room Fires. *Anesthesiology*. 2013;118(2):271-290.)

SPECIAL CONSIDERATIONS: LASER PROCEDURES AND AIRWAY FIRES

Laser procedures, especially in and around the airway, are now common, which means they are an increasing source of OR fires. Given their power, OR fires caused by lasers are often more severe and life-threatening. Open communication among team members before the start of a laser procedure must include discussion about preventative measures and management of a potential fire. Intubation should utilize a special laser-resistant endotracheal tube in which the tracheal cuff is filled with saline plus an indicator dye. The anesthesiologist should discontinue the use of nitrous oxide and decrease the delivered oxygen concentration to the lowest possible level several minutes before the laser is activated. These steps also apply to other procedures involving an ignition source for surgery inside the airway. If it is not possible to avoid entering the airway with an ignition source, a scavenging system may possibly lower the oxidizer concentration in the airway.

If a fire does occur in the airway or the breathing circuit, immediately remove the endotracheal tube and simultaneously stop all airway gas flow. After removing all flammable and burning material, pour saline or water into the patient's airway to extinguish the fire. Then initiate ventilation by face mask while avoiding the use of supplemental oxygen and nitrous oxide if possible. Examine the endotracheal tube to determine if any fragments are remaining in the patient's airway. Rigid bronchoscopy should be performed to remove any debris and to assess for injury before further airway management resumes.

SUGGESTED READINGS

Apfelbaum JL, Caplan RA, Barker SJ, et al. Practice advisory for the prevention and management of operating room fires: an updated report by the American Society of Anesthesiologists Task Force on Operating Room Fires. *Anesthesiology.* 2013;118:271-290.

Mehta SP, Bhananker SM, Posner KL, Domino KB. Operating room fires: a closed claims analysis. *Anesthesiology.* 2013;118:1133-1139.

C H A P T E R

101

Chronic Environmental Exposure to Inhalation Agents

Amanda Hopkins, MD, and Michael J. Berrigan, MD, PhD

Anesthesiologists and other operating room (OR) personnel are chronically exposed to trace amounts of waste anesthetics gases, including nitrous oxide (N_2O) and halogenated agents (halothane, isoflurane, desflurane, sevoflurane, etc) throughout their careers. Since the 1960s, various studies have implicated this chronic exposure as causing numerous adverse health effects, though no definitive link has been established. Though it has not been definitively proved that trace amounts of waste anesthetic gases are detrimental, it is nevertheless reasonable to be aware of possible effects and to take appropriate precautions to limit exposure. By remaining diligent of contamination sources and taking appropriate measures to minimize the concentrations of waste anesthetic gases, anesthesiologists can protect themselves and other OR personnel from potential harm.

EPIDEMIOLOGICAL STUDIES AND EXPOSURE LIMIT RECOMMENDATIONS

In 1967, A. Vaisman published the results of a survey of 15% of the anesthesiologists in the Soviet Union. The survey suggested that anesthesiologists more frequently experienced fatigue, exhaustion, and headache and that female anesthesiologists had higher rates of spontaneous abortion than other physicians. Several papers followed, with some reporting increased rates of spontaneous abortion, congenital abnormalities, and cancers among health-care personnel exposed to waste anesthetic gases, while other studies found no such increased risk.

Due to rising concerns over the possible deleterious effects of chronic waste anesthetic gas exposure, in 1972, the American Society of Anesthesiologists (ASA) Ad Hoc Committee on Adverse Reactions to Anesthetic Agents met with the National Institute of Occupational Safety and Health (NIOSH) to review the literature and retrospectively survey OR personnel. The survey, published in 1974, demonstrated increased risk of spontaneous abortion, congenital abnormalities, cancer, and hepatic and renal disease among female OR personnel. This data resulted in an NIOSH recommendation to scavenge all waste anesthetic gases, a practice which had not previously been a standard. NIOSH also issued the following recommended exposure limits for waste

anesthetic gases, given in parts per million (ppm) and measured as a time–weight average during the period of anesthetic administration:

- N_2O: 25 ppm
- Any halogenated agent used alone: 2 ppm
- Any halogenated agent used in combination with N_2O: 0.5 ppm

These recommendations, which remain in effect today, were somewhat arbitrarily derived from a 1974 study conducted by D.L. Bruce. The study looked at the effect of exposure to anesthetic gases on the cognitive and motor skills of 40 male volunteers. Their performance was significantly reduced after exposure to 500 ppm N_2O with or without 15 ppm halothane. However, no effect was seen with exposure to 25 ppm nitrous oxide with 0.5 ppm halothane.

Throughout the 1980s, the ASA continued to work toward uncovering possible effects of waste anesthetic gases. In 1985, an ASA-commissioned study analyzed the data from six prior investigations and was unable to establish an increase in relative risk for any evaluated outcome. An independent review conducted in the same year found that the studies which had asserted increased rates of spontaneous abortion and congenital abnormalities were significantly flawed in design and methodology, rendering the conclusions of those studies invalid. Both reviews suggested that further prospective studies were needed before trace anesthetics could be considered harmful.

In the UK, efforts for a prospective study were already underway. From 1977 to 1984, Spence et al. surveyed 11 500 female medical school graduates who were aged 40 or less and working in hospitals. The study, which considered various lifestyle, work, and medical factors, concluded that female anesthesiologists had no increased risk of infertility, spontaneous abortion, congenital abnormalities, cancer, or neuropathy compared to other physicians.

Given the criticisms of the studies, asserting harm from trace anesthetic gases, and the failure of more recent studies to establish increased risk, it does not appear that trace anesthetic gases are hazardous to health-care personnel. Additionally, many of the early studies predated the routine use

TABLE 101-1   ASA Task Force on Trace Anesthetic Gases Recommendations Summary

- Waste anesthetic gases should be scavenged.
- Appropriate work practices should be used to minimize exposure to waste anesthetic gases. Personnel working in areas where waste anesthetic gases may be present should be educated regarding current studies on health effects of exposure to waste anesthetic gases, appropriate work practices to minimize exposure, and machine checkout and maintenance procedures.
- There is insufficient evidence to recommend routine monitoring of trace levels of waste anesthetic gases in the OR and PACU.
- There is insufficient evidence to recommend routine medical surveillance of personnel exposed to trace concentrations of waste anesthetic gases, although each institution should have a mechanism for employees to report suspected work-related health problems.

of scavenging systems, the use of which has been shown to result in large reductions in exposure levels. Regardless, it is the position of the ASA, NIOSH, and the Occupational Safety and Health Administration, that anesthesiologists take reasonable precautions to reduce their exposure to trace anesthetic gases (Table 101-1).

PREVENTIVE MEASURES

Despite the standard use and effectiveness of scavenging systems, recent studies suggest that NIOSH standards for waste gas concentration are commonly violated. Multiple factors are thought to contribute to higher than anticipated levels of waste anesthetic gases. In particular, "flushing" the system and the use of mask induction, laryngeal mask airways, and cuff-less endotracheal tubes increases the waste gas concentration. Anesthesiologists should be aware of these sources of contamination and use reasonable methods to minimize them. Additionally, scavenging system disconnects, which anesthesia machines are not equipped to recognize, contribute heavily to environmental contamination. One study reported environmental contamination as high as 3000 ppm N_2O and

TABLE 101-2   NIOSH Work Practices to Maintain Minimum Waste Gas Concentrations

- Waste anesthetic gas disposal systems are in place prior to starting an anesthetic.
- A face mask shall provide as effective a seal as possible against leakage during anesthetic administration.
- Vaporizers shall be filled in a ventilated area and turned to OFF position when not in use.
- Leak tests shall be performed on both high- and low-pressure components so that waste anesthetic gas levels are maintained at a minimum. Low-pressure leaks occurring in the patient circuit or its components shall be <100 mL per minute at 30 cm H_2O pressure. High-pressure leaks from the gas supply (cylinder to pipeline) to the flow control valve should be a maximum of 10 mL per minute.
- Anesthetic gas flows shall not be started prior to induction of anesthesia.
- Anesthetic flowmeters (ie, flow control valves) shall be turned off or the Y-piece sealed when the breathing circuit is disconnected from the patient after administration of the anesthetic agent has started.
- Before the breathing bag (reservoir) is disconnected from the anesthetic delivery system, it shall be emptied into the scavenging system.
- Appropriate disposal procedures for spills of any anesthetic agent are necessary.

50 ppm halogenated anesthetic when scavenging was not used. Scavenging system disconnects are generally due to human error rather than equipment failure, so diligence on the part of the anesthetist can eliminate this contamination source.

The NIOSH has published a set of recommended work practices to maintain minimum waste anesthetic gas concentrations (Table 101-2).

SUGGESTED READING

Task Force on Trace Anesthetic Gases: Waste anesthetic gases: Information for management in anesthetizing areas and the postanesthesia care unit (PACU). http://ecommerce.asahq.org/publicationsAndServices/wasteanes.pdf.

Hypothermia

Ronak Patel, MD, and Katrina Hawkins, MD

Perioperative hypothermia has been associated with an increase in morbidity and mortality. Central blood temperature, also known as core body temperature, ranges on average from 36 to 37°C. Throughout the day, due to the circadian cycle, core body temperature typically varies by 1°C, with a peak arising in the mid-afternoon and the nadir ensuing in the early morning.

General hypothermia (which can be categorized into mild, moderate, or severe) is defined as a 1°C decline from normal body temperature; that is, a core body temperature less than 35°C. More specifically, mild hypothermia is defined as a core body temperature 32°C-35°C, with moderate hypothermia being 28°C-32°C, and severe hypothermia being characterized by less than 28°C.

Hypothermia is caused by (1) heat loss, (2) a decrease in heat production, or (3) inhibition of the body's innate thermoregulatory mechanisms. All three of these mechanisms can occur during general or regional anesthesia, resulting in the common occurrence of hypothermia during surgery.

The human body naturally auto-regulates its own temperature. Thermoregulatory receptors in the body relay information to the hypothalamus, the main area in the brain that activates varied thermogenesis mechanisms. These mechanisms include shivering, vasoconstriction, and piloerection. Shivering produces heat by continual muscle contraction. Neonates, however, who are unable to shiver effectively, depend on nonshivering thermogenesis via metabolism of brown fat or dietary thermogenesis to stay warm. Vasoconstriction can help prevent cutaneous heat loss by allowing heat to be maintained in the core compartment of the body. However, hyperthermia causes sweating and vasodilatation to dissipate heat. Piloerection aids in preventing air, and thus heat, from escaping the body.

General anesthesia interferes with hypothalamic thermoregulation via centrally and peripherally acting mechanisms. For example, volatile anesthetics (propofol and older opioids) foster heat loss through vasodilation. In addition, these drugs interfere with thermoregulation at the level of the hypothalamus. Regional anesthetics can similarly lead to hypothermia by causing vasodilatation and subsequent redistribution of heat. Thermoregulatory impairment in the hypothalamus also occurs because of altered dermatome perception. Through all of these mechanisms, anesthesia affects the body's capability to auto-regulate its own temperature, predisposing to perioperative hypothermia.

PERIOPERATIVE HYPOTHERMIA

The operating room environment, surgical procedure, and anesthetic drugs all contribute to perioperative hypothermia. Operating rooms are often kept cold for surgeon comfort. Once in the operating room, a large portion of the patient's body surface area is often exposed. Depending on the surgery, exposed viscera can also lead to substantial heat loss. Large amounts of cold antiseptic, intravenous, and irrigating solutions can likewise lower the core body temperature. Cool anesthetic gases inspired by the patient during the surgery constantly cause heat loss (as the body loses heat to the cold vapors) unless preventive measures are taken. Furthermore, anesthetic drugs such as volatile anesthetics can cause vasodilation, causing heat to be transferred from the core compartment of the body to the periphery. Most importantly, as mentioned previously, anesthetics interfere with hypothalamic thermoregulatory mechanisms.

The patient undergoing surgery has a decline in core body temperature that occurs via five mechanisms: (1) redistribution, (2) radiation, (3) conduction, (4) convection, and (5) evaporation. Redistribution is the transfer of heat from the peripheral compartments of the body to the central core. Radiation is the dissipation of heat to cooler surroundings, for example, from the warm patient to the cooler operating room. Redistribution and radiation often account for the major temperature fluctuations that occur during surgery. Conduction is the dissipation of heat resulting from direct contact of cool objects, as occurs when the patient's skin contacts with cold in the operating room. Convection is heat loss to airflow that surrounds the patient. Evaporation is the loss of heat through vaporization, as occurs when the patient exhales gases or has exposed viscera. Prevention of perioperative hypothermia is aimed at preventing heat loss via these different mechanisms.

Each of the above mechanisms contributes to the three-phase temperature decline that is seen with anesthesia.

During the first hour of general anesthesia, the core temperature decreases by 1°C-2°C (phase I). Phase one occurs largely because of redistribution of heat from central to peripheral compartments. A more gradual decline in temperature then occurs over the next 3 to 4 hours, wherein heat is lost to the environment (phase II). This is largely a result of radiation. Lastly, a steady state is reached wherein heat loss equals metabolic heat production (phase III). Depending on the length of the surgery, each phase may or may not be seen during an operation.

Neurologic Effects

A temperature decline causes a decrease in cerebral metabolic activity. This allows for a decrease in oxygen and other nutrient utilization in the brain during times of decreased cerebral blood flow. Anaerobic metabolism (and its anaerobic byproducts) is minimized, and there is a decrease in production of excitatory neurotransmitters and proinflammatory cytokines during hypothermia. For these reasons, hypothermia can actually be beneficial for the neurologic system in times of cerebral hypoxia. On the other hand, extreme hypothermia can cause a decrease in cerebral blood flow so great that detrimental ischemia may occur. In addition, delayed emergence from anesthesia is observed when the patient is not normothermic.

Cardiovascular Effects

The cardiovascular system is perhaps the most important system affected by hypothermia. Hypothermia causes peripheral vasoconstriction, which causes an elevation in blood pressure and an increase in myocardial afterload. This increase in myocardial afterload can cause conduction and contractility disturbances, which may manifest as bradycardia. Under severe hypothermia, arrhythmias and ventricular fibrillation are seen. Hypothermia, moreover, causes an increase in coronary vascular resistance. Myocardial oxygen demand is increased by shivering as well as by adrenergic and metabolic processes (cortisol and norepinephrine release). Oxygen consumption is increased up to fivefold during vigorous shivering. This can lead to myocardial ischemia in the susceptible patient. Just as it does in the brain, hypothermia reduces metabolic oxygen requirements (outside of shivering) and can be protective during times of cardiac ischemia.

Respiratory, Renal, and Hepatic Effects

Although hypothermia can be helpful at times for the neurologic and cardiovascular systems, it is harmful to many other organ systems. A decline in temperature causes the respiratory system to hyperventilate before eventually settling to a state of hypoventilation. Hypothermia causes a leftward shift in the oxygen–hemoglobin dissociation curve. Hemoglobin, thus, has a greater affinity for oxygen and does not release it as readily as compared to the normothermic patient. These principles can lead to hypoxia, anaerobic metabolism, and lactic acidosis.

Bronchial artery blood flow is correspondingly decreased, leading to diminution in oxygen uptake and delivery.

The kidneys are also affected by hypothermia. There is a decrease in glomerular filtration rate and a rise in blood urea nitrogen and creatinine. Hepatic and pancreatic functions are also decreased, resulting in slowed metabolism of medications such as muscle relaxants. This can contribute to delayed emergence. Glucose metabolism is also impaired leading to hyperglycemia.

Hematologic Effects

Temperature declines cause coagulopathy. Clotting factor enzymes are temperature dependent and do not function as well under hypothermic conditions. Prothrombin and partial thromboplastin times are elevated, but may return to normal because blood samples may be heated to 37°C before tests are run. Platelet dysfunction occurs by alteration of thromboxane A-2 (TXA2), which normally serves to activate the aggregation of platelets. This dysfunction is reversible and temporary if the patient is subsequently rewarmed. While under surgery, the hypothermic patient has an increased risk of developing a deep vein thrombosis because blood viscosity, stasis, and peripheral vascular resistance increase while perfusion to the extremities is decreased. Lastly, surgical wound healing is delayed and infection rates are increased in the hypothermic patient. Vasoconstriction causes less oxygen, nutrients, and leukocytes to migrate to wound sites. This, coupled with a decline in immune function and macrophage phagocytosis, allows bacteria to overwhelm fresh surgical sites.

Temperature Monitoring

Proper measurement of core body temperature should guide therapy. There are several techniques available to measure a patient's temperature, however they are not all equally accurate and some do not reflect central blood temperature. Tympanic membrane thermometers can reflect brain temperature because auditory canal blood supply derives from the external carotid artery (posterior auricular and internal maxillary artery branches). However, trauma can occur with the use of such devices and cerumen can obscure values. Nasopharyngeal thermometers can be accurate when placed next to the nasopharyngeal mucosa (reflecting carotid blood passing) but again can cause trauma via epistaxis. A pulmonary artery catheter thermometer is perhaps the most accurate means of obtaining a core body temperature, but they are not routinely available and carry their own risks. Axillary temperature varies according to skin perfusion at that time, as does liquid crystal adhesive thermometers. Rectal, oral, and bladder temperatures have a slow response to actual core temperatures. Esophageal temperature is perhaps the most commonly used intraoperatively. It provides accurate measurements when placed in the lower third of the esophagus behind the heart. Regardless, when treating hypothermia one must make sure that accurate temperature measurements are being taken so that overheating does not occur.

Prevention of Perioperative Hypothermia

Prevention is an active process. Methods to allow the patient to remain warm include increased ambient room temperature, active rewarming via humidified air, low flow anesthesia (to allow the patient to rebreathe heated vapor), warm intravenous fluids, heating mattresses, and convective forced air-warming blankets. Thirty minutes of prewarming prior to induction can prevent the initial phase I temperature decline due to redistribution. Special care must be taken in the elderly. Decrease in muscle mass and adipose tissue, and dysfunction of thermoregulatory mechanisms in the elderly make them especially prone to temperature declines. Children and neonates also fall into this category because of their increased body surface to mass ratio. Trauma, hypothyroid, burn, spinal cord injury, and malnourished patients need particular attention, as they are prone to hypothermia.

SUGGESTED READING

Kurz A, Sessler DI, Lenhardt R. "Perioperative normothermia to reduce the incidence of surgical-wound infection and shorten hospitalization." In: The Study of Wound Infection and Temperature Group. *N Engl J Med.* 1996;334:1209-1216. DOI: 10.1056/NEJM199605093341901.

Nonmalignant Hyperthermia

Christopher Edwards, MD

Heat results from the human body's natural metabolic processes, such as ATP breakdown, protein synthesis, and most other homeostasis reactions. Heat released during these reactions needs to be removed from the body in an efficient and timely fashion to maintain normothermia because most physiologic processes within a cell function within a narrow temperature range. Small derangements in temperature, high or low, can lead to organ system failure. Key mechanisms employed to dissipate excess heat are radiation, conduction, convection, and evaporation.

Hyperthermia and fever are different terms. Hyperthermia is an increase in temperature while fever is the body's controlled increase of its thermoregulatory system (Table 103-1).

The primary causes of nonmalignant hyperthermia are as listed.

Drug Reactions

a. *Serotonin syndrome*—This is caused by exposure to medications, including *SSRI, MAOI, tryptophan, and amphetamines*. These reactions range from mild to life threatening. The classic trait associated with serotonin syndrome includes hyperthermia, altered mental status, neuromuscular excitation (lead-pipe rigidity), and autonomic instability. Treatment involves supportive care, withdrawal of the offending agent and potential sedation, and muscle relaxation.

b. *Neuroleptic malignant syndrome*—A potentially life-threatening complication associated with use of *antipsychotic* medications. The clinical symptoms consist of hyperthermia, severe muscle rigidity, autonomic instability, and altered mental status.

c. *Sympathomimetic toxicity*—Leads to hyperthermia associated with the use of *amphetamines, cocaine, and amphetamine derivatives*. Other clinical signs include agitation,

hypertensive crisis, coronary or cerebral vasospasm, dysrhythmias, acidosis, seizures, and hyperkalemia.

d. *Anticholinergic syndrome*—A condition associated with *antihistamines, antipsychotics, TCAs, and anticholinergic plants*. Hallmark symptoms include hyperthermia, tachycardia, blurry vision, dry skin, urinary retention, lethargy, and hallucinations. Treatment includes increasing acetylcholine via an anticholinesterase medication.

Blood Product and Infectious Reactions

a. *Transfusion reactions*—There are a variety of transfusion reactions that can lead to hyperthermia as well as other sequela. These reactions include, but are not limited to, febrile nonhemolytic, ABO incompatibility, and transfusion-associated lung injury.

b. *Infection*—Infections can lead to a febrile reaction, including abscess, sepsis, respiratory, cellulitis, meningitis, or any other infection. Fever is the body's response to infection, which needs to be diagnosed and treated appropriately with antibiotics and supportive therapies.

Exogenous Heating Sources

Forced air warming, fluid warming devices, cardiopulmonary bypass machines, closed anesthesia circuits, humidity moisture exchangers, and other warming devices warm patients intraoperatively. If the devices malfunction or are not monitored closely, unintentional hyperthermia may result.

System-Based Considerations

a. *Endocrine system*—The endocrine system often controls metabolic activity. Various pathologic hypermetabolic states may lead to hyperthermia if left untreated: thyroid storm, pheochromocytoma, and adrenal insufficiency are several examples.

b. *Pulmonary*—Numerous pulmonary processes lead to hyperthermia such as aspiration, atelectasis, pulmonary embolism, or DVT.

c. *Central nervous system*—Seizures can lead to increased metabolic rate and hyperthermia.

TABLE 103-1 Temperature Ranges

Hypothermia	< 36°C
Normothermia	36-38°C
Hyperthermia	> 38°C

MANAGEMENT OF NONMALIGNANT HYPERTHERMIA

The prompt recognition and treatment of hyperthermia is vitally important to providing sound medical care during delivery of an anesthetic. While many initial therapies focus on returning the body to normothermia, the underlying cause must be addressed. First-line treatment includes removing external warming devices and attempting active cooling strategies (ice, forced air cooling, fluid infusions). After initial therapies have been initiated, a thorough review of patient history and pertinent events may provide insight into a potential diagnosis leading to a focused treatment regimen.

Bronchospasm

Brian S. Freeman, MD

Bronchospasm is a reversible reflex constriction of the smooth muscle lining the bronchioles. It usually occurs as a result of worsening of underlying airway reactivity. Transient increases in airway resistance lead to an obstruction of both expiratory and inspiratory airflow. The inability to ventilate a patient despite the presence of a properly positioned endotracheal tube is life threatening. In the perioperative course, this serious event typically occurs during induction of anesthesia, but may present during maintenance and emergence. Immediate diagnosis and management are critical to prevent hypoxemia, brain damage, and death.

The overall incidence of bronchospasm during general anesthesia is approximately 0.2%. However, the incidence of bronchospasm is highest (about 6%) in asthmatic patients receiving general endotracheal anesthesia. Regardless, life-threatening bronchospasm can still occur in healthy patients without any underlying pulmonary pathology. In fact, of the cases of bronchospasm in settled malpractice claims reported by the ASA Closed Claims study, only half of patients had any history of reactive airway disease (whether asthma or chronic pulmonary disease [COPD]).

PATHOPHYSIOLOGY

Perioperative bronchospasm is a reflex that is mediated by the vagus nerve. A noxious stimulus, such as endotracheal intubation, activates afferent sensory fibers in the vagus nerve that stimulate neurons within the nucleus of the solitary tract. These neurons then stimulate efferent fibers through the vagus nerve to bronchiolar smooth muscle. Released acetylcholine neurotransmitters then bind to the M3 muscarinic receptor, resulting in an increase in cyclic guanosine monophosphate and inducing bronchiolar smooth muscle contraction. Other mediators that may participate in this reflex include histamine, tachykinins, vasoactive intestinal peptide, and calcitonin gene-related peptide.

ETIOLOGY AND DIFFERENTIAL DIAGNOSIS

Bronchospasm may occur in isolation or as one of several manifestations of a more serious underlying perioperative problem. Most causes of perioperative bronchospasm involve a nonallergic mechanism. The most common precipitating factor is airway irritation in patients known to be at higher risk of bronchial hyperreactivity, such as those with poorly controlled reactive airway disease (asthma and COPD), an upper respiratory tract infection, and history of smoking. In these at-risk patients, there are pharmacological causes of bronchospasm: desflurane, β-blockers, NSAIDs, cholinesterase inhibitors (neostigmine), and histamine-releasing drugs (atracurium, mivacurium, sodium thiopental, morphine). The bronchospasm reflex also highly depends on the depth of anesthesia. Therefore, surgical stimulation or mechanical manipulation of the airway (especially endotracheal intubation), in conjunction with an inadequate depth of anesthesia, significantly increases the chance of bronchospasm.

Bronchospasm that occurs after induction in a patient without risk factors for airway hyperreactivity may be the result of pulmonary aspiration of gastric contents. Aspiration may involve active vomiting or passive regurgitation. In addition to the classic signs of bronchospasm (bilateral expiratory wheezing, increased peak inspiratory pressures), the patient who aspirated typically develops hypoxemia. Aspiration can occur in a patient receiving general anesthesia with a face mask, laryngeal mask, and endotracheal tube.

At any stage of anesthesia, bronchospasm may be one of several manifestations of a serious allergic reaction or anaphylactic shock. Bronchospasm can represent either an anaphylactoid reaction or IgE-mediated anaphylaxis. The most common allergens responsible are muscle relaxants (rocuronium, succinylcholine), antibiotics (penicillins, cephalosporins), latex, and blood products (red blood cells, fresh frozen plasma). In addition to the usual presentation of bronchospasm, anaphylaxis typically includes cutaneous signs such as an urticarial rash and angioedema as well as severe hemodynamic aberrations (tachycardia, hypotension, circulatory collapse).

Although patients who develop bronchospasm will typically have expiratory wheezing, not all wheezes represent bronchospasm. In fact, the differential diagnosis for intraoperative bronchospasm includes numerous pathologies that need to be properly diagnosed and distinguished from simple bronchospasm. Without rapid recognition and treatment, life-threatening consequences may result. These situations include:

- Problems with the endotracheal tube:
  - Malpositioned (endobronchial, esophageal, abutting the carina)
  - Obstructed (mucous plug, foreign body, cuff herniation)
  - Kinked
- Obstruction in the breathing circuit;
- Pulmonary edema;
- Pulmonary embolism;
- Tension pneumothorax;
- Foreign body in the tracheobronchial tree;
- Laryngospasm in the nonintubated patient.

PRESENTATION

In a patient receiving general anesthesia and mechanical ventilation, the respiratory manifestations of bronchospasm are fairly consistent, no matter the etiology:

a. **Rapid increase in peak inspiratory airway pressure—** Plateau airway pressures are typically unchanged.

b. **Decreased exhaled tidal volume.**

c. **Bilateral expiratory wheezes—**If bronchospasm is severe, breath sounds may be diminished or absent due to the reduction in airflow.

d. **Altered capnograph waveform—**Because of the obstruction to expiratory airflow from the narrowed bronchioles, the capnograph produces a delayed rise in end-tidal carbon dioxide, seen as a slowly increasing wave that appears like a "shark fin."

e. **Auto-PEEP—**Patients with narrowed bronchioles require a longer period of expiration for complete alveolar emptying. If the ventilator delivers a breath before expiration that is complete, the patient can develop intrinsic **Positive End-Expiratory Pressure (PEEP)** due to the stacking of breaths and lung hyperinflation. Auto-PEEP will be evident when the patient's expiratory flow curve does not return to baseline before the next breath begins, as seen on the flow-time scalar display or flow-volume loop. Significant auto-PEEP may increase intrathoracic pressures to the point where venous return is compromised, resulting in a decrease in cardiac output.

f. *Hypoxemia,* if gas exchange is severely impaired (V/Q mismatch).

MANAGEMENT

To restore adequate ventilation (and therefore, oxygenation), intraoperative bronchospasm should be treated expeditiously while simultaneously investigating the underlying cause. The goals are to relieve the obstruction to airflow and reverse hypoxemia before irreversible ischemia results.

Primary Management

1. Increase inspired oxygen concentration to 100%.
2. Increase inspired concentration of inhalation anesthetic. The potent volatile anesthetics have bronchodilating properties. Sevoflurane and isoflurane are preferred over desflurane because of its airway resistance effects. If bronchospasm is severe enough to impair delivery of the gases, then an intravenous anesthetic such as propofol may be necessary to achieve a rapid increase in the depth of anesthesia. Both propofol and sevoflurane may promote GABA-ergic inhibitory interneurons in the NST to suppress the bronchospasm reflex. Ketamine is the only intravenous anesthetic agent with bronchodilating properties.
3. Institute manual ventilation (by circle system, self-inflating bag, or Mapleson circuit) to evaluate pulmonary compliance and to rule out occlusions of the breathing circuit.
4. Administration of bronchodilator therapy. Note that nondepolarizing muscle relaxants relax skeletal muscle only and, therefore, have no role in the management of bronchospasm.
   a. **β_2-adrenergic receptor agonists—**Rapidly acting drugs such as albuterol can be delivered through the inspiratory limb of the circuit either via a nebulizer or metered dose inhaler. If the bronchospasm responds poorly to β_2-agonists, inhaled anti-muscarinic agents such as ipratropium bromide may be considered. If the severity of bronchospasm prohibits delivery of inhaled β-agonists, consider giving an IM or SC dose of β_2-agonists such as terbutaline.
   b. **Magnesium—**A single intravenous dose (2 g) of magnesium may help resolve bronchoconstriction in asthmatics.
   c. **Epinephrine—**For severe bronchospasm refractory to all other modalities, especially when associated with hypotension or anaphylactic shock, epinephrine is the rescue drug of choice. Escalating systemic doses, starting at 10 mcg IV, should be titrated for patients in extremis. Epinephrine achieves bronchodilation by binding to and activating β_2-adrenergic receptors.

Secondary Management

1. Address the underlying cause and reconsider alternative diagnoses. For instance, thoroughly inspect the endotracheal tube to rule out an obstructed, kinked, or malpositioned tube. If bronchospasm is suspected due to an allergic reaction or anaphylaxis, expose and examine the patient for cutaneous and cardiovascular signs, review medications, and stop administration of suspected drugs or blood products.
2. Change ventilator settings to improve gas exchange. It may be necessary to decrease tidal volumes to lower high peak airway pressures and prevent barotrauma. Permissive hypercapnia should be well tolerated as long as there is no severe respiratory acidosis and adequate oxygenation. In addition, slow respiratory rates (4-10) and

inspiratory: expiratory time ratios of at least 1:2 to 1:3 will help prolong the expiratory rate. This allows the patient with narrowed bronchioles to have more complete exhalation and minimize breath stacking and development of auto-PEEP.

3. Administration of systemic corticosteroids. Intravenous glucocorticoids such as methylprednisolone are important in decreasing the degree of airway inflammation. The anti-inflammatory benefit takes several hours, however, they are most helpful in preventing recurrences of bronchospasm.

4. If ventilation and oxygenation remains difficult, consider postponement of elective surgery.

5. Prepare for potential bronchospasm reoccurrence during emergence and postoperative period. Consider additional administration of bronchodilating drugs. Administer neostigmine carefully. The patient's oropharynx should be thoroughly suctioned of secretions, and consideration should be given to deep extubation of the trachea. If bronchospasm persists in the recovery period, continued administration of regular therapy (bronchodilators, corticosteroids, chest physiotherapy) should be arranged.

PREVENTION

Patient risk factors for the development of intraoperative bronchospasm include reactive airway disease (asthma, COPD), history of smoking, and recent upper respiratory tract infections. A complete preoperative evaluation of asthma and COPD, including auscultation of active wheezing and assessing the degree of medical optimization and disease control, should be performed. Smokers should abstain from smoking at least 6 to 8 weeks before surgery to significantly reduce the risk of bronchospasm. An upper respiratory tract infection generally takes about 2 weeks for the associated airway hyperreactivity to resolve.

Measures to lower the risk of precipitating intraoperative bronchospasm include:

- Administration of preoperative inhaled bronchodilators (β_2 adrenergic agonists) and steroids (inhaled and IV) about 30 minutes prior to surgery.
- Use of regional techniques where appropriate can avoid the need for general anesthesia and intubation.
- Ensure adequate depth of anesthesia before airway instrumentation.
- Consider the use of a laryngeal mask airway rather than endotracheal intubation.
- Consider the use of ketamine.
- Avoid drugs that cause histamine release.
- Consider topical lidocaine to the airway.
- Consider deep extubation.

SUGGESTED READINGS

Dewachter P, Mouton-Faivre C, Emala CW, Beloucif S. Case scenario: bronchospasm during anesthetic induction. *Anesthesiology* 2011;114:1200-1210.

Woods BD, Sladen RN. Perioperative considerations for the patient with asthma and bronchospasm. *Br J Anaesth.* 2009;103:57-65.

105

Anaphylaxis

Brian A. Kim and Seol W. Yang, MD

Allergic, hypersensitivity reactions are amplified immunologic responses triggered by allergen, or antigen stimulation in previously sensitized individuals. The sensitization occurs from the identical antigen that triggers future allergic reaction, or from a different antigen sharing similar molecular structures.

Four main hypersensitivity reactions are classified by the immune system components involved:

- Type I reactions are anaphylactic or immediate-type hypersensitivity reactions. Antigens bind to and cross-link IgE antibodies, causing mast cells to release inflammatory mediators. Examples of Type I reactions include anaphylaxis, allergic rhinitis, and asthma.
- Type II reactions involve the activation of the classic complement system by IgG or IgM antibodies, which causes lysis and destruction of cells. Examples include ABO incompatibility, drug-induced hemolytic anemia, and heparin-induced thrombocytopenia.
- Type III reactions primarily involve immune complexes of antigens and antibodies bound together. Deposition of immune complexes in tissues activates neutrophils and triggers the complement system. An example of Type III reaction is serum sickness.
- Type IV reactions, or delayed hypersensitivity reactions, are characterized by antigen-to-lymphocyte binding. They primarily result in proliferation of cytotoxic T lymphocytes with the purpose of extinguishing antigen-bearing triggering cell. These particular reactions occur within 24 hours, peak from 40-80 hours and resolve by 96 hours. Examples include graft-versus-host reactions, tuberculin immunity as well as contact dermatitis.

ANAPHYLAXIS: PATHOPHYSIOLOGY

Type I immediate hypersensitivity reactions begin when a susceptible individual is exposed to an antigen. During primary exposure, antigen is processed by the antigen-presenting cell (APC). APC then presents antigen's processed peptide to CD4+ T cells, inducing CD4+ T cell production of IL-4, IL-5, IL-6, IL-10, and granulocyte-macrophage colony-stimulating factor (GM-CSF). These factors stimulate B cells to switch their immunoglobulin production to peptide-specific IgE.

Newly produced IgE antibodies are released from B cells and bind to IgE receptors on mast cells and basophils in peripheral tissue and circulation. The IgE antibodies are fixated on the membrane of basophils and mast cells by the Fc receptors. Upon secondary exposure, the allergen binds to IgE, causes cross-linking, and stimulates the basophils and mast cells to degranulate and release their inflammatory vasoactive mediators—prostaglandins, leukotrienes, histamines, and tryptase. The sudden release of these mediators causes arteriolar vasodilatation with increased vascular permeability, bronchiolar smooth muscle constriction, and increased mucus secretions. The degree of immediate hypersensitivity responses varies from mild allergic rhinitis or atopic dermatitis to life-threatening angioedema and anaphylaxis.

Anaphylaxis is a severe, unanticipated, Type I reaction with a variety of respiratory, cardiovascular, gastrointestinal, and cutaneous signs and symptoms (Table 105-1). These manifestations are driven by active mediators, including histamines, released by antigen-IgE stimulated basophils and mast cells, which cause smooth muscle contraction, vascular permeability, and leukocyte and platelet aggregation. Severe symptoms include cardiovascular collapse and pulmonary edema.

Intraoperatively, the most common identifiable features are hypotension, tachycardia, and bronchospasm. The timing of symptoms plays a vital role in clinical suspicion and diagnosis. Anaphylactic reactions typically occur within 2-20 minutes ("rule of 2's") of antigen exposure and occur more frequently with parenteral, antigen administration.

TABLE 105-1 Clinical Manifestations of Anaphylaxis

System	Signs and Symptoms
Cardiovascular	Tachycardia, hypotension, dysrhythmias
Respiratory	Bronchospasm/wheezing, dyspnea, laryngeal edema, hypoxemia, pulmonary edema
Dermatologic	Urticarial rash, facial edema

TABLE 105-2   Common Causes of Perioperative Allergic Reactions

Anaphylactic reactions	Antibiotics (penicillins, cephalosporins, sulfa drugs) Local anesthetics Latex Disinfectants (chlorhexidine) Enzymes (trypsin, streptokinase) Human proteins (insulin, corticotrophin)
Anaphylactoid reactions	Muscle relaxants (succinylcholine, rocuronium) Opioids (morphine, meperidine) Radio contrast dye Anesthetics (propofol, thiopental) NSAIDs Protamine Dextran Preservatives (sulfites)

Perioperative triggers for anaphylaxis are the tertiary and quaternary ammonium groups found in muscle relaxants. Not surprisingly, significant cross-sensitivity between succinylcholine and nondepolarizing muscle relaxants exists. The second most common intraoperative allergen is latex. Latex allergies commonly occur in patients with spina bifida, urogenital abnormalities, and health-care workers.

Allergic reactions occur with antibiotics, blood products, colloids, and NSAIDs, but may be elicited by any substance (Table 105-2). Antibiotics most likely to instigate an anaphylactic response are β-lactam antibiotics, including penicillins and cephalosporins. Carbapenem and cephalosporins are antibiotics with penicillin cross-reactivity. About 2% of the general population has penicillin allergy, but only 0.01% of penicillin administrations result in an anaphylactic reaction. Medical history of atopy, allergy, or asthma makes life-threatening allergic reactions more likely albeit still rare. These symptoms do not warrant perioperative medical pretreatment or drug avoidance. However, allergic workup should be considered with an unknown trigger of a past anaphylaxis event.

ANAPHYLACTOID REACTIONS

Anaphylactoid reactions are nonimmune mediated but still cause mast cell and basophil release of inflammatory mediators that symptomatically approximate anaphylaxis. Anaphylactoid reactions causing the nonimmune mediated release of histamines may be caused by several mechanisms, which include stimulation by drugs or substance *P*. These substances can trigger the calcium-induced degranulation of histamines without the involvement of any surface antibodies, including IgE antibodies—mandatory in true allergic type I hypersensitivity reactions. The clinical presentation is identical to true allergic reactions with the most dangerous manifestations

being respiratory and cardiovascular collapse. Nonimmunologic, histamine-releasing drugs include antibiotics, basic compounds, hyperosmotic agents, muscle relaxants, opioids, and barbiturates. Antibiotics that are most likely to induce an anaphylactoid reaction are vancomycin ("red man syndrome") and pentamidine.

MANAGEMENT

Initial therapy should be executed promptly to avoid severe cardiovascular collapse and death. The first interventions include:

1. Discontinue administration of the suspected antigen.
2. Administer 100% O_2 and maintain a patent airway.
3. Discontinue all anesthetic agents, if appropriate.
4. Begin IV volume expansion with crystalloid and colloid to treat hypotension.
5. Administer epinephrine (5-10 μg IV bolus and titrate as needed (0.1-1.0 mg IV for severe cardiovascular collapse).

Epinephrine treatment causes α-adrenergic stimulation, leading to vasoconstriction. Epinephrine's $β_2$-agonist activity causes bronchodilation, reversing bronchospasm. Furthermore, epinephrine stabilizes mast cell membranes, preventing degranulation of histamine and inflammatory mediators.

Secondary treatment options include:

1. Antihistamines (0.5-1 mg/kg diphenhydramine).
2. Adrenergic/catecholamine infusions: epinephrine, norepinephrine, or isoproterenol titrated as needed.
3. Bronchodilators (albuterol, terbutaline).
4. Corticosteroids (0.25-1 gm hydrocortisone; 1-2 gm methylprednisolone).
5. Sodium bicarbonate (0.1-1 mEq/kg for hypotension and acidosis).
6. Vasopressin for refractory shock.

Unpredictable, adverse drug reactions activate a cascade of immune-mediated activity that is typically dose-independent and unrelated to a drug's pharmacological activity. All patients with anaphylaxis receive at least 24 hours of intensive care unit monitoring, as hypersensitivity reactions may recur following initially successful treatment.

Over 80% of adverse drug effects ("side effects") are predictable; however, often mistaken for an allergy or hypersensitivity reactions. Adverse effects are dose-dependent and manifest a known pharmacological action.

SUGGESTED READING

Hepner DL, Castells MC. Anaphylaxis during the perioperative period. *Anesth Analg.* 2003;97:1381-1396.

Laryngospasm

Adrian M. Ionescu, MD, and Sudha Ved, MD

Laryngospasm refers to the phenomenon that involves the involuntary and forceful contraction of laryngeal muscles, which results from the depolarization of the *superior laryngeal nerve*. Contraction of the laryngeal muscles results in vocal cord adduction, complete airway obstruction, and impaired ventilation. Incidence of laryngospasm is higher in children and hypoxia develops more quickly compared to adults, requiring vigilance and prompt treatment.

Three structures are involved in the laryngospasm reflex: aryepiglottic folds, false vocal cords, and true vocal cords. The muscles most involved in the laryngospasm are the lateral cricoarytenoid and the thyroarytenoids (adductors of the glottis) and the cricothyroid (a tensor of the vocal cord). During laryngospasm, either the true vocal cords alone or the true and false vocal cords both become apposed in the midline and close the glottis. Folding in of the aryepiglottic folds results in a true ball-valve closure of the larynx and involves contraction of the infrahyoid ("strap") muscles of the neck (sternohyoid, sternothyroid, thyrohyoid, and omohyoid muscles).

ETIOLOGY

Stimuli that may trigger laryngospasm include "light" anesthesia, irritant volatile anesthetics or failure of the anesthesia delivery system, regurgitation of enteric contents into the oropharynx and oropharyngeal secretions or blood contacting adjacent laryngeal structures, the contact of the endotracheal tube with laryngeal structures during tracheal intubation/extubation causing airway irritation as well as the presence of nociceptive stimuli during surgical stimulation. Laryngospasm is more common after upper airway procedures, particularly ENT procedures in which blood, secretions, and surgical debris are present.

SIGNS AND SYMPTOMS

Laryngospasm may manifest with inspiratory stridor, increased inspiratory efforts (ie, tracheal tug), paradoxical chest and abdominal movements that can quickly progress to complete airway obstruction, desaturation, bradycardia, and central cyanosis.

PREVENTION

Different approaches that may be used in preventing laryngospasm under anesthesia include intravenous lidocaine, topical lidocaine, intravenous magnesium, and "deep" extubation.

TREATMENT

Early management of laryngospasm includes clearing blood and secretions from the airway and applying chin lift and jaw thrust, and insertion of an oral-pharyngeal airway followed by the application of end-expiratory pressure (PEEP) or continuous airway pressure (CPAP) via a tight-fitting mask and 100% oxygen to aid in splinting open the laryngeal musculature. The cricothyroid muscle is the only tensor of the vocal cords and a gentle stretching of this muscle may overcome moderate laryngospasm. Jaw thrust will aid in lifting up the tongue and unfurling of the aryepiglottic fold, and opening of the anterior commissure to allow passage of some flow with CPAP.

The laryngospasm notch, also called Larson point, is located behind the lobule of the pinna of each ear (Figure 106-1). Firm digital pressure is applied at the most superior portion of the laryngospasm notch inward, toward the base of the

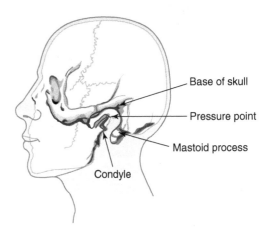

FIGURE 106-1 The laryngospasm notch. (Reproduced with permission from Larson PC Jr. Laryngospasm—the best treatment. *Anesthesiology*, 1998,89(5):1293-1294.)

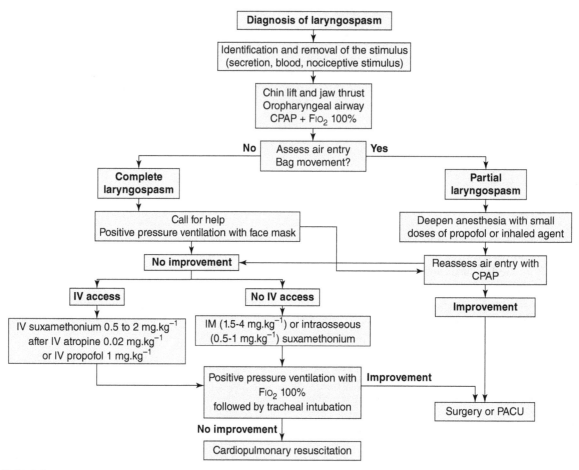

FIGURE 106-2 Diagnosis and treatment of laryngospasm algorithm (Reproduced with permission from Orliaguet, GA, Gall, O, Savoldelli, GL, et al. Case scenario: perianesthetic management of laryngospasm in children. *Anesthesiology.* 2012;116(2):458-471.) CPAP, continuous positive airway pressure; F_{IO_2}, fraction of inspired oxygen; IV, intravenous; IM, intramuscular; PACU, postanesthesia care unit.

skull with both fingers and simultaneously the mandible is lifted at right angle to the body, as in jaw thrust. This will resolve the laryngospasm to unobstructed breathing within a few breaths. According to Larson, it is very reliable and superior to other treatments mentioned above. There are two possible reasons why this works: (1) forward displacement of the mandible as in jaw thrust, and (2) severe painful stimulus relaxes the vocal folds and vocal cords by way of either the parasympathetic or sympathetic nervous systems.

If continuous oxygen desaturation occurs, increase depth of anesthesia with intravenous lidocaine (dose 1 mg/kg), intravenous propofol (dose 1 mg/kg), and continue attempts at PEEP, CPAP, and positive pressure ventilation (PPV). If laryngospasm continues, the definitive treatment is with intravenous succinylcholine (dose 0.5-2 mg/kg) and atropine (0.02 mg/kg) which acts rapidly to relax the laryngeal

musculature (ie, cricothyroid muscle). If intravenous access is not available, succinylcholine can be administered via the intramuscular route (IM dose 1.5-4 mg/kg) or via the intraosseous route (IO dose 0.5-1 mg/kg). An algorithm for the diagnosis and treatment of laryngospasm is further detailed in Figure 106-2.

SUGGESTED READINGS

Fink BR. The etiology and treatment of laryngeal spasm. *Anesthesiology* 1956;17:569-577.

Larson PC Jr. Laryngospasm—the best treatment [Correspondence] *Anesthesiology* 1998;89:1293-1294.

Orliaguet, GA, Gall, O, Savoldelli, GL, et al. Case scenario: perianesthetic management of laryngospasm in children. *Anesthesiology* 2012;116(2):458-471.

107

Postobstructive Pulmonary Edema

Adrian M. Ionescu, MD, and Sudha Ved, MD

Postobstructive pulmonary edema, also known as negative-pressure pulmonary edema (NPPE), is a serious, potentially fatal condition which commonly results from upper airway obstruction. More specifically, forced inspiration against an obstructed upper airway generates a large intrathoracic pressure gradient, an increased pulmonary vascular volume, and subsequently a significant increase in the pulmonary capillary transmural pressure, which produces a significant disruption of the capillary alveolar membrane. The movement of fluid across the pulmonary capillary bed can be further summarized by the Starling equation: $Q = K \times [(P_c - P_i) - \sigma (\pi_c - \pi_i)]$ (Q, flow across the pulmonary capillary bed; P_c, capillary hydrostatic pressure; P_i, interstitial hydrostatic pressure; π_c, capillary oncotic pressure, and π_i, interstitial oncotic pressure).

Negative-pressure pulmonary edema has been reported in the literature to occur in approximately 0.1% of anesthetic cases. NPPE can be further classified as either Type I or Type II. Generally, Type I NPPE results *immediately* after an episode of acute airway obstruction, most often caused by laryngospasm. Other causes of Type I NPPE include upper airway tumors, foreign bodies, drowning, endotracheal tube obstruction, epiglottitis, and croup. Type II NPPE usually develops as a *delayed* response, following the relief of chronic upper airway obstruction, commonly caused by tonsillar, adenoid, or uvular hypertrophy (Table 107-1).

TABLE 107-1 Types of Negative-Pressure Pulmonary Edema

Type I NPPE	Type II NPPE
Postextubation laryngospasm	Post-tonsillectomy/ adenoidectomy
Croup	
Epiglottitis	Postoperative removal of upper airway tumor
Foreign body in the airway	
Endotracheal tube obstruction	Hypertrophic uvula
LMA obstruction	Choanal stenosis
Laryngeal mass	
Goiter	
Postoperative vocal cord paralysis	

PATHOPHYSIOLOGY

The mechanism underlying NPPE is usually triggered following an obstruction of the upper airway, which generates a negative intraalveolar pressure with the resultant transmural pressure gradient causing a fluid shift from the pulmonary capillary bed into the interstitial and alveolar spaces.

There are four basic mechanisms that account for an increased level of pulmonary fluid in the interstitial compartment: (1) increased hydrostatic pressure in the capillary bed; (2) decreased plasma oncotic pressure; (3) capillary alveolar membrane disruption leading to increased permeability; and (4) decreased lymphatic return to the venous circulation.

Under normal physiologic conditions, intrathoracic pressure ranges from –3 to –10 cm H_2O, but highly negative intrathoracic pressures (> –50 cm H_2O) can produce a significant increase in venous return of blood, thus substantially increasing the left ventricular end-diastolic volume and subsequently the end-diastolic pressure. The combination of low intrathoracic pressure and high left ventricular end-diastolic pressure favors the formation of a transmural pressure gradient. This pressure gradient results in the accumulation of fluid in the alveolar and interstitial compartments, with concomitant significant pulmonary edema. The sudden increase in venous return combined with a decrease in cardiac output (resulting from severe hypoxemia) reduces the pulmonary venous drainage into the left atrium. The net result is an increase in the pulmonary capillary pressure and disruption of the capillary alveolar membrane. Disruption of the capillary alveolar membrane accounts for the additional fluid accumulation in the alveolar and interstitial compartments.

SIGNS AND SYMPTOMS

The initial signs of NPPE include oxygen desaturation, hypoxemia, agitation, tachypnea, tachycardia, pink frothy sputum, diffuse crackles on auscultation, diffuse interstitial infiltrates on chest X-ray, and ground-glass opacities (indicative of hemorrhage) on chest CT scan. Negative-pressure pulmonary edema requires prompt intervention as symptoms usually develop within the first hour following the inciting event.

TREATMENT AND MANAGEMENT

The priority in the treatment of NPPE should initially target relieving the airway obstruction as a means of improving ventilation and oxygenation. Following the establishment of a patent airway, the treatment of NPPE includes supplemental oxygen, mask ventilation, continuous positive airway pressure, and positive end-expiratory pressure for the treatment of severe hypoxemia. Intravenous diuretics (furosemide 50 mg) may also be utilized to address the pulmonary edema. In situations where the airway obstruction persists, endotracheal intubation and mechanical ventilation may be necessary to correct the severe hypoxemia. Steroids, however, do not have a role in the management of NPPE.

If untreated, NPPE can quickly progress with worsening hypoxemia, respiratory failure, adult respiratory distress syndrome, and eventually death. Therefore, prompt diagnosis and treatment of NPPE is necessary to avoid life-threatening complications. If recognition is delayed, mortality from NPPE can be as high as 40%, but in patients where NPPE is appropriately recognized and treated, symptoms usually resolve within 24 hours.

Aspiration of Gastric Contents

Alan Kim, MD, and Medhat Hannallah, MD

Aspiration of gastric contents is a rare but significant concern during the perioperative period. The incidence of pulmonary aspiration ranges between 0.7 and 4.7 per 10 000 administered anesthetics in nonpregnant adults, 5.3 per 10 000 anesthetics in pregnant patients, and 3.8 and 10.2 per 10 000 anesthetics in children. Pulmonary aspiration increases the risk of perioperative morbidity (ARDS, prolonged intubation, infection) and mortality (3.8%-4.6% in the general population, 0%-12% in the obstetric patients).

General anesthesia increases the risk of aspiration. Patients with certain comorbidities are at higher risk for pulmonary aspiration than the general population. Appropriate identification of these high-risk patients, as well as the implementation of risk-reduction interventions, are important for the safe delivery of anesthesia.

PATHOPHYSIOLOGY OF ASPIRATION

Natural barriers to aspiration include the lower esophageal sphincter, the upper esophageal sphincter, and the intrinsic protective airway reflexes.

Lower Esophageal Sphincter

The lower esophageal sphincter (LES) is a complex anatomic region which combines both circular and longitudinal fibers, and forms a barrier between the esophagus and the stomach. The left border of the esophagus aligns with the gastric fundus. The right crus of the diaphragm forms a sling around the abdominal esophagus, forming the "extrinsic LES." The intrinsic LES is the band of circular muscle fibers that lie deeper into this extrinsic LES.

Gastroesophageal reflux is caused by a defect in the combined LES tone with transient relaxation of its tone that allows transit of gastric contents into the distal esophagus. Anesthetic agents and techniques can further exacerbate such a defect (Table 108-1). The net effect of a standard IV induction is a decrease in the LES tone. Conditions associated with chronic increased intraabdominal pressure, such as obesity and pregnancy, are associated with a high incidence of gastroesophageal reflux.

TABLE 108-1 **Factors Affecting LES Tone**

Lower LES Tone	Increased LES Tone	No Effect on LES Tone
Anticholinergic agents	Antiemetics	Atracurium
Opioids	Succinylcholine	Vecuronium
Thiopental	NMBD	H_2 antagonists
Propofol	Cholinergic agents	Sleep
Inhaled anesthetics	Antacids	
Cricoid pressure		
NG tube		
Alkalinization		
Protein feeding		

Upper Esophageal Sphincter

Once gastric contents are present in the esophagus, the upper esophageal sphincter (UES) presents the next barrier to pulmonary aspiration. The cricopharyngeus muscle acts as a functional UES, assisting the actual UES to maintain a barrier between the hypopharynx and the proximal esophagus. Its tone is reduced during both general anesthesia and normal sleep. In fact, with the exception of ketamine, most anesthetic agents will cause relaxation of the UES.

Intrinsic Protective Airway Reflexes

If gastric contents make it past the UES, four reflexes help mitigate aspiration: apnea with laryngospasm, coughing, expiration, and spasmodic panting. Laryngospasm initially adducts both true and false vocal cords. If the laryngospasm is prolonged, then the false cords open, while the true vocal cords remain adducted. Coughing and expiration attempt to expel any foreign objects from the upper trachea. Spasmodic panting consists of breathing at 60 breaths per minute, with rapidly opening and closing vocal cords. Expiration is the most commonly triggered reflex, while laryngospasm is the hardest reflex to abolish. Triggers for these reflexes are present on the larynx, trachea, bronchus, and esophagus. These triggers lose their sensitivity with age.

The protective airway reflexes are diminished in the perioperative period. Depending on the anesthetic technique used, this decrease may unexpectedly persist. In a recent study of same-day surgery patients, the auditory reaction time (a measure of recovery from general anesthesia) was normal in spite of persistently depressed airway reflexes. Accordingly, care should be taken to avoid sources of aspiration in the postextubation postanesthesia care unit stay as well.

Factors that Increase Aspiration Risk (Table 108-2)

A. Surgical Factors

Trauma, emergency, abdominal, and gastrointestinal surgery, as well as surgery performed in the lithotomy or the Trendelenburg positions are all associated with increased risk of pulmonary aspiration.

Patients undergoing emergency surgery may have recent food intake. They frequently have increased sympathetic tone from anxiety or pain; and may have some degree of intraabdominal pathology associated with peritoneal irritation and ileus. The use of opiates in these patients can also decrease gastric emptying.

Abdominal and gastrointestinal surgeries are associated with a higher rate of postoperative ileus.

The lithotomy and the Trendelenburg positions increase the intraabdominal and intragastric pressures leading to increased risk of regurgitation and aspiration of gastric contents.

Trauma patients are at an especially high risk of aspiration. Since they are likely to need emergency surgery, these

TABLE 108-2   Risk Factors for Pulmonary Aspiration

Surgical Factors	Patient-Related Factors	Anesthesia-Related Factors
Trauma	Diabetes	General anesthesia
Emergency	Bowel obstruction	Positive pressure ventilation
Abdominal	Dysfunctional swallowing	Inadequate sedation
Gastrointestinal	Gastroesophageal reflux	Inadequate relaxation
Lithotomy	Obesity	Opiate use
Trendelenburg	Pregnancy	
	Increased ICP	
	Altered mental status	
	Age	
	Increased sympathetic tone	
	Anxiety	

patients are unlikely to fulfill the nil per os (NPO) recommendations. Furthermore, the associated increased sympathetic tone and the use of opiates result in gastric stasis and increased residual gastric volume which can last for a prolonged period after the initial trauma. Trauma patients may also present with altered level of consciousness as a result of head injury or blood loss, or from the use of sedative and analgesic medications to treat pain. The resulting compromise of the intrinsic airway protective mechanisms increases aspiration risk.

B. Patient Factors

Diseases that affect gastrointestinal tract function increase the risk of pulmonary aspiration. Stroke may result in dysfunctional swallowing mechanism and decreased ability to clear hypopharyngeal secretions.

Conditions associated with decreased gastric motility such as diabetes (due to autonomic neuropathy), pregnancy (progesterone-mediated), bowel obstruction (duodenal distention inhibiting gastric emptying), advanced age (associated with progressive decline in gastric motility), and high sympathetic tone (hyperactivity of the celiac plexus) can also contribute to an increased risk of aspiration.

Other contributing factors include gastroesophageal reflux (decreased LES tone with an increase in intraesophageal contents), increased intraabdominal pressure (obesity, pregnancy), increased nausea (pregnancy, increased intracranial pressure [ICP]), or decreased level of consciousness.

C. Anesthesia Factors

General anesthesia is associated with a higher risk of aspiration relative to regional anesthesia. High levels of positive pressure ventilation cause gastric insufflation. The resulting increased intragastric pressure can lead to regurgitation of gastric contents.

Opiate use for pain control can delay gastric motility and promote ileus. Airway instrumentation during inadequate muscle relaxation and/or depth of anesthesia can lead to bucking, increased intraabdominal, intragastric pressures, and increased risk of regurgitation.

Aspiration Risk Reduction Strategies

Strategies that are designed to reduce aspiration risk include reducing the volume and the acidity of gastric contents, utilizing physical barriers to aspiration, and using precautions during high-risk periods such as induction and laryngoscopy.

The volume, formulation, and acidity of gastric aspirates are thought to be related to the severity of lung injury.

Early animal studies, where different volumes at different pH were instilled directly into the lungs, identified a gastric volume greater than 0.4 mL/kg and a pH less than 2.5 as risk factors contributing to severe aspiration pneumonitis. Subsequent studies demonstrated that high gastric volumes did not necessarily correlate to high aspirated volumes. It is unlikely that the entire gastric contents will end up in the lungs.

In animal models, a 20.8 mL/kg gastric volume correlated to spontaneous gastric regurgitation, bypassing the LES and UES. This regurgitation could then increase the risk of pulmonary aspiration. This is well above the 0.4 mL/kg that was previously extrapolated. Furthermore, patients with known gastric volumes over 0.4 mL/kg have been anesthetized without evidence of aspiration, suggesting that the 0.4 mL/kg cutoff may be a conservative threshold in an otherwise healthy patient.

Gastric pH seems more closely associated with the severity of injury. In one study, smaller, more acidic aspirated volumes produced more severe injuries than larger, less acidic aspirated volumes. Both gastric volume and acidity should be addressed concomitantly.

A. Gastric Volume Reduction

Preoperative fasting is the main method of reducing gastric volume. If adherence to NPO status is not possible, alternatives include preinduction gastric decompression using a nasogastric tube, or the use of pharmacological enhancement of gastric emptying.

Following are the recommended fasting guidelines for an otherwise healthy patient.

Clear liquid: 2 hours (pediatric), 3 hours (adults)
Human milk: 4 hours
Nonhuman and formula milk: 6 hours
Light meal: 6 hours, Heavy meal: 8 hours

In patients with conditions known to potentially reduce GI motility and gastric emptying, a more conservative interpretation of these guidelines is required.

B. Gastric Decompression Using a Nasogastric Tube (NG Tube)

Prior to emergency surgery, decompression of the stomach using an NG tube should be considered prior to anesthesia induction. Although its presence may prevent the UES and LES from completely closing, the NG tube does not impair an effective application of cricoid pressure. Placement of an NG tube allows a rapid initial decompression of gastric contents. Since GI secretions are continuous, continuous drainage during the case and final suctioning prior to extubation is advisable. Furthermore, the NG tube acts as a path of low resistance for gastric contents if the intraabdominal pressure acutely rises, as is the case in retching, or emesis. This outlet may also decrease the potential for esophageal rupture in the face of such rapid rise of intragastric pressure during rapid sequence anesthesia induction with effective cricoid pressure.

A significant disadvantage of NG tubes is the fact that it leads to incomplete closures of the LES and UES, thus predisposing to active reflux and regurgitation. The size of the NG tube does not affect the degree of impairment. One study did not show a statistically significant difference in the rate of reflux and aspiration in patients with NG tube size 2.85 mm versus 6.0 mm.

Given the incompetence of the LES and UES in the presence of an NG tube, an NG tube with an inflatable gastric balloon that occludes the cardia of the stomach was created. This modified NG tube significantly reduces the incidence of regurgitation and protects against external gastric compression, induced emesis, and steep Trendelenburg positions.

C. Reducing the Acidity of Gastric Contents

High acidity of gastric contents was found to cause greater predisposition to lung injury than large gastric volume alone. Premedication with agents that reduce gastric pH may help reduce the severity of lung damage should aspiration occur. The agents that can be used to achieve this goal are:

1. **H_2 Antagonists**—H_2 antagonists bind directly to the histamine receptors on the gastric parietal basal cells that are primarily responsible for gastric acid production. Although both ranitidine and famotidine significantly increase gastric pH and decrease gastric volume, a side-by-side comparison demonstrated that famotidine was more efficacious in children. The drawbacks of H_2 antagonists include significant variability in the degree of acid inhibition, quick development of tolerance, and a lack of direct correlation between plasma concentration of the drug and the peak level of acid inhibition.

2. **Proton Pump Inhibitors**—Proton pump inhibitors (PPIs) bind and block the H+/K+ ATPase on the acidic luminal side of the gastric parietal cells. This prevents the influx of K and efflux of H+ needed to form acid. These drugs have significant first-pass metabolism, which prevents a reliable prediction of the degree of acid suppression.

   Rabeprazole, lansoprazole, and omeprazole are the most effective of the PPIs. For optimal preoperative acid suppression, these drugs should be given in two sequential doses, one dose on the night before surgery and the second dose on the morning of surgery to maximize their effect. If only one dose is possible, rabeprazole and lansoprazole should be given the morning of the surgery, while omeprazole should be given the night before the surgery. There is no direct relationship between peak plasma level of PPIs and peak acid inhibition. Acid inhibition may persist even after plasma levels of the drug become undetectable.

   There are a myriad of studies comparing H_2 antagonists and PPIs. In these reports, a single dose of ranitidine was found to be just as effective as the recommended two doses of PPIs in reducing gastric volume and increasing gastric pH in healthy patients. Consideration of existing comorbidities may influence the choice between the two agents. In patients with peptic ulcer, PPIs are more effective than H_2 antagonists in improving healing rates, providing symptomatic relief, and reducing recurrence rates.

3. **Antacids**—Antacids such as sodium citrate can be used to directly reduce acidity in the stomach. Their effect has a limited duration, requiring additional agents such as PPIs and H_2 antagonists to maintain perioperative control. These agents only address the acid that is already present in the stomach, without altering acid production. These agents are available in particulate and nonparticulate formulations. Only nonparticulate antacids are recommended since pulmonary aspiration of particulate material can potentially cause lung injury.

Although these drugs have a proven effect on the character of gastric contents, given the rarity of pulmonary aspiration, the ASA practice guidelines do not recommend their routine use in healthy patients.

D. Rapid Sequence Induction

Rapid sequence induction is the anesthesia induction sequence of choice for patients who are at higher risk of aspiration. It consists of rendering a patient unconscious with an intravenous induction agent such as propofol or etomidate, followed immediately by a rapidly acting paralytic agent such as succinylcholine or high-dose rocuronium, followed by endotracheal intubation without prior positive pressure ventilation. Cricoid pressure is initiated prior to induction and maintained until confirmation of correct endotracheal tube placement. It is important to establish that the patient is fully anesthetized and fully relaxed prior to instrumenting the airway to avoid the risk of bucking and gagging. Another important goal of the technique is to avoid positive pressure ventilation during the period between anesthesia induction and endotracheal intubation so as to avoid insufflating the stomach. Thorough preoxygenation is critical to achieving this goal since it will allow for much longer time to deal with unexpected airway difficulty without having to mask ventilate the patient. When breathing 100% oxygen, near-complete denitrogenation of the lungs is achievable after 3 minutes of normal breathing, or 6-8 vital capacity breaths.

E. Cricoid Pressure

Cricoid pressure is the application of 44 N of force on the cricoid cartilage, directed in a posterior and cephalad orientation. Premature application of cricoid pressure is associated with retching. It is recommended that the pressure gradually increase from 10 N preinduction to the full 30 N postinduction. Although it is widely employed for its theoretical reduction in the incidence of pulmonary aspiration during induction, its efficacy is controversial for several reasons:

1. The definition may be inaccurate. Several studies have shown adequate occlusion of the esophagus at pressures less than the 44 N.
2. The consistent and accurate application of cricoid pressure varies widely among practitioners, although standardized training methods may improve this deficiency.
3. Even if a practitioner is trained in the appropriate degree of force needed to occlude the esophagus, studies have

shown that it is only performed appropriately for a few minutes before lapses in pressure quality occur.
4. Imaging studies have shown that the cricoid cartilage does not consistently lie directly over the esophagus, and even when it does the application of cricoid pressure may displace the esophagus laterally, affording only a partial occlusion.

F. Endotracheal Intubation

An endotracheal tube placed during a rapid sequence induction technique is the gold standard for securing the airway from aspiration. However, the standard high-volume, low-pressure endotracheal tube cuff can allow trace amounts of fluid to leak past the balloon along the longitudinal tracks created by the folds in the cuff. A pressure-limited endotracheal tube cuff provides a more secure seal. Using lubricant can further help seal the area around the tracheal balloon.

MANAGEMENT OF ASPIRATION

To manage aspiration, one needs to distinguish between aspiration pneumonitis and aspiration pneumonia. The former is a physicochemical process, whereas the latter is an infectious process.

Aspiration Pneumonitis

Aspiration pneumonitis consists of local inflammatory damage, generally due to an inflammatory response to chemical or mechanical damage to the lung parenchyma. This process leads to local inflammation, pulmonary edema, and impaired gas exchange with potential progression to ARDS. Although infection may not be an initial part of this process, a concurrent pneumonia must be carefully considered.

Aspiration Pneumonia

Aspiration pneumonia should be treated with broad spectrum antibiotic coverage that focuses on ventilator associated pneumonia pathogens. Preemptive anaerobic coverage is not indicated, unless the patient presents with risk factors such as severe periodontal disease, necrotizing pneumonia, or lung abscesses. Cultures should be taken early, and antibiotic coverage should be narrowed down to the resulting pathogens as quickly as possible.

Suction

If the aspirate is a nonparticulate fluid, there is no indication for bronchoscopy as the fluid will quickly disperse. In particulate fluid aspiration, routine bronchoscopy or suctioning is not indicated, because there is a potential to push the aspirate more distally into the lungs and involve previously unaffected tissue. Lavage is also not routinely indicated for the same reason. However, if there is clear radiographic evidence of lobar collapse or severe atelectasis, or if there is a concern regarding antibiotic efficacy, a bronchoalveolar lavage may help open up these collapsed regions and also help identify the offending organism.

Antibiotics

Antibiotics are not routinely recommended for patients with pulmonary aspiration unless the aspirate is thought to be from a clearly infectious source. Gastric contents are generally sterile, but tracking along the hypopharynx can carry otherwise innocuous bacterial flora into the lungs. In immunocompromised patients, such an aspirate may require antibiotic intervention. Patients who aspirate nonsterile water, such as pond or river water during drowning, should be given an appropriate broad antibiotic coverage.

Steroids

No benefits have been shown from the use of large dose steroids and in one study there was a higher risk of gram-negative infection in a patient who had received steroid therapy.

Postoperative Pain Relief: Pharmacologic

Jessica Sumski, MD, Kelly Arwari, MD, and Tanya Lutzker, MD

Postoperative pain control begins in the preoperative period through careful assessment of the patient's medical history and anticipated procedure. A multimodal approach to pharmacological therapies should be considered, combining different medication to decrease overall pain scores.

OPIOIDS

Opioids act by G-protein coupled receptors. They work on nociceptive systems by mimicking endogenous ligands. Opioid receptor binding increases K^+ conductance, causing hyperpolarization and Ca^{2+} channel inactivation. This decreases neurotransmitter release. Opioids also inhibit gamma-aminobutyric acid (GABA) transmission, thus inhibiting descending pain pathways. Commonly used opioid medications are discussed below:

Morphine

Morphine is a hydrophilic, opioid receptor agonist with typical onset from 15 to 30 minutes and duration of action around 3-4 hours. Morphine undergoes hepatic glucuronidation, producing the active metabolite, morphine-6-glucuronide, which causes analgesia and respiratory depression. Morphine-3-glucuronide, another metabolite, is pharmacologically inactive but may cause agitation, myoclonus, delirium, and hyperalgesia. Morphine is metabolized by the liver and excreted renally. It can be associated with prolonged sedation and respiratory depression in renal failure patients.

Fentanyl

Intravenous (IV) fentanyl administration provides immediate onset with analgesia that lasts 30 minutes to 1 hour. Fentanyl is a lipid soluble selective mu receptor agonist. It is 80 times more potent than IV morphine. Fentanyl is metabolized by the liver into inactive metabolites and excreted in urine and bile. It is a good choice of analgesic in renal failure patients.

Sufentanil

Sufentanil has an immediate onset when delivered IV. Sufentanil can last 30 minutes to 1 hour. Sufentanil is 1000 times more potent than IV morphine. It is known for a smaller volume of distribution than fentanyl. Compared to fentanyl, sufentanil administration may be associated with higher rates of respiratory depression and bradycardia. It undergoes liver and small intestine metabolism.

Meperidine

Meperidine's typical onset is 5-7 minutes with duration of 2-4 hours. Meperidine is one-tenth as potent as morphine. It acts via mu, kappa, and delta receptor activation. It is typically used for short-term management of acute pain or for the treatment of postoperative shivering. It undergoes liver metabolism. Repetitive doses may cause buildup of the active metabolite normeperidine, which can cause seizures, myoclonus, and tremulousness. Meperidine should not be used with MAOIs, as it may cause *serotonin syndrome*. Also, meperidine is not used in renal or central nervous system (CNS) disease. Finally, meperidine administration may be associated with mild anticholinergic effects, such as increased heart rate and mydriasis.

Hydromorphone

Hydromorphone is 4-6 times more potent than morphine. It has a quick onset (15 minutes) and a long duration (4-5 hours). Hydromorphone is metabolized by the liver into active metabolites and excreted in urine. It is known to produce fewer opioid-related side effects than morphine.

Codeine

Codeine is another opioid analgesic with a rapid onset of 15 minutes to 1 hour, and a long duration of action 3-4 hours. It is used with caution in pediatric patients as it may cause respiratory depression. It is metabolized by liver and excreted in urine. The active metabolite of codeine is morphine.

Oxycodone

Oxycodone has an onset within 60 minutes. Its duration of action depends on preparation (immediate release vs extended release). Oxycodone is metabolized in the liver and excreted in urine. The active metabolite of oxycodone is oxymorphone.

Methadone

Methadone has a quick onset of 10-20 minutes when administered IV, and duration of 3-6 hours. It is a mu receptor agonist, NMDA receptor antagonist, and monoamine transmitter reuptake inhibitor. When given orally, it can be absorbed from gastrointestinal tract with 80% bioavailability. It is metabolized in the liver by cytochrome P450 to inactive metabolites. Methadone is excreted in urine and bile. It can be associated with cumulative toxicity; with repeated administration, it can accumulate in tissue and can be re-released.

DISSOCIATIVE ANALGESICS

Ketamine

Ketamine is a sedative-hypnotic, NMDA receptor antagonist. It acts as an Na^+ channel blocker, but also has effects on opioid receptors, cholinergic receptors, and monoaminergic receptors. Ketamine is highly lipid soluble. It has an onset in 30-60 seconds, and lasts 15-20 minutes. Ketamine is metabolized in the liver via N-demethylation by cytochrome P450, and it is excreted in urine. The active metabolite of ketamine is norketamine, which is less potent than ketamine. Ketamine administration results in a dissociative state, hallucinations, anesthesia, and analgesia. Ketamine is a sialagogue and bronchodilator, causing minimal respiratory depression.

NONSTEROIDAL ANTI-INFLAMMATORY DRUGS

Nonsteroidal anti-inflammatory agents (NSAIDs) provide anti-inflammatory action, analgesia, and antipyresis. They block COX-1 and COX-2 enzymes, preventing the conversion of arachidonic acid to prostaglandin. Peripherally, prostaglandins sensitize nociceptors to histamine and bradykinin, which lead to hyperalgesia. Centrally, prostaglandins enhance pain transmission through the dorsal horn. NSAIDs are not typically used in patients with renal disease, gastrointestinal bleeds, or platelet dysfunction. *Ketorolac* is an IV NSAID that has more analgesic than anti-inflammatory effects. It has an onset of 45 minutes to 1 hour, and duration of 2-6 hours. *Celecoxib* is COX-2 specific inhibitor and therefore does not inhibit platelet function. It should be avoided in patients with sulfa allergy and coronary disease.

OTHER DRUGS

Acetaminophen has analgesic and antipyretic properties. It works synergistically with other analgesics (Percocet, Vicodin, Tylenol #3). It inhibits COX-3, decreasing prostaglandin production in the CNS. The liver metabolizes acetaminophen. Acetaminophen has fewer gastrointestinal side effects than NSAIDs.

Calcium channel α-2-δ antagonists (gabapentin, pregabalin) are commonly used for neuropathic and postoperative pain. They prevent development of central excitability and have synergistic effects with NSAIDs. Side effects include somnolence, dizziness, confusion, and ataxia. The half-life is 5-7 hours and they are excreted in urine.

Cyclobenzaprine is a spasmolytic drug that has anticholinergic effect similar to TCAs. Cyclobenzaprine should not be administered with MAOIs. It undergoes liver metabolism and urinary excretion.

SUGGESTED READING

American Society of Anesthesiologists. Practice guidelines for acute pain management in the perioperative setting: an updated report by the American Society of Anesthesiologists Task Force on Acute Pain Management.

Postoperative Pain Relief: Routes

Jessica Sumski, MD, Kelly Arwari, MD, and Tanya Lutzker, MD

Route of administration is one of the determinants of effective postoperative analgesia. Each route has risks and benefits described below. The most widely used are intravenous and oral due to their greater predictability and ease of delivery. Other methods of treatment may become important when standard routes of administration are not available.

INTRAVENOUS

Intravenous (IV) medication administration is the most common approach to postoperative pain relief due to ease of delivery, speed of onset, and variety of medications available. Since most patients have an IV placed for their procedure, it is also a guaranteed access point for medications. If a patient does not have IV access, though, this may not be an option.

Pain medications can be delivered via IV either by healthcare team or through patient-controlled analgesia (PCA). PCA often results in improved patient satisfaction scoring due to the immediacy and control over the delivery of pain medication. Some studies have shown that PCA administration reduces total opioid administered. Nevertheless, patient pain scores are equivocal to nurse/staff administered IV pain medication.

Patient-controlled analgesia requires patient comprehension, cooperation, and physical ability to depress a button. Also, PCA introduces susceptibility to patient, family, or staff misuse. Finally, there is a risk of dosing errors if machines are not set properly.

Common drug choices for IV administration for postoperative pain include: fentanyl, sufentanil, morphine, meperidine, hydromorphone, methadone, Ketorolac, and acetaminophen.

ORAL (POSTOPERATIVE)

Orally administered medications are another commonly used method of postoperative (PO) pain control. The PO route is particularly useful in the ambulatory surgery setting. Administration by this route generally has a longer duration of action and allows patients to reach a comfortable state of pain control prior to discharge. This route is easy to use and can be used to control pain in patients without IV access.

The PO route is suboptimal for treatment of severe pain because of limited titration ability and prolonged time to peak effect. It is also not tolerated in patients with postoperative nausea or vomiting. Oral administration of medications may have low bioavailability, and increased side effects with the higher doses required for therapeutic effect.

Common drug choices for PO administration for postoperative pain include: morphine, meperidine, methadone, hydromorphone, oxycodone IR, NSAIDs, and acetaminophen.

INTRAMUSCULAR

The intramuscular (IM) route involves medication injection into the muscle body. The benefit of using this route is the ability to deliver medications without IV access. This route also works for patients unable to tolerate PO. Problems associated with IM administration are pain on injection as well as residual pain at the site of injection. The delivery system via this route is unpredictable because of wide swings in drug concentration, requiring frequent monitoring after administration.

Common drug choices include: fentanyl, morphine, and Ketorolac.

SUBCUTANEOUS

Administration via the subcutaneous route involves administration of drug directly under the dermal layer into subcutaneous fat for systemic absorption. Subcutaneous injection is less painful than an IM injection of medication. It is an option in patients without an IV who are unable to tolerate PO. This route has varied absorption and requires larger doses of medication for effect.

Common drug choices include: fentanyl, hydromorphone.

MUCOSAL ABSORPTION

Mucosal administration of pain medications involves the absorption of medication across mucus membranes into systemic circulation. Routes available for mucosal administration include per rectum (PR), transdermal, sublingual, and transmucosal. This route can be administered without IV or PO access. Absorption via this route can be slow, limiting the ability to provide immediate postoperative pain control. The amount of absorption and effect of the medications cannot be as easily predicted as IV administration.

Common drug choices for transmucosal administration include: fentanyl, hydromorphone, acetaminophen, fentanyl patch, and lidocaine patch.

NEURAXIAL BLOCKADE

Neuraxial blockade includes both epidural and intrathecal routes. Single shot intrathecal injection for postoperative pain control has limited use due to time-limited duration and inability to redose.

Epidural pain control, on the other hand, enjoys widespread use for postoperative pain control. Opioids administered via epidural directly target mu opioid receptors in the spinal cord's substantia gelatinosa. Epidural opioids also diffuse across the dura for systemic absorption with central effects. Typically, opioids administered via epidural are not associated with sympathetic denervation, skeletal muscle weakness, or loss of proprioception, thus allowing patients to ambulate while receiving pain control.

The level of analgesia provided depends on the amount of medication, rate of infusion, and catheter or injection level. Epidurals can be placed at caudal, lumbar, thoracic or, less commonly, cervical spinal levels. In general, patients have improved pain scores with the combination of epidural opioids and local anesthetics as compared to either alone.

Drawbacks to using neuraxial anesthesia for postoperative pain control are: procedural pain, difficult placement, positioning limitations, and anticoagulation requirements.

If a patient is expected to be on anticoagulation regimen in the postoperative period, the epidural injection, catheter placement and removal must be carefully timed with anticoagulant dosing to minimize hematoma risk. Side effects from epidural medicine administration are pruritus, nausea, urinary retention, and respiratory depression.

Common neuraxially administered drugs include: fentanyl, sufentanil, morphine, meperidine, hydromorphone, and local anesthetics.

PERIPHERAL NERVE BLOCKS

Nerve blocks are commonly administered in the preoperative setting to provide pain relief in the intraoperative as well as postoperative setting. They can be performed postoperatively as well. Local anesthetics are typically injected or infused, resulting in anesthesia in the distribution of the peripheral nerve blocked.

TRANSCUTANEOUS ELECTRICAL STIMULATION

Transcutaneous electrical stimulation (TENS) involves the placement of transcutaneous electrodes to deliver a current resulting in nerve excitation. Continuous excitation of electrode stimulated nerves results in overstimulation and downregulation of pain pathway impulse transmission.

TENS is associated with decreased postoperative analgesic agent use and is useful as an adjunct with other therapies. It can be administered without IV or PO access. The effectiveness of this method to reduce pain has been disputed. The actual electrical stimulation used during TENS can be quite painful to some patients.

Postoperative Pain Relief: Alternative Techniques

Nima Adimi, MD, Rohini Battu, MD, and Neil Lee, MD

NEURAXIAL BLOCKADE

Epidural or intrathecal injection of local anesthetic with or without opioid can control postoperative pain. Lumbar epidural placement can be used for postoperative pain control following major abdominal, pelvic, or lower extremity surgeries. Epidural medication can also be introduced via a catheter through the sacrococcygeal membrane using a caudal technique for groin, pelvic, or lower extremity surgeries. Thoracic epidurals can be used to control pain after thoracic surgery, upper and lower abdominal surgery, and after multiple rib fractures. Useful landmarks to help approximate the puncture site are the C7 spinous process, the scapular spine (T3), and the inferior border of the scapula (T7).

Epidural analgesia has been shown to decrease the incidence of venous and pulmonary thromboembolism, limit cardiac complications due to increased coronary blood flow, and improve myocardial oxygen balance. Epidural analgesia reduces the incidence of postoperative pneumonia, atelectasis, and respiratory depression. Patients also require less parenteral opioids, which decrease the risk of postoperative ileus and results in earlier return of gastrointestinal function.

Contraindications to Neuraxial Blockade

Since neuraxial blockade requires the cooperation of an "awake" patient, neuraxial blockade is contraindicated with uncooperative patients. In some cases, an exception may be made to perform neuraxial blockade under anesthesia. Local infection at the site of spinal or epidural placement is another contraindication. Spinal and epidural anesthesia frequently results in sympathetic blockade and subsequent hypotension. Therefore, neuraxial blockade should be avoided in patients with severe hypovolemia, sepsis, or aortic stenosis in which a precipitous reduction in afterload would exacerbate cardiac dysfunction. There is a risk of brainstem herniation in patients with increased intracranial pressure who receive neuraxial blockade; therefore, increased intracranial pressure should negate consideration of neuraxial blockade. Coagulopathy is a contraindication to neuraxial blockade due to the risk of neuraxial hematoma formation. It is important to check platelet levels, noting absolute number, rate of change, conditions that may affect platelet quality (ie, preeclampsia), and any anticoagulant medications or herbal remedies the patient is taking to properly assess for coagulopathy.

Anticoagulation and Neuraxial Blockade

Patients are frequently placed on anticoagulation while in the hospital for thromboprophylaxis. It is always important to document when a patient last received anticoagulation as there is a possible risk of neuraxial hematoma. The American Society of Regional Anesthesia and Pain Medicine's guidelines summarize the anticoagulation status and when to safely perform or discontinue neuraxial blockade.

Adjuncts to Local Anesthetic

Vasoconstrictors, such as epinephrine, can be added to the local anesthetic injectate. They help to decrease the uptake of the local anesthetic, thereby increasing the duration and density of the blockade.

Opioids can also be added to local anesthetic or can be the sole agent used for pain control. The most commonly used opioids are morphine and fentanyl. The time of onset and duration of action relates to an opioids' lipid solubility. Morphine is less lipophilic, extending the onset and duration of action on the mu opioid receptors in the dorsal horn. Morphine takes approximately 45 minutes until onset and can last for 18-24 hours. Fentanyl is more lipid soluble and thus has a more rapid onset and offset time than morphine.

PERIPHERAL NERVE BLOCKS

Upper Extremity Peripheral Nerve Blockade

Surgical anesthesia and postoperative analgesia of the upper extremity can be achieved by anesthetizing the brachial plexus. The brachial plexus comprises the ventral rami of the fifth cervical through first thoracic nerve roots. The nerves first converge to form trunks that pass between the anterior and middle scalene muscles, and are vertically arranged in a superior, middle, and inferior trunk. The trunks then pass over the lateral border of the first rib and under the clavicle where they divide into anterior and posterior divisions.

Interscalene Nerve Block

The interscalene nerve block is used primarily for procedures of the shoulder and upper arm. It targets brachial plexus roots and trunks, which pass between the anterior and middle scalene muscles. The C5-C6 nerve roots form the superior trunk of the brachial plexus, innervating a majority of the shoulder. Interscalene nerve block side effects include block of the stellate ganglion, phrenic nerve, and recurrent laryngeal nerve due to their proximity to the brachial plexus. Stellate ganglion anesthesia results in Horner syndrome: myosis, ptosis, and anhidrosis. Phrenic nerve (C3-C5) anesthesia results in unilateral diaphragmatic paralysis. Otherwise healthy individuals with phrenic nerve block may remain asymptomatic. However, those with poor pulmonary status may begin to exhibit dyspnea and respiratory failure. This procedure should not be done in patients with contralateral lung pathology (ie, pneumonia, pleural effusion, lobectomy). Recurrent laryngeal nerve anesthesia can lead to hoarseness and ipsilateral vocal cord paralysis. Contralateral vocal cord impairment or paralysis may occur with interscalene nerve block. The vertebral artery is in close proximity to this part of the brachial plexus. Inadvertent intraarterial local anesthetic injection at this location may produce seizures. Finally, pneumothorax is a potential complication of brachial plexus blockade.

Supraclavicular Nerve Block

The supraclavicular block approaches the brachial plexus at the level of the trunks where they are more closely packed together. This results in anesthesia of the entire arm. It is used for elbow, wrist, and hand surgery. The incidence of pneumothorax is higher with this block compared to others. The same complications discussed for interscalene blocks apply to supraclavicular blocks.

Infraclavicular Nerve Block

Infraclavicular block approaches the brachial plexus at the level of the cords and is used for surgery performed on the wrist and hand. Complications are the same as supraclavicular blocks, but less frequent.

Lower Extremity Peripheral Nerve Blockade

Three peripheral nerve blocks most commonly control postoperative pain in the lower extremity: femoral, sciatic (at the popliteal fossa), and ankle. Peripheral nerve blocks can be used to control pain, decrease oral and intravenous opioid requirements, and decrease the amount of time until ambulation.

Femoral Nerve Block

The femoral nerve block is commonly used to control pain after surgical procedures involving the knee, including arthroscopy, arthroplasty, and fracture repair. The femoral nerve originates from the posterior branches of L2 through L4 nerve roots. The nerve passes anterior to the iliopsoas muscle under the inguinal ligament and lateral to the femoral artery and nerve. It provides sensation to the anterior thigh and knee. The femoral nerve then gives rise to the saphenous nerve and provides sensation to the medial aspects of the calf, ankle, and foot. Thus, femoral nerve blocks frequently spare the posterior part of the knee.

Supine positioning is appropriate for this block. If nerve stimulation is used for placement, quadriceps femoris muscle response or patellar twitch is used to help guide accurate nerve localization. The femoral nerve's proximity to the femoral artery and vein introduces intravascular injection risk and systemic local anesthetic toxicity.

Sciatic Nerve Block

The popliteal fossa block targets the sciatic nerve, which is formed by the anterior rami of L4 to S3. The sciatic nerve provides almost complete sensation to the distal leg below the knee. It spares the medial portion of the leg and controls pain after foot and ankle procedures.

The sciatic nerve divides into two major branches at the popliteal fossa: common peroneal and tibial nerves. Proper popliteal block injects local anesthetic perineurally prior to sciatic nerve bifurcation into common peroneal and tibial nerves. If the block is performed from a posterior approach (prone position), the needle inserts approximately 7 cm superior to the popliteal crease and midpoint between the biceps femoris tendon laterally and the semitendinosus and semimembranosus muscles medially. The block can also be accomplished in the supine position with a lateral approach. Specific contraindications include preexisting sciatic neuropathy. Possible complications include infection, hematoma, intravascular injection, and neural injury with persistent foot drop.

Ankle Block

The ankle block is performed for foot procedures. It is mainly an infiltration block and does not require the facilitation of muscle twitch response. Motor blockade is not essential and less concentrated local anesthetics can be used. Also, epinephrine should not be used in conjunction with local anesthetics for the block due to the risk of vasoconstriction and ischemia. An adequate block anesthetizes the four branches of the sciatic nerve, femoral terminus, and the saphenous nerve. The four branches of the sciatic nerve are : (1) the deep peroneal nerve that provides sensation to the first web space of the foot; (2) the superficial peroneal nerve that provides sensation of the skin over the dorsum of the foot; (3) the posterior tibial nerve that provides sensation to the calcaneus and plantar surface of the foot; and (4) the sural nerve that provides cutaneous sensation to the lateral ankle and foot, and also the fifth digit. The saphenous nerve provides sensation to the medial aspect of the ankle and foot, and is a branch of the femoral nerve.

General Considerations, Complications, and Contraindications

With any peripheral nerve block, the use of ultrasonographic guidance and nerve stimulation result in improved nerve localization, local anesthesia delivery, and pain control while decreasing risks. All blocks discussed above with the exception of the ankle block can be performed as a single shot or a catheter can be placed for a continuous infusion.

General complications that apply to any peripheral nerve blockade include infection and abscess formation, bleeding and hematoma formation, intravascular injection, and possible intraneural injection with nerve injury. Contraindications to peripheral nerve blockade include infection at the site of placement, coagulopathy, and patient's inability to cooperate.

FIELD BLOCKS

Subpleural and subcutaneous catheters may be inserted to infuse local anesthetic solutions postoperatively. Typically, surgeons place catheters under direct visualization during wound closure.

Paravertebral Blocks

Paravertebral blocks are performed to control pain during breast surgery, thoracic surgery, hip surgery, and after rib fractures. Local anesthetic injected into the paravertebral space, which contains the spinal nerves as they exit the intervertebral foramina, results in ipsilateral somatic and sympathetic nerve blockade in a dermatomal distribution. They can be performed at any spinal level. Complications include pneumothorax, intravascular injection, and unintended epidural or intrathecal injection.

Transverse Abdominus Plane Blocks

Transverse abdominus plane (TAP) blocks are used to control pain after abdominal surgeries, including total abdominal hysterectomy, cesarean delivery, and laparotomy with bowel resection. Local anesthetic is delivered in the fascial plane between the transversus abdominis muscle and the internal oblique muscle, blocking somatic afferents from T8-L1 anterior abdominal wall dermatomes. Bilateral blocks provide optimum pain control for midline incisions. TAP blocks help to control somatic incisional pain, but additional oral and intravenous analgesics are required to control visceral pain from surgery. Specific complications for this block include bowel puncture. Reports of liver puncture have also been reported. The use of ultrasound guidance for this technique helps reduce the risk of intra-abdominal viscera puncture.

SUGGESTED READINGS

Fredrickson MJ, Krishnan S, Chen CY. Postoperative analgesia for shoulder surgery: a critical appraisal and review of current techniques. *Anaesthesia* 2010;65:608-624.

Rawal N. Epidural technique for postoperative pain: gold standard no more? *Reg Anesth Pain Med.* 2012;37:310-317.

Postoperative Respiratory Complications

Nima Adimi, MD, Rohini Battu, MD, and Neil Lee, MD

Postoperative pulmonary complications are the second most common complication, following nausea and vomiting, in the postanesthesia care unit (PACU). Anesthetic, surgical, and patient factors contribute to the likelihood of pulmonary complications. Hypoxia in the PACU can be divided into two categories: hypoventilation with a low PAO_2, or impaired O_2 exchange with a decreased alveolar-arterial gradient.

ATELECTASIS

Atelectasis due to anesthesia occurs in almost all patients. It leads to ventilation-perfusion mismatch or dead space ventilation and hypoxemia. Atelectasis occurs as a result of respiratory physiology changes caused by anesthetic medications, positioning, pain, and mechanical limitations imposed by surgery, pregnancy, or obesity. Loss of respiratory muscle coordination and tone leads to abnormal chest wall function, decreased lung volumes, and reduced capacities. Impaired gas exchange and surfactant function also lead to atelectasis. Atelectasis occurs in dependent lung fields.

Development of atelectasis can be decreased by using adequate positive-end expiratory pressure (PEEP) and by using recruitment maneuvers intraoperatively. In the PACU, use of incentive spirometry and noninvasive ventilation therapy such as continuous positive airway pressure (CPAP) limit atelectasis and hypoxemia.

BRONCHOSPASM

Bronchospasm and increased airway resistance are likely to occur in patients with reactive airways such as asthma or chronic pulmonary disease (COPD). Pharyngeal and tracheal stimulation from secretions, aspiration, or suctioning can trigger constriction of bronchial smooth muscle. In a patient who is intubated, bronchospasm will manifest as high peak airway pressures, low tidal volumes, and high end-tidal carbon dioxide. In a spontaneously ventilating patient, a patient will exhibit labored breathing with retraction of accessory muscles. Treatment is aimed at the underlying etiology and includes inhaled albuterol, intravenous anticholinergics, and though it does not act acutely, intravenous steroids. If treatment is resistant, then IV epinephrine should be administered.

PNEUMONIA

Anesthesia can decrease the lung's defense mechanisms and lead to pneumonia. Anesthetic changes in the lung include impaired cough, forced vital capacity, mucociliary clearance, surfactant function, and alveolar macrophage activity. Bacteria enter the airways via aspiration or endotracheal tube contamination as it passes through the oral cavity. Factors that increase pneumonia risk include intubation greater than 48 hours, age over 65 years, COPD, prolonged surgery, trauma or emergency surgery, and intraoperative transfusion.

HYPOVENTILATION

Hypoventilation can be defined as $Paco_2$ greater than 45 mm Hg. Severe hypoventilation with respiratory acidosis causing circulatory depression occurs with $Paco_2$ levels greater than 60 or pH less than 7.25. Conditions leading to hypoventilation include:

Obstruction

The most common cause of airway obstruction in the PACU is relaxation and weakness of pharyngeal muscles due to residual anesthetic, neuromuscular blockade, or opioids. Patients with obstructive sleep apnea (OSA) are more prone to obstruction and high dosages of sedating medications should be used cautiously. Maneuvers such as jaw thrust and chin lift help bring the base of the tongue anterior, alleviating supraglottic inlet obstruction. Patients with OSA may require CPAP while in the PACU to prevent obstruction.

Other causes of obstruction include laryngospasm (children > adults, electrolyte abnormalities), airway edema (due to airway manipulation, head down positioning, extensive fluid therapy), hematoma, and foreign bodies such as surgical packs.

CO_2 and Opioid Narcosis

Volatile anesthetics and opioids decrease CO_2 sensitivity in the brain's respiratory center, which diminishes respiratory drive and results in decreased respiratory rate and tidal volume. Opioid-induced narcosis can be reversed with 0.04 mg of naloxone every 5 minutes. Treatment also includes supportive care with noninvasive positive pressure ventilation such as CPAP.

Neuromuscular Weakness

Prolonged neuromuscular relaxation or inadequate reversal can lead to residual paralysis manifested as airway obstruction, inability to overcome airway resistance, decreased airway protection, and inability to clear secretions. Prior to extubation, patients' strength should be tested via sustained head lift, adequate tidal volumes, negative inspiratory pressure of 25 cm H_2O and train-of-four testing. Patients not meeting these criteria should remain intubated until muscular blockade has worn off or can be appropriately reversed. Prolonged muscular blockade may be due to early reversal administration, pseudocholinesterase deficiency, or renal failure. Patients with neuromuscular disorders such as myasthenia gravis or muscular dystrophy are more sensitive to muscle relaxants, and often have decreased ventilatory status without the use of muscle relaxants.

PULMONARY EMBOLUS

Pulmonary embolus (PE) is usually rare in the immediate postoperative period, but should always be included in the differential in patients with symptomatic hypoventilation. PE results from deep vein thrombosis, fat emboli after long bone surgery, or amniotic fluid emboli following childbirth. Signs include hypoxia, tachycardia, chest pain and, if severe, right heart failure.

SUGGESTED READINGS

Cook M, Lisco S. Prevention of postoperative pulmonary complications. *Int Anesthesiol Clin.* 2009;47:65-88.

Gerardo T, Bohm S, Warner D, Sprung J. Atelectasis and perioperative pulmonary complications in high-risk patients. *Current Opin Anesth.* 2012;25:1-10.

Postoperative Cardiovascular Complications

Nima Adimi, MD, Rohini Battu, MD, and Neil Lee, MD

Cardiac complications occurring in the postanesthetic care unit (PACU) are typically due to hypotension, hypertension, and dysrhythmias. Patients with known coronary artery disease or congestive heart failure are more prone to these complications after surgical procedure.

HYPOTENSION

Decreased intravascular volume, or hypovolemia is due to inadequate intravenous fluid administration or blood loss. Patients can be resuscitated with crystalloids, colloids, and various blood products. If fluid resuscitation is inadequate to perfuse end organs, then vasopressors and inotropes should be added.

Myocardial ischemia with acute heart failure and ventricular or valvular dysfunction can also lead to hypotension. This may be associated with tachycardia and ST segment changes on electrocardiogram. A history of coronary artery disease predisposes patients to these complications and should be noted on preoperative evaluation. Drug-eluting stents typically require antiplatelet therapy for surgical procedures; if antiplatelet therapy is halted, patients may be at increased risk for acute coronary events. Suspected coronary thrombosis requires immediate evaluation for cardiac catheterization.

Decreased systemic vascular resistance in the PACU setting is usually iatrogenic and leads to hypotension. Disease states that cause decreased SVR include sepsis, spinal shock from spinal cord injury, and histamine release during anaphylactic reactions. While supportive measures are instituted, the underlying cause should be identified and treated. Residual effects of anesthetics, including inhalational, intravenous, and neuraxial agents, also produce hypotension. Treatment is indicated if mean arterial pressure is 20% less than baseline.

HYPERTENSION

Pain is a common cause of hypertension in the PACU. Surgical trauma and pain cause increased sympathetic tone leading to hypertension and tachycardia. Multimodal pain management strategies are preferable.

Hypercarbia from respiratory failure also leads to hypertension. Treatment includes promoting effective gas exchange via invasive or noninvasive, positive pressure ventilation.

Urinary retention and bladder distention are a common cause of hypertension in the PACU. It is more common after inguinal hernia repair, neuraxial anesthesia, and in elderly men with prostatic obstruction. Patients may require bladder catheterization.

Patients who remain intubated in the PACU, if not adequately sedated, may become hypertensive from irritation of the endotracheal tube.

ARRHYTHMIAS

Arrhythmias occur often in the PACU and some can be life threatening. If cardiac arrest should occur, PACU treatment may have to be tailored to accommodate surgical incisions. Thorough review of current Advance Cardiac Life Support (ACLS) algorithms should be reviewed.

Bradycardia in the PACU can be due to vasovagal reflexes, residual effects of anticholinesterases, β-blockers, or opioids. Bradycardia may also result from severe myocardial infarction with complete heart block. The ACLS algorithm should be consulted for unstable bradycardia. Anticholinergic medications and pacing options must be readily available.

Sinus tachycardia can be due to pain, hypovolemia, fever, sepsis, or certain drugs such as albuterol or anticholinergics.

Atrial fibrillation commonly occurs in patients after cardiac or thoracic surgery. Either rhythm control, using drugs such as amiodarone, or rate control using β-blockers or nondihydropyridine Ca^{2+} channel blockers may be used for management. Unstable blood pressure requires cardioversion.

Premature ventricle contractions are usually due to electrolyte abnormalities, which should be corrected.

Tachydysrhythmias (ventricular fibrillation and ventricular tachycardia) and pulseless electrical activity should be treated according to current ACLS guidelines. However, the differential diagnosis for cardiac arrest remains unchanged and includes: hypoxia, hypovolemia, hyperkalemia, hypokalemia, hydrogen ions (acidosis), hypoglycemia, toxins (anaphylaxis, anesthetics), tension pneumothorax, thrombus, tamponade, QT prolongation, and pulmonary hypertension.

Postoperative Neuromuscular Complications

114

Nima Adimi, MD, Rohini Battu, MD, and Neil Lee, MD

The use of paralytics has become common in modern surgical care; yet these drugs pose risk, particularly during the recovery process. To minimize the duration of acute adverse effects, it is important to consider certain factors that may amplify or prolong the effects of paralytic agent postsurgery. These factors include: (1) residual blockade; (2) preexisting neuromuscular diseases; and (3) conditions that may mimic residual blockade.

RESIDUAL BLOCKADE

Residual blockade is the most common neuromuscular complication encountered during a patient's postanesthetic care unit (PACU) course. Each case varies in severity and has a multitude of factors influencing the outcome. Some stem from the types of paralytic used (mechanism of action), others from inadequate reversal administration and/or suboptimal monitoring throughout the procedure. In general, residual blockade can cause serious complications, which include, but are not limited to: hypoxemia, upper airway obstruction, prolonged PACU visit, prolonged ventilator time, and postoperative pulmonary complications.

DEPOLARIZING VERSUS NONDEPOLARIZING AGENTS

There are two main types of paralytics used in anesthesia. Depolarizing agents (ie, succinylcholine) are direct acetylcholine receptor agonists that bind to the acetylcholine receptor and propagate action potentials. Since they are not metabolized by acetylcholinesterase, prolonged depolarization occurs, leaving the end plate unable to repolarize, which in turn causes Phase I blockade. Eventually, the depolarizing agent leaves the neuromuscular junction and becomes metabolized by pseudocholinesterase in the plasma. The nondepolarizing agents (ie, rocuronium, veruronium) act as competitive antagonists at the acetylcholine receptor site. They block the binding of acetylcholine to its receptor, preventing an action potential from occurring. The nondepolarizing agent's reversal is dictated by the rate of redistribution and metabolism, making its half-life longer than that of a depolarizing agent.

REVERSAL

Due to the mechanism of action, nondepolarizing agent more commonly causes residual neuromuscular blockade in the PACU than depolarizing agent. This complication can be avoided by administering the appropriate amount of reversal prior to emergence. The most common reversal agents used are cholinesterase inhibitors (ie, neostigmine, pyridostigmine). These are routinely administered with anticholinergic agents (eg, glycopyrrolate, atropine) to reduce the cholinergic effects.

MONITORING

The most common method of monitoring neuromuscular blockade in the operating room is train-of-four (ToF). ToF nerve stimulation consists of four supramaximal stimuli delivered in 0.5 seconds intervals. The degree of muscle response to the stimulation determines the level of blockade. The level of fade is directly proportional to the level of neuromuscular blockade, making ToF the gold standard of monitoring. The addition of ToF monitoring has significantly reduced the amount of residual blockade seen in the PACU. There are also secondary measures of neuromuscular blockade used such as: five-second head lift, grip testing, or eye opening. These are less reliable, but still used in addition to ToF monitoring.

EXISTING NEUROMUSCULAR DISEASE

Patients with existing neuromuscular diseases require special considerations when undergoing neuromuscular blockade. These diseases include, but are not limited to: multiple sclerosis, seizure disorders, Guillain–Barré syndrome, Parkinson disease, Alzheimer disease, autonomic dysfunction, and syringomyelia.

Multiple Sclerosis

In a case involving multiple sclerosis, it is important to avoid depolarizing agents such as succinylcholine to avoid hyperkalemia. This is particularly important in patients with paralysis or paresis, as the upregulation of extra-junctional receptors may cause hyperkalemic arrest.

Seizure Disorders

For cases involving seizure disorders, it is important to inquire regarding a patient's current medications list. Many antiepileptic medications increase the rate of metabolism of nondepolarizing agents. Consequently, frequent redosing might be required to maintain adequate blockade.

Guillain–Barré Syndrome

As in multiple sclerosis, when managing a case with Guillain–Barré, one should avoid using depolarizing agents such as succinylcholine because of possible hyperkalemia.

Parkinson Disease

In general, patients with Parkinson disease tolerate neuromuscular blockade without complications. Although rare, use of succinylcholine should still be avoided due to theoretical hyperkalemia.

Alzheimer Disease

No special consideration is needed with Alzheimer patients for neuromuscular blockade. When using reversal agents, glycopyrrolate is preferred to atropine since atropine is centrally acting and can lead to postoperative confusion. Glycopyrrolate does not cross the blood–brain barrier.

Autonomic Dysfunction

No special consideration needs to be taken in terms of neuromuscular blockade.

Syringomyelia

Many patients with syringomyelia have existing neurologic deficits as well as pulmonary compromise. Therefore, adequate reversal of neuromuscular blockade is especially important in cases involving this disease. As in most neuromuscular diseases, succinylcholine should be avoided due to hyperkalemia.

ELECTROLYTE MIMICRY OF RESIDUAL BLOCKADE

Hypercalcemia/Hypocalcemia

Hypercalcemia and to a lesser extent hypocalcemia can cause weakness, mimicking residual neuromuscular blockade. In a setting where this is anticipated, point-of-care measurement of ionized Ca^{2+} should be checked.

Magnesium Derangements

Both hypomagnesemia and hypermagnesemia can cause general weakness. These should be included in a differential for postoperative weakness.

SUGGESTED READINGS

Murphy GS, Brull SJ. Residual neuromuscular block: lessons unlearned. Part I: definitions, incidence, and adverse physiological effects of residual neuromuscular block. *Anesth Anal.* 2010;111:120-128.

Plaud B, Debaene B, Donati F, Marty J. Residual paralysis after emergence from anesthesia. *Anesthesiology* 2010;112:1013-1022.

Postoperative Nausea and Vomiting

Christopher Potestio, MD, and Lisa Bellil, MD

Postoperative nausea and vomiting (PONV) is a common complication of anesthesia, affecting 71 million patients per year. Without prophylactic treatment, PONV occurs in 20%-30% of the general population and up to 70%-80% of high-risk surgical patients. Because of its high prevalence, identifying risk factors for PONV and optimizing treatment is essential to the practice of operative anesthesia.

IDENTIFYING PONV

Patient Risks

Although many studies have aimed to identify risk factors for PONV, only a few baseline risk factors have been consistently identified: female gender, nonsmoking, and history of PONV or motion sickness. Additional risk factors that are less reliable include migraine, young age, anxiety, and low ASA risk classification.

In addition to these, many patient factors augment risk of PONV but are not actually independent risk factors. Factors that augment risk for PONV include obesity, anxiety, and antagonizing neuromuscular blockade with acetylcholinesterase inhibitors such as neostigmine.

Procedure Risks

Postoperative nausea and vomiting has also been associated with particular anesthesia techniques, including anesthesia with volatile anesthetics, nitrous oxide, and the use of postoperative opioids. These effects are dose-related, so longer procedures increase risk and so does increased postoperative opioid consumption. In fact, each 30 minute increase in duration of surgery increases PONV risk by 60%.

Type or surgery also correlates with incidence of PONV; however, it is unclear if this is a causal relationship. Abdominal and gynecological surgeries are often implicated, especially laparoscopic procedures where insufflation of the abdomen may play a role in increasing risk. The risk of PONV may also be increased during ear, nose, and throat surgeries where the eye is manipulated causing transient increase in intracranial pressure.

PREVENTION OF PONV

Avoiding Triggers of PONV

Limiting exposure to volatile anesthetics, nitrous oxide, and opioids in any manner will theoretically decrease risk. Patients receiving regional anesthesia are nine times less likely to experience PONV. Use of propofol for induction and maintenance of anesthesia decreases PONV during the first 6 hours of recovery. Avoiding nitrous oxide altogether can decrease incidence of PONV, and is a rather easy strategy in patients with risk factors considering other viable alternatives.

Tailoring a pain management plan to decrease opiate use can also minimize risk. Nonsteroidal anti-inflammatory drugs, cyclooxygenase-2 inhibitors, and gabapentinoids have been shown to have a morphine-sparing effect in the postoperative period and may help limit PONV related to opioid use.

Limiting reversal of neostigmine may possibly decrease risk of PONV, although the effect of neostigmine on PONV is not well established. The patient, surgical and anesthesia factors that increase the risk for PONV are listed in Table 115-1.

TABLE 115-1   Risk Factors for PONV

Patient factors (strong independent)	Female gender, nonsmoker, history of PONV or motion sickness
Patient factors (weak independent)	Migraine, young age, anxiety, and low ASA risk classification
Patient factors (not independent, but augment risk)	Obesity, anxiety
Surgical factors	Length of procedure > 30 min, laparoscopy, laparotomy, breast, strabismus, plastic surgery, maxillofacial, gynecological, abdominal, neurologic, ophthalmologic, urologic
Anesthesia factors	Volatile anesthetics, nitrous oxide, opioids, reversal with acetylcholinesterase inhibitor

Administration of Pharmacological Agents for PONV Prophylaxis

A. 5-HT3 Antagonists

First-line treatment for PONV prophylaxis is 5-hydroxytryptamine antagonists (5-HT3), the most common of which is ondansetron. Ondansetron has greater antivomiting than antinausea effects. At the recommended dose of 4 mg, the number needed to treat (NNT) to prevent vomiting is 6 and the NNT to prevent nausea is 7. Other 5-HT3 receptor antagonists include palonosetron, dolasetron, granisetron, and tropisetron. They are most effective when given at the end of surgery.

5-HT3 receptor antagonists have a favorable side effect profile, with headache, transaminitis, and constipation as the most common side effects. There are few contraindications, but 5-HT3 receptor antagonists should be avoided in patients with carcinoid tumors or patients taking SSRIs, as these medications are active in the serotonin system and have been implicated as a cause of serotonin syndrome when given with other serotonin modulating drugs. In addition, 5-HT3 receptor antagonists have been known to prolong QTc and should be avoided in patients with atrioventricular (AV) blocks.

B. Butyrophenones

Droperidol at recommended prophylactic dose of 0.625-1.25 mg IV has similar efficacy to ondansetron and dexamethasone and has an NNT of 5 to prevent PONV in the first 24 hours after surgery. Droperidol is most effective when administered at the end of surgery. A very effective antiemetic, droperidol has unfortunately fallen out of favor due to an FDA "black box" warning that restricts its use due to its association with significant cardiovascular events at higher doses. At doses used for PONV prophylaxis, droperidol is very unlikely to be associated with cardiovascular events.

Low dose haloperidol has been investigated as an alternative to droperidol for PONV prophylaxis. At doses of 0.5-2 mg, haloperidol reduces PONV risk with NNT around 5. No cardiovascular risk has been reported at this dose and there is a very low incidence of extrapyramidal symptoms.

C. Steroids

Dexamethasone, at the recommended prophylactic dose of 4 mg IV, should be given at induction rather than at the end of surgery. It has equivalent antinausea and antiemetic effect when compared to ondansetron 4 mg IV and droperidol 1.25 mg IV. No adverse events have been attributed to this single dose of dexamethasone.

D. Anticholinergics

Transdermal scopolamine has been established as a useful adjunct to other antiemetic therapies. For prevention of PONV with a scopolamine patch, the NNT is 6. Efficacy is best when applied the night before or 4 hours before the end of surgery due to its 2-4 hour onset. Scopolamine has a side effect profile similar to other anticholinergic medications, with most common side effects being visual disturbance, dry mouth, and dizziness.

E. Other Options

Phenothiazines (promethazine, prochlorperazine) and antihistamines (dimenhydrinate) are also used as PONV prophylaxis, but are not extensively studied, so optimal timing and dose has not been established.

Providing Prophylaxis for PONV

Patient risk factors can help identify patients in whom PONV prophylaxis is warranted. Using a model for predicting PONV can help establish whether a patient is high, medium, or low risk for PONV. Simplified risk scores by Apfel et al. provide simple, yet reliable prediction for adults and children, respectively (Figure 115-1). Similar models exist for PONV in children. These models are based on patient groups and not individual risk, so clinical judgment must guide assessment of risk.

By using simplified risk scores, it is easy to estimate risk. A patient with no risk factors has a 10% chance of developing PONV. Each additional risk factor discussed above adds roughly 10%-20% increase in risk of developing PONV.

For the low-risk adult population, no PONV prophylaxis is necessary. For medium-risk patients with 1-2 risk factors, one or two prophylaxis medications should be administered. For high-risk patients with more than two risk factors, a multimodal approach is warranted.

Multimodal Approach for High-Risk Patients

To maximize prophylaxis for high-risk patients, antiemetics from different classes should be combined. Dual therapy with a combination of 5-HT3 receptor antagonists, dexamethasone, and droperidol has been shown to be superior to monotherapy, with no combination superior to the others.

Anesthetic technique should be modified to minimize risk factors. Regional anesthesia should be considered, volatile agents, nitrous oxide, opiates, and neuromuscular blockers should be avoided if possible. Other strategies which have not been systematically reviewed but can be considered

Risk Points	Estimated Risk of PONV
1	20%
2	40%
3	60%
4	80%

FIGURE 115-1 Model for predicting PONV. 1 point given for statistically significant risk factors: female gender, nonsmoker, postoperative opioid use, previous PONV, or motion sickness.

include aggressive hydration, oxygen therapy, TIVA with propofol and remifentanil.

Strategies for Failed Prophylaxis or Absence of Prophylaxis

When PONV occurs, treatment should consist of an antiemetic from a pharmacological class different than the prophylactic drug given. Repeating the same medication given for PONV prophylaxis adds no additional benefit.

If no prophylaxis was given and the patient is experiencing PONV, then 5-HT3 antagonists are recommended at doses lower than those used for prophylaxis (eg, 1 mg of ondansetron is recommended for treatment of PONV, much less than the prophylactic dose of 4 mg). For other pharmacological classes, "rescue" doses are similar to prophylactic doses: dexamethasone 2-4 mg IV, droperidol 0.625 mg IV, promethazine 6.25-12.5 mg IV. Propofol 20 mg IV is equivalent to ondansetron and can be considered a rescue therapy.

Opioids for postoperative pain lead to nausea in one-third of patients. Adding 2.5 mg droperidol for every 100 mg morphine in a PCA was effective in reducing PONV. Also, many nonopioids have been shown to have opiate sparing effect, such as IV acetaminophen, Ketorolac, celecoxib, and pregabalin. These agents can be used to decrease risk of PONV by decreasing postoperative opiate use.

With the growing field of ambulatory surgery, postdischarge nausea and vomiting has become an increasing concern; 17% of patients experience nausea and 8% of patients vomit after discharge. Administration of prophylaxis may be warranted in high-risk groups, although no guidelines have been established.

SPECIAL CONSIDERATIONS IN CHILDREN

In children, the term postoperative vomiting (POV) is used because evaluation and measurement of nausea is difficult in nonverbal children. For children at risk for POV, guidelines suggest a more aggressive approach. Children are twice as likely to incur POV and therefore need a lower threshold for prophylaxis. Children who are at moderate or high risk for POV should receive combination therapy with two or three prophylactic drugs from different classes.

Ondansetron is the only 5-HT3 antagonist approved for pediatric age less than 2 years. Dolasetron is also recommended, but only for children older than 2 years of age. Dexamethasone, droperidol, dimenhydrinate, and perphenazine among other agents, have also been studied in children, although 5HT-3 antagonists have proved superior in meta-analysis and single studies.

SUGGESTED READINGS

Apfel CC. Philip BK, Cakmakkaya OS. Who is at risk for post-discharge nausea and vomiting after ambulatory surgery? *Anesthesiology* 2012;117;475-486.

Apfel CC, Kranke P, Eberhart LHJ, Roos A, Roewer N. Comparison of predictive models for postoperative nausea and vomiting. Br *J Anaesth*. 2002;88:234-240.

C H A P T E R

116

Cerebral Cortex and Subcortical Areas

Sarah Uddeen, MD, and Gregory Moy, MD

The brain is a highly complex and integrated organ that integrates and processes sensory and motor input. The brain can be categorized into the forebrain (prosencephalon), midbrain (mesencephalon), and hindbrain (rhombencephalon). The forebrain is further broken into the cerebral hemispheres, thalamus, and basal nuclei. The cerebral hemispheres have three layers which include the cerebral cortex, subcortical white matter (largely the internal capsule), and the basal ganglia.

The cerebral cortex is made up of gray matter and is a covering over the cerebral hemispheres. It is known as the center for higher intellectual processes. Sulci, or fissures, separate the cortex into the frontal, parietal, temporal, and occipital lobes. To increase the amount of surface area, the cortex has many gyri, or folds. There are many different types of nerve cells as well as layers of the cerebral cortex. Functionally, the cerebral cortex is divided into 47 different Brodmann areas.

MOTOR

The areas involved in motor movement include the primary motor cortex (Brodmann area 4), which is somatotopically organized as the motor homunculus. This area occupies the precentral gyrus. The area involved for each body part is proportional to the amount of complexity involved in movement, with the face, eyes, lips, mouth, and nose taking up at least half of the area. This area is responsible for voluntary movement on the opposite side of the body. Secondary areas involved in motor movement include the premotor cortex, supplementary motor area, frontal eye field, and posterior parietal motor area. All of these areas help prime and mediate complex

movements, which are eventually relayed and carried out by the primary motor complex.

SENSORY

The primary somatosensory cortex (Brodmann areas 3, 1, and 2) is responsible for receiving sensory information from the opposite side of the body. It is located in the postcentral gyrus and, like the primary motor cortex, is somatotopically arranged as a homunculus.

Vision input from the lateral geniculate nucleus goes to the primary visual cortex, which helps in processing color, motion, and three-dimensional vision. It is located on the lateral surface of the occipital lobe by the calcarine fissure. The primary visual cortex then sends signals to the visual association cortex, which helps in identifying objects, determining location, and determining visual significance based on prior experiences.

The primary auditory cortex receives information from both ears from the medial geniculate body of the thalamus. It helps detect pattern alteration and location of sound. It also receives information from the lateral geniculate nucleus and is arranged in a tonotopic manner in regard to frequencies, with higher frequencies being located more caudally. Sensory association areas help integrate sensory information from various systems.

SPEECH

Wernicke and Broca areas are the two areas that are involved with language. They are interconnected by the arcuate fasciculus, which is imperative for communication. In most people, the left hemisphere is dominant as far as language function. Wernicke area is part of the auditory association cortex and is known as the sensory language area. It is important for comprehending and formulating speech. Broca area is the motor speech area and communicates with the primary motor complex as well as supplementary motor area to initiate and produce speech as well as have an impact on individual expression of speech.

PREFRONTAL CORTEX

The prefrontal cortex is involved with forming an individual's personality. It functions to help regulate emotion, judgment, depth of feeling, working memory, and intelligence.

SUBCORTICAL AREAS

There are various structures below the cerebral cortex that are involved in brain function, called subcortical areas. These areas can be divided up and categorized by location as the forebrain, midbrain, and hindbrain.

The subcortical areas in the forebrain include the thalamus, hypothalamus, epithalamus, basal ganglia, and limbic system. The thalamus is made up of numerous nuclei that act as a relay station for processing a wide variety of information from motor, sensory, limbic, auditory, and visual systems. It also plays a large role in arousal. The hypothalamus is involved in controlling the autonomic nervous system (both sympathetic and parasympathetic), endocrine functions (pituitary), endocrinological responses, thermoregulation, and circadian rhythms. It also plays a role with the limbic system with memory. The epithalamus contains the pineal gland (produces melatonin) involved in the sleep–wake cycle. The basal ganglia mediate movement. Parkinson disease occurs when there is degeneration of dopaminergic neurons in the substantia nigra portion of the basal ganglia, causing hypokinesia, akinesia, shuffling gait, and rigidity. Huntington disease involves degeneration of the caudate and putamen portions of the basal ganglia, resulting in a hyperkinetic disorder (choreiform movements) and progressive dementia. The hippocampus and amygdala are both part of the limbic system. The hippocampus is involved with memory and learning. The amygdala determines how emotions, such as fear, affect memory and learning.

The brainstem is made up of the midbrain and hindbrain, which includes the medulla, pons, and cerebellum. These areas are involved in relaying sensory and motor information via tracts. They also contain some of the cranial nuclei. The medulla is involved in mediating respiration, circulation, and gastrointestinal motility through autonomic centers. Finally, the cerebellum is an area of the brain involved in numerous functions, including coordination, learning movement, posture, muscle tone, position of head in space, and eye movements. It is located infratentorially between the temporal and occipital lobes and the brainstem.

Cerebral Blood Flow: Determinants

Choy R.A. Lewis, MD

Cerebral blood flow (CBF), defined as the volume of blood (mL)/100 g of brain tissue/min, is primarily determined by autoregulation, cerebral perfusion pressure (CPP), CO_2 reactivity, O_2 reactivity, cerebral metabolic rate of O_2 ($CMRO_2$) coupling, temperature, viscosity, and some autonomic influences. Normal CBF is 45-60 mL/100 g/min.

AUTOREGULATION

Through autoregulation, the CBF is kept constant despite changes in CPP or mean arterial pressure (MAP). This feature enables the normal brain to tolerate large swings in blood pressure. Autoregulation occurs between MAP of 50 and 150 mm Hg (Figure 117-1).

Any decrease in CPP or MAP leads to cerebral vasodilation and increase in CPP or MAP leads to cerebral vasoconstriction. Outside of these limits, CBF is pressure dependent. High MAPs could greatly increase CBF and lead to cerebral edema or hemorrhage. Low MAPs may greatly decrease CBF and lead to injury from hypoxia/anoxia.

In patients who are chronically hypertensive, the cerebral autoregulation curve is shifted to the right for both the lower and upper limits. Some studies suggest it may be possible to restore normal cerebral autoregulatory limits with chronic antihypertensive therapy.

CEREBRAL PERFUSION PRESSURE

Cerebral perfusion pressure determines CBF at the extremes of MAP where there is no cerebral autoregulation or in situations where cerebral autoregulation has been compromised (Traumatic brain injury [TBI], increased intracranial pressure [ICP], tumor, meningitis, etc). Cerebral perfusion pressure is MAP - ICP or central venous pressure (CVP) or cerebral venous pressure (cVP), whichever is greatest. Because the ICP, CVP, and cVP are usually less than 10 mm Hg, CPP is primarily determined by MAP.

Normal CPP is approximately 80-100 mm Hg. Cerebral perfusion pressure progressively decreases as ICP or CVP increases until the body's compensatory sympathetic nervous system begins to activate. Likewise, CPP decreases as MAP decreases. CPP less than 50 mm Hg shows slowing on EEG, CPP of 25-40 mm Hg shows flat EEG, and CPP sustained at less than 25 mm Hg results in irreversible brain damage.

CARBON DIOXIDE

Cerebral blood flow changes proportionately to changes in Pa_{CO_2} (1-2 mL/100 g/min per mm Hg change in Pa_{CO_2} (Figure 117-2). This effect is thought to be due to CO_2 diffusing across the blood–brain barrier (BBB) and inducing changes in the pH of the CSF and the cerebral tissue. This feature is referred to as CO_2 reactivity. Immediate changes with metabolic acidosis are not evident because bicarbonate and other ions do not cross the BBB easily.

OXYGEN

Unlike the vigorous reactivity to changes in CO_2, CBF is only altered when there are extreme changes in Pa_{O_2}. There is a minor change in CBF with hyperoxia. On the other hand, severe hypoxia (Pa_{O_2} <50 mm Hg) causes marked increase in CBF (Figure 117-2). O_2 reactivity.

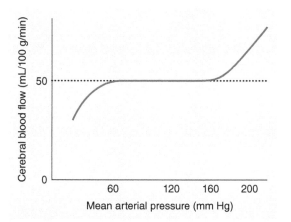

FIGURE 117-1 Autoregulation of cerebral blood flow. (Reproduced with permission from Butterworth JF, Mackey DC, *Wasnick JD, Morgan and Mikhail's Clinical Anesthesiology*, 5th ed. McGraw-Hill; 2013.)

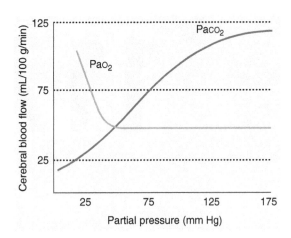

FIGURE 117-2 Relationship between cerebral blood flow and blood gas partial pressures. (Reproduced with permission from Butterworth JF, Mackey DC, Wasnick JD, *Morgan and Mikhail's Clinical Anesthesiology*, 5th ed. McGraw-Hill; 2013.)

CEREBRAL METABOLIC RATE

There are regional variations in CBF, which are primarily due to differences in $CMRO_2$ in sections of the brain. Cerebral blood flow is coupled to $CMRO_2$ such that blood flow increases or is greatest where $CMRO_2$ is greatest. This safety mechanism provides protection against hypoxia and anoxia.

TEMPERATURE

Cerebral blood flow changes 5%-7% per degree centigrade change in temperature. Both $CMRO_2$ and CBF increase as the temperature increases. A decrease in temperature leads to decrease in $CMRO_2$ and corresponding decrease in CBF. Of note, at about 20°C, the EEG becomes isoelectric but any further decrease in temperature will cause continued decrease in $CMRO_2$.

VISCOSITY

Changes in viscosity may alter CBF. Decreased viscosity seen with low hematocrit (HCT) does not appreciably alter CBF. To the contrary, CBF is reduced in states of increased viscosity as in polycythemia.

AUTONOMIC NERVOUS SYSTEM

Intracranial vessels are innervated by parasympathetic (vasodilatory), sympathetic (vasoconstricting), and nonadrenergic fibers. The exact function is unknown. Nonetheless during periods of intense or prolonged sympathetic drive the vessels may vasconstrict and restrict CBF.

EFFECT OF ANESTHETIC AGENTS ON CBF

Intravenous agents—IV induction agents generally decrease CBF. Ketamine is the only exception in that it increases CBF.

Opioids—Opioids generally either have no effect or decrease CBF. Remifentanil increases CBF at low sedative doses.

Benzodiazepines—Benzodiazepines reduce CBF.

Volatile anesthetics—Volatile inhaled anesthetics increase CBF at greater than or equal to 1 minimum alveolar concentration (MAC) (halothane > enflurane > desflurane = isoflurane > sevoflurane).

Nitrous oxide—Nitrous oxide increases CBF. The effect is exaggerated when used in conjunction with volatile agents and less when used with intravenous induction agents other than ketamine.

Cerebral Blood Flow: Autoregulation

Choy R.A. Lewis, MD

Autoregulation is the maintenance of constant cerebral blood flow (CBF) over a range of cerebral perfusion pressure (CPP). Cerebral perfusion pressure is defined as mean arterial pressure (MAP)–central venous pressure (CVP) or intracranial pressure (ICP) or cerebral venous pressure (cVP), whichever is greatest. Because ICP, CVP, and cVP are usually less than 10 mm Hg in the healthy brain, MAP is the main driving force for CPP. In light of this, autoregulation is often depicted as maintenance of constant CBF over range of MAP usually 50-150 mm Hg (Figure 118-1).

To keep CBF constant, compensatory changes in vasomotor tone are made in response to changes in CPP or MAP. When CPP increases, cerebral vascular resistance increases. Likewise, when CPP decreases, cerebral vascular resistance decreases. It may take up to a minute for these compensatory changes to initiate. Hence, for brief periods there may be changes in CBF with swings in blood pressure even within the limits where there is usually autoregulation.

For individuals who are chronically hypertensive, the autoregulatory curve is shifted to the right for both the upper and lower limits. These individuals are at risk of experiencing cerebral hypoperfusion and ischemia with blood pressures that would be considered acceptable for individuals without hypertension.

Autoregulation may be impaired or nonexistent in or around areas of the brain with relative ischemia, surrounding mass lesions, following brain injury, during the postictal state, or during periods of hypoxemia, or hypercarbia. Patients are susceptible to new or worsening injuries from swings in blood pressure.

EFFECTS OF ANESTHETIC AGENTS

The degree to which the cerebral vasculature tone can be altered to facilitate autoregulation while under anesthesia is influenced by background factors that also alter vascular tone. Such factors include hypercapnea, hypocapnea, temperature, cerebral metabolic rate, and neuronal activation. All of these factors must be taken into consideration when assessing the effect of anesthesia on cerebral autoregulation. For example, when administered alone, volatile anesthetics impair cerebral autoregulation in a dose-dependent manner such that as the dose of the anesthetic is increased the level of impairment increases. Autoregulation may be completely abolished at very high doses. The effect is different for each agent. Nitrous oxide causes significant cerebral vasodilation and increase in CBF. This effect can be attenuated by other anesthetic agents or by hyperventilation. Cerebral autoregulation is preserved with intravenous induction agents. Opioids generally do not affect cerebral autoregulation

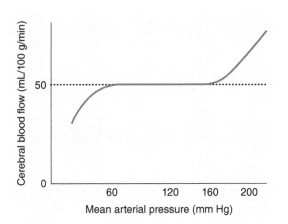

FIGURE 118-1 Relationship between CBF and MAP. (Reproduced with permission from Butterworth JF, Mackey DC, Wasnick JD, *Morgan and Mikhail's Clinical Anesthesiology*, 5th ed. McGraw-Hill; 2013.)

Pathophysiology of Cerebral Ischemia

Mohebat Taheripour, MD

Stroke is the third most common cause of death in most industrialized countries with an estimated global mortality of 4.7 million per year. Each year, about 700 000 people suffer new or recurrent stroke. It is the major cause of serious, long-term disability, with more than 1 100 000 American adults reporting functional limitations resulting from stroke. Also, recent evidence suggests that the presence of small strokes or of local chronic ischemia may be much more common in aging populations than previously thought.

Stroke is more common in men than women, although at older ages the incidence is higher in women than in men. Unlike traumatic brain injury (TBI), there is one treatment that is somewhat successful in a subpopulation of stroke victims. The thrombolytic, tissue plasminogen activator (tPA) has been proved to be effective in treating stroke when given within 3 hours after onset of neurologic symptoms. Although stroke and traumatic brain primarily affects different age groups, both result in a significant number of individuals with long-term deficits.

PATHOPHYSIOLOGY OF FOCAL ISCHEMIA

Normal cerebral blood flow (CBF) in man is typically in the range of 45-50 mL/min/100 g between a mean arterial pressure (MAP) of 60 and 130 mm Hg. When CBF falls below 20-30 mL/min/100 g, marked disturbances in brain metabolism begin to occur, such as water and electrolyte shifts and regional areas of the cerebral cortex experience failed perfusion. At blood flow rates below 10 mL/min/100 g, sudden depolarization of the neurons occurs with rapid loss of intracellular potassium to the extracellular space.

Ischemic and traumatic brain injury results from the interaction of complex pathophysiologic processes that are activated by ischemic or traumatic events. In both injury settings, areas of risk are present that may be salvaged by specific treatment strategies. Although each of these pathophysiologic mechanisms is a target for therapeutic interventions, the complex interaction of these pathomechanisms may make it difficult for targeted pharmacological agents to protect the brain long-term and improve behavioral outcome. Also tissue responses to different injury severities and types (ie, ischemic vs traumatic) may differ and, therefore, complicate treatment strategies not tailored to individual cases.

Current knowledge regarding the pathophysiology of cerebral ischemia and brain trauma indicates that similar mechanisms contribute to loss of cellular integrity and tissue destruction. Mechanisms of cell damage include excitotoxicity, oxidative stress, free radical production, apoptosis, and inflammation. Genetic and gender factors have also been shown to be important mediators of pathomechanisms present in both injury settings. However, the fact that these injuries arise from different types of primary insults leads to diverse cellular vulnerability patterns as well as a spectrum of injury processes.

Blunt head trauma produces shear forces that result in primary membrane damage to neuronal cell bodies, white matter structures, and vascular beds as well as secondary injury mechanisms. Severe cerebral ischemic insults lead to metabolic stress, ionic perturbations, and a complex cascade of biochemical and molecular events ultimately causing neuronal death. Similarities in the pathogenesis of these cerebral injuries may indicate that protective therapeutic strategies following ischemia may also be beneficial after trauma.

PRIMARY INSULTS

Stroke and traumatic injuries arise from very different initial insults. There are three major categories of stroke:

- Subarachnoid hemorrhage
- Intracerebral hemorrhage
- Ischemic stroke

The most common types of stroke are atherothrombotic brain infarction (61%) and cerebral ischemia (24%).

Cerebral ischemia results from severe reductions in CBF, after cardiac arrest, the occlusion of cerebral and extracerebral vessels supplying nervous tissues, or periods of prolonged systemic hypotension. Severe and/or prolonged reductions in CBF lead to deprivations in oxygen and glucose delivery as well as the buildup of potentially toxic substances. Because nerve cells do not store alternative energy sources, these hemodynamic reductions can result in the reduction in metabolites such as adenosine triphosphate (ATP), leading to metabolic stress, energy failure, ionic perturbations, and ischemic injury.

Ischemic insults can be either focal or global, as well as permanent or transient, leading to reperfusion of postischemic areas. Depending on how early reperfusion is initiated, metabolic and ionic homeostasis can return and cell survival maintained.

BIOCHEMICAL EVENTS

Within 20 seconds of interruption of blood flow to the mammalian brain under conditions of normothermia, the EEG disappears, probably as a result of the failure of high-energy metabolism. Within 5 minutes, high-energy phosphate levels virtually disappear (ATP depletion), and profound disturbances in cell electrolyte balance begin to occur.

Potassium begins to leak rapidly from the intracellular compartment and sodium and calcium begin to enter the cells. Sodium influx results in a marked increase in cellular water content, particularly in the astrocytes.

CELLULAR VULNERABILITY

In both cerebral ischemic and traumatic insults, patterns of neuronal vulnerability are well described. The neuron has classically been shown to be very sensitive to periods of cerebral ischemia. Flow reductions reaching 25 mL/100 g/min in rodents are considered severe enough to lead to eventual cell death.

In addition to the severity of the ischemic insult, the duration of ischemia also determines vulnerability patterns. For example, a brief period of severe ischemia may lead to selective neuronal damage, with minor cellular changes observed in glia and blood vessels. However, with longer ischemic periods, other cellular responses can be observed, ultimately producing ischemic infarction.

With reperfusion injury, damage to cerebral blood vessels and the activation of inflammatory processes can produce hemorrhagic transformation of infarcted tissue and severe brain swelling.

Severe injuries can lead to damage of glial cells, including astrocytes and oligodendrocytes. Indeed, one of the earliest cellular changes observed after contusion injury is glial swelling. In both cerebral ischemia and trauma, abnormalities in vascular permeability participate in the early pathogenesis of these insults.

PLATELET AGGREGATION

In clinical stroke, platelet aggregation leading to vascular thrombosis and subsequent embolization are common mechanisms involved in the production of ischemic insult.

Abnormal platelet function is seen in patients at risk for stroke and following transient ischemic events. Platelets may accumulate in areas of abnormal flow characteristics, including heart valves and specific cerebral arterial branch points. Platelet events can lead to severe but transient hemodynamic perturbations that may result in mild, moderate, or severe morphologic changes.

Transient platelet accumulation can also lead to vascular perturbations, including leakage of blood-brain barrier (BBB) and abnormalities in vascular reactivity. In stroke, the thrombolytic agent, tPA, is currently the only therapeutic strategy shown to be beneficial in acute stroke therapy.

CELL DEATH MECHANISMS

Both necrotic and apoptotic cell death mechanisms have been implicated in the pathogenesis of ischemia. The brain is vulnerable to oxidative stress due to its high rate of oxidative metabolic activity. Oxidative stress leading to calcium accumulation, mitochondrial dysfunction, and the production of reactive oxygen radicals is an important mechanism of cell death following both ischemic and traumatic insults. After cerebral ischemia and trauma, evidence for the generation of reactive oxygen species has been demonstrated in a variety of injury models.

The exact percentage of cells dying of apoptosis versus necrosis depends upon several factors, including ischemic severity and duration. Importantly, whereas necrotic neuronal damage is commonly observed early after severe ischemic insults, apoptotic cell death may occur with more mild insults and with longer survival periods.

INFLAMMATION

Inflammation, a host defense mechanism that is initiated by injury or infection, is a process through which blood-leukocytes (neutrophils, monocytes/macrophages, T cells) and soluble factors (cytokines, chemokines, complement, lipid by-products) attempt to restore tissue homeostasis. The inflammatory response in the CNS may have various consequences on outcome, depending upon the degree of inflammatory response and when it occurs. Both acute and chronic inflammatory processes have been shown to influence outcome in various experimental models of cerebral ischemia and trauma. Whereas acute inflammatory events may participate in secondary injury processes, more delayed inflammatory events may be reparative. Thus, the importance of the inflammatory response to functional outcome is an area of active investigation.

Cerebrospinal Fluid

Taghreed Alshaeri, MD, and Marianne D. David, MD

Cerebrospinal fluid (CSF) surrounds the brain and spinal cord in the subarachnoid space. It primarily protects these structures as a cushion and mechanical barrier. Although composed of 99% water, CSF contains glucose, proteins, and lipids to provide nutrition to the central nervous system. Moreover, as part of the blood–CSF barrier, it serves as an excretory pathway to remove waste products by tightly regulating the brain's extracellular ionic milieu.

Production of CSF occurs in the lateral cerebral ventricles by the choroid plexus. About 20 mL/h (500 mL/day) is produced, but absorption at arachnoid villi in cerebral venous sinuses maintains total CSF volume at 100-150 mL. The entire CSF volume is replaced about 3-4 times daily. Cerebrospinal fluid flow proceeds from lateral ventricles to the third ventricle through the intraventricular foramina, and then enters the fourth ventricle via the cerebral aqueduct. From the fourth ventricle, CSF reaches the subarachnoid space to surround the brain and the spinal cord (Figure 120-1).

Excess CSF results in increased intracranial pressure and hydrocephalus, most commonly through obstructed CSF circulation and noncommunicating hydrocephalus. Overproduction or underabsorption, communicating hydrocephalus, rarely occurs as well. A shunt or drain can surgically displace CSF. Cerebrospinal fluid production can be decreased pharmacologically as well, using osmotic (ie, mannitol) or loop diuretics (ie, furosemide). The least invasive means of lowering CSF are patient positioning (ie, elevated head of bed by 30 degrees) and short-term hyperventilation, either via encouragement of spontaneous respirations or positive pressure ventilation.

Certain medications and anesthetics interfere with CSF production. Carbonic anhydrase inhibitors (ie, acetazolamide), furosemide, and thiopental decrease CSF production, whereas desflurane, halothane, and ketamine increase CSF production.

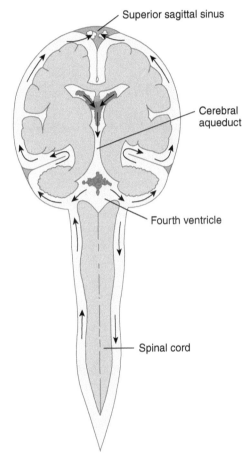

FIGURE 120-1 The flow of CSF in the central nervous system. (Reproduced with permission from Waxman SG, *Clinical Neuroanatomy*, 27th ed. McGraw-Hill Companies, Inc. 2013. All rights reserved.)

Cerebral Protection

Taghreed Alshaeri, MD, and Marianne D. David, MD

CEREBRAL METABOLISM AND ISCHEMIA

The cerebral metabolic rate of O_2 ($CMRO_2$) is 3-3.8 mL/100 mg/min. Cerebral metabolism has two basic components: neuronal activity and cellular integrity. The brain depends on aerobic glucose metabolism; hence, large O_2 demand consumes 20% of total body O_2 to maintain neuronal activity for adenosine triphosphate (ATP) generation.

Cerebral ischemia occurs when metabolic demand exceeds tissue O_2 supply. Ischemia can be either global or focal. Cerebral protection limits brain tissue injury. Maximizing O_2 delivery and decreasing cerebral metabolism achieve protective goals. Clinical strategies for cerebral protection include physiologic and medical interventions.

CEREBRAL PROTECTION

Physiologic Interventions

1. **Temperature control**—Hypothermia decreases both the brain's neuronal activity and cellular integrity. Profound hypothermia or deep hypothermic circulatory arrest (DHCA) at 15-18°C decreases cerebral metabolic and electrical requirements, with proven benefits for cardiac arrest lasting 30 minutes to 1 hour with adverse neurologic effects. Mild hypothermia at 33-35°C is also neuroprotective by decreasing the $CMRO_2$ and attenuating inflammatory responses to an ischemic insult. Potential complications from induced hypothermia include coagulopathy and cardiac dysrhythmias.
2. **Glycemic control**—Hyperglycemia adversely affects neurologic outcomes during cerebral ischemia in the ICU setting, especially for prolonged hospitalizations.
3. **Hemodilution**—Whereas optimizing hemoglobin level maximizes O_2-carrying capacity, hemodilution to decrease blood viscosity, thereby increasing O_2 delivery, may provide cerebral protection.
4. **Blood pressure control**—Cerebral profusion pressure (CPP) = mean arterial pressure (MAP)–intracranial pressure (ICP). Maintaining MAP also maintains CPP. Critical CPP to avoid ischemic brain injury is greater than 50 mm Hg.
5. Avoidance of hypoxia and hypercapnia.

Medical Interventions

1. **Anesthetic agents**—Volatile and intravenous anesthetics can be used for cerebral protection by influencing brain neuronal activity and inducing an isoelectric EEG. Anesthetic agents are not protective against global insults. Barbiturates protect against focal ischemia by decreasing $CMRO_2$. Propofol, etomidate, and inhalational agents (ie, isoflurane) similarly may protect against focal ischemia.
2. **Steroids**—Dexamethasone reduces brain tissue edema surrounding tumors. Otherwise, steroids are not neuroprotective following ischemic insult.
3. **Ca^{2+} channel blockers**—No impact on neurologic outcome after cerebral ischemia, but nimodipine decreases cerebral vasospasm after injury.

SUGGESTED READING

Fukuda S, Warner DS. Cerebral protection. *Br J Anaesth.* 2007;99:10-17.

Spinal Cord: Organization and Tracts

Sarah Uddeen, MD, and Gregory Moy, MD

The spinal cord is made of both gray and white matter. Gray matter consists of neurons, neuronal processes, and neuroglia. It is butterfly or H-shaped. White matter surrounds gray matter and is made up of neuronal processes (myelinated and unmyelinated), neuroglia, and blood vessels. The proportion of gray to white matter varies at different levels of the spinal cord. The ratio of gray to white matter is greatest at the cervical and lumbar regions.

GRAY MATTER

Gray matter can be categorized into columns (or horns) and laminae (Figure 122-1). The columns include a ventral (or anterior) column, which contains motor neurons, and an intermediolateral gray column, which contains preganglionic cells for the autonomic nervous system. The intermediolateral gray column contains preganglionic sympathetic neurons from T1-L2 and contains parasympathetic neurons at S2-S4. In addition, a dorsal (or posterior) gray column is involved in sensory processing. Lissauer tract lies in this area and is part of

the pain pathway. The anterior and posterior horns are united by a gray commissure that contains a small, central canal.

There are 10 laminae (layers of nerve cells), also known as Rexed laminae that make up the gray matter. Each of these laminae is involved in sensory or motor pathways (Table 122-1).

TABLE 122-1 Laminae (Gray Matter)

Laminae	Sensory or Motor	Other Info/Function
I	Sensory	Respond to noxious stimuli—mediate pain, temperature, and touch. Substance P found in high concentrations
II	Sensory	Substantia gelatinosa. Responds to noxious stimuli—pain and temperature. Substance P and glutamate found in high concentrations
III and IV	Sensory	Together known as nucleus proprius. Convey position and light sense
V	Sensory	Respond to noxious and visceral afferent stimuli
VI	Sensory	Respond to mechanical signals from joints and skin. Located only in cervical and lumbar spinal segments
VII	Motor, autonomic	Contains cells of dorsal nucleus, which give rise to posterior spinocerebellar tract. Also contains intermediolateral nucleus (intermediolateral cell column) in thoracic and lumbar regions which contains sympathetic fibers
VIII and IX	Motor	Medial and lateral components. Medial—axial muscles. Lateral—distal muscles. Flexor muscles innervated by motor neurons closer to central canal (more ventral)
X	Autonomic	Small neurons/remnants around central canal

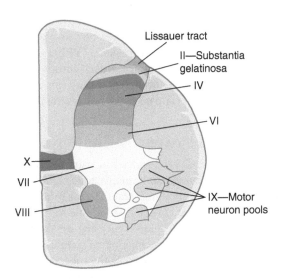

FIGURE 122-1 Laminae of spinal cord gray matter. (Reproduced with permission from Waxman SG, *Clinical Neuroanatomy*, 27th ed. McGraw-Hill Companies, Inc. 2013. All rights reserved.)

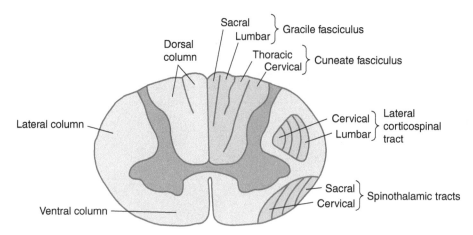

FIGURE 122-2 Spinal cord tracts. (Reproduced from Waxman SG, *Clinical Neuroanatomy*, 27th ed. McGraw-Hill. All rights reserved.)

WHITE MATTER

The white matter is divided into columns, including the dorsal, lateral, and ventral columns (Figure 122-2). Each column contains tracts, which are groups of nerve fibers that have similar destinations in relaying sensory and motor information. For instance, the dorsal column can be divided into a medial tract (fasciculus gracilis) and a lateral tract (fasciculus cuneatus) in the cervical and upper thoracic regions of the spinal cord. The fasciculus gracilis and fasciculus cuneatus are somatotopically arranged, with the former sending sensory information from the lower body below T6 and the latter sending sensory information from the upper half of the body above T6.

ASCENDING TRACTS OF THE SPINAL CORD

The white matter of the spinal cord has several ascending and descending tracts that either relay sensory information to higher centers (the former) or relay information from higher centers to the periphery to influence motor movement (the latter).

The ascending tracts contain nerve bundles that generally communicate through a three-neuron system (Table 122-2). The first-order neuron has a sensory receptor ending and cell body in the dorsal root ganglion (DRG) of the spinal nerve. It synapses with a second-order neuron in the dorsal horn, which then crosses the spinal cord to the opposite side as it ascends to higher levels. Finally, the third-order neuron is generally located in the thalamus, which then projects to sensory areas in the sensory cortex.

Dorsal Column/Medial Lemniscus Pathway

This pathway carries fibers that control fine touch, vibration, proprioception, and pressure. The initial sensory receptors include those located in Meissner corpuscles, Pacinian corpuscles, muscle stretch receptors, and golgi tendon organs. The first cell body is located in the DRG. The fibers travel up

TABLE 122-2   Ascending Tracts

Name of Tract	Function
Spinothalamic	Lateral—pain and temperature, itch Anterior—light touch and pressure
Dorsal column	Joint, muscle sensation. Proprioception, vibration. Two-point discrimination
Dorsal and ventral spinocerebellar	Unconscious proprioceptive information regarding lower extremity
Cuneocerebellar	Unconscious proprioceptive information regarding upper extremity
Spinotectal	Reflexes involved with movements of eye and head
Spinoreticular	Levels of consciousness

fasciculus gracilis (below T6) or fasciculus cuneatus (C2-T6) and terminate at the cell body (second-order neuron) of either the nucleus gracilis or nucleus cuneatus. The fibers then decussate at the contralateral medial lemniscus and ascend until they terminate in the ventral posterior lateral (VPL) nucleus of the thalamus. This is where the third-order neurons are located. Finally, the fibers travel through the posterior limb of the internal capsule and terminate in the postcentral gyrus.

Anterolateral System

This system carries fibers involved in pain and temperature sensation, as well as nondiscriminative touch. The majority of fibers follow the **spinothalamic tract**. Axons from the periphery travel to the spinal cord and travel one to two segments higher in Lissauer tract before synapsing on the first-order cell body in the DRG. These fibers then terminate where the second-order cell body is located in the substantia gelatinosa and nucleus proprius. The fibers then decussate in the anterior white commissure and ascend one to three spinal segments. These fibers then ascend to the thalamus and are somatotopically arranged; the lateral portion carries fibers from the lower extremities and the medial portion carries fibers from the upper extremities. The third-order neuron cell body lies in the VPL of the thalamus. Once the fibers reach the thalamus, they travel through the posterior limb of the internal capsule and corona radiata and terminate at the postcentral gyrus. Other tracts involved in processing pain and temperature sensations include the spinoreticular, spinomesencephalic, spinohypothalamic, and spinobulbar tracts.

Other major ascending pathways include the **spinocerebellar tracts,** which help send information regarding proprioception and movement to the cerebellum.

DESCENDING TRACTS OF THE SPINAL CORD

The descending motor tracts originate in either the cerebral cortex or brainstem (Table 122-3). The neurons that initially descend in the tract can be referred to as **upper motor neurons**. These fibers target **lower motor neurons** of the spinal cord or cranial nerves to assist with voluntary movement. Similar to the ascending tracts, these pathways are generally made of a three-neuron system. For those tracts originating in the cortex that travel to the spinal cord, the first-order neuron is in the cerebral cortex, which then synapses with a second-order neuron (usually an interneuron) located in the anterior gray column of the spinal cord. Finally, the third-order neuron, or the lower motor neuron, is the final destination that causes motor activity. Somatosensory fibers influence the majority of these descending pathways. Injuries to upper motor neurons, either in the cerebral cortex or descending fibers, cause a spastic paralysis and hyperactive deep tendon reflexes, a classic sign being a positive Babinski sign (extensor plantar reflex). Injuries to lower motor neurons cause a flaccid paralysis, diminished or absent deep tendon reflexes, muscle atrophy, and possible fasciculations.

TABLE 122-3   Descending Tracts

Name of Tract	Function
Corticospinal	Voluntary movement of lower extremities (lateral) and proximal extremities (anterior)
Reticulospinal	Influence voluntary movement and reflexes. Involved in hypothalamic control of autonomic activity
Tectospinal	Reflex postural movements in response to visual stimuli
Rubrospinal	Activates flexor muscles and inhibits activity of extensor muscles
Vestibulospinal	Medial—responds to changes in balance. Lateral—facilitates flexors, inhibits extensors, responds to changes in balance

Corticospinal Tract

These fibers start in the precentral gyrus and ultimately end in the ventral horn of the spinal cord. In the ventral horn, axons synapse with interneurons as well as alpha and gamma motor neurons, which innervate skeletal muscle and muscle stretch receptors, respectively. The corticospinal tract has fibers that divide into the lateral corticospinal tract and the anterior corticospinal tract. They share the initial pathway. One-third of fibers arise from Brodmann area 4 of the precentral gyrus, whereas the other fibers arise from frontal and parietal areas of the brain. These are upper motor neurons that then descend by traveling through the corona radiata and posterior limb of the internal capsule. As the fibers descend they take up the middle-third of the cerebral peduncles and then continue through the basal pons.

Of these fibers, 85%-95% then decussates in the caudal medulla where they form the pyramids and continue to descend as the **lateral corticospinal tract** in the lateral funiculus. They terminate in the cervical, lumbar, and sacral gray matter (lateral intermediate gray zone and anterior horn gray matter) and synapse with interneurons. These excitatory and inhibitory interneurons then synapse with lower motor neurons, which in turn cause muscle contraction or relaxation, respectively. The lateral corticospinal tract is involved with mediating rapid and skin voluntary movement of distal muscles of the upper and lower extremities.

Instead of decussating at the pyramids, the other 10%-15% of fibers continues to descend ipsilaterally as the **anterior corticospinal tract**. They descend the anterior funiculus and decussate at the anterior white commissure near their termination site at the anterior horn in the cervical and upper thoracic levels. In the anterior horn they synapse with interneurons. The anterior corticospinal tract is involved with mediating axial and proximal (girdle) muscles.

Corticobulbar Tract

This tract is involved in voluntary movement of muscles involved with motor nuclei (cranial nerves). Similar to the corticospinal tract, fibers arise from the precentral gyrus in areas somatotopically related in the head and face. They then descend through the corona radiata, genu of the internal capsule, and cerebral peduncles. At this point, they break off from the corticospinal tract and terminate on various motor nuclei. The majority of fibers synapse with interneurons initially, which then synapse with motor neurons of the cranial nerve motor nuclei. The cranial nerves involved include CN III (oculomotor), CN IV (trochlear), CN V (trigeminal), CN VI (abducens), CN II (facial), CN IX (glossopharyngeal), CN X (vagus), CN XI (spinal accessory), and CN XII (hypoglossal). Hence, this pathway is involved in mediating extraocular muscles, muscles of facial expression, mastication, intrinsic and extrinsic muscles of the tongue, and muscles of the larynx, pharynx, and soft palate. The majority of fibers project bilaterally, except for CN VII and CN XII.

Other descending tracts include the rubrospinal, reticulospinal, descending autonomic, tectospinal, and medial longitudinal fasciculus.

Spinal Cord Evoked Potentials

Sarah Uddeen, MD, and Gregory Moy, MD

The spinal cord is a complex portion of the nervous system involved in receiving, sending, and processing information from the outside world to the brain and vice versa. Many neurologic monitoring modalities exist to aid in the preservation of spinal cord integrity during surgical intervention. One of these modalities is spinal cord evoked potentials. Spinal cord evoked potentials are electrical activity generated in response to either a sensory or motor stimulus: hence, they are categorized as sensory evoked potentials and motor evoked potentials (MEPs). Monitoring requires special training, as well as appropriate equipment and sufficient operating room space.

SENSORY EVOKED POTENTIALS

Somatosensory evoked potentials require electrodes placed near peripheral nerves. An electric signal stimulates the electrodes that are transmitted to the sensory cortex where electrodes placed in the scalp measure the potential. Sensory evoked potentials measure the integrity of the dorsal columns.

MOTOR EVOKED POTENTIALS

With MEPs, electric or magnetic signals are sent through transcranial stimulation or stimulation directly on the spinal cord to peripheral nerves, spinal column, or muscle, where the potential is measured. Motor evoked potentials measure the integrity of the ventral column and associated motor pathways. Transcranial stimulation can involve electric or magnetic stimulation. Electric stimulation consists of electrodes being placed in the scalp over the motor cortex, whereas magnetic stimulation consists of a magnetic stimulator being placed over the motor cortex.

CLINICAL APPLICATION

Both sensory and motor potentials are measured in terms of latency and amplitude. Latency is the time period from the stimulus to the measured response, and amplitude is a measurement of the voltage of the response. Monitoring of spinal cord evoked potentials can be beneficial in numerous surgeries, including spinal fusion with instrumentation, spinal cord resection, cerebral tumor resection, thoracoabdominal aortic aneurysm repair, epilepsy surgery, and brachial plexus surgery.

Anesthetic Agents and Evoked Potentials

Because multiple anesthetic agents can affect the parameters measured (latency and amplitude), anesthesia management and technique is usually modified during evoked potential monitoring. Volatile agents, such as sevoflurane, desflurane, and isoflurane, cause a dose-dependent decrease in amplitude and increase the latency in somatosensory evoked potentials (SSEPs). When monitoring is being used, a minimum alveolar concentration (MAC) of 0.5-0.75 is ideal. Nitrous oxide can further interfere with monitoring and is typically avoided. In general, the intravenous anesthetic agents also decrease amplitude and increase latency in SSEPs, except for etomidate and ketamine, which can increase amplitude. Opioids, when given in large doses, can cause a transient interference with signal transmission. However, the clinical doses of intravenous agents and opioids, particularly when given as infusions, have negligible effects on electrophysiologic (EP) monitoring. Balanced anesthetic techniques using IV agents (eg, propofol) and opioids should be considered when developing the anesthetic plan. Clonidine and dexmedetomidine have negligible effects on EP monitoring and can be used to decrease anesthetic requirements.

Motor evoked potentials are similar in their sensitivity to IV agents, but are extremely sensitive to volatile agents. A total IV technique or a balanced anesthetic technique with less than 0.5 MAC of volatile agent should be considered in the anesthetic plan. Muscle paralysis is generally not used or is titrated to maintain one or two twitches on train-of-four when MEPs are monitored.

CHAPTER

124

Anatomy of the Neuromuscular Junction

Sarah Uddeen, MD, and Gregory Moy, MD

The neuromuscular junction is an anatomic location in which signals are transmitted from a motor neuron to a muscle fiber via neurotransmitters (acetylcholine) which diffuse across a synapse. These signals cause muscle contraction.

COMPONENTS

The neuromuscular junction consists of several components that allow for transmission of signals from the motor neuron to motor end plate. The motor neuron is made up of a cell body that has dendritic branches and contains a nucleus. The cell body connects to a myelin-covered axon composed of Schwann cells, which allows for faster impulse conduction. As the axon ends, it becomes the axon terminal that branches into processes. Each axonal process has a prejunctional motor nerve ending that innervates one muscle fiber. Mitochondria, voltage-gated calcium channels, and presynaptic vesicles containing acetylcholine reside in the motor nerve ending.

The synaptic cleft of the neuromuscular junction is the area 30-50 nm wide that connects the basement membranes of the prejunctional motor nerve ending and the postjunctional muscle fiber. This cleft is a chemical synapse in which neurotransmitters, specifically acetylcholine, are released from the motor nerve ending to attach to receptors on the postjunctional muscle fiber.

The postjunctional membrane of the muscle fiber consists of junctional folds that maximize surface area (Figure 124-1). Here, nicotinic acetylcholine receptors (sodium channels) as well as voltage-gated calcium channels reside. When an action potential travels along the axon and depolarizes the presynaptic/prejunctional nerve ending, acetylcholine is released and diffuses across the synaptic cleft. Once acetylcholine binds the acetylcholine receptors it causes an action potential in the muscle fiber, resulting in muscle movement.

ACETYLCHOLINE AND ACETYLCHOLINE RECEPTORS

Acetylcholine was the first neurotransmitter discovered. It is highly involved in transmission of signals in the parasympathetic

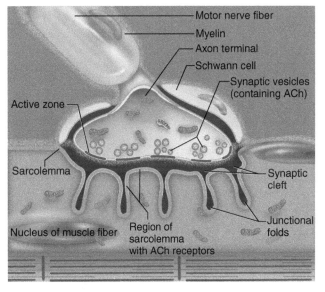

FIGURE 124-1 Neuromuscular junction. (Reproduced with permission from Barrett KE, Barman SM, Boltano S, Brooks HL. *Ganong's Review of Medical Physiology*, 24th ed. McGraw-Hill Companies, Inc. All rights reserved.)

and sympathetic nervous systems as well as at the neuromuscular junction. Acetylcholine binds acetylcholine receptors, which can be classified as either nicotinic or muscarinic receptors. At the neuromuscular junction, acetylcholine binds to nicotinic receptors. The receptor consists of five subunits (two alpha subunits and a single beta, gamma, and delta subunit) that form a channel, allowing ion flow.

Acetylcholine is only capable of binding the alpha subunits. Acetylcholine must occupy both alpha subunit sites for a conformational change to occur, which then leads to an action potential. Acetylcholine is broken down into acetate and choline by acetylcholinesterase. This process occurs via hydrolysis. Acetylcholinesterase is located at the motor end plate adjacent to the acetylcholine receptors. The choline undergoes reuptake by the presynaptic nerve cell and, together with acetyl-CoA, acetylcholine is synthesized and stored into vesicles.

EXTRAJUNCTIONAL RECEPTORS

Extrajunctional receptors are located throughout skeletal muscle. In contrast, postjunctional receptors are specifically located across the prejunctional motor neuron. Extrajunctional receptors further differ from postjunctional receptors in that an epsilon subunit replaces the delta subunit. These receptors are usually suppressed; however, they are upregulated in instances of prolonged activity, burns, and sepsis. When extrajunctional receptors are activated they tend to stay open for a longer period of time, which can lead to hyperkalemia.

Physiology of Neuromuscular Transmission

125

Sarah Uddeen, MD, and Gregory Moy, MD

Signals from the motor neuron cross a chemical synapse, the neuromuscular junction, to the muscle fiber to produce muscle contraction. This complex process involves action potentials, numerous ion channels, the neurotransmitter acetylcholine (ACh), and receptors. Several medications, toxins, and disease states affect the integrity of transmission.

TRANSMISSION AT THE MOTOR NEURON

The motor neuron's axon receives an action potential leading to depolarization of the presynaptic terminal. "Active zones" of the presynaptic terminal contain high concentrations of voltage-dependent Ca^{2+} channels, mitochondria, and presynaptic vesicles containing ACh. Upon depolarization, these voltage-gated Ca^{2+} channels open, causing an influx of calcium into the nerve terminal. Ca^{2+} influx induces the cascade that begins with phosphorylation of proteins called synapsins, which keep vesicles containing ACh in a presynaptic actin network. Once this cascade starts, presynaptic vesicle release from the actin network begins, allowing presynaptic membrane fusion. Vesicle contents, which include ACh, are subsequently released into the synaptic cleft via exocytosis.

TRANSMISSION AT THE SYNAPSE

Acetylcholine diffuses across the 30-50 nm synaptic cleft to reach its target, nicotinic receptors, on the postjunctional muscle fiber. Some of the neurotransmitter is lost and some is inactivated before reaching the postjunctional membrane.

TRANSMISSION AT THE MUSCLE FIBER

Once ACh reaches the postjunctional membrane, it binds to nicotinic ACh receptors, which are permeable to Na^+ and Ca^{2+}. Binding of ACh to these receptors causes a conformational change, allowing Na^+ and Ca^{2+} influx into the cell. These receptors are also permeable to K^+ (although to a lesser extent), which flows out of the cell. Acetylcholine binding

cation influx causes a miniature end-plate potential (MEPP) in which the cell starts to become depolarized. If several vesicles are released, the MEPPs summate to generate an end-plate potential of the muscle fiber that leads to an action potential if large enough. This action potential spreads among the plasma membrane and T-tubule system, causing release of Ca^{2+} from the sarcoplasmic reticulum and ultimately muscle contraction.

Acetylcholine is rapidly degraded by acetylcholinesterase to prevent reexcitation of muscle. The ion channels on the postsynaptic membrane close following ACh reduction, thus repolarizing the cell and causing muscle relaxation.

MEDICATIONS AND TOXINS

Curare was the first muscle relaxant to be introduced. Since then, synthetic compounds derived from curare have been used for muscle relaxation in surgical settings. Curare works by binding ACh receptors and preventing ACh from acting upon them. Both nondepolarizing and depolarizing muscle relaxants work at the neuromuscular junction. Nondepolarizing agents work by competitively binding either one or both of the alpha subunits on the ACh receptor located on the postjunctional membrane. This prevents receptor opening and depolarization. Depolarizing agents, namely succinylcholine, work by binding the alpha subunits and mimicking ACh to prolong the depolarized state. This causes muscle relaxation because the muscle fiber cannot repolarize to start the cascade of events that lead to muscle contraction.

Cholinesterase inhibitors, such as those used to reverse neuromuscular blockade, work by decreasing the activity of acetylcholinesterase, resulting in increased ACh in the nerve terminal. Organophosphates are toxins whose mechanism of action is to irreversibly inhibit anticholinesterase, leading to exceedingly high ACh levels at the neuromuscular junction, which leads to a cholinergic toxidrome. Symptoms include those that result from muscarinic and nicotinic receptor activation. Management strategies include intubation, fluids, atropine, and pralidoxime. Pralidoxime requires concomitant atropine administration.

Botulinum toxin is an exotoxin from the bacterium *Clostridium botulinum*. It prevents ACh release from the presynaptic nerve terminal. It does so by membrane binding and interfering with the docking of ACh-filled vesicles. This causes flaccid paralysis.

Lastly, abnormalities in Mg^{2+} and Ca^{2+} can cause inhibition of ACh release. High levels of Mg^{2+}, such as when administered to preeclamptic parturients, block Ca^{2+} channels and decrease ACh released.

DISEASE STATES

Myasthenia gravis is an autoimmune disorder that produces antibody against the ACh receptor. Antibodies bind these receptors, rendering them nonfunctional. The disease is characterized by extreme muscle weakness, particularly limb, eye, and oropharyngeal muscles. Treatment for myasthenia typically involves anticholinesterase inhibitors to increase the amount of ACh at the synapse. Receptor downregulation makes these patients more resistant to depolarizing agents and more sensitive to nondepolarizing agents.

Similarly, Lambert–Eaton syndrome is an autoimmune disorder in which antibodies attack the Ca^{2+} channel located on the presynaptic membrane. This subsequently causes decreased ACh release, leading to muscle weakness, particularly proximal muscles. Neuromyotonia, also known as Isaacs disease, involves hyperactivity at the prejunctional membrane, which causes repetitive muscle activity and symptoms such as fasciculations, myotonia, stiffness, excessive sweating, and muscle cramps. Most cases are autoimmune related with antibodies targeted against K^+ channels. Anticonvulsants, such as carbamazepine and phenytoin have been used to provide some degree of symptomatic relief.

Skeletal Muscle Contraction

126

Matthew de Jesus, MD

Voluntary skeletal muscle contraction occurs when an electrical signal (action potential) travels via somatic nerves to the synaptic cleft. Here, the electrical action potential opens voltage-gated calcium channels, and calcium causes the release of acetylcholine (ACh) into the synaptic cleft. The ACh travels across the synaptic cleft binding to nicotinic ACh receptors, which when activated, allow an influx of sodium ions into the muscle fiber membrane. The intracellular voltage change from the influx of sodium transmits an action potential via T-tubules to the center of the muscle cell, where upon reaching the sarcoplasmic reticulum, calcium ions are released, enabling muscle fibers to contract.

Skeletal muscle is composed of muscle fascicles, which in turn comprises a group of muscle fibers. A muscle fiber has thick filaments made of myosin, and thin filaments made of actin, troponin, and tropomyosin. Myosin heads have two types of binding sites; actin and adenosine triphosphate (ATP). For contraction to occur, both must be occupied. Binding sites on actin unit are blocked by the protein tropomyosin. The inflowing calcium from the sarcoplasmic reticulum binds to troponin, which changes conformation of tropomyosin, thus exposing actin binding sites, and ultimately allowing myosin to bind to actin. Relaxation requires sequestration of calcium back into the sarcoplasmic reticulum, as well as an additional molecule of ATP.

Muscle contraction can be inhibited by blocking postsynaptic ACh receptors. Nondepolarizing muscle relaxants are competitive antagonists of ACh, whereas succinylcholine is a competitive agonist. Both bind to the postsynaptic nicotinic ACh receptor. Succinylcholine causes a depolarization of the muscle, seen clinically as muscle fasciculation.

CONDITIONS RELATED TO SKELETAL MUSCLE CONTRACTION

Malignant hyperthermia manifests when a triggering agent (inhalational agents, succinylcholine) causes massive release of calcium from the sarcoplasmic reticulum in susceptible individuals. This results in gross uncoordinated muscle fasciculation, and generates heat, raising body temperature. Muscle breakdown can result in rhabdomyolysis, and myoglobin released from damaged muscle can lead to renal failure. Treatment of a malignant hyperthermic episode includes dantrolene, which depresses excitation–contraction coupling of skeletal muscle.

Myasthenia gravis is an autoimmune disease where antibodies destroy nicotinic ACh receptors in the neuromuscular junction, leading to fluctuating muscle weakness, and increased muscle fatigue after activity.

Lambert–Eaton myasthenic syndrome is also an autoimmune disease, where antibodies are developed against presynaptic voltage-gated calcium channels. It manifests as limb weakness that improves with activity.

Pain Mechanisms and Pathways

Elvis W. Rema, MD

Pain serves an important role in providing essential protective mechanisms against injury. The International Association for the Study of Pain defines pain as "an unpleasant sensory and emotional experience associated with actual or potential tissue damage, or described in terms of such damage." This definition infers that pain has both sensory as well as affective and cognitive consequences.

NOCICEPTORS

Nociceptors are specialized sensory receptors with the ability to detect noxious stimuli and transform the stimuli into electrical signals that the central nervous system interprets. The free nerve endings of primary afferent A delta and C fibers are responsible for nociception (Table 127-1). Nociceptors respond to intense heat, cold, mechanical, and chemical stimuli. The axons of the A delta are thinly myelinated with a faster conduction speed of 5-15 m/s in contrast to the unmyelinated C fibers with a conduction speed of 1-2 m/s. A delta fibers respond to mechanical and thermal stimuli. They carry rapid, sharp pain and are responsible for the initial reflex response to acute pain. C fibers are polymodal, responding to chemical, mechanical, and thermal stimuli. The C fiber activation leads to slow, dull pain.

TABLE 127-1   Comparison of Pain Fibers

	A delta Fibers	C Fibers
Diameter	2-5 μm	<2 μm
Myelination	Thinly	None
Conduction velocity	5-15 m/s	<2 m/s
Receptor activation threshold	High and low	High
Sensation on stimulation	Rapid, sharp, localized pain	Slow, diffuse, dull pain

NOCICEPTION

Nociception is defined as the neural occurrences of encoding and processing noxious stimuli. It is the afferent activity produced in the peripheral and central nervous systems by stimuli that have the potential to damage tissue. The succession by which a stimulus is perceived as noxious comprises the following four processes:

Transduction

Transduction is the process where nociceptors convert different forms of noxious energy to electrical activity or action potentials that can be recognized by the central nervous system.

Transmission

Transmission is the process by which the electrical activity created by nociceptors is conducted to the central nervous system. There are three components to this process: (1) the peripheral sensory cells in the dorsal root ganglia transmit signals from the site of transduction to the spinal cord; (2) spinal neurons send projections to the brain stem; and (3) neurons of the brainstem project to various cortical sites.

Modulation

Modulation involves changing or inhibiting transmission of pain impulses in the spinal cord. The multiple, complex pathways involved in the modulation of pain are referred to as the descending modulatory pain pathways and these can lead to either an increase in the transmission of pain impulses (excitatory) or a decrease in transmission (inhibition).

Perception

Perception is the end result of the neuronal activity of pain transmission where pain becomes a conscious multidimensional experience. The somatosensory cortex is responsible for the perception and interpretation of sensations. It identifies the intensity, type, and location of the pain sensation. The limbic system is responsible for the emotional and behavioral responses to pain. The reticular system is responsible for the autonomic and motor response to pain.

DORSAL HORN OF THE SPINAL CORD

The dorsal horn can be divided histologically into 10 layers called the Rexed laminae (see Chapter 122). A delta and C fibers synapse with secondary afferent neurons in the dorsal horn of the spinal cord and transmit information to nociceptive specific neurons in laminae I, II, III, and V. Primary afferent terminals release a number of excitatory neurotransmitters that include glutamate and substance P. Intricate interactions occur in the dorsal horn between afferent neurons, interneurons, and descending modulatory pathways, which will determine the activity of secondary afferent neurons. Glycine and gamma-aminobutyric acid are the neurotransmitters acting as inhibitory mediators.

ASCENDING TRACTS IN THE SPINAL CORD

There are two main pathways that carry nociceptive signals to higher centers in the brain.

Spinothalamic Tract

The spinothalamic tract carries secondary afferent neurons which decussate within a few segments of the level of entry into the spinal cord and ascend in the contralateral spinothalamic tract to nuclei within the thalamus. Third-order neurons then ascend to terminate in the somatosensory cortex. The spinothalamic tract transmits signals that are important for pain localization.

Spinoreticular Tract

The spinoreticular tract also decussates and ascends the contralateral cord to reach the brainstem reticular formation, before projecting to the thalamus and hypothalamus. There are also many further projections to the cortex. This pathway is involved in the affective aspects of pain.

DESCENDING INHIBITORY PAIN PATHWAY

The periaqueductal gray in the midbrain and the rostral ventromedial medulla are two important areas of the brain involved in descending inhibitory modulation. These areas contain opioid receptors and endogenous opioids that project to the dorsal horn of the spinal cord to inhibit pain transmission. Also involved in the descending inhibitory pathway are the neurotransmitters norepinephrine and serotonin.

Sympathetic Nervous System

128

George Hwang, MD

Understanding the autonomic nervous system (ANS) is critical in anesthetic management, as many disease states have profound ANS effects. In addition, many of the pharmacological interventions commonly implemented by anesthesiologists have direct effects on the ANS—leading some to state that anesthesiology is the practice of autonomic medicine.

The ANS is instrumental in the control of many of the body's organ systems below the conscious level, including central nervous system (CNS) and peripheral nervous system regulation of cardiac muscle, smooth muscle, and visceral functions. The ANS is predominantly an efferent system, consisting of the sympathetic nervous system (SNS) and parasympathetic nervous system (PSNS). The ANS also has an afferent component, transmitting information from the periphery to the CNS. Examples of this include the baroreceptors and chemoreceptors in the carotid sinus and aortic arch or the vasovagal response.

ANATOMY OF THE SYMPATHETIC NERVOUS SYSTEM

The SNS and PSNS innervate most organs, providing opposing yet complementary effects. The anatomy of the efferent ANS is characteristically different than the somatic and ANS afferent pathways. The ANS efferents consist of a two-neuron chain from the CNS to the ANS ganglion (via preganglionic fibers) to the effector organ (via postganglionic fibers). This organization contrasts with the somatic afferent and efferent system, which consists of one neuron from the CNS making direct contact with the effector organ.

The preganglionic fibers of the SNS (thoracolumbar division) originate in the intermediolateral column (lateral horn) of the gray matter in the spinal cord between the first thoracic and second lumbar vertebrae (Figure 128-1). The myelinated axons of these nerve cells leave the spinal cord with the motor fibers to form the white (myelinated) communicating rami. The rami enter one of the paired 22 sympathetic ganglia at their respective segmental levels. The preganglionic fiber enters the rami and proceeds by either synapsing with postganglionic fibers in the ganglia at the level of exit, traversing

cephalad or caudad in the SNS chain to synapse in ganglia at other levels, or tracking through the SNS chain at variable distances and exiting without synapsing to terminate in an outlying, unpaired SNS collateral ganglion. The exception is the adrenal gland, where preganglionic fibers pass directly into the organ without synapsing in a ganglion.

The SNS postganglionic neuronal cell bodies are located in ganglia of the paired lateral SNS chain or unpaired collateral ganglia (such as the celiac and inferior mesenteric ganglia). The SNS ganglia are typically closer to the spinal cord than the effector organ; thus, the SNS postganglionic neuron can originate in either the paired lateral paravertebral SNS ganglia or one of the unpaired collateral ganglia. The postganglionic fiber proceeds from the ganglia to terminate within the effector organ. In general, SNS preganglionic fibers are short, and postganglionic fibers tend to be long.

Of note, some postganglionic fibers pass from the lateral SNS chain back into the spinal nerves forming the gray communicating rami, which are distributed distally to sweat glands, pilomotor muscle and blood vessels of the skin and muscle. These unmyelinated nerves are called C-type fibers and are carried within somatic nerves.

The superior cervical, middle cervical, and cervicothoracic (stellate) ganglia are formed from the first four or five thoracic preganglionic fibers. The stellate ganglion is formed by the fusion of the inferior cervical and first thoracic SNS ganglia. These three special ganglia provide sympathetic innervation of the head, neck, upper extremities, heart, and lungs.

SYNTHESIS AND RELEASE OF NEUROTRANSMITTERS

The effects of the ANS are mediated by the release of neurotransmitters. Preganglionic fibers of both PSNS and SNS secrete acetylcholine (ACh). Sympathetic nervous system postganglionic fibers are mostly adrenergic and thus secrete the catecholamines, epinephrine (EPI) and norepinephrine (NE). Norepinephrine synthesis occurs in or near postganglionic nerve endings. The nerve terminal axoplasm takes up

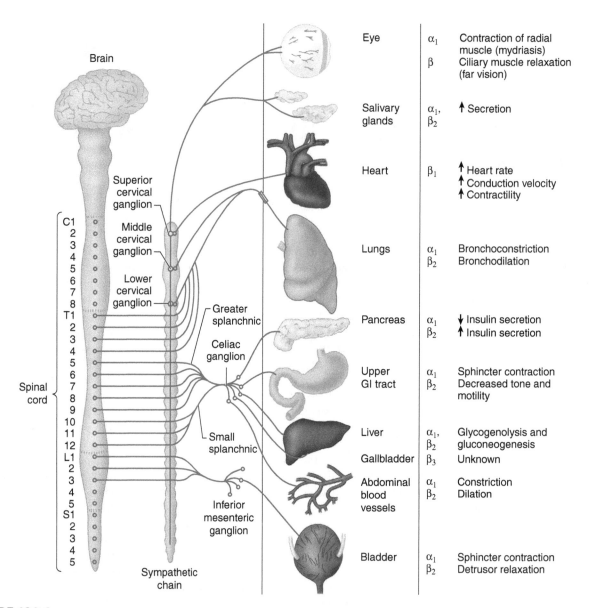

FIGURE 128-1 The sympathetic nervous system. (Reproduced with permission from Butterworth JF, Mackey DC, Wasnick JD, *Morgan and Mikhail's Clinical Anesthesiology*, 5th ed. McGraw-Hill; 2013.)

phenylalanine or tyrosine, which is then synthesized into either NE or EPI. The rate-limiting step is tyrosine conversion to dihydroxyphenylalanine via tyrosine hydroxylase, and it is mediated through feedback inhibition. Dopamine synthesis occurs in the neuronal cytoplasm, and is converted to NE via dopamine beta–hydroxylase.

The effect of postganglionic nerve stimulation depends on the receptors present at the effector site—usually alpha or beta adrenoreceptors. Termination of action is due to NE reuptake into the presynaptic nerve ending where it is inactivated by the enzyme monoamine oxidase (MAO) in the mitochondria or metabolized locally by the enzyme catechol-O-methyltransferase (COMT).

Again, the exception to the rule is the adrenal medulla, where the organ responds to impulses in the SNS cholinergic preganglionic fibers by transforming the neural impulses into hormonal secretion. There is no sympathetic chain synapse, thus the nerve reaching the adrenal medulla is strictly preganglionic, where ACh is the neurotransmitter leading to EPI and NE release. Chromaffin cells take the place of postganglionic neurons. In addition, the SNS postganglionic fibers supplying the sweat glands secrete ACh and exert their effects via muscarinic receptors.

Adrenoreceptors are subdivided into alpha and beta receptors, which are then further subdivided into subgroups alpha-1 and alpha-2 and beta-1, beta–2, and beta-3.

Alpha receptors are G protein-linked receptors, and generally lead to excitatory effects. Alpha-1 receptors are predominant in the peripheral vasculature, and stimulation causes vasoconstriction. Alpha-2 receptors are largely presynaptic and act via G protein subgroup Gi, inhibiting adenylate cyclase, reducing cyclic AMP (cAMP) and calcium levels. The net effect is downregulation of the SNS response. Alpha-2 receptors are also present in the CNS, specifically the locus ceruleus in the floor of the fourth ventricle with the effect of analgesia, anesthesia, and hypotension.

Beta receptors are also G protein linked, but unlike alpha-2 stimulation, adenylate cyclase activity is increased, leading to increased intracellular cAMP. There are three major subgroups of beta receptors: beta-1, beta-2, and beta-3. Beta-1 receptors have classically been viewed as cardiac, where stimulation leads to increased heart rate and positive inotropy. The renin–angiotensin–aldosterone axis is activated as well, leading to release of renin from the juxtaglomerular apparatus. Beta-2 receptor stimulation causes relaxation of bronchial and uterine smooth muscle, vasodilatation in the pulmonary, coronary, and skeletal muscle vascular beds, and some positive inotropy and chronotropy. Beta-3 receptors are in adipose tissue and may be involved with regulating metabolism, thermogenesis, and body fat.

PHYSIOLOGY OF THE SYMPATHETIC NERVOUS SYSTEM

In the heart, the vagus nerve is a mixed nerve containing both PSNS and SNS fibers. The SNS has more ventricular distribution than the PSNS despite having similar supraventricular distribution. The SNS fibers traverse through paired stellate ganglia. Right stellate ganglion stimulation leads to increased heart rate and decreased systolic time, whereas left stellate ganglion stimulation leads to increased inotropy and mean arterial pressure with little change in chronotropy.

Peripheral circulation is mediated by the SNS to a much larger extent compared to the PSNS. The main SNS effect on vessels is vasoconstriction, and is greatest in the vascular beds of skin, kidneys, and spleen, with less effect in organs such as the heart, brain, and muscle. Basal vasomotor tone is mediated by the medulla oblongata, which continuously transmits impulses via the SNS.

In the lungs, SNS fibers from the stellate ganglia innervate the bronchial and pulmonary blood vessel smooth muscle, resulting in bronchodilation and pulmonary vasoconstriction, respectively. Other SNS effects include decreased gastrointestinal motility, sphincter contraction, glycogenolysis, gluconeogenesis, lipolysis, renin secretion, uterus contraction or relaxation, and pupillary dilation.

Parasympathetic Nervous System

George Hwang, MD

ANATOMY OF THE PARASYMPATHETIC NERVOUS SYSTEM

Like the sympathetic nervous system (SNS), the parasympathetic nervous system (PSNS) also begins with unmyelinated preganglionic neurons and ends with myelinated postganglionic neurons. Parasympathetic preganglionic fibers leave the central nervous system (CNS) in both cranial and sacral nerves. Cranial fibers arise from specific parasympathetic brainstem motor nuclei of cranial nerves III, VII, IX, and X, traveling with the main body of fibers within the cranial nerves to ganglia that are generally distant to the CNS and close to the target organ. Sacral outflow originates in the intermediolateral gray horns of the second, third, and fourth sacral nerves.

Cranial nerve X (vagus) accounts for more than 75% of PSNS activity, innervating the heart, lungs, esophagus, stomach, small intestine, proximal half of the colon, liver, gall bladder, pancreas, and upper portions of the ureters. The sacral nerves form the pelvic visceral nerves, which supply the descending colon, rectum, uterus, bladder, and lower portions of the ureters.

In contrast to the SNS, preganglionic PSNS fibers are generally long and pass directly to the effector organ, whereas postganglionic fibers are short and are situated near or within the innervated viscera. The ratio of postganglionic to preganglionic neurons is also much smaller in the PSNS (3:1) when compared to the SNS (20:1). The decreased number of preganglionic to postganglionic synapses may explain the discrete and limited effect of PSNS, such as vagal bradycardia occurring without concomitant change in intestinal motility.

PHYSIOLOGY OF THE PARASYMPATHETIC NERVOUS SYSTEM

Parasympathetic effects are generally mediated by muscarinic acetylcholine (ACh) receptors, with termination of action due to ACh hydrolysis. Similar to adrenoreceptors, they are G protein-linked receptors classified as M1-M5. M1 receptors are found on gastric parietal cells stimulating acid secretion; M2 receptors are found in the heart and decrease the heart rate; M3 receptors contract smooth muscle in the gut; M4 receptors cause epinephrine (EPI) release from the adrenal medulla with SNS stimulation; and M5 receptors have a CNS effect that is not well understood.

In the heart, the PSNS fibers travel via the vagus nerve, which also contains some SNS fibers to primarily control chronotropy. The majority of cardiac PSNS fibers are distributed to the sinoatrial and atrioventricular nodes, with some distribution to the atria and very little distribution to the ventricles. Vagal stimulation leads to decreased sinoatrial (SA) node discharge and decreased atrioventricular (AV) excitability, ultimately leading to decreased ventricular conduction and bradycardia. The PSNS effect on contractility is relatively negligible compared to its profound chronotropic effects.

The lungs are also innervated by the PSNS via the vagus nerve. Pulmonary vasculature is poorly responsive to vagal stimulation, especially when compared to the SNS effect. However, vagal stimulation causes intense bronchoconstriction and bronchial secretion. Vagal stimulation in the alveolar ducts also controls the reflex regulation of the ventilatory cycle.

The PSNS also controls peripheral circulation, but to a much lesser extent compared to the SNS. The PSNS dilates vessels, but only in specific regions such as the genitals. Other PSNS effects include increased gastrointestinal motility, sphincter relaxation, glycogen synthesis, and pupillary constriction.

CHAPTER 130

Temperature Regulation

Jason Hoefling, MD

The primary reason to maintain normothermia is to improve patient outcomes, both clinically and financially. With medical reimbursement in the balance, maintaining normothermia is becoming an important part of the surgical process. Patients have numerous disadvantages that contribute to the stress response, including preoperative anxiety, prolonged fasting, and arriving in a cold operating room in a thin backless gown.

Perioperative hypothermia is associated with increased surgical site infection, increased intraoperative bleeding, prolonged stay in recovery room, increased cardiac morbidity and mortality, and increased requirements for postoperative mechanical ventilation.

DEFINITIONS

Normothermia—Core body temperature −36°C to 38°C (96.8°F-100.4°F)

Hypothermia—Core body temperature below 36°C (96.8°F)

Ideal thermic state—Near 37.0°C (98.6°F)

Conduction—Direct transfer of energy between two materials in contact with each other

Convection—Dispersion of heat via currents of air or fluid

Radiation—Infrared emission of heat

Evaporation—Phase change where heat is lost (liquid to gas)

Core temperature—The thermal compartment of the body composed of highly perfused tissues where the temperature is uniform

Ambient temperature—The temperature of the surrounding environment

Passive insulation—Containing body heat and insulating the body from heat loss via radiation

Active warming—Application of conductive, convective, or radiation to the skin

PHYSIOLOGY

Skin temperature fluctuates with patient's surroundings, whereas core temperature remains relatively constant at 98.0°F to 98.6°F (37°C). In fact, core temperature normally remains between 97°F and 100°F even while environmental temperatures fluctuate from as low as 55°F to as high as 130°F. The "interthreshold range" is the narrow limit above and below the body's normothermic state of 37.0°C (±0.2°C) and temperatures below the lower limit trigger the body's cold responses of thermoregulation.

Thermal-sensitive cells (cold receptors) are triggered by temperatures below a set threshold and generate impulses that travel mainly via A delta nerve fibers. Temperatures above threshold excite heat receptors that generate impulses along unmyelinated C fibers which also conduct pain sensation. Afferent information is integrated at several levels within the spinal cord and brain. Although some temperature regulation occurs in the spinal cord, the hypothalamus integrates most afferent input and produces efferent outputs to maintain normothermia. Additional factors known to alter temperature thresholds include circadian rhythm, food intake, infection, and drugs.

The efferent response is modulated by neurotransmitters, including norepinephrine, dopamine, serotonin, and acetylcholine. Thermogenesis is accomplished by piloerection, shivering, vasoconstriction, decreased sweating, and increased metabolic rate.

Development of intraoperative hypothermia occurs in distinct stages. During the first 40 minutes the body loses heat due to the lowered threshold vasodilation and redistribution via radiation. This results in a rapid decrease in core temperature of up to 1-2°C. Over the next 2-3 hours heat loss outpaces production in a linear fashion. After a 3-hour loss, it matches production as vasoconstrictive thermoregulation commences resulting in a stabilization of core temperature.

RISK FACTORS FOR INTRAOPERATIVE HYPOTHERMIA

- Extremes in patient age
- Female sex
- Low ambient room temperatures
- Length and type of surgical procedure
- Amount of body fat

- Preexisting conditions (*peripheral vascular disease, endocrine disease, pregnancy, burns, open wounds, etc*)
- Significant fluid shifts
- Use of cold irrigation

ADVERSE EFFECTS

- Shivering
- Cold diuresis
- Hypertension
- Tachycardia
- Hyperglycemia
- Tachypnea
- Hepatic dysfunction
- Vasoconstriction
- Decreased metabolism alters pharmacokinetics
- Increased need for postoperative mechanical ventilation

One significant long-term sequela of hypothermia is the potential for increased surgical site infection. In the perioperative period, decreased perfusion at the wound site inhibits both antibiotic and phagocytic penetration. The problem is compounded by directly impaired immune function (neutrophils become less effective) as well as protein wasting and decreased collagen synthesis.

Increased surgical bleeding is a potentially catastrophic complication resulting from the decreased activation of coagulation cascade as well as altered and reduced platelet function. This may result in the increased need for transfusion of red blood cells, platelets, and plasma.

Postoperative hypothermia disposes a patient to an increased risk for adverse cardiac events, including ischemia and dysrhythmias. This is mediated by the increased oxygen consumption due to shivering (400%-500%) coupled with vasoconstriction.

ANESTHESIA AND NORMOTHERMIA

The overall effect of general anesthesia is the induced inhibition of thermoregulation as well as a decrease in metabolic heat production. The resulting redistribution of heat within the body coupled with increased environmental heat loss leads to a drop in core temperature. Specifically, volatile anesthetics and propofol result in vasodilation and decreased metabolic rate, whereas neuromuscular blockade agents prevent shivering. As a class, opioids, especially morphine and meperidine, lead to vasodilation. In addition, opioids widen the normal threshold range from approximately 0.2°C to as much as 4°C and diminish the threshold for cold response. Fentanyl and its derivatives directly impair hypothalamic thermoregulation.

Regional anesthesia produces similar patterns of heat loss and hypothermia as those produced by general anesthesia. Hypothermia following spinal and epidural anesthesia results from the blockade of afferent fibers from preventing cold input to the hypothalamus. Although local anesthetics have no direct action on the hypothalamus, the thermoregulatory center nevertheless becomes impaired as it incorrectly judges skin temperature in blocked regions to be abnormally elevated. The net result is that the threshold range increases 3-4 times and despite a drop in core temperature, patients generally feel warm and may even become hypothermic enough to commence shivering. The concomitant use of sedation not only compounds the depression of thermoregulation but also obtunds the patient's subjective sensations.

MANAGEMENT

Hypothermia is easier to prevent than to treat, and prewarming patients can reduce core temperature drop by "banking" heat. A 30-minute period of prewarming reduces infection rates from 14% to 5% with no adverse effects. Intraoperative measures include increasing ambient temperature (room or heat lamps,) surface warming using forced air or warm fluid blankets, warming fluids (IV and surgical irrigation), and warming of anesthetic gasses. Postoperative management should consist of warm blankets and/or forced air device depending on patient core temperature as well as maintaining ambient room temperature at a minimum of 75°F.

Intraoperative hypothermia has clinical consequences that extend well into the postoperative period. Understanding the physiology of thermoregulation and managing patient temperature can have significant positive effects on patient outcome.

Anatomy of the Brain and Cranial Nerves

Mohebat Taheripour, MD

ANATOMY OF THE BRAIN

Cerebrum

The cerebrum contains 83% of the brain tissue and consists of two hemispheres. The thick folds of the cerebrum are *gyri*, whereas the shallow grooves are *sulci*. Longitudinal fissures separate the two hemispheres. The corpus callosum, located at the bottom of the longitudinal fissure, is a bundle of nerve fibers that connects the hemispheres.

The cerebral cortex is a 2- to 3-mm thick layer of tissue covering the cerebrum, which contains about 40% of the brain mass. The cerebral cortex has six layers known as the neocortex. The layers are numbered I-VI, with VI being the innermost layer. Layer VI is thickest in sensory regions, whereas layer V is thickest in motor regions. All axons that leave the cortex, and enter the white matter, arise from layers III, V, and VI.

The cerebral cortex is divided into lobes:

- The *frontal lobe* is the site for voluntary and planned motor behaviors. The motor speech area (Broca area) is usually in the frontal lobe of the left hemisphere, regardless of which hemisphere is dominant. It is also the lobe responsible for sensory reception and integration of taste and some visual information. When the cortical control of movements is considered, the left frontal lobe controls the right side of the body, whereas the right frontal lobe controls the left side.
- The *parietal lobe* is concerned with sensory reception and integration of somesthetic (touch, pressure, heat, cold, pain, stretch, movement), taste, and some visual information. Damage to the right parietal lobe can cause visual–spatial deficits. Damage to the left parietal lobe may disrupt a patient's ability to understand spoken or written language.
- Various parts of the *temporal lobe* are important for the sense of hearing, certain aspects of memory, and emotional behavior. The right temporal lobe is mainly involved in visual memory, whereas the left temporal lobe is mainly involved in verbal memory.
- The *occipital lobe* is crucial for the sense of sight.
- The *insular lobe* is located within the cerebral cortex, under the frontal, parietal, and temporal lobes. It plays a role in emotion and homeostasis.

Basal Ganglia

The basal ganglia are a group of nuclei lying deep in the subcortical white matter of the frontal lobes. It organizes the muscle-driven motor movements of the body behavior. Its major components are the caudate, putamen, and globus pallidus nuclei. The basal ganglia are functionally associated with the substantia nigra.

Cerebellum

The cerebellum consists of two cerebellar hemispheres connected by a narrow bridge-like vermis. Three pairs of cerebellar peduncles connect it to the brainstem (inferior peduncle to the medulla oblongata, middle peduncle to the pons, and superior peduncle to the midbrain). The cerebellum receives most of the information from the pons. Spinocerebellar tracts enter through the inferior peduncle. Motor outputs leave the cerebellum through the superior peduncle.

Thalamus

The thalamus is a major relay center to the cortex for all sensations except for smell. It consists of many nuclei, including the lateral geniculate nucleus (visual information) and the medial geniculate nucleus (auditory information).

Hypothalamus

The hypothalamus lies just inferior to the thalamus. It controls the pituitary gland and integrates autonomic and endocrine functions with behavior.

ANATOMY OF THE CRANIAL NERVES

There are 12 cranial nerves (CN I-CN XII) that leave the brain and pass through foramina in the skull (Table 131-1 and Figure 131-1). All the nerves are distributed in the head and neck, except the 10th, which also supplies structures in the thorax and abdomen. For each CN, the motor or efferent fibers arise from a group of neurons in the brain. The sensory or afferent fibers arise from a group of neurons outside the brain.

TABLE 131-1   Cranial Nerves

CN	Name	Function
I	Olfactory	Sensory
II	Optic	Sensory
III	Oculomotor	Motor
IV	Trochlear	Motor
V	Trigeminal	Mixed
VI	Abducens	Motor
VII	Facial	Mixed
VIII	Vestibulocochlear	Sensory
IX	Glossopharyngeal	Mixed
X	Vagus	Mixed
XI	Accessory	Motor
XII	Hypoglossal	Motor

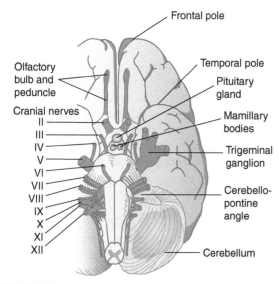

FIGURE 131-1 Ventral view of the brainstem with CNs. (Reproduced with permission from Waxman SG, *Clinical Neuroanatomy*, 27th ed. McGraw-Hill Companies, Inc. 2013. All rights reserved.)

Olfactory Nerve

The olfactory nerve serves the sense of smell. Bipolar cells in receptors carry the impulse to the olfactory nerve fibers through cribriform plate, olfactory bulb, olfactory tract, and enter the cortex and brainstem. In severe head injuries involving the anterior cranial fossa, anosmia or loss of olfaction is produced.

Optic Nerve

The optic nerve, mediating vision, is distributed to the eyeball. This nerve arises from retina and converges on the optic disc, which will then pass the optic canal and create the optic chiasma. The optic tract receives these fibers and sends impulses via the lateral geniculate body to the visual cortex (as optic radiation). A complete lesion of optic nerve leads to complete blindness. Compression of optic chiasma produces bitemporal hemianopia. Lesions of the optic tract and optic radiation cause contralateral temporal hemianopia.

Oculomotor Nerve

Oculomotor nerve supplies all the extraocular muscles of the eyeball except lateral rectus and superior oblique muscles. Complete lesion of CN III results in ptosis, a drooping of the eyelid due to paralysis of the levator palpebrae muscle. External strabismus is caused by unopposed action of the lateral rectus and superior oblique muscles. Injuries to CN III can also result in the loss of accommodation and light reflex as well as internal or external ophthalmoplegia.

Trochlear Nerve

Trochlear nerve, which is the thinnest, supplies the extraocular superior oblique muscle after passing through the lateral wall of cavernous sinus. Injury to this nerve causes the eye to rotate medially leading to diplopia.

Trigeminal Nerve

As the largest CN, CN V is responsible for the sensory supply to the face, the greater part of the scalp, teeth, oral, and nasal cavities. It carries motor fibers to the muscles of mastication. The ophthalmic division (V1) provides the sensation of the upper eye lid, conjunctivae, skin of forehead, and lacrimal gland. The maxillary division (V2) supplies the lower eye lid, skin of midface, nose, upperlip, soft palate, hard palate, and nasopharynx. Mandibular division (V3) provides sensation to a small area of cheek skin, vestibular gum, floor of mouth, and salivary glands. Trigeminal neuralgia is characterized by pain in the distribution of any of the branches of CN V.

Abducens Nerve

Abducens nerve supplies only the lateral rectus muscle of the eye and passes through the cavernous sinus. Lesion of CN VI causes internal strabismus, since the unopposed medial rectus muscle pulls the eye medially.

Facial Nerve

Cranial nerve VII provides the primary motor innervation to muscles of the face as well as the stapedius and stylohyoid muscles. It provides taste fibers to the anterior two-thirds of the tongue, and innervation of salivary and lacrimal glands. Its primary branches are the posterior auricular, greater petrosal, and chorda tympani nerves. Lesions to CN VII can result in loss of facial sensation, loss of taste from the anterior part of the tongue, sensitivity to sound in one ear, ipsilateral deafness, and facial paralysis. Bell palsy is caused by inflammation of facial nerve near the stylomastoid foramen. Patients with Bell palsy have facial asymmetry and paralysis, drooping eyebrows, widened palpebral fissures, and poor control of tears and saliva.

Vestibulocochlear Nerve

Cranial nerve VIII is the main sensory supply of the internal ear. It carries two major sets of fibers: the vestibular nerve (arising from the vestibular ganglion) and the cochlear nerve (arising from the cochlear ganglion). Damage to the vestibular branch results in vertigo and nystagmus, whereas lesions to the cochlear branch cause deafness and tinnitus.

Glossopharyngeal Nerve

Cranial nerve IX carries both motor and sensory fibers. It supplies motor innervation to the stylopharyngeus muscle, parasympathetic innervation to the parotid gland, and sensory innervation to the tonsils, pharynx, and posterior one-third of the tongue. Isolated nerve damage is extremely rare.

Vagus Nerve

Cranial nerve X contains motor, sensory, and parasympathetic fibers. It has a more extensive course and distribution than any other CN, traversing the neck, thorax, and abdomen. Various branches of the vagus nerve are affected due to lesions. Recurrent laryngeal nerve palsy is the most common due to malignancies and surgical traumas. Lesions on the left side are more frequent, and it causes difficulty in swallowing and vocal cord defects. Lesions to the superior laryngeal nerve branch lead to palsy of the cricothyroid muscle.

Accessory Nerve

This nerve is formed by the union of its spinal and cranial roots. It provides motor function for the trapezius and sternocleidomastoid muscle. Lesions of the spinal root will cause paralysis of these muscles.

Hypoglossal Nerve

Cranial nerve XII is the main motor supply of tongue, except for the palatoglossus muscle. Complete lesion of this nerve causes unilateral lingual paralysis and hemiatrophy.

Anatomy of the Spinal Cord

132

Christopher Edwards, MD

Anatomy of the spinal cord is often broken down by associated vertebral level. The various functions of the spinal cord depend on whether it is cervical, thoracic, lumbar, or sacral. The spinal cord is generally divided into a posterior sensory portion and an anterior motor portion.

VERTEBRAL AND SPINAL CORD ANATOMY

The spinal cord is housed within the vertebral canal. The anatomic boundaries of the canal are:

- Superior—Foramen magnum
- Inferior—Coccyx
- Lateral—Neural foramen
- Posterior—Ligamentum flavum
- Anterior—Posterior spinal ligament and vertebral bodies

The spinal cord is made up of gray and white matter. The internal gray matter is made up of cell bodies, whereas the surrounding white matter consists of axons organized into various spinal tracts. Tracts are continuations of cell bodies and axons that originate in the brainstem and cerebral cortex. Each tract has specific functions, ranging from controlling motor and sensory inputs and outputs to transmitting temperature and pain signals from periphery to brain.

The spinal cord is organized and named according to its corresponding vertebral level and consists of the *cervical, thoracic, lumbar,* and *sacral* levels. Each vertebral body has an associated spinal nerve consisting of both sensory and motor nerve roots which exit through its corresponding neural foramen. There are 7 cervical, 12 thoracic, 5 lumbar, and 5 sacral vertebral bodies and 31 spinal nerves, including the coccygeal nerve. Spinal nerves from C1 to C7 emerge *above* the corresponding vertebral level, and spinal nerves from C8 to S5 emerge *below* the corresponding vertebral level. Consequently, there are eight cervical nerves, but only seven cervical vertebrae. C8 emerges below C7 and from there, on all nerves exit below their corresponding level.

SPINAL CORD MOTOR AND SENSORY DISTRIBUTION

C1-C4 form nerves that provide both sensory and motor innervation to the head and neck. The phrenic nerve (C3-C5) supplies the diaphragm. C5-T1 supply upper extremity innervation. T1-T12 provide motor control to the thoracoabdominal musculature. L2-S2 provide lower extremity motor control.

The clinically important dermatome levels include: C5, shoulder; C6, thumb; C7, index and middle fingers; C7–C8, ring finger; C8, little finger; T1, medial forearm; T2, medial, upper arm; L1, anterior, upper, medial thigh; L2, anterior, upper thigh; L3, knee; L4, medial malleolus; L5, dorsum of foot and toes 1-3; S1, toes 4-5 and lateral malleolus; S3-C1, anus; T4, nipple; and T10, umbilicus.

The spinal cord extends from the transition between the upper cervical cord and lower medulla to its terminal end, which in the adult is the L1-L2 vertebral body. In the infant, the spinal cord extends to as low as L3-L4, but rises until adulthood due to vertebral growth with development. As the spinal cord terminates at the L1-L2 level, spinal nerves continue caudally and exit with their corresponding vertebral level. This collection of spinal nerves is referred to as the *cauda equina*. The spinal cord ends as a fibrous extension of the cord called the *conus medullaris*. The conus medullaris has a terminal extension of pia mater called the *filum terminale*, which ultimately inserts into the coccyx.

VASCULAR SUPPLY

Perfusion of the spinal cord divides into both anterior and posterior blood supplies. The anterior spinal artery supplies the anterior portion of the spinal cord and the two posterior spinal arteries supply the posterior spinal cord. Both the anterior and posterior descending spinal arteries originate from vertebral arteries and run caudally to the spinal cord's medullary cone. Segmental arteries arise from cervical, deep cervical, intercostals, and lumbar arteries. Segmental arteries reinforce the blood supply from spinal arteries and enter the cord via corresponding neural foramens. In particular, the *artery of Adamkiewicz* provides a large portion of blood supply to the anterior lumbar cord. It arises from the aorta between T8 and L1. Damage to this artery leads to anterior spinal cord syndrome. The spinal cord has two anatomic enlargements, one in the cervical and one in the lumbar region. These larger areas are prone to ischemia during a vascular insult.

Both anterior and posterior longitudinal veins accomplish venous drainage of the spinal cord. These veins exit the spinal space in the neural foramen and join the systemic venous circulation via larger thoracic, abdominal, and intercostal veins.

Anatomy of the Meninges

Mohebat Taheripour, MD

The brain, as well as the spinal cord, is surrounded by three layers of membranes: a tough outer layer (**dura mater**); a delicate, middle layer (**arachnoid mater**); and an inner layer, firmly attached to the surface of the brain (**pia mater**). Figure 133-1 illustrates these relationships. The cranial meninges are continuous with, and similar to, the spinal meninges through the foramen magnum. However, there is one important distinction: The cranial dura mater consists of two layers, and only one of these is continuous through the foramen magnum.

DURA MATER

This outermost layer consists of an outer periosteal layer and an inner meningeal layer. The outer *periosteal* layer is firmly attached to the skull, is the periosteum of the cranial cavity, and contains the meningeal arteries. This layer is continuous with the periosteum on the outer surface of the skull at the foramen magnum. The inner *meningeal* layer is in close contact with the arachnoid mater and is continuous with the spinal dura matter through the foramen magnum.

There are four dural partitions that project inward and incompletely separate parts of the brain:

1. **Falx cerebri**—The falx cerebri, is a crescent-shaped projection of meningeal dura mater that passes between the two

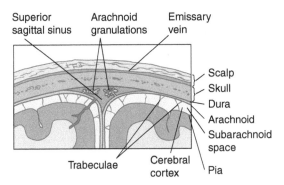

FIGURE 133-1 Coronal section through brain and meninges. (Reproduced with permission from Waxman SG, *Clinical Neuroanatomy*, 27th ed. McGraw-Hill Companies, Inc. 2013. All rights reserved.)

cerebral hemispheres. It is attached anteriorly to the crista galli of the ethmoid bone and frontal crest of the frontal bone.

2. **Falx cerebelli**—The falx cerebelli is a small midline projection of meningeal dura mater in the posterior cranial fossa. It is attached posteriorly to the internal occipital crest.
3. **Tentorium cerebelli**—This layer is a projection of the dura mater that covers and separates the cerebellum in the posterior cranial fossa from the posterior parts of the cerebral hemispheres.
4. **Diaphragma sellae**—This small shelf of the meningeal dura mater covers the hypophysial fossa in the sella turcica of the sphenoid bone. There is an opening in the center of the diaphragm sellae through which passes the infundibulum, connecting the pituitary gland with the base of the brain.

The arterial supply to the dura mater travels in the outer periosteal layer of the dura. It consists of:

- Anterior meningeal arteries. Located in the anterior cranial fossa, the anterior meningeal arteries are branches of the ethmoidal arteries.
- Middle and accessory meningeal arteries. Located in the middle cranial fossa, the middle meningeal artery is a branch of the maxillary artery. It enters the middle cranial fossa through the foramen spinosum and divides into anterior and posterior branches.
- Posterior meningeal artery and other meningeal branches. Located in the posterior cranial fossa, these arteries come from several sources.

All vessels are small arteries except for the middle meningeal artery, which is much larger and supplies the greatest part of the dura.

The innervation of the dura mater is by small meningeal branches of all three divisions of the trigeminal nerve (V1, V2, and V3), the vagus nerve, and the first, second, and third cranial nerves.

ARACHNOID MATER

The arachnoid mater is a thin, avascular membrane that lines, but is not adherent to, the inner surface of the dura mater. From its inner surface, the arachnoid mater extends downward, crosses the subarachnoid space, and become continuous with the pia mater. Unlike the pia mater, the arachnoid mater does not enter the grooves or fissures of the brain, except for the longitudinal fissure between the two cerebral hemispheres.

PIA MATER

The pia mater is a thin, delicate vascular membrane that closely invests the surface of the brain. It follows the contours of the brain, entering the grooves and fissures on its surface, and is closely applied to the roots of the cranial nerves at the origin.

The cranial pia mater invests the entire surface of the brain, dips between the cerebral gyri and cerebellar laminae. It forms the choroid plexuses of the third and lateral ventricles, and the roof of the fourth ventricle.

In contrast, the spinal pia mater is thicker and less vascular because it is composed of bundles of connective tissue fibers. Below the conus medullaris, the pia mater is continued as a long slender filament called *filum terminale*.

ARRANGEMENT OF MENINGES AND SPACES

There is a unique arrangement of meninges, coupled with real and potential spaces, within the cranial cavity. A potential space is related to the dura mater, whereas a real space exists between the arachnoid mater and the pia mater.

The spinal dura mater is separated from the arachnoid by a potential cavity, the *subdural cavity*. The two membranes are, in fact, in contact with each other, except where they are separated by a minute quantity of fluid, which serves to moisten the surfaces. It is separated from the wall of the vertebral canal by a space, the *epidural space*, which contains a venous plexus, and loose areolar tissue.

The subarachnoid cavity is the interval between the arachnoid and pia mater and contains the subarachnoid fluid.

Carotid and Aortic Bodies

Jessica Sumski, MD, and Seol W. Yang, MD

The control of ventilation is achieved by regulating and processing complex inputs from central and peripheral chemoreceptors to the central nervous system. The main peripheral chemoreceptors in the body are the carotid bodies and the aortic bodies.

ANATOMY AND PHYSIOLOGY

The carotid body is a collection of sensory chemoreceptors located near the common carotid artery bifurcation. Its primary role is to detect changes in the composition of arterial blood such as oxygen tension, CO_2 tension, pH, and temperature, and relay the information to the central respiratory center. The carotid body is composed of glomus cells, which exist in two types: type I and type II. After sensing changes in the arterial blood, type I glomus cells release neurotransmitters, acetylcholine, adenosine triphosphate (ATP), and dopamine, which generate an action potential that travels via glossopharyngeal nerve (CN IX) to the central respiratory center. Type II glomus cells are supporting cells that do not participate directly in respiratory regulation.

Whereas central chemoreceptors largely respond to changes in H^+ concentration in direct correlation with $Paco_2$, carotid body chemoreceptors respond mainly to changes in arterial oxygen tension, Pao_2. The action potential output of type I glomus cells is minimal when Pao_2 remains greater than 100 mm Hg. When Pao_2 is less than 100 mm Hg, the glomus cells respond by releasing stored neurotransmitters, resulting in immediate information relay to the central respiratory center. The degree of response is exponential, as Pao_2 continues to fall below 100 mm Hg. Changes in $Paco_2$, pH, and temperature in the arterial blood are also able to elicit the glomus cell's response, albeit not to the level of Pao_2.

Although the carotid body is not believed to directly initiate a modulatory response, a fall in Pao_2 will increase the ventilatory drive. When the carotid body is activated, a reflex increase in minute volume ventilation promotes CO_2 removal from alveoli and decreased alveolar $Paco_2$ ensues. This reduction in alveolar $Paco_2$, along with increased alveolar and arterial Po_2, minimizes hypoxia. Consequently, adequate tissue oxygen supply is maintained. The response of carotid bodies to the combination of hypoxemia and hypercapnia is greater than the sum of the individual responses to each

component. Notably, separate carotid baroreceptors modulate cardiovascular response to changes in blood pressure.

Aortic bodies are sensory chemoreceptors and baroreceptors scattered throughout the aortic arch and its branches. Similar to the carotid body, aortic body chemoreceptors sense changes in Pao_2, $Paco_2$, and pH in the arterial blood. Signals from aortic body chemoreceptors travel via the vagus nerve (CN X) to the medulla where respiratory centers are stimulated, increasing ventilatory drive.

CELLULAR MECHANISMS

The cellular mechanism by which the carotid body responds to stimulation has not been resolved, but there are a few leading theories to consider. It is proposed that hypoxia causes glomus cell depolarization, leading to activation of voltage-gated Ca^{2+} influx and enhanced excitatory transmitter secretion. Initial depolarization may be mediated by hypoxia-sensitive K^+ channels. Another hypothesis posits that carbonic anhydrase in the glomus cells of the carotid body plays an important role in the initial response to CO_2 stimulus. As CO_2 increases, it diffuses into the cell where it increases concentrations of carbonic anhydrase. H_2CO_3 forms following the equation: $CO_2 + H_2O \Leftrightarrow H_2CO_3$. H_2CO_3 further dissociates into H^+ and HCO_3^{-2}. These ions participate in the intracellular pH regulation. Inhibition of carbonic anhydrase activity reduces the carotid chemosensory responses to CO_2 and O_2.

The mechanism by which aortic bodies respond to hypoxia, hypercapnia, and acidosis is even less understood than that of the carotid body. Chemostimulation from acidosis, hypercapnia, or hypoxia causes a rise in intracellular Ca^{2+} in aortic body cells. This rise in intracellular Ca^{2+} activates aortic body receptors, increasing medullary stimulation to increase minute ventilation.

EFFECT OF MEDICATIONS

Inhaled anesthetics—Potent inhaled anesthetics depress the hypoxic ventilatory response by depressing carotid and aortic body response to hypoxemia. This results in a decreased stimulation and release of neurotransmitters with the onset of arterial hypoxemia during general anesthesia or anesthetic recovery.

Narcotics—Narcotics decrease minute ventilation and respiratory drive through depression of central chemoreceptors. Increased CO_2 stimulates the carotid bodies, but they are unable to properly compensate.

Benzodiazepines—These agents result in a depression of hypoxic ventilatory drive through depression of peripheral chemoreceptor activity. The effects from these medications can only be partially reversed by administration of flumazenil. Tolerance to the respiratory depressant effects of diazepam is possible.

Chemoreceptor stimulants—Cyanide will stimulate the carotid receptors through blockade of the cytochrome electron transport system, which prevents oxidative metabolism. As a result, patients with cyanide toxicity will have increased minute ventilation. Nicotine, through sympathetic ganglion stimulation, as well as acetylcholine will result in carotid body activity and an increase in minute ventilation.

ANESTHETIC CONSIDERATIONS

Patients who are dependent on hypoxic ventilatory drive have Pao_2 values below 60 mm Hg. Once Pao_2 values exceed 60-65 mm Hg, ventilator drive diminishes and Pao_2 falls until ventilation is stimulated again by arterial hypoxemia. This is observed clinically as periods of apnea.

Carotid body denervation may occur in patients who have had a carotid endarterectomy (CEA) for atherosclerotic disease. If one carotid body has been lost, ventilator response to mild hypoxemia may be impaired. Bilateral loss of carotid bodies is associated with loss of normal ventilatory and arterial pressure responses to acute hypoxia and an increase in resting partial pressure of $Paco_2$. In these patients, central chemoreceptors primarily maintain ventilation and severe respiratory depression following opioid administration is possible, especially in the postoperative period.

The clinical significance of aortic body chemoreceptors is limited as they are mainly active in infancy and childhood and then become relatively quiescent in adults.

Lung Volumes and Spirometry

Lorenzo De Marchi, MD

Lung volumes are divided into two categories (Figure 135-1). Static lung volumes are measured with slow breathing, whereas dynamic lung volumes are measured with fast or forced breaths. The lung volumes and capacities measured during spirometry are compared with theoretical values that reference values relative to the height, age, and sex of the subject in whom lung volumes are measured.

STATIC LUNG VOLUMES AND CAPACITIES

The "static lung volumes" are individual volumes that cannot be further divided (Table 135-1):

- **Tidal volume**—The amount of air that is mobilized with each unforced breath (300-500 mL). To find out how much air arrives to the alveoli (and therefore participates in the gas exchange), one must calculate the alveolar volume, subtracting the anatomical dead space from the tidal volume. The anatomical dead space is given by

TABLE 135-1   Lung Volumes and Capacities

Measurement	Definition	Average Adult Values (mL)
Tidal volume (V_T)	Each normal breath	500
Inspiratory reserve volume (IRV)	Maximal additional volume that can be inspired above V_T	3000
Expiratory reserve volume (ERV)	Maximal volume that can be expired below V_T	1100
Residual volume (RV)	Volume remaining after maximal exhalation	1200
Total lung capacity (TLC)	RV + ERV + V_T + IRV	5800
Functional residual capacity (FRC)	RV + ERV	2300

(Reproduced from *Morgan & Mikhail's Clinical Anesthesiology*, 5th ed. McGraw-Hill. Table 23-1.)

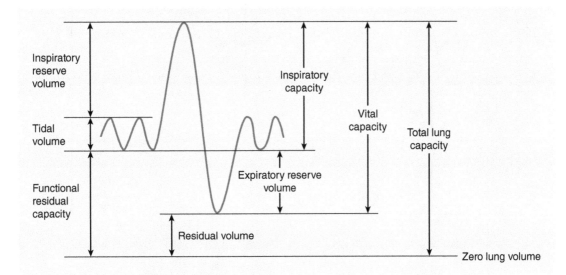

FIGURE 135-1 Spirogram showing static lung volumes. (Reproduced from *Morgan & Mikhail's Clinical Anesthesiology*, 5th ed. McGraw-Hill. Figure 23-5.)

the initial portion of the airways (from the mouth to the terminal bronchioles). Anatomical dead space does not participate in the exchange of O_2 and CO_2 between air and blood, but has only one function to bring the air to the alveoli. The dead space volume is on average 150 cc, and it can be calculated approximately by multiplying the weight in kilograms by 2.

- **Inspiratory reserve volume**—The maximum amount of air that, after normal inspiration, may still be forcibly introduced in the lungs.
- **Expiratory reserve volume**—The maximum amount of air that, after a normal expiration, can still be expelled with a forced exhalation.
- **Residual volume**—The air that remains in the lungs after a forced exhalation. This volume cannot be measured directly and is calculated using various methods: plethysmography, helium mixing, nitrogen washout. Increased residual volume is a sign of lung hyperinflation due to bronchoconstriction or pulmonary emphysema. It is also very important in forensic medicine, because the absence of this residual air is an indication of death by suffocation.

The lung capacities are sums of volumes:

- **Vital capacity (VC)**—The sum of *tidal volume* plus *inspiratory reserve* and *expiratory reserve* volumes. Vital capacity corresponds to the maximum amount of air that can be moved with single breath, forced inspiration

starting from maximal inhalation and arriving to a maximal exhalation.

- **Total lung capacity (TLC)**—The sum of the *VC* and *residual volume*. Total lung capacity corresponds to the maximum amount of air that can be contained in the lungs.
- **Inspiratory capacity (IC)**—The sum of *tidal volume* plus *inspiratory reserve volume*. Inspiratory capacity is the maximum amount of air that can be drawn into the lungs after normal expiration.
- **Functional residual capacity (FRC)**—Corresponds to the sum of the *expiratory reserve volume* and the *residual volume*. Functional residual capacity is the volume of air that remains in the lungs at the end of passive exhalation. At this volume, the respiratory system is in equilibrium.

The "Motley index" is the ratio of residual volume to the TLC (RV/TLC%). Normal index is about 20%. An increase in this index is a sign of lung hyperinflation, secondary to bronchoconstriction or pulmonary emphysema.

DYNAMIC LUNG VOLUMES

Dynamic lung volumes are indicative of the increased flow resistance in the airways and reduced lung recoil (Figure 135-2). The main dynamic lung volume is the *forced expiratory volume at 1 second* (FEV_1). The forced expiratory volume at 1 second is determined by the amount of air exhaled in the first second of forced expiration. The "Tiffeneau index" is the ratio of FEV_1

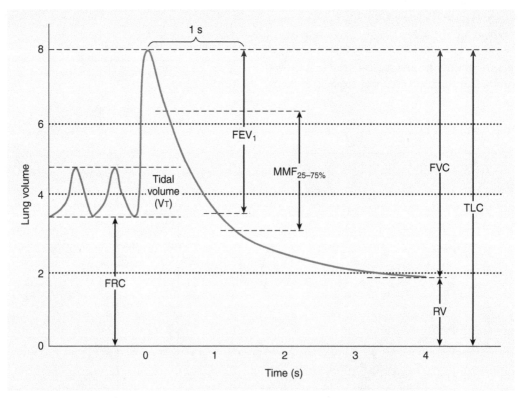

FIGURE 135-2 The normal forced exhalation curve. $FEF_{25-75\%}$ is also called the maximum midexpiratory flow rate ($MMF_{25-75\%}$). FRC, functional residual capacity; FEV_1, forced expiratory volume in 1 second; FVC, forced vital capacity; RV, residual volume; TLC, total lung capacity. (Reproduced from *Morgan & Mikhail's Clinical Anesthesiology*. 5th ed. McGraw-Hill. Figure 23-10.)

to the forced VC (FEV_1/FVC%). This ratio represents the proportion of a person's VC that is exhaled in the first second of expiration. A reduction of FEV_1 or FEV_1/FVC less than 70% indicates bronchoconstriction with expiratory difficulties (asthma, chronic obstructive pulmonary disease) and/or a reduction of recoil capacity of the lung (emphysema).

Another dynamic volume measured during pulmonary function testing is the maximum voluntary ventilation. This test measures the maximum amount of air that can be inhaled and exhaled in 1 minute of breathing. It provides an assessment of the maximum ventilatory capacity of the individual.

136

Lung Mechanics

Alex Pitts-Kiefer, MD, and Lorenzo De Marchi, MD

COMPLIANCE OF THE RESPIRATORY SYSTEM

Compliance is a mechanical property used to describe the elastic behavior of the lung, chest wall, or respiratory system as a whole. It is defined as a change in volume (ΔV) divided by the change in pressure (ΔP) needed to cause the change in volume, and can be expressed mathematically as:

$$\text{compliance} = \frac{\Delta V}{\Delta P}$$

If a patient who is breathing spontaneously inhales 500 mL of air and has an intrapleural pressure of –5 cm H_2O prior to inhalation and an intrapleural pressure of –10 cm H_2O following inhalation, the compliance of the respiratory system (both lung and chest wall) can be calculated as follows:

$$\text{compliance} = \frac{\Delta V}{\Delta P} = \frac{500 \text{ mL}}{(-5 \text{ cm } H_2O)(-10 \text{ cm } H_2O)}$$
$$= 100 \text{ mL} \times \text{cm } H_2O^{-1}$$

It should be noted that transpulmonary pressure (intrapleural pressure minus alveolar pressure) is generally used to calculate total pulmonary compliance during spontaneous ventilation. Intrapleural pressure was used in this example because alveolar pressure remains constant during spontaneous ventilation without obstruction of the airway.

Lung compliance in a healthy adult is normally 150-200 ml × cm H_2O^{-1}, chest wall compliance in a healthy adult is normally 200 ml × cm H_2O^{-1}, and total compliance of the chest wall and lungs together is normally 100 ml × cm H_2O^{-1}. The relationship between separate lung and chest wall compliances and total respiratory compliance can be expressed as:

$$\frac{1}{\text{Total compliance}} = \frac{1}{\text{Chest wall compliance}} + \frac{1}{\text{Lung compliance}}$$

Compliance is the inverse of elastance. If a lung has high elastance, it will by definition have a low compliance. It can also be helpful to think of compliance as the inverse of "stiffness." A "stiff" tissue will have a low compliance.

STATIC AND DYNAMIC COMPLIANCE

In anesthesiology practice, the concept of compliance is most often encountered during positive pressure ventilation of a patient where information provided by the ventilator can be used to calculate compliances. Static compliance is defined as pulmonary compliance without the presence of gas flow. The plateau pressure during an inspiratory hold maneuver minus the peak end-expiratory pressure (PEEP) can be used as the ΔP to calculate static compliance. Dynamic compliance is defined as pulmonary compliance during gas flow. The peak inspiratory pressure (PIP) minus PEEP can be used as the ΔP to calculate dynamic compliance.

Compliance is affected by the factors listed in Table 136-1.

Pressure–volume curves can be created to better understand compliance over the range of lung volumes. Multiple pressure–volume curves are demonstrated in Figure 136-1. The slope of the curve represents compliance. As lung volume increases, compliance is decreased based on the elastic properties of the tissue. Notice the decreased slope for fibrosis and an increased curve for emphysema. Also note the parallel left shift in the curve of a patient with asthma or bronchitis, which shows that lung volumes may change but compliance remains the same.

TABLE 136-1 Factors Affecting Compliance

Causes of Increased Compliance	Causes of Decreased Compliance
COPD/emphysema[a]	Idiopathic fibrosis
Normal aging	Alveolar proteinosis
Use of neuromuscular blocking (NMB) agents	Sarcoidosis
	Interstitial and alveolar edema
	Supine position
	Insufflation of abdomen
	Restrictive lung pathologies
	Hydrothorax
	Pneumothorax
	Lack of lung surfactant
	Obesity
	Opioid-induced rigidity
	endotracheal (ET) tube/breathing circuit obstruction

[a]In emphysema, static compliance is increased secondary to loss of elastic tissue but dynamic compliance is decreased secondary to compression of the airway (Bernoulli's Principle).

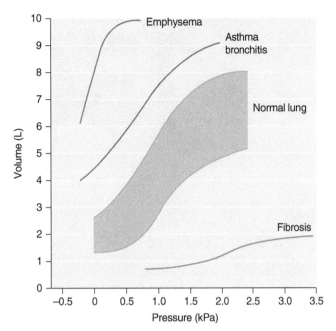

FIGURE 136-1 Effects of lung pathology on pressure–volume curve and compliance. (Reproduced with permission from Miller RD, *Miller's Anesthesia*, 7th ed. Philadelphia, PA: Churchill Livingstone/Elsevier; 2010.)

RESISTANCE OF THE RESPIRATORY SYSTEM

Elastic and nonelastic types of resistance contribute to the total resistance of the respiratory system. Elastic resistance is related to the compliance of the respiratory system as well as surface tension forces at the gas–fluid interface in alveoli. These surface tension forces result in an "inward" pressure in the alveoli that creates a tendency to collapse. This pressure is inversely proportional to alveolar radius and directly proportional to surface tension, which is expressed by Laplace's law:

$$\text{Alveolar pressure} = \frac{2 \times \text{Surface tension}}{\text{Radius of alveoli}}$$

This law demonstrates the importance of pulmonary surfactant, which decreases surface tension. The amount of reduction in surface tension is directly proportional to its concentration in the alveolus. Smaller alveoli will have a higher concentration of surfactant than larger alveoli. This increased concentration can moderate the inward pressure resulting from the smaller radius.

In addition to the resistance caused by the tissues of the respiratory system and the surface tension forces in the alveoli, airway resistance to gas flow contributes to the total resistance of the pulmonary system. Laminar flow is airflow that is streamlined and travels in parallel layers without disruption of the layers. Velocity is highest in the center of the flow and decreases as the wall of the airway is approached. Laminar flow principally occurs in the small peripheral airways.

Turbulent flow is characterized by a chaotic, random flow of air, and is more difficult to model mathematically.

Resistance is not constant during turbulent flow but is directly proportional to gas flow and gas density, and is inversely proportional to the fifth power of the radius. Turbulent flow occurs in larger airways, at high velocities, and at transition points from larger to smaller airways.

Total airway resistance in healthy adults is 0.5-2 cm H_2O/L/s. Most airway resistance is produced in the medium-sized bronchi. Although resistance in each individual small airway is high, the large number of these airways results in a large cross-sectional area, resulting in a small contribution to total airway resistance. Large airways have low resistance secondary to their large diameters. Common causes of increased airway resistance include airway collapse, bronchospasm, edema, and secretions.

WORK OF BREATHING

Respiratory work is measured as the product of pressure and volume, and is the work required to move the chest wall and lungs during inspiration and expiration. Both nonelastic resistance (resistance to airflow) and elastic resistance (compliance and surface tension forces) must be overcome by work. In Figure 136-2, the shaded areas to the left of the curves represent the work performed. As a patient inspires, airway resistance and elastic recoil (related to compliance) must be overcome by inspiratory muscle effort. This kinetic energy is stored as potential energy. During expiration, this stored energy is used to overcome expiratory resistances and perform expiratory work.

Because the work performed during both inspiration and expiration is performed by the inspiratory muscles, there

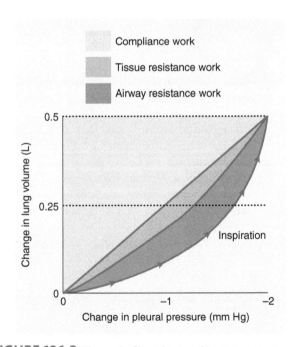

FIGURE 136-2 The work of breathing and its components during inspiration. (Reproduced with permission from Butterworth JF, Mackey DC, Wasnick JD, Morgan and Mikhail's Clinical Anesthesiology, 5th ed. McGraw-Hill; 2013.)

is increased work performed by the inspiratory muscles when either inspiratory or expiratory resistances increase. In the case of increased expiratory resistance, the need for increased potential energy to be stored as greater elastic recoil is provided for by a larger tidal volume, which decreases compliance and increases elastance of the respiratory system.

Tidal volume and respiratory rate are physiologically altered to minimize work of breathing. In patients with decreased compliance, total work will be decreased by lowering tidal volume and increasing respiratory rate. In patients with increased resistance to airflow, the respiratory rate will be decreased and the tidal volume will be increased.

Ventilation and Perfusion

Howard Lee and Christopher Monahan, MD

MINUTE AND ALVEOLAR VENTILATION

Minute ventilation (MV) is the amount of air inspired in one breath (tidal volume = V_T) multiplied by respiratory rate (RR), where:

$$MV = V_T \times RR$$

Ventilation can also be expressed as alveolar ventilation, or the amount of air that enters the alveoli and is thus available for gas exchange. Alveolar ventilation can be expressed as:

$$V_A = (V_T - V_D) \times RR \qquad \text{where } V_D \text{ is dead space ventilation}$$

or

$$V_A = V_{CO_2}/PA_{CO_2}$$

This equation states that alveolar P_{CO_2} (PA_{CO_2}) is directly proportional to the amount of CO_2 produced by metabolism and delivered to the lungs (V_{CO_2}) and inversely proportional to the alveolar ventilation (V_A).

VENTILATION/PERFUSION

Ventilation can be described as the amount of air that reaches the alveoli. *Perfusion* is the amount of blood that reaches the alveoli. Ideally, ventilation matches perfusion, which allows equal exchange of O_2 and CO_2. In reality, different anatomic regions of the lung receive unbalanced perfusion and ventilation due to gravitational and nongravitational forces.

Zones of Lung

An understanding of the west zones of the lung is essential to comprehend both lung perfusion and ventilation. West zones describe areas of the lung based upon variations in pulmonary arterial pressure (PAP), pulmonary venous pressure (PVP), and alveolar pressure (AP). These differences result from a 20 mm Hg increase in blood flow found in the base of the lung relative to

the apex as a result of gravity in an upright patient. While this pressure gradient is less apparent in the supine position, gravitational forces still lead to a greater degree of perfusion in the posterior lung than the anterior aspect (Figure 137-1).

Although gravity has a major impact on regional lung perfusion differences, recent research has highlighted the influence of nongravitational forces. Specifically, intrinsic features of the lung during inspiration also play a role in altering lung perfusion. Extraalveolar vasculature expands with inspiration due to radial traction, which may lead to increased blood flow even as alveolar pressure increases.

The perfusion dynamics of each zone are as follows:

Zone 1: AP > PAP > PVP

Zone 2: PAP > AP > PVP

Zone 3: PAP > PVP > AP

where AP = arterial pressure; PAP = pulmonary artery pressure; PVP = pulmonary vein pressure.

Zone 1 is defined by high AP, which may compress both arterial and capillary vessels. Generally, Zone 1 is associated

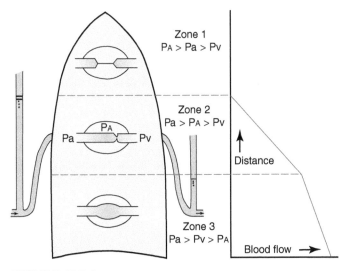

FIGURE 137-1 West zones in the upright patient. (Reproduced with permission from Levitsky MG, *Pulmonary Physiology*, 8th ed. New York: McGraw-Hill; 2013.)

with the lung's apex. In reality, alveolar pressure is never truly great enough to completely prevent blood flow. Moving toward the base of the lung, the effect of gravity begins to become more apparent in Zone 2 where the flow of blood within the pulmonary vasculature is driven by the ability of arterial pressure to overcome alveolar pressure. In Zone 3 (the base of the lung), gravity plays an even greater role, as pulmonary blood flow is dictated by arterial pressure in relation to venous pressure, both of which are consistently greater than alveolar pressure.

Variations in Ventilation and Perfusion

Although alveolar pressure is higher than both arterial and venous pressures in the apex of the lung, apical ventilation is not greater (Zone 1). Greater negative intrapleural pressure and larger transmural pressure gradient exist in Zone 1. These factors lead to less compliant alveoli, limiting further alveolar expansion necessary for improved ventilation. By contrast, the lung base (Zone 3) has greater ventilation due to more compliant alveoli, which readily expand in the setting of more negative intrapleural pressure and a smaller transmural pressure gradient. Thus, ventilation improves from the apex (Zone 1) to the base (Zone 3) of the lung.

Lung perfusion balances intravascular pressures, vasculature recruitment, pulmonary vascular resistance (PVR), and blood flow. The apex of the lung has lower intravascular pressures, less vascular recruitment, greater PVR, and less blood flow; while the lung base has higher intravascular pressures, greater vascular recruitment, lower PVR, and higher blood flow. Thus perfusion, similar to ventilation, improves from the apex to the base of the lung.

Even though ventilation and perfusion are both greater in the base of the lung relative to the apex, regions exist where the two are not equal. Ventilation and perfusion (V/Q) mismatch is the most important aspect of inadequate gas exchange. V/Q mismatch is the result of: (1) airway obstruction (Shunt) or (2) physiologic dead space.

A. Shunt

Airway obstruction leads to inadequate ventilation in a region that otherwise has adequate perfusion, thus making the V/Q ratio near zero. The resultant shunt does not allow for gas exchange. Examples of shunts include disease processes that limit ventilation without perfusion effects, such as atelectasis, pneumonia, bronchospasm, and pulmonary edema. Positive end-expiratory pressure (PEEP) ventilation strategies can overcome airway obstructions, such as atelectasis, by maintaining alveolar patency and limiting V/Q mismatch. Shunt can be quantified as the amount of cardiac output (CO) that is not ventilated, or the shunt fraction:

$$\text{Shunt fraction} = Q_s/Q_t = (Cc_{O_2} - Ca_{O_2})/(Cc_{O_2} - Cv_{O_2})$$

where Q_s = shunted cardiac output; Q_t = total cardiac output; Cc_{O_2} = end-capillary O_2 content; Ca_{O_2} = arterial O_2 content; and Cv_{O_2} = mixed venous O_2 content.

Generally, a normal individual has a shunt fraction of 2%-3% due to bronchial veins, which drain deoxygenated blood into pulmonary veins. As the shunt fraction increases in the lung region, 100% O_2 supplementation does not improve Pa_{O_2} due to poor gas exchange. This will be reflected by a wider alveolar–arterial, or A-gradient.

B. Dead Space

Whereas shunt describes regions of the lung with adequate perfusion and inadequate ventilation, physiologic dead space describes adequate ventilation but insufficient perfusion. In this case, the V/Q ratio approaches infinity. Hundred percent O_2 supplementation improves Pa_{O_2} if any perfusion is maintained. Examples of physiologic dead space include pulmonary embolism and hypovolemia. Dead space and resultant hypoxia in the lungs leads to pulmonary vasoconstriction (HPV). Vasoconstriction physiologically reduces dead space and optimizes ventilation and perfusion. This allows blood flow to be diverted away from poorly ventilated areas of the lung to better-ventilated lung regions.

Pulmonary Diffusion

Mandeep Grewal, MD, and Seol W. Yang, MD

Diffusion is a net movement of gas molecules from an area of high partial pressure to low partial pressure. Pulmonary diffusion largely refers to the passive movement of O_2 and CO_2 along their pressure gradients in the lungs. At the level of the alveolus, where pulmonary diffusion occurs, inhaled anesthetic agents move according to partial pressure differences.

ANATOMY

Lung respiratory zones include bronchioles leading to alveolar ducts, then sacs, and finally alveoli. The alveolus is composed of three primary cell types: Type 1 cells, Type 2 cells, and alveolar macrophages. Type 1 pneumocytes cover 95% of the alveolar septal surface and join one another by tight junctions. They are approximately 0.3-0.4 μm thick and allow for gas exchange between the alveolus and the pulmonary capillaries. Type 2 pneumocytes contain characteristic lamellar inclusions for surfactant production. Surfactant is responsible for decreasing pulmonary surface tension. These cells are also mitotically active and can differentiate into Type 1 cells. Lastly, Type 2 cells secrete a variety of substances in defense of the structure, including fibronectin and alpha1-antitrypsin. The third type of cells is macrophages that perform cleansing and defense functions.

ATMOSPHERE

The atmosphere is composed of permanent gases whose percentage remains relatively constant, and variable gases which change in concentration over time. Table 138-1 indicates typical values for atmospheric gases.

ALVEOLI

Alveolar air differs in composition of gases from the atmosphere. Alveolar air is only partially replaced with atmospheric air with each breath (Table 138-2). Oxygen is constantly being absorbed into the pulmonary bloodstream from alveolar air, while CO_2 moves down its concentration gradient from bloodstream to alveolus.

TABLE 138-1   Atmospheric Gases

Type	Gas	Percentage
Permanent	Nitrogen	78.1
	Oxygen	20.9
	Argon	0.9
	Neon	0.002
	Helium	0.0005
	Krypton	0.0001
	Hydrogen	0.00005
Variable	Water vapor	0-4
	Carbon dioxide	0.035
	Methane	0.0002
	Ozone	0.000004

Another important factor contributing to the difference between alveolar and atmospheric air is humidification. Atmospheric air becomes 100% humidified by the time it reaches the alveolus. The partial pressure of water vapor at the normal body temperature of 37°C is 47 mm Hg, the partial pressure of water vapor in alveolar air. Total pressure in the alveoli can never be greater than atmospheric pressure. Therefore, alveolar water vapor dilutes all inspired gases, and partial pressure of O_2 and CO_2 in the alveolus is about 149 and 0.3 mm Hg, respectively.

VENOUS BLOOD

Partial pressure of CO_2 in mixed venous blood and pulmonary capillary blood are similar, about 50 mm Hg. Partial pressure of O_2 in mixed venous blood is 40-50 mm Hg and it further decreases to 20-40 mm Hg in pulmonary capillary blood.

DIFFUSION

Diffusion across the blood–gas membrane in the lungs is passive (no active transporters involved) and is governed by Fick's law of diffusion. This law states that the rate of transfer of a gas through tissue is proportional to the tissue area and the difference in the gas partial pressure between the two sides, and

TABLE 138-2   Respiratory Gas Composition

	Atmospheric air (mm Hg)	Alveolar humidified air prior to gas exchange (mm Hg)	Alveolar air after gas exchange (mm Hg)	Expired air (mm Hg)
N_2	597.0 (78.62%)	563.4 (74.09%)	569.0 (74.9%)	566.0 (74.5%)
O_2	159.0 (20.84%)	149.3 (19.67%)	104.0 (13.6%)	120.0 (15.7%)
CO_2	0.3 (0.04%)	0.3 (0.04%)	40.0 (5.3%)	27.0 (3.6%)
H_2O	3.7 (0.50%)	47 (6.20%)	47.0 (6.2%)	47.0 (6.2%)
Total	760.0 (100%)	760.0 (100%)	760.0 (100%)	760.0 (100%)

inversely proportional to the tissue thickness. The equation is as below:

$$\text{Volume of gas (per unit time)} = \text{Area/thickness} \times \text{diffusion constant} \times (PP_1 - PP_2)$$

The law predicts that O_2 will diffuse along its gradient from alveolus to pulmonary capillary blood (from 149 mm Hg to 20-40 mm Hg) and CO_2 will diffuse along its gradient from capillary blood to alveolus (from 40 mm Hg to 0.3 mm Hg).

Diffusion Capacity of Lung for Carbon Monoxide

Diffusion capacity of lung for carbon monoxide (DLCO) is designed to test lung parenchymal function, namely O_2 exchange via lung tissues. It measures the difference between inspired and expired carbon monoxide concentration and relies on strong affinity of hemoglobin in red blood cells to bind carbon monoxide, thus making its uptake in blood less dependent on cardiac output. A low DLCO indicates damage to lung parenchyma and decreased oxygen exchange. Predicted postoperative DLCO less than 40% is related to higher pulmonary complication rates, indicating that other clinical tests and predictors are warranted in overall consideration of patient's condition and perioperative planning.

Factors Affecting Diffusion

Factors that decrease diffusion:

- Changes in alveolar cell membrane (fibrosis, alveolitis, vasculitis)
- Restrictive lung disease
- Emphysema
- Pulmonary embolism
- Decreased cardiac output
- Pulmonary hypertension
- Anemia
- Drugs (bleomycin)

Factors that increase diffusion:

- Polycythemia
- Asthma (DLCO can remain normal)
- Increased pulmonary blood volume

Oxygen Transport

Ramon Go, MD, and Seol W. Yang, MD

Oxygen molecules (O_2) take advantage of two important properties that facilitate its bodily transport. First, O_2 is lipid soluble and crosses cell membranes without the aide of membrane transporters. Second, the free movement across cell membranes relies on a partial pressure gradient for diffusion according to Fick's law. When O_2 reaches the alveolar capillary blood, it diffuses into erythrocytes and bonds to hemoglobin where the interaction is governed by the oxyhemoglobin dissociation curve.

OXYGEN UPTAKE

Oxygen exerts a partial pressure of 160 mm Hg in the atmosphere at sea level. In the alveolus, water vapor and carbon dioxide dilute atmospheric gas, slightly decreasing the partial pressure of O_2 to 150 mm Hg. Pulmonary arterial blood in alveolus capillaries has O_2 partial pressure of 20-40 mm Hg. According to this decreasing pressure gradient from atmosphere to alveolar capillaries, O_2 easily diffuses into erythrocytes. Increasing FIO_2 to 100% O_2 increases alveolar partial pressure of O_2 and creates a larger gradient, aiding in O_2 diffusion. Several variables affect oxygen uptake (Table 139-1).

TABLE 139-1   Factors Affecting Oxygen Uptake

Increases Oxygen Uptake	Decreases Oxygen Uptake
Left shift in oxyhemoglobin dissociation curve	Anemia
Blood transfusion	Blood dyscrasias
Increased alveolar ventilation	Dead space
Increased FIO_2	V/Q mismatch
	Chronic obstructive lung disease
	Diffusion limitation (ie, pulmonary edema or interstitial lung disease)

TABLE 139-2   Factors Affecting Oxygen Carrying Capacity

Increases Hgb Oxygen Carrying Capacity	Decreases Hgb Oxygen Carrying Capacity
Left shift in oxyhemoglobin dissociation curve	Right shift in oxyhemoglobin dissociation curve
Blood transfusion	Anemia
Alkalosis	Acidosis
	Genetics (ie, Sickle cell disease or thalassemia)

HEMOGLOBIN

In erythrocytes, O_2 is readily taken up by hemoglobin. Hemoglobin is a tetrameric metalloprotein that acts as an O_2 carrier, increasing O_2 carrying capacity of blood by seven times when compared to dissolved O_2 alone. A normal hemoglobin protein has the capability of carrying 1.34 mL of oxygen per gram of hemoglobin. This protein consists of four subunits, two alpha subunits and two beta subunits, each with an iron-containing heme moiety. The iron ion functions as a site of reversible binding for oxygen molecules and exists as ferrous iron (Fe^{2+}) or ferric (Fe^{3+}) when oxidized. As one O_2 binds to a heme group, molecular conformational changes occur causing other heme groups to increase their O_2 affinity. This is known as *cooperativity*. Several variables affect the carrying capacity of hemoglobin for oxygen (Table 139-2). The degree of O_2–hemoglobin binding (O_2 saturation) is represented by the oxygen–hemoglobin dissociation curve. At an O_2 partial pressure of 80 mm Hg, 95.8% of hemoglobin is saturated with O_2. After O_2 diffusion has occurred from alveoli, pulmonary arterial blood partial pressure of O_2 is 100 mm Hg, an almost 100% saturation of hemoglobin.

OXYHEMOGLOBIN DISSOCIATION CURVE

The oxyhemoglobin dissociation curve displays the relationship between hemoglobin–oxygen saturation and varying O_2 partial pressures. At a PaO_2 of 50 mm Hg, 80% of hemoglobin

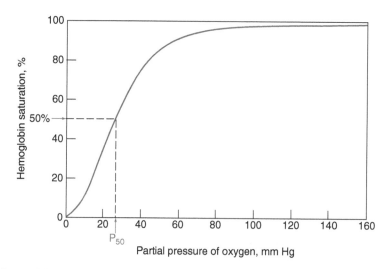

FIGURE 139-1 Adult oxyhemoglobin dissociation curve. (Reproduced with permission from Levitsky MG, *Pulmonary Physiology* , 8th ed. New York: McGraw-Hill; 2013.)

TABLE 139-3   Factors Affecting the Oxy-Hgb Dissociation Curve

Left Shift	Right Shift
Alkalosis	Acidosis
Hypothermia	Hyperthermia
Decreased 2,3-DPG levels	Increased 2,3-DPG levels
Fetal-hemoglobin	Beta and alpha thalassemia
Carboxyhemoglobin	Increased CO_2 levels
Methemoglobin	

is saturated. P_{50}, the partial pressure at which 50% of hemoglobin is saturated, is normally 26.7 mm Hg. The oxyhemoglobin dissociation curve shows the important relationship between hemoglobin and oxygen saturation by plotting the hemoglobin saturation at varying oxygen concentrations (Figure 139-1).

Factors Influencing Oxygen–Hemoglobin Dissociation Curve

There are several variables that affect the oxyhemoglobin dissociation curve (Table 139-3). A left shift in the curve indicates higher affinity of hemoglobin for oxygen, whereas a right shift suggests lower affinity. Left shift is associated with alkalosis, decreased 2,3-diphosphoglycerate (DPG), methemoglobinemia, and hypothermia.

OXYGEN CONTENT

About 98% of O_2 in arterial blood exists as oxyhemoglobin and less than 2% is dissolved in plasma. Oxygen content is calculated by the sum of oxyhemoglobin and dissolved oxygen in the blood. The amount of oxygen bound to hemoglobin is determined by the concentration of hemoglobin and the percent saturation, while the dissolved oxygen is measured using

arterial blood gas analysis. Hence, total oxygen content (CaO_2) can be calculated by the following equation:

$$CaO_2 = (Hgb \times 1.39 \times SaO_2/100) + (Pao_2 \times 0.003)$$

The constant 1.39 represents the amount of O_2 (at 1 atmosphere) bound per gram of hemoglobin or simply the coefficient for hemoglobin–oxygen capacity. The constant 0.003 represents the amount of dissolved oxygen in blood. Note that dissolved oxygen contributes little to the oxygen content. Several variables affect the level of oxygen content (Table 139-4).

Oxygen Delivery

Delivery of O_2 rich blood to end organs relies on cardiac output for circulation along with oxygen content (CaO_2); as either component increases, the delivery of oxygen also increases.

The product of the two variables will give the total O_2 delivery in mL/min, resulting in the equation:

$$Do_2 = CaO_2 \times CO$$

Stroke volume and heart rate thus affects oxygen delivery and tissue O_2 exchange. During cardiogenic shock, CO is not maintained, resulting in decreased O_2 delivery anaerobic metabolism. Pressors, such as epinephrine and norepinephrine, can increase adrenergic activity thereby providing cardiac support to allow end organ perfusion. Oxygen content consists of both oxyhemoglobin and dissolved oxygen, with

TABLE 139-4   Factors Affecting Oxygen Content

Increases Oxygen Content	Decreases Oxygen Content
Impaired oxygen extraction from tissues	Anemia
Increased RBC (ie, transfusions or polycythemia)	Hypoxia
Increased Fio_2	Poor oxygen uptake from alveolus

TABLE 139-5 **Factors Affecting Oxygen Delivery**

Increases Oxygen Delivery	Decreases Oxygen Delivery
Increased cardiac output	Anemia and blood dyscrasias
RBC transfusion	Impaired cardiac output (ie, heart failure)
Increased F_{IO_2}	Methemoglobinemia
Increased oxygen gradient between plasma and tissues	Poor oxygen uptake from alveolus

the former consisting of the majority of oxygen content. With higher O_2 saturation and hemoglobin concentration, CaO_2 increases, subsequently resulting in higher oxygen delivery. Several variables affect oxygen delivery (Table 139-5).

FICK PRINCIPLE

Oxygen consumption can be calculated using the Fick principle that describes the relationship between O_2 flow as a function of cardiac output and O_2 consumption with the equation:

$$Vo_2 = Q \times (aO_2 - VO_2)$$

The result is expressed in L/min. In a healthy adult, oxygen consumption (Vo_2) is approximately 0.25 L/min. During rest, the CO is 5 L/min and the arterial-venous O_2 content difference is 5 mL O_2/100 mL of blood. The volume of oxygen consumed at rest is, therefore, 0.25 L of O_2/min.

O_2 consumption can also be measured by oximetry. Oxygen consumption as a fraction of the oxygen delivery provides the extraction ratio, with a normal value of 25%. Mixed venous saturation is the sum of the oxygen not extracted by tissues and is best measured from pulmonary artery blood sampling. Normal mixed venous saturation is greater than 65%.

In severe sepsis, mixed venous saturation may be low. This suggests that metabolic demand of organ systems is greater than O_2 supply. However, high mixed venous saturation can also indicate that tissues are failing to extract oxygen, indicating the absence of cellular metabolism as seen in multisystem organ failure.

SUGGESTED READING

McLellan S, Walsh T. Oxygen delivery and haemoglobin. *Br J Anesth, Crit Care Pain* 2004;4.

140

Hypoxemia and Hyperoxia

Eric Pan, MD, and Darin Zimmerman, MD

Hypoxemia is defined as low oxygen content in the blood, with a Pao_2 of less than 60 mm Hg or Spo_2 of less than 90%. The main causes of hypoxemia include:

1. **V/Q mismatch**—The most common etiology for hypoxemia is V/Q mismatch. Dead space is ventilation without perfusion, as seen with pulmonary embolism. Shunt is perfusion without ventilation, as seen with pneumothorax. Hypoxic pulmonary vasoconstriction improves V/Q matching by reducing shunt as poorly oxygenated areas of the lung vasoconstrict, diverting blood to more oxygenated regions.

   Functional residual capacity (FRC) is the volume remaining in the lung after normal exhalation. Closing capacity (CC) is the lung volume at which small airways without cartilaginous support close. If CC exceeds FRC, atelectasis occurs. Atelectasis commonly occurs in the postoperative period during anesthetic recovery as a result of inadequate tidal volumes. Pneumonia and bronchospasm can also cause V/Q mismatch in the perioperative setting.

2. **Hypoventilation**—Hypoventilation leads to hypoxemia by reducing fresh O_2-rich gas from entering the alveolar space, resulting in the accumulation of CO_2. If hypoventilation is left uncorrected, hypoxemia rapidly develops. Use of respiratory depressants such as narcotics and benzodiazepines during anesthesia predisposes patients to hypoventilation. Residual neuromuscular blockade can decrease tidal volume and minute ventilation, and lead to airway obstruction. Intraoperatively, ventilator failure or disconnect can cause hypoventilation.

3. **Low Fio_2**—Alveolar oxygen content is dependent on Fio_2, which is tightly controlled perioperatively. Patients may require increased Fio_2 with V/Q mismatch or hypoventilation. Inadequate Fio_2 can occur from failure to recognize increased patient O_2 demand or equipment malfunction. If mechanical failure is suspected, an immediate change to an alternative O_2 source is indicated.

4. **Right-to-left shunts**—Right-to-left shunting of blood permits deoxygenated venous blood to bypass the lungs and enter systemic circulation. Intracardiac right-to-left shunt lesions include: Tetralogy of Fallot, pulmonary stenosis with atrial-septal defect, transposition of the great vessels,

and Eisenmenger syndrome. Other important causes of right-to-left shunting include states of hyperdynamic circulation such as sepsis and liver failure, where transit time through the lungs is reduced.

5. **Diffusion impairment**—Patients with interstitial lung disease have impaired gas exchange across their pulmonary capillary beds. Increased cardiac output during exercise or times of stress worsens diffusion impairment because blood spends less time at the alveolar:pulmonary capillary interface; thereby, limiting time for gas exchange.

6. **Impaired oxygen-carrying capacity**—Oxygen is transported to tissues by hemoglobin. Anemia leads to decreased global oxygen carrying capacity. Functional impairment of hemoglobin such as carbon monoxide poisoning, methemoglobinemia, and hemoglobinopathies prevents normal binding and unbinding of oxygen, and can lead to tissue hypoxemia.

7. **Impaired oxygen delivery**—Tissue hypoxia can result from impaired delivery of oxygen. Low cardiac output and low circulating blood volumes are the most common causes. Pulmonary thromboembolism and air embolism can cause a rapid drop in venous return and cardiac output, impairing O_2 delivery to tissue.

INVESTIGATION AND TREATMENT OF INTRAOPERATIVE HYPOXEMIA

A systematic and organized approach is necessary to quickly and accurately evaluate, diagnose, and treat a hypoxemic patient (Table 140-1). Hypoxemia can develop rapidly intraoperatively, so efforts to correct the hypoxia must be undertaken while etiology is investigated. Communication with the surgical team should be ongoing as hypoxemia may require interventions (auscultation, bronchoscopy, replacement of the airway, etc) that interrupt surgery. Requesting the second opinion of an anesthesiologist should be considered for persistent hypoxemia.

Pulse oximetry can detect hypoxemia, however, there are several causes of inaccurate readings on the pulse oximeter, including: (1) excessive ambient light; (2) patient motion; (3) sensor malposition; (4) hypoperfusion; (5) blue-colored

TABLE 140-1   Approach to Hypoxemic Patient

Inspect pulse oximeter position and waveform
Alert the surgeon
Auscultate lungs
Inspect ETT position
Check all machine connections, flow-volume loops, CO_2 absorbent
Switch to hand ventilation and evaluate for equal chest excursion and compliance
Suction airway
Check labs—ABG, CBC
Bronchoscopy
Request backup support

nail polish; (6) methemoglobinemia which causes a falsely low Sao_2 of 85% (despite an actual Sao_2 of >85%); and (7) pulseless states (ie, cardiopulmonary bypass or LVAD).

A quick inspection of the endotracheal tube (ETT), circuit, and all machine connections rules out mechanical causes of hypoxemia. Disconnecting the circuit from patient commonly causes intraoperative hypoxemia and can be corrected by reconnecting patient to breathing circuit. A kink in the ETT or circuit can lead to high airway pressures and hypoventilation. Cracks in the plastic tubing at junctions in the circuit can lead to significant air leak, causing hypoventilation.

Auscultation of the lungs can reveal the cause of hypoxemia. If a patient is intubated, absence of breath sounds over a single lung field can indicate a malpositioned ETT (ie, right mainstem bronchus intubation), and absence of breath sounds bilaterally can indicate esophageal intubation. Mainstem intubation can lead to atelectasis and collapse of the nonventilated lung, causing shunt and hypoxemia. Pneumothorax should be suspected in patients with absent breath sounds, tachycardia, hypotension, and high peak airway pressures. Wheezing is often present during periods of bronchospasm, but if severe, breath sounds might not be heard and airway pressures will be elevated. A mucous plug must also be considered with decreased lung sounds; ETT suctioning should be attempted if mucous is suspected.

Switching off the ventilator and hand-bagging the patient with 100% Fio_2 is useful. Normal lungs are compliant and easy to ventilate. High resistance to ventilation is abnormal. Common causes are: (1) severe bronchospasm; (2) mainstem intubation; or (3) kinked ETT. A recruitment breath can be administered to reinflate atelectatic lung; which is accomplished by holding a pressure of 30-40 cm H_2O for 30 seconds with 100% Fio_2. During these maneuvers, the patient is inspected to verify equal, bilateral chest rise.

There are certain clinical situations where bronchoscopy will be beneficial in evaluating the cause of hypoxemia. During cases involving a double-lumen endotracheal tube (DLT), the DLT can become malpositioned with relatively minor changes in patient positioning or table adjustment. Bronchoscopy should also be used if it is suspected that the ETT may have migrated above the vocal cords, or if endobronchial obstruction is suspected due to mucous, mass, or foreign body.

HYPEROXIA

Tissue exposure to high partial pressures of O_2 can lead to toxicity. Toxicity develops from the excessive production of oxygen free radicals, including: superoxide anion, hydroxyl radicals, and singlet oxygen species, which are cytotoxic and cause damage to the alveolar-capillary membrane. In addition, high O_2 predisposes patients to mucous plugging and atelectasis. Acute respiratory distress syndrome can develop with extended periods of hyperoxia.

Retinopathy of prematurity, or retrolental hyperplasia, occurs most commonly in infants born at less than 28 weeks gestational age. Development of fibrous scar tissue in the maturing retinal vasculature of premature infants leads to retinal detachment and subsequent retinopathy. Supplemental oxygen therapy has been identified as a risk factor for the development of this disease. It is appropriate to maintain Pao_2 50-80 mm Hg or Spo_2 88%-93%, unless cardiopulmonary deficits require higher O_2 levels.

Hyperbaric oxygen therapy can produce oxygen toxicity, which manifests as tracheobronchial irritation, coughing, and chest pain. Neurotoxicity due to hyperoxia leads to nausea, vomiting, numbness, twitching, dizziness, and possible seizures. Seizure risk related to oxygen toxicity directly relates to increasing PO_2 and exposure period. Treat with immediate reduction of inspired PO_2 until seizing ceases. Ocular toxicity can also occur with hyperbaric oxygen therapy leading to a reversible condition called hyperoxic myopia. Symptoms indicate ongoing toxicity.

Carbon Dioxide Transport

Andrew Winn and Brian S. Freeman, MD

In the human body, carbon dioxide (CO_2) is a metabolic waste product of aerobic metabolism. Specifically, two catabolic processes, pyruvate decarboxylation and the Kreb's cycle, both of which occur in the mitochondria of cells, produce CO_2. As a result of these processes, the concentration of CO_2 increases proportionally to metabolic activity within tissues, leading to an increased partial pressure of carbon dioxide (Pco_2). This pressure gradient drives CO_2, a highly lipid-soluble molecule, out of tissues, across cell membranes, and into the blood of systemic capillaries. Once it has diffused into the capillaries, CO_2 is transported to the lungs by three mechanisms.

The majority ($\approx 70\%$) of CO_2 is transported to the lungs in the form of bicarbonate (HCO_3^-), a process known as *isohydric transport*. Upon entering red blood cells, CO_2 rapidly combines with water (H_2O) to form carbonic acid (H_2CO_3) via the reversible enzyme *carbonic anhydrase*. Just as rapidly as it is produced, carbonic acid releases hydrogen ion (H^+) and forms bicarbonate (HCO_3^-). This reversible reaction is represented below:

$$CO_2 + H_2O \leftarrow(\text{carbonic anhydrase})\rightarrow H_2CO_3 \longleftrightarrow HCO_3^- + H^+$$

The proton released from carbonic acid is buffered by binding to histidine residues on hemoglobin. Simultaneously, the bicarbonate ion diffuses out of the cell in exchange for a chloride ion via a bicarbonate-chloride carrier protein embedded in the membrane of the red blood cell. This exchange of bicarbonate for chloride maintains the electric neutrality within the cell and leads to an increase in chloride within blood cells of the venous system, as well as a decreased concentration of chloride in venous blood, referred to as the *chloride shift*, or *Hamburger shift*.

Approximately 23% of CO_2 is carried to the lungs, bound to hemoglobin and other plasma proteins. Hemoglobin possesses four N-terminal amino groups, each of which can bind CO_2 to form *carbaminohemoglobin*. During the reaction, a proton is released, which eventually leads to a decrease in the pH of surrounding tissues and concomitant release of O_2 from hemoglobin. The reaction is represented by the following equation.

$$CO_2 + Hb-NH_2 \longleftrightarrow H^+ + Hb-NH-COO^-$$

A small percentage of CO_2 binds to amino groups on the polypeptide chains of plasma proteins.

Finally, the remaining 7% of CO_2 produced in tissues travels to the lungs dissolved in plasma. A negligible portion of CO_2 dissolved in plasma combines with water to form carbonic acid, with immediate release of a proton to form bicarbonate. This reaction is identical to that which occurs in red blood cells. However, it should be noted that carbonic anhydrase is not present in the plasma and thus, the reaction takes place at a rate approximately equal to 1/1000 of the same reaction catalyzed by carbonic anhydrase within red blood cells.

In summary, the three primary mechanisms of CO_2 transport from the tissues to the lungs are:

1. 70% in the form of bicarbonate
2. 23% bound to hemoglobin (carbaminohemoglobin) and plasma proteins
3. 7% dissolved in plasma

Venous blood carrying CO_2 arrives at the lungs, with an oxygen saturation (O_2 sat) of approximately equal to 75%, partial pressure of oxygen (Po_2) of approximately equal to 40 mm Hg, and with hydrogen ions bound to histidine residues on the hemoglobin molecule.

The high Po_2 in alveoli, relative to venous blood, causes oxygen to diffuse down its pressure gradient, across the alveolar-capillary membrane, and into red blood cells where it binds to hemoglobin. This binding of oxygen to hemoglobin causes a conformational change in hemoglobin from the T (tense) state to the R (relaxed) state that promotes release of CO_2. This release of CO_2 that results from oxygen binding to hemoglobin is termed the *Haldane effect*. In the R state, hemoglobin tends to release protons. These released protons combine with bicarbonate in the plasma to form carbonic acid. The carbonic acid, a neutral molecule, diffuses into red blood cells where it is converted back into carbon dioxide and water via carbonic anhydrase. Carbon dioxide diffuses down its concentration gradient, out of the red blood cell, into the alveolus, where it is exhaled from the body. This process, represented by the equation below, is the reverse of that which occurs in the tissues.

$$CO_2 + H_2O \leftarrow(\text{carbonic anhydrase})\rightarrow H_2CO_3 \longleftrightarrow HCO_3^- + H^+$$

According to Le Chatelier's principle, increased concentrations of bicarbonate and protons (released by hemoglobin) in the lungs lead to increased formation of carbonic acid, followed by breakdown via carbonic anhydrase into carbon dioxide and water.

Hypocarbia and Hypercarbia

Brian S. Freeman, MD

For most patients receiving general or regional anesthesia, the arterial carbon dioxide tension ($Paco_2$) should be maintained within normal physiologic limits (35-45 mm Hg). Alterations in homeostasis may lead to hypercarbia or hypocarbia.

HYPOCARBIA

Presentation

Hypocarbia, or hypocapnia, occurs when levels of CO_2 in the blood become abnormally low ($Paco_2$ <35 mm Hg). Hypocarbia is confirmed by arterial blood gas analysis. Hypocarbia, especially if only transient, is usually well tolerated by patients. Deliberate hyperventilation, leading to hypocarbia, is often used to decrease intracranial pressure in neurosurgical patients.

Causes

A. Increased Carbon Dioxide Elimination

1. Hyperventilation
   - Excessive minute ventilation in mechanically ventilated patients
   - Increased minute ventilation in spontaneously ventilating patients
     ○ Response to metabolic acidosis
     ○ Pain
     ○ Pregnancy
     ○ CNS pathology (infection, tumors)
2. Decreased dead space ventilation
3. Decreased CO_2 rebreathing

B. Decreased Pulmonary Perfusion

1. Decreased cardiac output
   - Hypovolemia
   - Hypotension
   - Cardiac arrest
2. Pulmonary embolism

C. Decreased Carbon Dioxide Production

1. Hypothermia
2. Deep anesthesia

3. Hypothyroidism
4. Decreased metabolism

D. Airway/Equipment Problems

1. Esophageal intubation
2. Accidental extubation or circuit disconnection
3. Air entrainment (eg, cuff leaks)
4. Dilution with circuit gases

Physiologic Effects

1. Cardiovascular:
   - Decreased myocardial oxygen supply
   - Increased coronary vascular resistance
   - Increased risk of coronary artery vasospasm
   - Increased coronary microvascular leakage
   - Increased myocardial oxygen demand
2. Neurologic:
   - Decreased cerebral blood flow
   - Decreased cerebral oxygen delivery
   - Decreased cerebral blood volume
   - Decreased intracranial pressure
3. Metabolic/hematologic:
   - Respiratory alkalosis
   - Increased intracellular calcium concentration
   - Increased platelet count and aggregation

Management

1. Assess oxygenation status
2. Obtain arterial blood gas to confirm capnography results
3. Since the most common cause of hypocarbia during surgery is iatrogenic hyperventilation, the first step in management should focus on decreasing minute ventilation
4. Assess and restore circulation if the problem involves decreased cardiac output

HYPERCARBIA

Presentation

Hypercarbia, or hypercapnia, occurs when levels of CO_2 in the blood become abnormally high ($Paco_2$ >45 mm Hg).

Hypercarbia is confirmed by arterial blood gas analysis. When using capnography to approximate $Paco_2$, remember that the normal arterial–end-tidal carbon dioxide gradient is roughly 5 mm Hg. Hypercarbia, therefore, occurs when $PETco_2$ is greater than 40 mm Hg.

In the awake or sedated patient, signs and symptoms include dyspnea, sweating, muscle tremors, flushed skin, headache, lethargy, and confusion. Spontaneously breathing patients develop tachypnea while mechanically ventilated patients may overbreathe the ventilator.

In patients breathing room air or low inspired oxygen concentrations, severe hypercarbia leads to severe hypoxemia. According to the alveolar gas equation, a patient breathing room air with $Paco_2$ of 90 mm Hg would have significant hypoxia (PAo_2 37 mm Hg).

Causes

A. Increased CO_2 Production

1. Hyperthermia
   - Malignant hyperthermia
   - Fever, sepsis
2. Thyrotoxicosis
3. Shivering
4. Seizures
5. Compensation for metabolic alkalosis
6. Exogenous or iatrogenic:
   - Intravenous sodium bicarbonate administration
   - Total parenteral nutrition with excessive carbohydrate content
   - CO_2 insufflation (laparoscopy)
   - Release of extremity tourniquets
   - Removal of vascular cross-clamps

B. Decreased CO_2 Elimination

1. Hypoventilation
   - Inadequate minute ventilation in mechanically ventilated patients
   - Altered respiratory mechanics in spontaneously ventilating patients
     - Decreased pulmonary compliance (eg, Trendelenburg positioning)
     - Increased airway resistance (eg, bronchospasm, endobronchial intubation)
     - Pharmacological-induced decrease in respiratory drive
   - Upper airway obstruction
   - Neuromuscular depression (eg, residual neuromuscular blockade, high spinal anesthesia)
   - Equipment problems
     - Ventilator malfunction
     - Leak in breathing circuit
   - Primary CNS pathology (eg, ischemia, tumor, edema)
   - Splinting from pain due to upper abdominal and thoracic incisions

2. Increased dead space ventilation
   - Lung pathology (COPD, pulmonary embolus, ARDS)
   - Decrease in pulmonary artery pressure (eg deliberate hypotension)
   - Application of positive end-expiratory pressure
   - Mechanical disruption of pulmonary arterial blood flow
3. Rebreathing of carbon dioxide
   - Stuck expiratory valve
   - Inadequate fresh gas flow
   - Exhausted CO_2 absorber
   - Excessive circuit dead space

C. Increased Carbon Dioxide Delivery to the Lungs

1. Increased cardiac output
2. Right-to-left shunts

Physiologic Effects

1. Cardiovascular
   - Systemic hypertension (peripheral vasoconstriction)
   - Tachycardia
   - Dysrhythmias (PVCs)
   - Pulmonary hypertension
   - Hypotension (if $Paco_2$ is very high)
2. Pulmonary
   - Tachypnea ($Paco_2$ 45-90 mm Hg)
   - Respiratory depression ($Paco_2$ >90 mm Hg)
   - Bronchodilation
3. Neurologic
   - Increased cerebral blood flow
   - Increased intracranial pressure
   - Obtundation
   - Central depression (if $Paco_2$ is very high)
4. Metabolic
   - Acidosis (intracellular and respiratory)
   - Compensatory metabolic alkalosis from chronic hypercarbia
   - Hyperkalemia
   - Depression of intracellular metabolism
   - Right shift of oxyhemoglobin dissociation curve

Management

- Assess oxygenation and airway
- Restore appropriate ventilation, if impaired or inadequate
- Obtain arterial blood gas to confirm capnography
- Treat secondary causes, such as shivering, malignant hyperthermia, and thyroid storm
- Administer antihypertensive and antidysrhythmic drugs, if necessary
- Examine and correct problems with anesthesia equipment
  - Replace CO_2 absorbers
  - Increase fresh gas flow
  - Remove excessive dead space apparatus

Control of Ventilation

Johan P. Suyderhoud, MD

The anatomic location of the neural elements involved in the control of breathing and ventilation reside primarily in **medullary** and **pontine** structures of the brainstem. In the **medulla**, two groups exist: a dorsal respiratory group lying in close proximity to the nucleus *tractus solitarius* and the fourth ventricle, and a ventral respiratory group located in the ventral medullary reticular formation, each richly cross-innervated. The dorsal respiratory group is involved mainly with timing and initiation of the respiratory cycle and can be thought of as the pacemaker for breathing, while the ventral group modulates the function of breathing, such as modulating and inhibiting pacemaker signaling to allow for cessation of inspiratory effort and eventual exhalation, controlling the force of contraction of inspiratory muscles, and dilator functions of the larynx and pharynx. Of note, generation of the medullary drive requires no afferent input from other parts of the body, be it lungs or otherwise. In the **pons**, neural activity can be thought of as processing medullary afferents involved in both inspiratory and expiratory activities. The pneumotaxic respiratory center of the rostral pons is not, as was earlier thought, involved with respiratory rhythmicity but with limiting inspiratory lung volumes, or apneusis (cessation of ventilation effort at TLC).

Other brain and/or neural structures contribute to ventilatory control. Stimulation of the reticular activating system will increase the frequency and depth of breathing. The cerebral cortex can interrupt and modulate ventilator effort required for such actions as talking, singing, coughing, and various expulsive efforts. Stimulation of carotid sinus will decrease both vascular tone and respiratory effort, while carotid body activation will have the opposite effect. A variety of above-brainstem structures will also assist and inhibit medullary output in the performance of sneezing, coughing, and swallowing, but these mechanisms are poorly defined.

Chemical control of breathing and ventilation occurs at both the peripheral and central nervous system levels via peripheral and central chemoreceptors (Figure 143-1). **Central chemoreceptors** can be thought mainly to be responsive to changes in Pco_2, pH, and acid–base parameters. Around 80%-85% of the ventilatory response to inhaled carbon dioxide originates within the central medullary chemoreceptors. These receptors lie very close to the anterolateral surface of the medulla close to both the glossopharyngeal and vagus nerves,

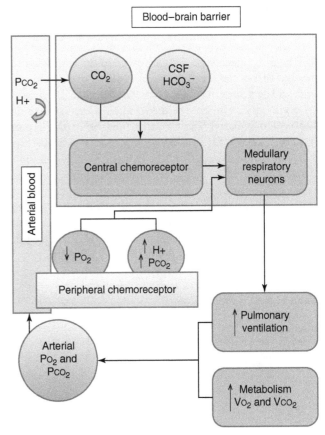

FIGURE 143-1 Schematic overview of the chemical control of ventilation. Peripheral chemoreceptors (carotid and aortic bodies) send afferent input via both glossopharyngeal and vagus nerves to modulate medullary pacemaker output. CO_2 diffusing across the blood–brain barrier is converted to carbonic acid, which ionizes and then effects pH sensors of the central chemoreceptors.

and are overlaid by the anterior inferior cerebellar arteries, allowing CO_2 to diffuse rapidly across the blood–brain barrier at this location. The rise in brain tissue and CSF CO_2 will lead to a corresponding increase in carbonic acid, whose ionization will then increase H^+ ion concentration, and decrease pH. It is the resulting change in pH that stimulates the firing rate of the medullary ventilation pacemaker neurons. As a result, increases in ventilatory rates are more responsive to respiratory acidosis than metabolic acidosis at similar blood pH, and for several reasons. First, changes in blood pH will be counteracted rapidly by multiple buffering mechanisms, whereas CSF buffering is far less robust. Hydrogen ions do not cross the blood–brain barrier. Increased levels of CSF CO_2 will thus generate higher levels of CSF H^+ ion production. Finally, CSF and brain tissue CO_2 levels are found to be about 10 mm Hg higher than in arterial blood.

Changes in $Paco_2$ will lead to rapid changes in minute ventilation. If $Paco_2$ elevation persists, these changes will gradually return to normal as compensatory mechanisms restore CSF bicarbonate levels, due to both active and passive transport of bicarbonate into the CSF. Similar changes in CSF bicarbonate will result from hyperventilation of a patient, leading to decreases in CSF bicarbonate that may take hours to readjust, leading to increases in minute volumes and rates until CSF bicarbonate levels are restored to homeostatic levels. The same mechanisms are involved in the compensatory changes that occur due to hypoxia at altitude, where hypoxemia and decreases in Pao_2 leads to stimulation of the hypoxic drive via the carotid bodies, inducing a respiratory alkalosis leading to decreased CSF CO_2 that then limits the hypoxic drive increase. In this case, $Paco_2$ falls more slowly over time than one would expect from the hypoxic stimulation alone; providing supplemental O_2 will only partially ablate this hypoxic stimulation to return ventilation parameters to resting states because a compensatory CSF acidosis still exists in response to the respiratory alkalosis. Humans who have acclimated to altitude, then, will continue to hyperventilate until CSF, brain tissue bicarbonate, and pH re-equilibrates.

Finally, central chemoreceptors are not stimulated by hypoxia, and in fact are depressed, probably as a result of both ischemia and hypoxemia.

Peripheral chemoreceptors are rapid responders to decreases in arterial Po_2, increases in Pco_2 and H^+, and decreases in perfusion pressure. The carotid bodies are located at the bifurcation of the common carotid arteries and are entirely responsible for the hypoxic drive to ventilation, exerted via afferents through the glossopharyngeal nerve; the aortic bodies are located throughout the aortic arch and its branches, and mainly modulate circulatory functions.

The carotid bodies are comprised primarily of glomus cells and have extensive sinusoids, allowing for much higher rates of perfusion in relation to their intrinsic, and already very elevated, metabolic rate. These tissues, thus, sense true decreases in arterial Po_2, not tissue Po_2, within 1-3 seconds. Stimulation occurs when Pao_2 is at or falls below 100 mm Hg, becomes parabolic as it falls below 60 mm Hg (and begins to increase minute ventilation), and is maximal at 32 mm Hg; below this level there is no further stimulation effect as ventilatory efforts has reached its physiologic limit (Figure 143-2). The carotid bodies are responsible for about 30% of the total ventilatory drive in normoxic patients. These receptors do not respond to anemia, carboxyhemoglobinemia, or methemoglobinemia, thus to decreases in either Sao_2 or Cao_2. Stimulation also occurs with decreases in pH or increases in $Paco_2$, but these are much less robust than hypoxic stimulation. In addition, hypoperfusion and hypotension will cause carotid body stimulation as a result of tissue hypoxia. Increases in pressure at both carotid and aortic body baroreceptors can cause respiratory depression and even apnea, such as engendered with large doses of catecholamines.

Hemodynamic effects from peripheral chemoreceptors include bradycardia, hypertension, increases in bronchomotor tone, and adrenal gland output. Catecholamines such as norepinephrine and epinephrine will increase the

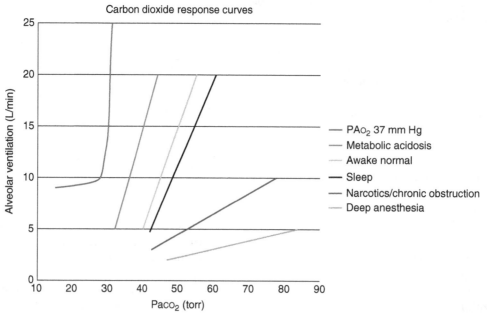

FIGURE 143-2 Ventilatory response to increasing concentrations of CO_2. Note the synergistic effect of hypoxia on CO_2 responsiveness as manifested by both a left and upward shift of the curve. The effect of exercise is similar to the curve for metabolic acidosis.

responsiveness to stimulation, but exogenous dopamine, which is secreted by the glomus cells, will inhibit their response. Nondepolarizing neuromuscular blocking agents inhibit carotid body sensitivity to hypoxia in direct relation to their degree of neuromuscular blockade. Together, these profound pulmonary and circulatory effects have led the carotid body to be called *ultimum moriens* (last to die).

Interaction between the peripheral and central chemoreceptors is synergistic; the slope of the hypoxic response curve is steeper in the presence of hypercarbia just as the slope of the hypercarbic responsive curve is increased with concomitant hypoxia. This modulation is mostly a function of the peripheral chemoreceptors.

Anesthetic agents can affect both the hypoxic and hypercarbic drives to ventilation. The centrally mediated hypercarbic drive is blunted by all inhalation agents in a dose-dependent fashion. More profound is the near-complete ablation of the carotid body-mediated hypoxic drives by very small subanesthetic doses of inhalation agents; 0.1 MAC concentrations will cause a 90% reduction in their output. Residual anesthetic gas concentrations in the immediate postoperative period could place patients at risk whose primary drive to respiration is O_2-dependent, whether by pulmonary pathophysiology or with primary alveolar hypoventilation,

as occurs in poliomyelitis or Pickwickian/obstructive sleep apnea syndromes. Likewise, sedatives and narcotics will shift the CO_2 response curve downward and to the right, whereas exercise, academia, and hypoxia will cause an upwards left shift (Figure 143-2).

Mechanical, or reflex, control of ventilation also plays an important role. Stretch receptors in the smooth muscle of the conducting airways provide feedback of increased airway pressure to limit inspiratory effort. Tendon spindles within the intercostal muscles likewise provide proprioceptive information about chest wall expansion. These reflexes have been thought to participate in the *Hering-Breuer* reflex, in which increased stretch and pulmonary transmural pressure gradient in a sustained inflation leads to apnea. However, this has only been proven true for lower mammals, where low levels of CPAP cause apnea; in humans, ventilatory efforts will persist even at CPAP levels above 40 cm H_2O.

Conscious efforts to control ventilation by breath holding result in consistent breaking points in all humans for both $Paco_2$ and Pao_2, both around 50 mm Hg after 60-90 seconds of apnea. Prebreath holding supplemental 100% O_2 administration and hyperventilation to a $Paco_2$ of less than 20 mm Hg may allow for as many as 6 or more minutes of voluntary apnea.

Nonrespiratory Functions of the Lung

144

Amir Manoochehri and Marian Sherman, MD

While the primary function of the respiratory system is gas exchange, the lungs serve several additional physiologic roles. Some of the nonrespiratory functions of the lungs include defense against inhaled particles and pathogens, filtration of blood-borne substances, metabolism of endogenous and exogenous substances, and provision of a vascular reservoir.

CLEARANCE

Inhaled particle size determines lung removal method. Larger particles (>3 μm) are captured within the airway's mucus layers. These particles are propelled away from the lungs by cilia and later expectorated or swallowed. Smaller particles are removed by exhalation or macrophage ingestion. Smoking, dry gas inspiration, extreme temperature exposure, dehydration, inhaled anesthetics, opioids, atropine, and alcohol decrease cilia activity. High-dose ketamine and fentanyl have been shown to increase cilia activity.

PROTECTION AGAINST INFECTION

Multiple defense mechanisms against pathogen inhalation exist. Like inhaled particles, pathogens may be directly captured by the pulmonary mucous membrane, propelled cephalically by cilia, then expectorated or swallowed. For pathogens that escape the mucus membrane, chemical inactivation is used to render pathogens harmless. Type II alveolar epithelial cells produce surfactant, which increases bacterial cell wall permeability, leading to pathogen death. Additionally, surfactant stimulates macrophage migration, production of reactive oxygen species, and synthesis of immunoglobulin and cytokines. Lactoferrin contributes to bacterial destruction by blocking iron uptake and impairing proliferation of bacteria. Defensins are peptides that cause bacterial cell wall defects and stimulate respiratory epithelium chemokine release. If pathogens escape direct and chemical removal, the humoral and cellular immune systems are the final line of respiratory defense. The humoral immune system consists of IgA in the upper respiratory tracts and IgG in the lower respiratory tracts. IgA is responsible for preventing bacterial binding and invasion in the respiratory mucosa. IgG surrounds the pathogen and enhances phagocytosis by macrophages. The cellular immune response increases pathogen phagocytosis by respiratory endothelial release of adhesion molecules, chemokines, cytokines, growth factors, and extracellular matrix proteins.

FILTRATION

The lungs filter systemic venous return of blood and prevent the passage of endogenous and exogenous substances to systemic circulation. The lungs prevent passage of most microemboli to the arterial system while maintaining gas exchange for moderate to small clots. Abundant anastamoses throughout the pulmonary circulation maintain gas exchange despite the microemboli present. Inefficiencies in filtration lead to thrombi bypassing the lungs, such as when a patient has a patent foramen ovale. The pulmonary endothelium produces substances that both lyse clots and promote clot formation. The lung is rich in plasmin activator, which catalyzes the conversion of plasminogen to plasmin, which then promotes the conversion of fibrin to fibrin degradation products. The lung contains heparin, which prevents future clot formation. Additionally, the lung contains prothrombotic agents such as thromboplastin, which converts prothrombin to thrombin.

METABOLISM

The lungs facilitate many metabolic processes. The lungs metabolize noradrenaline, serotonin, atrial natriuretic peptide, and endothelins, but do not affect epinephrine, histamine, and dopamine metabolism. Approximately 33% of noradrenaline that passes through the lungs is metabolized. Monoamine oxidase and catechol-*O*-methyl transferase breakdown noradrenaline after it is actively transported into the endothelial cells. Approximately 98% of serotonin that passes through the lungs is metabolized. Similar to noradrenaline, serotonin is removed from the circulation by active transport and breakdown by monoamine oxidase.

One of the metabolic functions of the lung is the conversion of angiotensin I to angiotensin II by angiotensin-converting

401

enzyme (ACE). Approximately 80% of the angiotensin I that circulates through the lungs is converted. Once converted to angiotensin II, this substance causes vasoconstriction and release of aldosterone from the zona glomerulosa. Though ACE can be elsewhere in the body, such as in the plasma, the highest concentration of ACE is found within the lungs. ACE also functions to inactivate bradykinin, a vasodilator; thus, ACE functions to preserve vascular tone. ACE inhibitors cause an increase in bradykinin levels, resulting in hypotension and cough side effects.

The pulmonary epithelium releases pulmonary activating factor (PAF), which increases inflammatory cell migration, platelet aggregation, and pulmonary hypertension. The primary site of action for PAF includes leucocytes and platelets, but PAF also plays an important function in the lungs. PAF is thought to be a mediator for chronic obstructive pulmonary disease. Adenosine, a purine derivative, acts in the lungs as a cell signaler and as a cellular energy source. The lung controls the local and systemic concentrations of adenosine through selective release and metabolism of adenosine. For example, when an allergen is inhaled, the lungs release adenosine and cause systemic vasodilation. Additional factors released by the lungs in response to inhaled allergens are histamine, endothelin, serotonin, platelet-activating factor, and eicosanoids.

First Pass Metabolism

The lung has the unique ability to metabolize both inhaled and intravenous drugs. Inhaled anesthetics such as methoxyflurane and halothane undergo metabolism in the lungs by cytochrome P450 enzymes. Intravenous administration of drugs such as local anesthetics, sedative hypnotics, and opioids are taken up by the lungs and slowly released back into the circulation. This controlled reentry into the circulation helps maintain a constant, steady state concentration of such drugs. When lidocaine is administered intravenously and bypasses lung metabolism, as in the case of severe right-to-left shunting, lidocaine toxicity may occur. The lungs can also activate certain inhaled pro-drugs through the action of esterases found in the lung (ie, beclomethasone dipropionate). This is beneficial because the less potent steroid pro-drug is far less likely to cause side effects when inhaled.

BLOOD RESERVOIR

The lungs provide the body with a 500-1000 mL blood reservoir in their vasculature. This reservoir is particularly helpful during hemodynamically challenging situations such as postural changes and hemorrhage. For example, when changing from supine to upright position, approximately 400 mL of blood is directed out of the pulmonary vasculature and into systemic circulation to maintain perfusion. In contrast, during physical activity and its concomitant increase in oxygen demand, the pulmonary vasculature dilates to accommodate and oxygenate a larger volume of blood. The amount of blood in the pulmonary vasculature can double during forced inspiration.

PLATELET FORMATION

It is thought that fragmented lung megakaryocytes create platelets for systemic circulation. The exact amount of platelet formation and platelet function within the lungs is not known, but it is known that the pulmonary vein contains a higher concentration of platelets than the pulmonary artery.

SUGGESTED READINGS

Deepak J, Raju P, Hari K. Non-respiratory functions of the lung. *Cont Educ Anaesth, CC, and Pain,* 2013;13:98-102.

Airway and Pulmonary Anatomy

CHAPTER 145

Catherine Cleland, MD, and Christopher Jackson, MD

The term "airway" refers to the nasal and oral cavities, pharynx, larynx, trachea, and principal bronchi.

NASAL CAVITY

The nasal cavities are divided by the nasal septum. The roof of the nasal cavity is the cribriform plate. The lateral wall is the origin of the turbinates. Openings in the lateral wall communicate with paranasal sinuses. The greater and lesser palatine nerves innervate the turbinates and most of the nasal septum, and the anterior ethmoid nerve. The ethmoid nerve provides sensation to the nares and the anterior third of the nasal septum. The palatine nerves arise from the sphenopalatine ganglion.

ORAL CAVITY

The roof of the mouth consists of the hard palate anteriorly and the soft palate posteriorly. The tongue makes up most of the mouth floor. Temporomandibular joint (TMJ) rotation initiates mouth opening, followed by sliding of mandibular condyles within the TMJ.

PHARYNX

The pharynx is a fibromuscular tube that extends from the base of the skull to the lower border of the cricoid cartilage. The oropharynx is innervated by branches of the vagus, facial, and glossopharyngeal nerves. The glossopharyngeal nerve gives sensory innervation to the posterior third of the tongue, vallecula, anterior surface of the epiglottis, walls of the pharynx, and tonsils.

LARYNX

As seen in Figure 145-1, the larynx consists of nine cartilages: three single (thyroid, cricoid, and epiglottic) and three paired (arytenoid, corniculate, and cuneiform). Together, these house the vocal cords. The thyroid cartilage helps to protect the vocal cords. The intrinsic and extrinsic muscles of the larynx control

Posterior view

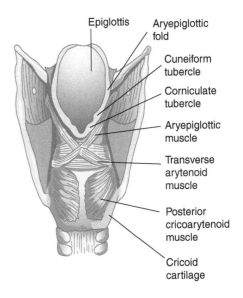

Lateral view

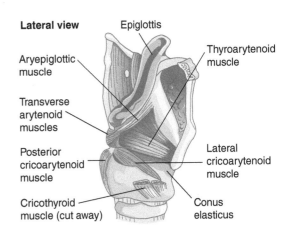

FIGURE 145-1 Anatomy of the larynx. (Reproduced with permission from Lalwani AK. *CURRENT Diagnosis & Treatment in Otolaryngology–Head & Neck Surgery,* 3rd ed. New York: McGraw-Hill; 2012.)

the laryngeal structures. The superior laryngeal nerve and the recurrent laryngeal nerve, both branches of the vagus nerve, innervate the larynx. The recurrent laryngeal nerves supply all the intrinsic muscles of the larynx except the cricothyroid muscle. The superior laryngeal nerve provides sensory innervation to the base of the tongue, epiglottis, aryepiglottic folds, and the arytenoids, as well as motor innervation to the cricothyroid muscle. The cricothyroid membrane is located anteriorly between the thyroid and cricoid cartilages, directly subcutaneous to the skin. Any needle punctures or incisions made to this membrane should be made in the inferior third because the superior cricothyroid arteries course through the upper two-thirds.

In adults, the trachea is approximately 15 cm with 17-18 C-shaped cartilages supporting its structure anteriorly, and a membranous portion overlying the esophagus posteriorly, the trachealis muscle. The first tracheal ring is anterior to the C6 vertebra. The trachea ends at the carina, at the level of the T5 vertebra, where it bifurcates into the right and left bronchus. The right bronchus comes off at a less acute angle from the trachea than the left, thus making it more susceptible to aspiration and mainstem bronchial intubation. The recurrent laryngeal nerve provides sensory innervation of the vocal folds and trachea.

Bronchodilators

Catherine Cleland, MD, and Christopher Jackson, MD

Bronchoconstriction during anesthesia occurs in patients with preexisting conditions such as reactive airway disease, but it also occurs from noxious stimulation of tracheal and laryngeal structures that activate vagal afferent nerves and from histamine-releasing drugs. Bronchoconstriction is more pronounced in smokers, or lightly anesthetized patients.

If a patient wheezes on expiration with auscultation prior to surgery, it is necessary to postpone surgery until the patient returns to normal condition. With chronic wheezing, such as chronic obstructive pulmonary disease (COPD), the patient must be optimized before elective surgery. Wheezing in patients with COPD results from gas flow obstruction due to smooth muscle contraction, secretions, and mucosal edema. Bronchodilators reverse the bronchospastic component of obstructive disease.

SYMPATHOMIMETIC DRUGS

Sympathomimetic drugs are either mixed beta-1 and beta-2 adrenergic receptor agonists or selective beta-2 receptor agonists. These drugs increase the formation of cyclic adenosine monophosphate (cAMP) by activating adenylate cyclase. Adenylate cyclase converts ATP to cAMP, which is responsible for bronchodilation. Conversely, cyclic guanosine monophosphate (cGMP) causes bronchoconstriction. The balance between these two molecules relaxes or constricts bronchial smooth muscle cells.

The mixed sympathomimetic agents are epinephrine, isoproterenol, and isoetharine. Their beta-1 adrenergic effects stimulate cardiac muscle and therefore must be used cautiously in patients with cardiac conditions. The physiologic effects of beta-1 receptor stimulation include increased heart rate, contractility, and myocardial oxygen consumption. These agents produce tachyphylaxis with chronic usage. Epinephrine can be given intravenously, subcutaneously, or via endotracheal tube. The subcutaneous dose is 0.3-0.5 mg for bronchospasm, with peak effect seen in 5-25 minutes. Isoproterenol is effective via inhalation or intravenous routes.

Selective beta-2 receptor agonists avoid cardiac stimulation. These drugs include albuterol, terbutaline, and metaproterenol, which can be administered by aerosol or metered dose inhaler. These agents promote bronchodilation if wheezing is present. Albuterol reduces airway resistance for 4-6 hours with minimal cardiac effects. Terbutaline is given subcutaneously 0.25 mg, although some beta-1 effect occurs. Metaproterenol is given via inhaler and lasts 1-4 hours.

PHOSPHODIESTERASE INHIBITORS

Phosphodiesterase inhibitors inhibit cAMP breakdown by suppressing the action of phosphodiesterase in the cytoplasm. Increased cAMP levels lead to increased bronchial smooth muscle relaxation. Methylxanthines (aminophylline, theophylline) are the most common phosphodiesterase inhibitors, although the entire class is rarely prescribed due to a narrow therapeutic window. Aminophylline is given intravenously or orally. It stimulates the diaphragm, improving contractility at the expense of diaphragmatic fatigue. Aminophylline also induces catecholamine release and blocks histamine release. It may cause ventricular dysrhythmias. Smokers exhibit induced metabolism, while heart failure, liver disease, and COPD patients risk toxicity due to reduced drug metabolism.

Theophylline reduces obstruction in asthmatics in a dose-dependent manner. It also decreases pulmonary vascular resistance, with a therapeutic range of 10-20 µg/mL. It stimulates cardiac receptors, increasing cardiac output. Side effects include nausea and vomiting, seizures (>40 µg/mL), tachycardia, and dysrhythmias.

STEROIDS

Glucocorticoids are used for maintenance therapy to prevent bronchoconstriction, based on anti-inflammatory and membrane stabilizing properties. Common steroids are beclomethasone, triamcinolone, fluticasone, and budesonide. They are given by metered dose inhaler. Steroids may suppress the adrenal. In an acute, severe attack, hydrocortisone or methyl-prednisolone can be used intravenously followed by a tapering dose of oral prednisone. Steroids may take several hours to effectively treat airway reactivity.

PARASYMPATHOLYTIC DRUGS

Parasympatholytic drugs are antimuscarinic and block the formation of cGMP. These drugs bronchodilate and block reflex bronchoconstriction. They are used to treat chronic bronchitis and emphysema, and can be given by a metered dose inhaler or aerosol. Common parasympatholytics are atropine and ipratropium. The administration routes include aerosolization and nebulizer. Ipratropium, unlike atropine, does not exhibit systemic anticholinergic effects.

VOLATILE ANESTHETICS

Airway smooth muscle continues until terminal bronchioles, and is controlled by parasympathetic and sympathetic nerves. Parasympathetic nerves mediate airway tone and bronchoconstriction. The parasympathetic receptors responsible for bronchoconstriction are the M2 and M3 receptors. When activated, these receptors increase cGMP levels. Volatile agents relax smooth muscle by directly decreasing smooth muscle contractility. Direct action depends on bronchial epithelium; therefore, epithelial inflammation decreases smooth muscle relaxation. Volatile agents also act indirectly by inhibiting reflex neural pathways. Other mechanisms have been posited as well.

Desflurane may increase airway resistance in lightly anesthetized patients due to its pungency. These effects are more pronounced in smokers; whereas sevoflurane has a well-tolerated odor.

Anti-inflammatory Pulmonary Drugs

Camille Rowe, MD, and Marian Sherman, MD

Chronic inflammatory diseases of the lungs, including asthma and chronic obstructive pulmonary disease (COPD), are common pulmonary causes of morbidity and mortality. Although triggered by somewhat different mechanisms, both result in cell-mediated inflammation in the lungs (predominantly, eosinophilic in asthma and neutrophilic in COPD), leading to manifestations of increased bronchial smooth muscle tone, increased bronchial wall thickness, excess secretion of mucus, and (in the case of COPD) loss of elasticity of lung parenchyma. Chronic inflammatory disease patients experience the typical symptoms of cough and dyspnea. Various medications are used both singly and in combination to reduce chronic inflammation, and thereby relieve symptoms associated with asthma and COPD.

CORTICOSTEROIDS

This group of medications includes oral steroids (eg, prednisone, prednisolone), inhaled steroids (budesonide, fluticasone, flunisolide, beclomethasone), and parenteral steroids (methylprednisolone). Corticosteroids are potent suppressants of markers of inflammation including interleukins, chemokines, and TNF-alpha.

Inhaled corticosteroids are used for maintenance treatment of asthma and COPD, while oral and IV steroids are generally reserved for treatment of exacerbations. Routine use of inhaled corticosteroids helps to decrease airway inflammation and reactivity; over time this can improve symptoms as well as lung function. Inhaled agents are commonly used in management of mild to moderate asthma and also in COPD, although steroids have been noted to be less effective in COPD patients. According to findings of prior studies, it is possible that this is due to several mechanisms of corticosteroid resistance at the cellular level.

ANTICHOLINERGICS

Anticholinergics include the short-acting drug ipratropium bromide (Atrovent) and the long-acting drug tiotropium bromide (Spiriva). They relax bronchial smooth muscle to produce bronchodilation. They mostly affect the larger, central airways in the lung.

Anticholinergics are often used in conjunction with beta-2 adrenergic agonists, as this combination has shown to be more effective than either agent used alone. Anticholinergics have a slower time to onset but a longer duration of action than beta-2 agonists.

LEUKOTRIENE MODULATORS

These drugs fall into two categories: leukotriene receptor antagonists and leukotriene synthesis inhibitors. Montelukast (Singulair) and zafirlukast are both receptor antagonists while zileuton is a synthesis inhibitor.

Leukotrienes are potent bronchoconstrictors (1000 times greater than histamine); thus blocking their actions would have a benefit in opening tight airways. Leukotriene modulators have been used as an adjunct treatment for moderate to severe asthma.

METHYLXANTHINES

Theophylline is the best-known drug of this class. Methylxanthines inhibit bronchoconstriction mediated by cyclic adenosine monophosphate (cAMP); they are nonspecific phosphodiesterase inhibitors.

These medications were once commonly used, but have fallen out of favor due to their narrow therapeutic window (requiring frequent blood level monitoring) and numerous side effects, including abdominal pain, nausea, vomiting, diarrhea, headaches, arrhythmias, palpitations, tremor, and seizures. Occasionally, these drugs are used as adjunct medication for more severe asthma and COPD.

MAST CELL STABILIZERS

These include cromolyn sodium and nedocromil sodium. They act by stabilizing mast cells to prevent IgE-mediated release of the inflammatory substances histamine and leukotrienes.

These agents are only useful as prophylactic agents in asthma; they have no effect in acute exacerbation.

IMMUNOMODULATORS

The main drug of this class is omalizumab, a biologic agent (anti-IgE antibody) that inhibits activation of IgE receptors on mast cells triggered by inhaled allergens. This is used as an adjunct in the treatment of severe allergic asthma.

NOVEL THERAPIES—SELECTIVE PHOSPHODIESTERASE-4 INHIBITORS

Newer medications have been developed for the treatment of chronic inflammatory lung disease, targeting a particular enzyme called phosphodiesterase-4 (PDE-4), which is commonly expressed in inflammatory cells such as neutrophils, macrophages, and T-lymphocytes (and is over-expressed in patients with asthma and COPD). PDE-4 and other phosphodiesterases catalyze the breakdown of cAMP to inactive AMP. Inhibitors of PDE-4, in contrast, act by increasing the intracellular concentration of cAMP, which: (1) has a broad range of anti-inflammatory effects on many of the cellular mediators which cause asthma and COPD; and (2) reduces bronchoconstriction by relaxing bronchial smooth muscle. Studies have shown that these drugs reduce absolute counts of inflammatory cells, improve postbronchodilator FEV_1 values, and reduce exacerbations. Greater clinical benefit was observed with their use in combination with salmeterol and tiotropium.

Cilomilast (Ariflo) and roflumilast (Daxas) are the two flagship agents of the PDE-4 class. Cilomilast has been FDA approved for treatment of COPD and asthma, while roflumilast is still in development.

SUGGESTED READINGS

Hakim A, Adcock IM, Usmani OS. Corticosteroid resistance and novel anti-inflammatory therapies in chronic obstructive pulmonary disease. *Drugs*. 2012;72:1299-1312.

Koziol-White CJ, Damera G, Panettieri RA Jr. Targeting airway smooth muscle in airways diseases: an old concept with new twists. *Expert Rev Respir Med*. 2011;5:767-777.

Roche N, Marthan R, Berger P, et al. Beyond corticosteroids: future prospects in the management of inflammation in COPD. *Eur Respir Rev*. 2011;20:175-182.

148

Cardiac Cycle

Matthew Haight, DO, and Vinh Nguyen, DO

The cardiac cycle describes a sequence of mechanical and electrical events that cause a cardiac contraction and ejection (ventricular systole), and relaxation or filling (ventricular diastole). In general, a pressure gradient develops between the chambers, which leads to ejection of the stroke volume (SV) and forward flow of blood through the body. Therefore, the cardiac cycle is made up of four main phases: filling phase, isovolumetric contraction, ejection phase, and isovolumetric relaxation (Figure 148-1).

THE FOUR PHASES OF THE CARDIAC CYCLE

Isovolumetric Contraction Phase

This phase represents the beginning stage of systole, with an increase in ventricular pressure. The rapid increase in ventricular pressure exceeds atrial pressure and forces the atrioventricular (AV) valve to close due to the reversed pressure gradient. On the venous pulse tracing, the "c" wave is displayed due to the bulging of the AV valve into the atria. During its contraction, the ventricular architecture changes but not the volume. The blood volume prior to ejection represents the *end-diastolic volume* (EDV). On the ECG, this can be seen as the QRS complex.

Ejection Phase

This phase begins when the ventricular pressure exceeds the resting pressure of the aorta or pulmonary artery. Due to the pressure gradient, blood moves forward across the valve leaflets. During the first part of the ejection, the rapid ejection causes the ventricular pressure to rise and then rapidly decline as volume decreases. This is considered the *stroke* or *systolic volume* (SV), while the blood remaining in the ventricle is considered the *end-systolic volume* (ESV). Stroke volume can be indirectly calculated using EDV and ESV.

$$SV = EDV - ESV$$

Ejection phase is complete with closure of the semilunar valves and the start of the relaxation phase. On the ECG, this represents the ST segment.

Isovolumetric Relaxation Phase

This is the phase in which the ventricle returns to the precontractile configuration. At the end of systole, ventricle pressure declines rapidly and the pressure gradient allows the closure of the semilunar valves. The AV valve closes as well because of the lower atria pressure relative to the ventricle pressure. Again, the blood left over after ejection equals the ESV. On the venous pulse tracing, "v" wave is displayed at the end of isovolumetric relaxation due to the blood filling the atria and increasing its pressure. A dicrotic notch would be detected on the arterial waveform to indicate the closure of the aortic valve. On the ECG, this represents the end of the T-wave.

Filling Phase (Diastolic Filling)

When the buildup of atrial pressure from the influx of blood from the superior and inferior vena cava exceeds ventricular pressure, this promotes ventricular filling. The AV valve opens and blood flows to the ventricle. There are two phases to this flow: (1) rapid phase based on the pressure gradient comprising 75% of blood volume, and (2) the slower active atrial systole phase ("atrial kick") accounting for the remaining (25%) blood volume. Although ventricle volume increases, the pressure is relatively constant during this process. In the venous pulse tracing, a "y" wave descent represents blood evacuation from the atria to the ventricles. At the end of diastolic filling, the slow filling "atrial kick" represents the "a" wave on the venous pulse tracing.

THE CARDIAC CYCLE AND CARDIAC OUTPUT

Cardiac output, which reflects the amount of blood flowing into circulation per unit time, is calculated as:

$$CO = SV \times HR$$

During the systolic function of the cardiac cycle, adequate blood ejection from the heart depends on extrinsic as well as intrinsic factors. Preload and afterload are the primary

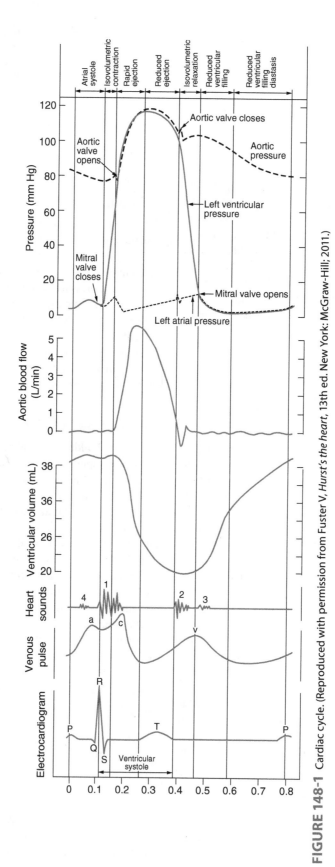

FIGURE 148-1 Cardiac cycle. (Reproduced with permission from Fuster V, *Hurst's the heart*, 13th ed. New York: McGraw-Hill; 2011.)

extrinsic factors coupled with the cardiac cycle. Intrinsic factors include myocardial contractility and heart rate.

Preload is the degree of stretch on the relaxed muscle fibers just before they contract and is thus related to left ventricular end-diastolic volume (LVEDV). LVEDV is difficult to measure clinically but surrogate representatives of LVEDV are often used clinically to assess preload (such as pulmonary wedge pressure or central venous pressure). Echocardiography has also been used with great accuracy.

Afterload is the second major extrinsic determinant of the mechanical properties of cardiac performance. It is considered as an impedance of forces on the systemic circulation opposing ventricular ejection. As a result, SV is dependent on the compliance and resistance of the arterial system (SVR). SVR can be calculated using the analog of Ohm's law:

$$SVR = \{MAP - CVP\}/CO$$

where SVR = systemic venous resistance; MAP = mean arterial pressure; CVP = central venous pressure; CO = cardiac output.

The intrinsic determinants of myocardial contractility are dependent on the availability of intracellular calcium. Drugs that have positive inotropic property will generally increase intracellular calcium to cause an increase in contractility. Although difficult to measure, the most common noninvasive index of ventricular contraction is the ejection fraction.

$$EF = SV/EDV$$

where EF = ejection fraction; SV = stroke volume; EDV = end-diastolic volume.

Heart rate is primarily influenced by the autonomic nervous system and represents the other major intrinsic factor that affects cardiac output.

149

Cardiac Electrophysiology

Matthew Haight, DO, and Vinh Nguyen, DO

Cardiac muscle, like skeletal muscle, contains myosin, actin, tropomyosin, and troponin in various isoforms. Even though cardiac muscle fibers resemble skeletal muscle fibers in that they are striated, they differ in that they form a functional syncytium, which means that all fibers are electrically connected via gap junctions. Pacemaker cells of the electrical conduction system can initiate depolarization, and thus contraction, throughout the myocardium without external neurohormonal control.

The cardiac conduction system consists of the sinoatrial (SA) node, atrioventricular (AV) nodes, AV bundle (Bundle of His), and left and right bundle branches and Purkinje fibers (Figure 149-1). A normal electrical impulse generally starts at the SA node and produces an action potential by allowing ions to cross the cell membrane to increase the resting membrane potential. As a result, electrical activation will cause adjacent myocardium to produce an action potential along the conduction pathway to elicit a normal heartbeat.

ELECTRICAL ACTIVITY AND ACTION POTENTIAL OF THE HEART

Cardiac muscle cells have a resting potential of −90 mV, with the inside of cell being negatively charged and the outside being positively charged. Ions flow in and out of the cell by a concentration gradient, electrical gradient, or permeability of the membrane. Potassium is higher inside the cell (140 mmol/L) than outside (4 mmol/L), and has the highest permeability (more than sodium or chloride). Thus, potassium is the major determinant of the resting membrane potential.

During a depolarization episode, the inside of the cell becomes less negative (increase in the membrane potential) due to the influx of ions (Table 149-1). Two distinct action potentials are recognized as either *fast* action potentials or *slow* action potentials (Figure 149-1B). A fast action potential utilized by cardiac ventricular myocytes is divided into five phases. Each phase depends on the type of ions that cross the membrane and the availability or activation of the ion channel. When myocytes reach about −70 mV ("threshold"), fast sodium channels open and an influx of sodium ions increase the membrane potential to +30 mV (phase 0).

A slight repolarization occurs when sodium channels are closed and potassium diffuse out of the cell (phase 1). Potassium diffusion is counterbalanced by the influx of calcium ions via the active calcium channels, creating a plateau phase (phase 2). Repolarization of the cell to resting potential follows when calcium channels close but potassium channels remain open for the outflow of potassium (phase 3). Ultimately, restoration of the resting potential commences the cycle and finishes with the next activation (phase 4). On the other hand, *slow* action potentials utilized by cells of the SA or AV node yield a similar result but lack the phase 1 and 2 components.

CARDIAC CONDUCTION AND HEART RATE

The SA node is the key pacemaker to initiate a regular rhythm. It inhibits the pacemaker function of the AV node, thus allowing itself to pace at its own intrinsic rate. SA and AV nodes can be indirectly controlled by the autonomic nervous system and circulating epinephrine. Parasympathetic stimulation causes a large release of acetylcholine, which binds to muscarinic receptors of the SA and AV nodes. The cells become more permeable to potassium and the cell membrane becomes hyperpolarized. This causes the intracellular membrane to be more negative and reduces the slope of phase 4. As a result, heart rate is slower and conduction is delayed through the AV node. During sympathetic response, beta-1 adrenergic receptors cause a decrease in potassium permeability but an increase in sodium and calcium permeabilities. These changes lead to an increase in the slope of phase 4 and reduce the extent of repolarization.

SPECIAL CHANNEL AND SIGNALING CONSIDERATIONS

Sodium (Na⁺) Channels

Ion channels are the fundamental units of cardiac excitation. They are the pores through which individual ions move from one side of the cell membrane to the other to generate

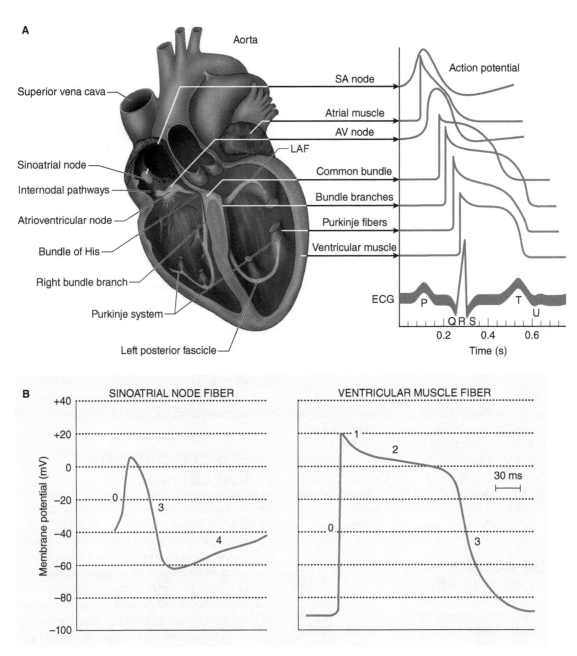

FIGURE 149-1 A, B: Cardiac conduction system. (Reproduced with permission from Butterworth JF, Mackey DC, Wasnick JD, *Morgan and Mikhail's Clinical Anesthesiology*, 5th ed. McGraw-Hill; 2013.)

TABLE 149-1   Cardiac Action Potential Components

Action Potential	Phases	Mechanism	Cardiac Myocytes	SA & AV Nodes
Depolarization	0	Rapid influx of Na$^+$	Present	Present
Slight repolarization	1	Na$^+$ channel closed, efflux of K$^+$	Present	Absent
Plateau	2	Influx of Ca^{2+}, efflux of K$^+$	Present	Absent
Repolarization	3	Efflux of K$^+$ continued, Ca^{2-} channel closed	Present	Present
Resting membrane	4	K$^+$ channel closed	Present	Present

an action potential. The cell membrane potential derives from an unequal distribution of ions across a semipermeable membrane. Sodium (Na^+) ion channels are present in all cardiac myocytes and are the site of action of all three types of Na^+ channel blocking antiarrhythmic agents. Genetic mutations in Na^+ channels cause two diseases associated with sudden death: one form of congenital long QT syndrome and the Brugada syndrome.

Na^+–K^+ ATPase

The unequal distribution of sodium ions (Na^+, greater concentration outside the cell) and potassium ions (K^+, greater concentration inside the cell) is generated by the energy requiring Na^+–K^+ ATPase pump. For each ATP, three Na^+ are pumped out of the cell and two K^+ are transported into the cell. Clinically, Na^+–K^+ ATPase is the only known receptor for digitalis glycosides.

Excitation–Contraction Coupling

Electrical activation of the myocardium releases calcium ions (Ca^{2+}) from intracellular stores in the sarcoplasmic reticulum to generate mechanical systole. The process by which mechanical shortening is transduced from an electrical signal is called excitation–contraction coupling. Long-lasting (L-type) Ca^{2+} channels located in t-tubule membranes are the main portals for Ca^{2+} entry into the cell, which then triggers the secondary release of Ca^{2+} from the sarcoplasmic reticulum. This is known as the calcium-induced calcium release (CICR), mechanism and is unique to cardiac muscle. L-type Ca^{2+} channel ligand antagonists include dihydropyridines (nifedipine and nitrendipine), phenylalkylamines (verapamil), and benzothiazepines (diltiazem).

Second Messengers

Ion channel gating refers to the mechanism whereby an ion channel protein undergoes transitions among conformations that correspond to open, closed, and inactivated states. Second messengers are produced intracellularly after agonist binding to a receptor on the cell membrane. The B1 receptor acts via a second messenger mechanism. B1 activates the membrane associated enzyme adenylate cyclase. This enzyme catalyzes the production of second messenger cAMP, which binds to the regulatory domain of protein kinase A (PKA) to release the active catalytic subunit. PKA phosphorylates L-type Ca^{2+}, Na^+, CL^-, and K^+ channels. Phosphorylation of L-type Ca^{2+} channels increases the probability of a gating transition to the open state. Agonist binding to the B1 receptor can activate additional intracellular second messengers via activation of phospholipase C (generating inositol 1, 4, 5-triphosphate).

G proteins are membrane-associated proteins that bind Guanine nucleotides. G proteins can affect ion channel function by: activating second messenger systems (cAMP), activating phospholipase C, and directly acting with ion channel proteins through cell membrane pathways. G-protein coupling is essential in muscarinic inhibition of L-type Ca^{2+} channels. For many of the cardiac ion channels, the gating process is not only driven by the cell membrane potential (voltage-dependent gating) but is also influenced by ion channel phosphorylation, ligand binding, and G-protein coupled interactions with ion channels.

ROLE OF THE AUTONOMIC NERVOUS SYSTEM

Heart rate is controlled by a combination of intrinsic (automatic) depolarization and external neurohumoral control. The resting heart rate in adults is around 70 beats/minute and this reflects a basic parasympathetic neural dominance at the SA node. At rest, sympathetic neural activity to the SA node is largely absent but during exercise as the parasympathetic tone is withdrawn, the sympathetic neuronal activity allows the heart rate to rise above 100 beats/minute.

Sympathetic innervation of the heart arises from the cervical and upper thoracic ganglia. Postganglionic nerve cells of the sympathetic nervous system are located in the grey matter of the lateral horn at levels T1–T4. The right sympathetic nerve fibers predominantly innervate the SA node and the left sympathetic nerves mainly innervate the AV node and ventricles. The sympathetic nervous system (SNS) acts through β_1-adrenergic receptors, which act upon potassium channels in the membrane of pacemaker tissue.

The parasympathetic nervous system (PNS) consists of two parts: the cranial (brainstem) and sacral (spinal cord level S2-S4) regions. The PNS innervates the heart via the vagus nerve. The parasympathetic innervation is denser in the SA and AV nodes than in the surrounding myocardium, and the right and left vagal nerves both provide bilateral innervation of the SA and AV nodes. The actions of the PNS are mediated through muscarinic cholinergic receptors (mAChR), which are stimulated by acetylcholine released from postganglionic fibers in the PNS.

Frank–Starling Law

Adrian M. Ionescu, MD, and Kerry DeGroot, MD

Cardiac output (CO) is dependent on the product of two variables, heart rate (HR) and stroke volume (SV), or the volume pumped by the heart with each contraction. The relationship between CO, HR, and SV can be summarized by the following equation: $CO = SV \times HR$. While the intrinsic HR is dependent on the depolarization of the sinoatrial (SA) node, SV is dependent on three factors: ventricular preload, aortic afterload, and the strength of the myocardial contraction.

THE FRANK–STARLING LAW

Left ventricular filling determines the left ventricular end-diastolic volume (LVEDV), which is generally directly proportional to left ventricular preload and CO. The *Frank–Starling Law* describes the relationship between LVEDV and CO. According to the *Starling Law*, CO increases with increasing left ventricular preload until the left ventricle reaches excessive end-diastolic volumes. With excessive end-diastolic volumes, the CO does not change and may actually decrease. The Frank–Starling Law is further described schematically in Figure 150-1.

Factors Affecting Frank–Starling Physiology

Left ventricular preload and therefore, LVEDV are directly affected by changes in the filling of the left ventricle. Left ventricular filling, in turn, is affected by changes in intravascular volume as well as venous tone.

Factors leading to an *increase* in LVEDV and CO, thus shifting the Starling curve *up and left*, include:

1. volume expansion of the intravascular compartment (with administration of crystalloid, colloid, or blood components);
2. avoiding increases in the intrathoracic pressure (from positive pressure ventilation or tension pneumothorax) or increases in the pericardial pressure (from effusions or tamponade physiology); and
3. augmenting venous tone and venous return to the heart.

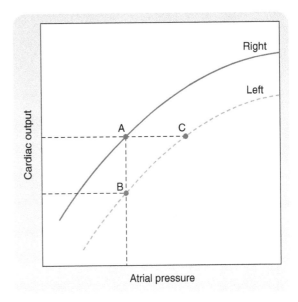

FIGURE 150-1 Relationships between the output of the right and left ventricles and mean pressure in the right and left atria, respectively. At any given level of cardiac output, mean left atrial pressure (eg, point C) exceeds mean right atrial pressure (point A). (Reproduced with permission from Koeppen BM, Stanton BA, Berne RM, *Berne and Levy Physiology*, 6th ed. Philadelphia, PA: Mosby/Elsevier; 2010.)

In contrast, factors leading to a *decrease* in LVEDV and CO, thus shifting the Starling curve *down* and *right*, include:

1. volume contraction of the intravascular space;
2. increases in the intrathoracic pressure (from positive pressure ventilation or tension pneumothorax) or increases in the pericardial pressure (from tamponade physiology); and
3. decreases in venous tone and venous return to the heart.

In addition to the effect of *LVEDV* on the shift of the Starling curve, *left ventricular contractility* is an additionally important factor with a profound impact on myocardial physiology. Myocardial contractility (inotropy) is influenced by the rate of myocardial fiber shortening (dependent on the concentration of intracellular calcium) as well as by neural and pharmacological factors. Sympathetic adrenergic fibers innervate atria, ventricles, and rate-setting nodes, and therefore the sympathetic nervous system has the greatest impact on myocardial contractility. It is important to note that catecholamines (epinephrine and norepinephrine) have positive chronotropic as well as inotropic effects (increased contractility via beta-1 receptor agonist activity) and thus shift the Frank–Starling curve *up and left* (increased CO).

Ventricular Function

Adrian M. Ionescu, MD, and Kerry DeGroot, MD

The cardiac cycle can be divided into alternating periods of myocardial contraction, or *systole*, and periods of myocardial relaxation, or *diastole*. Ventricular systolic function is best understood quantitatively in terms of cardiac output (CO) and ejection fraction (EF), whereas the diastolic component of ventricular function relates to the ventricular isovolumetric relaxation time and ventricular capacitance during filling.

VENTRICULAR FUNCTION CURVES

Ventricular function can also be summarized diagrammatically via *ventricular pressure–volume diagrams*, by plotting ventricular volume on the *x*-axis and ventricular pressure on the *y*-axis. There are primarily two points of interest: (1) the *end-diastolic volume* (EDV), which reflects diastolic function, including the ability of the ventricular myocardium to

relax to fill with blood; and (2) the *end-systolic volume* (ESV), which reflects systolic function, including the ability of the ventricular myocardium to contract to eject a fraction of the end diastolic ventricular volume. The relationships between ventricular filling, EDV, ventricular ejection, and ESV are depicted in Figure 151-1.

VENTRICULAR SYSTOLIC FUNCTION

One parametric measurement of ventricular systolic function is CO, which refers to the volume of blood pumped by the heart each minute. Generally, as both the right and left ventricle depolarize in synchronous fashion, the pulmonary and systemic COs generated are usually equal. Cardiac output can also be defined mathematically as the product of heart rate (HR) and stroke volume (SV), which is the volume of blood

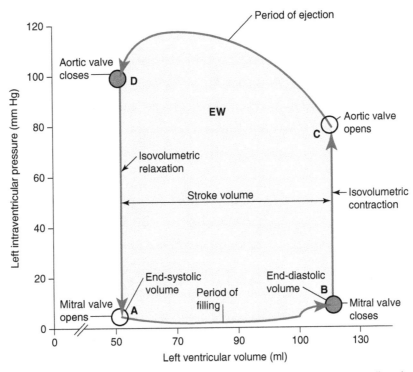

FIGURE 151-1 The cardiac cycle. (Reproduced with permission from Hall JE, Guyton AC, *Guyton and Hall Textbook of Medical Physiology,* 12th ed. Philadelphia, PA: Saunders/Elsevier; 2011.)

pumped by each ventricle with every depolarization of the myocardium. The following equation summarizes the relationship between CO, HR, and SV: $CO = HR \times SV$. Cardiac output can also be expressed as a cardiac index (CI), to account for individual body size differences and body surface area (BSA) variability, according to the following equation: $CI = CO/BSA$. The normal range for CI is usually 2.5-4.2 L/min/m².

A second parametric measurement of ventricular systolic function is the EF, which refers to the percentage of the EDV that is ejected from each ventricle with every depolarization of the myocardium. This relationship can be expressed as a function of the ventricular EDV and ESV according to the following equation: $EF = \{[EDV - ESV]/[EDV]\} \times 100$. The normal range for the left ventricular EF is usually 59%-75%.

The effect of ventricular systolic failure can be plotted on a ventricular pressure–volume loop. As the systolic function of the ventricle is failing, there is an increase in EDV and ESV because EF (the ability of the ventricle to eject a fraction of the EDV) is significantly reduced. The overall net effect of systolic failure translates into a *down and right* shift of the pressure–volume loop (*negative inotropy*). In contrast, *systolic augmentation* (*positive inotropy*) shifts the pressure volume loop *up and left*.

VENTRICULAR DIASTOLIC FUNCTION

One measurement of ventricular diastolic function reflects in the ability of the ventricle to relax (*ventricular capacitance*) to accommodate the blood volume delivered by the atria. The ventricular capacitance can be estimated via transesophageal echocardiography by assessment of the ventricular *isovolumetric relaxation time* and the *flow velocity* across the mitral valve during diastole (ventricular filling). Prolonged isovolumetric relaxation times and high flow velocities across the mitral valve correspond with a stiff and less compliant ventricle. As the diastolic function of the ventricle is failing, the EDV of the ventricle decreases and the less-compliant ventricle becomes unable to accommodate the blood volume delivered by the atrial depolarization. The effect of ventricular diastolic dysfunction can be plotted on a ventricular pressure–volume loop. The overall net effect of diastolic failure translates into a *downward shift* of the pressure–volume loop, as the decreased EDV contributes to a decreased SV and subsequently to a decreased CO. In contrast, a compliant ventricle is able to accommodate a larger EDV and augments SV and CO, thus shifting the loop *up and left*.

Myocardial Contractility

Adrian M. Ionescu, MD, and
Johan P. Suyderhoud, MD

The heart is made up of striated muscle of both atria and ventricles, along with the pacemaker and action-potential conducting tissue. The pacemaker cells of the myocardium have a unique, self-excitatory property, which allows myocardial contractility to occur independently of sympathetic or parasympathetic nervous system input. The intercalated discs allow the fast, uniform, and sequential transmission of electrical activity (action potentials) between myocytes to generate an effective cardiac output to perfuse vital tissue.

Myocardial contraction occurs as a result of cross-bridge formation between two contractile proteins, actin (thin filaments) and myosin (thick filaments). Contractility refers to the rate of myocyte shortening, which occurs when actin and myosin slide to form cross-bridges (Figure 152-1).

The intracellular release of calcium from the sarcoplasmic reticulum facilitates the conformational change in two regulatory proteins (troponin and tropomyosin) to allow the cross-bridge formation between actin and myosin. The initial calcium release from the sarcoplasmic reticulum is triggered by the electrical depolarization of dihydropyridine, voltage-gated calcium channels. As the intracellular calcium concentration increases, it triggers an even greater release of calcium

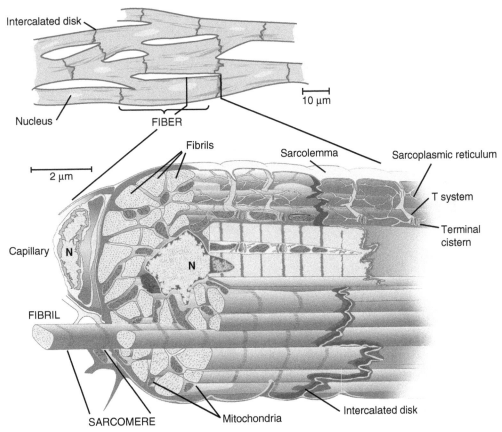

FIGURE 152-1 Cardiac muscle. (Reproduced with permission from Barrett KE, Barman SM, Boitano S, *Ganong's Review of Medical Physiology*, 24th ed. McGraw-Hill Medical; 2012.)

from the sarcoplasmic reticulum via ryanodine, nonvoltage-gated calcium channels.

The overall calcium concentration and rate of release from the sarcoplasmic reticulum determine the strength as well as rate of the contraction. Sympathetic nervous system stimulation (via norepinephrine) activates beta-1 adrenergic receptors, leading to an increase in the intracellular calcium concentration and strength of contraction. In contrast, parasympathetic nervous system stimulation (via acetylcholine) activates M_2 cholinergic receptors, which enhance the Ca^{2+}-ATPase activity to pump calcium back into the sarcoplasmic reticulum, thus effectively lowering the intracellular calcium concentration and decreasing the strength and rate of the myocardial contraction.

Cardiac Output

Adrian M. Ionescu, MD, and
Johan P. Suyderhoud, MD

Cardiac output (CO) is defined as the volume of blood pumped systemically by the left ventricle each minute. Physiologically, *CO* is a function of *heart rate* (HR) and *stroke volume* (SV), according to the following equation: $CO = HR \times SV$. The SV usually ranges between 70 and 120 mL, thus producing a resting CO of 5.6 L/min in men and 4.9 L/min in women. Alternatively, to compensate for variability in body weight and body surface area (BSA), CO can also be expressed as the *cardiac index* (CI), according to the following equation: $CI = CO/BSA$. The normal range for an individual's CI is usually between 2.5 and 4.2 L/min/m^2.

Both HR and SV are directly proportional to CO, such that increases in either the HR or the SV produce an increase in CO. While the HR is controlled by the spontaneous depolarization of the sinoatrial (SA) node (which is controlled by the autonomic nervous system), SV is a function of the following four factors: (1) preload; (2) afterload; (3) contractility; and (4) wall motion abnormalities.

CARDIAC OUTPUT PHYSIOLOGY

Heart Rate

The autonomic nervous system controls the automaticity and rate of spontaneous depolarization of the SA node, which in turn controls an individual's intrinsic HR (usually ranges between 60 and 90 beats/minute). The *sympathetic division* of the autonomic nervous system increases the HR via stimulation of *beta-1 adrenergic receptors*, while the *parasympathetic division* of the autonomic nervous system decreases the HR by stimulating muscarinic *M2 cholinergic receptors*.

Stroke Volume

Four major factors affect SV:

A. **Preload**—The most important factors contributing to the ventricular preload (synonymous with the ventricular end-diastolic volume, EDV) include *ventricular filling, ventricular compliance*, and *venous tone*. As the venous tone and ventricular compliance increase, the blood volume that the left ventricle is able to accommodate increases, thus resulting in an increased EDV, which subsequently contributes to an increased SV according to the *Frank–Starling Law* (Figure 153-1).

B. **Afterload**—Ventricular wall tension during systole approximates the ventricular afterload, which can be defined as the pressure the left ventricle must overcome to generate a particular ejection fraction. Stroke volume and afterload have an inversely proportional relationship—thus, as the afterload (synonymous with the aortic systolic pressure) increases, the ventricular wall tension increases, resulting in a decreased SV and CO. In contrast, as the afterload decreases, both SV and CO increase.

C. **Contractility**—Inotropism or contractility is affected by the rate of myofibril shortening as well as by the rate of calcium release from the smooth sarcoplasmic reticulum. Faster rates of myofibril shortening and calcium release into the intracellular space contribute to an increased strength of contractility and augmentation of SV and CO (Figure 153-2). The sympathetic nervous system has the most profound effect on myocardial contractility as the sympathetic adrenergic fibers release norepinephrine, which stimulates the myocardial beta-1 adrenergic receptors to enhance contractility and CO.

D. **Wall motion abnormalities**—Ischemia, alterations in conduction velocity, and myocardial remodeling may lead to impaired ventricular motion and contractility, which in turn reduce SV and CO. The various degrees of wall motion abnormalities range from hypokinesis, which refers to the diminished force of contractility, to dyskinesis, a paradoxical and asynchronous pattern of contraction, and finally to akinesis, which refers to the absence of contractility. It is important to note that wall motion abnormalities affect the ability of the left ventricle to adequately fill with the blood volume delivered by the atria, subsequently reducing its SV capacity and CO potential.

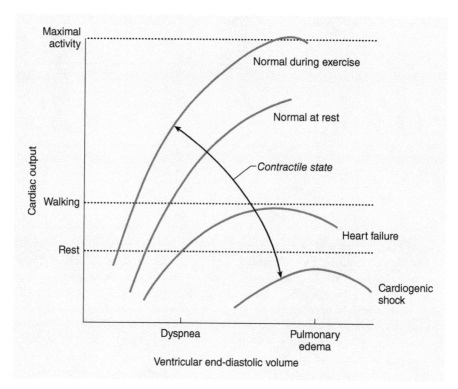

FIGURE 153-1 Starling's law of the heart. (Reproduced with permission from Butterworth JF, Mackey DC, Wasnick JD, *Morgan and Mikhail's Clinical Anesthesiology*, 5th ed. McGraw-Hill; 2013.)

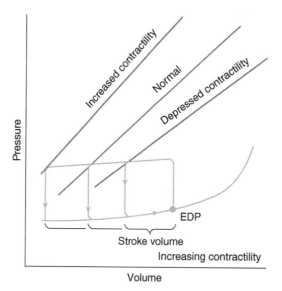

FIGURE 153-2 Increasing contractility with constant preload and afterload. EDP, end-diastolic point. (Reproduced with permission from Butterworth JF, Mackey DC, Wasnick JD, *Morgan and Mikhail's Clinical Anesthesiology*, 5th ed. McGraw-Hill; 2013.)

Myocardial Oxygen Utilization

154

Adrian M. Ionescu, MD, and Johan P. Suyderhoud, MD

The right and left coronary arteries are responsible for the delivery of oxygenated blood to the myocardium. The right coronary artery is responsible for supplying oxygen to the right atrium, the right ventricle, and the inferior portion of the left ventricle, sinoatrial and atrioventricular nodes. The distribution of the left coronary artery (LCA) includes the left atrium, the interventricular septum, and the anterolateral walls of the left ventricle. Branches of the LCA include the circumflex artery, which supplies the lateral wall of the left ventricle, and the left anterior descending artery (LAD), which supplies the anterior wall of the left ventricle as well as the interventricular septum. To supply the myocardium with oxygen, the blood flows from the epicardial vessels to the endocardial vessels, and then returns to the right atrium via the coronary sinus.

CORONARY CIRCULATION PHYSIOLOGY

The coronary perfusion pressure (CPP) is dependent on the difference between the aortic diastolic pressure (ADP) and the left ventricular end-diastolic pressure (LVEDP), according to the following equation: *CPP = ADP − LVEDP*. The LVEDP is an approximation of the resistance to coronary blood flow during diastole and is used because it can be inferred with standard invasive monitors such as pulmonary artery catheters. It should be recognized that there are other factors that can contribute to resistance to coronary artery blood flow besides LVEDP, such as intrinsic intramyocardial tissue pressures, that are not easily quantifiable with clinical monitors. As the left ventricle contracts during systole, it occludes the intramyocardial portion of the coronary arteries and results in intermittent perfusion of the left ventricle during diastole only, and actually some degree of retrograde coronary blood flow during systole (Figure 154-1). However, the right ventricle receives continuous perfusion during both systole and diastole.

To summarize, it is important to note that the effective CPP is directly proportional to ADP, but inversely proportional to LVEDP as well as heart rate (HR). The effective CPP *increases* with: (1) increases in ADP; (2) decreases in LVEDP; and (3) decreases in HR as the diastolic time extends, leading to prolongation of the time interval for left

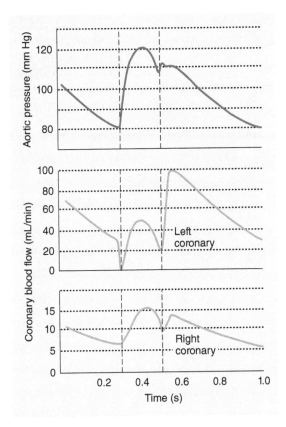

FIGURE 154-1 Coronary blood flow during the cardiac cycle. (Reproduced with permission from Butterworth JF, Mackey DC, Wasnick JD, *Morgan and Mikhail's Clinical Anesthesiology*, 5th ed. McGraw-Hill; 2013.)

ventricular coronary blood. In contrast, the CPP *decreases* with: (1) decreases in ADP; (2) increases in LVEDP; and (3) increases in HR.

MYOCARDIAL OXYGEN BALANCE

Effective CPP ranging from 50 to 120 mm Hg, produces coronary blood flows of 60-80 mL/100 g tissue/min in the average adult at rest. Myocardial oxygen consumption at rest is between 7 and 10 mL/100 g tissue/min; with exercise this can increase five- to sixfold. At the same time, coronary blood flow increases between four- and fivefold with exercise, with difference between supply and extraction being met with enhancements in extraction ratios (eg, shifts in the hemoglobin dissociation curve). In contrast to other organ beds, myocardial arterial oxygen extraction is quite high, about 70%-80%, compared to about 25% for the rest of the body. It is important to note that both hypoxic conditions as well as sympathetic nervous system activation produce coronary vasodilation, thus producing an increase in myocardial blood flow and oxygen supply. The parasympathetic nervous system has minimal effects on the tone of the coronary vasculature. Myocardial oxygen is utilized in the following manner: (1) pressure-related work (65%); (2) basal metabolism (20%); (3) volume-related work (15%); and (4) electrical activity (1%).

The important factors affecting myocardial oxygen *supply* are as follows: (1) HR (in particular, diastolic time); (2) CPP (as determined by ADP as well as by LVEDP); (3) arterial oxygen content (including both oxygen tension as well as hemoglobin concentration); and (4) coronary vessel diameter.

The rate of oxygen supply to the myocardium increases with increases in the diastolic time, increases in CPP, increases in oxygen and hemoglobin concentration, and coronary vasodilation. In contrast, the oxygen delivery to the myocardium decreases in the diastolic time, decreases in CPP, decreases in the oxygen and hemoglobin concentration, and coronary vasoconstriction.

Myocardial oxygen *demand* is affected by the following important factors: (1) HR; (2) ventricular wall tension

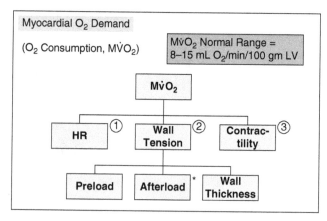

FIGURE 154-2 Myocardial oxygen demand. (Reproduced with permission from Barrett KE, Barman SM, Boitano S. *Ganong's Review of Medical Physiology*, 23rd ed. McGraw-Hill; 2008.)

(as determined by preload, afterload, and wall thickness); and (3) myocardial contractility (Figure 154-2).

The rate of myocardial oxygen consumption ($M\dot{v}O_2$) increases with increases in HR, increases in wall tension, and increases in contractility. In contrast, the rate of $M\dot{v}O_2$ generally decreases with a decreasing HR, decreasing wall tension, and decreasing contractility. As stated previously, the rate of myocardial oxygen extraction is quite high; further increases in metabolic demand are met primarily by an increase in coronary blood flow.

Venous Return

Gabrielle Brown, MD, and Tricia Desvarieux, MD

Venous return refers to the amount of blood and blood flow returned back to the heart from veins. The cardiovascular system, consisting of both systemic and pulmonary circulations, is a closed-loop system, with the right ventricle receiving blood from the systemic circulation and the left ventricle receiving blood from the pulmonary circulation. At steady state conditions, cardiac output (CO) equals venous return. If CO did not equal venous return, then blood volume would collect in one part of the circulation or another. Therefore, since CO is 5 L/min, venous return also equals 5 L/min.

VASCULAR FUNCTION RELATIONSHIP

Arthur Guyton correlated the relationship between mean systemic filling pressure (MSFP) and right atrial pressure (RAP) to control venous return. Baseline values are as follows:

MSFP	7 mm Hg
RAP	0 mm Hg
CO	5 L/min

A change in RAP (which is equivalent to central venous pressure [CVP]) is produced by a change in CO. As CO (or venous return) increases, CVP decreases and more blood is pumped from veins to the right atrium. Consequently, increases in MSFP or decreases in RAP lead to increased venous return.

Venous return increases as the pressure difference between RAP and MSFP increases. If RAP (or CVP) is low and MSFP high, then there will be a maximum change in pressure and a maximum venous return of blood to the right heart. On the other hand, if RAP increases, but there is no change in MSFP, then there will be a small difference between the two variables and venous return will decrease.

FACTORS AFFECTING VENOUS RETURN

Blood Volume

Increases in blood volume will increase MSFP. Higher blood volumes lead to greater vasculature stretch (preload) and end-diastolic volume, resulting in an increased gradient for flow

to the right atrium and venous return. Anything that causes volume retention increases MSFP. Examples include blood transfusion and fluid retention by renal mechanisms (ADH, renin-angiotensin, and aldosterone). Alternatively, situations that decrease blood volume, such as hemorrhage and dehydration, decrease MSFP and venous return.

Skeletal Muscle Contraction

During physical activity, venous pressure is increased due to muscle contraction, causing greater venous blood return to the heart. Peripheral veins have one-way valves that direct flow of blood away from the limbs and toward the heart. Muscle contraction causes venous compression, and muscle relaxation causes venous decompression. The alternative contraction and relaxation patterns cause blood to be pumped back to the heart, and unidirectional valves prevent blood from flowing back toward the limbs, enhancing venous return.

Respiratory Activity

As stated previously, venous return increases as the pressure difference between RAP and MSFP are increased. Respiratory activity influences venous return to the heart by augmenting the pressure difference between abdominal veins and the right atrium. Inspiration causes a decrease in intrathoracic pressure. As the chest wall expands, the diaphragm descends, which increases pressure in the abdominal contents and vessels while causing negative intrapleural pressure. This increases the pressure difference between the abdominal veins and right atrium, increasing venous return. When expiration occurs, the diaphragm ascends and causes an increase in intrathoracic pressure and a decrease in intraabdominal pressure, reducing the pressure difference between the right atrium and abdominal veins, therefore decreasing venous return. Atypical respiratory activity, such as positive pressure ventilation, impedes venous return by increasing intrathoracic pressure, decreasing blood volume contained within the thorax and venous return. Generally, anything that decreases intrathoracic pressure (such as inhalation) will increase venous return, while increasing intrathoracic pressure (expiration, PEEP) will decrease venous return.

Gravity and Body Position

When in a supine position, major systemic vessels are positioned close to the hydrostatic level of the heart, so distribution of blood volume between the head, legs, thorax, and abdomen is relatively uniform. However, when changing to a standing position, hydrostatic forces and gravity cause RAP to decrease and venous pressure in the limbs to increase as blood pools in the veins. In addition to the influence of gravity, blood pooling in veins occurs due to significant venous compliance, minor arterial compliance, shifting blood volumes to leg veins, and increasing venous pressure and volume. This decreases CVP, preload, and CO. Changing position from supine to standing activates baroreceptor reflexes, causing peripheral vasoconstriction and cardiac stimulation, which facilitate venous return and lowers venous pressures in dependent limbs, partially restoring CVP. Baroreceptor reflexes maintain blood pressure and venous return by increasing systemic vascular resistance and heart rate, preventing blood pressure from falling more than a few mm Hg and aiding venous return to help maintain CO.

Sympathetic Nervous System Activity

In comparison to arteries, veins are highly compliant, low-pressure vessels. Veins hold approximately 60% of total blood volume at rest. Since venous pressure is low, outside forces are needed to return blood back to the heart. Sympathetic stimulation of veins, also known as **venomotor tone**, decreases venous compliance by causing vasoconstriction, which increases CVP and promotes venous return. Vasoconstriction directly decreases the diameter of smooth muscles in the wall of veins, which increases MSFP, allowing greater blood return to the heart. Increased venous return increases CO and total blood flow through the circulatory system. Consequently, when sympathetic nervous system activity increases, the result is similar to that of an increase in blood volume.

Sympathetic activity does not affect veins more than arteries, meaning that increased activity will affect both arteries and veins equally. Nevertheless, increasing total peripheral resistance, which primarily affects arterioles, will decrease venous return. Blood volume becomes redistributed such that there is more blood in arteries than veins, subsequently decreasing venous return.

SUGGESTED READINGS

Greenway CV, Lautt WW. Blood volume, the venous system, preload, and cardiac output. *Can J Physiol Pharmacol.* 1986;64:383-387.

Guyton A. Determination of cardiac output by equating venous return curves with cardiac response curves. *Physiol Rev.* 1955;35:123-129.

Blood Pressures and Resistances

Gabrielle Brown, MD, and Tricia Desvarieux, MD

BLOOD PRESSURE

Blood pressure is the force exerted by blood against vessel walls. More specifically, blood pressure refers to the pressure of blood within the circulatory system's arteries. Arterial blood pressure is determined by the cardiac cycle's systole and diastole. During ventricular contraction, or systole, blood exits the heart's right and left ventricle into the pulmonary artery and aorta, causing pressures in these arteries to rise steeply. *Systolic blood pressure* (SBP) is the maximum pressure achieved during ventricular contraction. When ventricles relax during diastole, they fill with blood in preparation for the next contraction, and arterial blood pressure drops. *Diastolic blood pressure* (DBP) is the blood pressure following contraction of the heart, during heart chamber refilling, and represents the lowest arterial pressure prior to the next contraction cycle. The difference between systolic and diastolic pressures is the *pulse pressure*.

However, the primary pressure that drives blood flow in organs is the *mean arterial pressure* (MAP), which is determined from systolic and diastolic pressures. Mean arterial pressure drives blood flow to organs and tissues, and is the average pressure of several heartbeats over time. It can be determined by the following equation:

$$MAP = \frac{(2 \times DBP) + SBP}{3}$$

Diastole counts twice as much as systole since approximately two-third of the cardiac cycle is spent in diastole. The usual healthy range of MAP is 70-110, and an MAP of 60 is necessary to perfuse the body's vital organs and prevent ischemia.

Alternatively, cardiac output (CO), systemic vascular resistance (SVR), and central venous pressure (CVP) determine MAP, according to the equation:

$$MAP = (CO \times SVR) + CVP$$

Mean arterial pressure is proportional to the above variables. If CO and SVR change reciprocally, yet proportionately, MAP will remain the same.

PRESSURE, FLOW, AND RESISTANCE

Hemodynamics refers to the study of blood flow, and explains the physical laws that determine blood flow in vessels. Flow (Q) through a blood vessel is primarily determined by two factors: (1) the pressure gradient that pushes blood through the vessel (ΔP), and (2) the resistance of the vessel to blood flow (R). The pressure gradient (ΔP) is expressed as the difference between arterial and venous pressures. Flow is determined by the pressure gradient (ΔP) divided by resistance (R).

$$Q = \frac{\Delta P}{R}$$

Between the pressure gradient and resistance, flow is more dependent on resistance, since arterial and venous blood pressures are largely maintained within a narrow range. There are several factors that determine resistance to flow, including characteristics of blood (density or viscosity), blood flow (laminar or turbulent), vessels (length, radius), and vessel network organization (series or parallel).

The primary factors that determine resistance to blood flow are vessel length, vessel radius, and blood viscosity. The relationship is seen in the following equation, which is derived from Poiseuille's equation:

$$R \propto \frac{\eta \cdot L}{r^4}$$

where R = resistance; L = length; η = viscosity; r = radius

Vessel resistance is directly proportional to the length of vessel and viscosity of blood, and inversely proportional to the radius to the fourth power. Given the fact that any change in radius is able to alter resistance to the fourth power, vessel resistance is very sensitive to changes in radius, and consequently has a large effect on flow.

FACTORS AFFECTING RESISTANCE TO BLOOD FLOW

Changes in Vessel Size and Radius

Both extrinsic (neural and hormonal) and intrinsic factors affect resistance. Extrinsic vasoactive substances regulate blood flow by either constricting or dilating blood vessels. Sympathetic vascular tone via autonomic innervation works primarily through alpha adrenergic receptors to cause arterial and venous vasoconstriction, increasing resistance and decreasing blood flow. Removal of sympathetic stimulation causes vasodilation, decreasing resistance, and increasing blood flow. Extrinsic hormonal factors are circulating vasoactive hormones that work to constrict vessels and increase resistance (angiotensin II, epinephrine, norepinephrine, vasopressin), or to dilate vessels and decrease resistance (atrial natriuretic peptide, endothelin). Neural and hormonal factors work to regulate arterial pressure primarily by altering resistance to blood flow.

The intrinsic mechanism involved in local blood flow regulation is known as the myogenic mechanism. Myogenic mechanisms are intrinsic to vascular smooth muscle walls, particularly arteries and arterioles. With increasing pressure, the myogenic mechanism causes vasoconstriction and decreased blood flow, and also causes vasodilation with decreasing pressure, which increases blood flow. This intrinsic property most commonly reflects splanchnic and renal circulation.

Blood Viscosity

Viscosity refers to the internal friction of fluid levels sliding past one another. Given the heterogeneous nature of plasma (composed of cells, proteins, and electrolytes), plasma is 1.8 times more viscous than water. Red cells have the greatest effect on viscosity; hematocrit varies directly with viscosity. Patients with polycythemia—which causes an exaggerated increase in hematocrit—will have greater blood viscosity and resistance to flow. Increased resistance stresses the heart to pump, and risks inadequate end-organ perfusion over time.

Temperature varies inversely with viscosity, increasing viscosity by 2% per degree centigrade decrease in temperature. As blood cools, molecular interactions decrease and blood becomes thicker. Low flow states similarly increase viscosity, permitting molecular interactions between red cells.

Laminar Versus Turbulent Flow

Laminar flow is the normal condition for blood flow, and is characterized by concentric layers of blood moving in parallel through vessels. Laminar flow reduces energy loss in blood by decreasing viscosity. On the contrary, turbulent flow occurs when laminar flow becomes disrupted in areas of high flow such as the ascending aorta, stenotic lesions, and heart valves. Turbulence increases energy losses in the form of friction, thereby increasing energy required to drive flow. In comparison to laminar flow, turbulence decreases flow at any given perfusion pressure, increasing resistance to flow.

Series Versus Parallel Vascular Networks

In the body, vessels are arranged in both series and parallel arrangements, with major distributing arteries being in parallel with each other and most individual organs. Other organ systems (GI, hepatic) and capillaries have series connections. Overall, blood vessels travel along a length in series, branch out to smaller vessels in parallel, and regroup in series at end organs.

A. Series

For a series circulation, the total resistance equals the sum of all individual resistances. In a series circulation consisting of flow from a small artery (A) → arterioles (a) → capillaries (c) → venules (v) → veins (V), total resistance (R_T) is:

$$R_T = R_A + R_a + R_c + R_v + R_V$$

In series circulation, small arteries and arterioles have larger effects on total resistance than larger arteries. This is due to the greater quantity of small arteries and arterioles in circulation. Arteries and arterioles compose 70% of total vascular resistance. As an example, values for resistance are assigned to each of segment, with larger values assigned to segments that make up larger parts of the vascular system.

If $R_A = 10$; $R_a = 50$; $R_c = 20$; $R_v = 15$; $R_V = 5$

Then, $R_T = 10 + 50 + 20 + 15 + 5 = 100$

If R_v were doubled from 5 to 10, R_T would increase from 100 to 105, a 5% increase. However, if R_a is doubled from 50 to 100, R_T increases from 100 to 150, a 50% increase.

B. Parallel

Parallel vascular arrangement decreases R_T. For parallel vessels, the reciprocal of R_T is equal to the sum of the reciprocals of individual resistances. For a network of two parallel circulations, R_T is given by:

$$\frac{1}{R_T} = \frac{1}{R_1} + \frac{1}{R_2} \qquad \text{solving for } R_T, \qquad R_T = \frac{1}{\dfrac{1}{R_1} + \dfrac{1}{R_2}}$$

Given this reciprocal relationship, parallel arrangements reduce resistance to blood flow, as the R_T of a network of parallel vessels is less than the resistance of the lowest resistance vessel. Furthermore, when there are many parallel vessels, changing the resistances of a few vessels only minimally affects R_T for the segment. For example, even though capillaries, with small diameters have the highest resistance of all vessels, they minimally affect R_T.

SUGGESTED READING

Rose JC. Regulation of systemic vascular volume and venous return by sympathetic nervous system. *The Heart Bulletin;* 1959;8:98-100.

Baroreceptor Function

Brian S. Freeman, MD

Baroreceptors are specialized sensory neurons that enable the central nervous system (CNS) to maintain short-term control of blood pressure. These mechanoreceptors participate in a reflex (baroreceptor reflex, carotid sinus reflex) that regulates the mean arterial pressure, relatively constant at a preset value, usually around 100 mm Hg. In this negative feedback loop, a rise in blood pressure from baseline results in rapid signals from the baroreceptors to the CNS which then reduces MAP back down to normal level through the autonomic nervous system. A slight change in pressure causes a strong change in the baroreflex signal to readjust arterial pressure back toward normal. The arterial baroreceptor reflex serves as short-term blood pressure buffering system in response to relatively abrupt changes in blood volume, cardiac output, or peripheral resistance, such as during daily activities (posture changes, exercise) and during surgery (anesthesia, hemorrhage).

COMPONENTS OF THE BARORECEPTOR REFLEX

Baroreceptors

Baroreceptors are sensory neurons that can be divided into two types. High-pressure arterial baroreceptors are found clustered in abundance within the adventitia of the carotid sinus and in the aortic arch. The carotid sinus is the dilated root of the internal carotid artery, typically found where the common carotid artery bifurcates into the internal and external carotid arteries. These receptors participate in the classically described negative feedback reflex. In contrast, low-pressure cardiopulmonary baroreceptors are located in the right atrium (near the entrance of superior and inferior vena cavae) and left atrium (near the entrance of pulmonary veins). Unlike their counterparts in the carotid sinus, volume distension near these nerve endings will yield an increase in neuronal discharge.

The response rate of baroreceptors to changes in arterial blood pressure is rapid. They are mechanoreceptors with specialized nerve endings that get excited by stretch. Carotid sinus baroreceptors are not at all stimulated by pressures between 0 and 60 mm Hg. An increase in blood pressure causes stretching and distortion of the vascular wall, which

is sensed by the baroreceptor's specialized nerve endings. This will increase axonal depolarization and the frequency of action potential firing. As arterial pressure rises, impulse transmission progressively increases to a ceiling of around 180 mm Hg. Aortic arch baroreceptors are less sensitive than those in the carotid sinus and respond in a similar manner but function at pressure levels of about 30 mm Hg higher. Both types of baroreceptors can detect not only the rise of arterial pressure, but also the rate of change in pressure with each beat. Baroreceptors have higher impulse discharge rates when blood pressure increases rapidly as opposed to a simply stationary higher MAP (Figure 157-1).

Although the arterial baroreceptors provide powerful moment-to-moment control of arterial pressure, their importance in long-term blood pressure regulation has been controversial. Baroreceptors respond very quickly to higher pressures to maintain a stable blood pressure, but their responses diminish with time and thus, are most effective for conveying short-term pressure changes. After an initial high discharge rate, baroreceptor impulses tend to diminish to normal and "reset" in 1-2 days to the new arterial pressure level to which they are exposed.

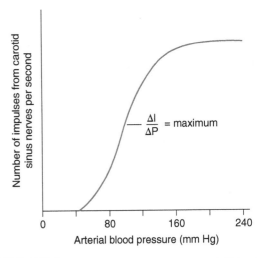

FIGURE 157-1 Baroreceptor activity versus arterial blood pressure. Reproduced with permission from Hall JE, Guyton AC, *Guyton and Hall Textbook of Medical Physiology*, 12th edition. Philadelphia, PA: Saunders/Elsevier; 2011.)

Cranial Nerves IX and X

Action potentials elicited by vascular stretch are sensed by the baroreceptors and transmitted to the brainstem through cranial nerves. Afferent impulses from baroreceptors located within the carotid sinus travel within Hering's nerve, a branch of the glossopharyngeal nerve (cranial nerve IX). Afferent impulses from baroreceptors located within the aortic arch are sent through the aortic nerve, a branch of the vagus nerve (cranial nerve X).

Nucleus Solitarius

Through CN IX and X, baroreceptor discharges eventually converge centrally on an area of the medulla known as the nucleus solitarius (nucleus of the solitary tract, nucleus tractus solitarii, NTS). The NTS is part of the cardiovascular center of the brainstem and has two anatomically different areas responsible for raising and lowering blood pressure. The cell bodies of the NTS integrate information received from the peripheral baroreceptors' firing rates.

Efferent Autonomic Response

Stimulation of the NTS by high baroreceptor firing rates brings blood pressure back to baseline through two mechanisms involving the cardiac autonomic nervous system. Neurons of the NTS send inhibitory signals to preganglionic sympathetic neurons in the spinal cord to decrease sympathetic nerve outflow to the peripheral blood vessels (depressor effect). The response of the depressor system includes decreased sympathetic activity leading to a decrease in cardiac contractility, heart rate, and systemic vascular resistance (SVR). In addition, the NTS sends excitatory signals to the nucleus of the vagus nerve, which promotes a parasympathetic response. The net effects are (1) vasodilation of the veins and arterioles throughout the peripheral circulatory system and (2) decreased heart rate and strength of heart contraction. Therefore, excitation of the baroreceptors by high pressure in the arteries causes the arterial pressure to decrease because of a decrease in peripheral resistance and cardiac output. Conversely, low pressure has opposite effects, causing the pressure to rise back to normal.

PERIOPERATIVE CONSIDERATIONS

Effects of Anesthetics

Both volatile and intravenous anesthetics cause a dose-dependent attenuation of baroreceptor activity, especially by inhibiting the efferent chronotropic component of this reflex arc. Halothane has been shown to have the most significant effects. The reflex is unaffected by low to moderate doses of opioids, but will be depressed by high doses.

Hypertension

In patients with long-standing essential hypertension, the carotid sinus stiffens because of the chronic exposure to high arterial pressures. As a result, baroreceptor sensitivity decreases, leading to a higher set point for the compensatory response to occur. For a given increase in transmural carotid sinus pressure, the reflex elicits a smaller drop in systemic arterial pressure than it does at a normal level of blood pressure. Patients with chronic hypertension often exhibit perioperative circulatory instability as a result of a decrease in their baroreceptor reflex response.

Carotid Endarterectomy

The surgical removal of an atheromatous plaque from the internal carotid artery can lead to hemodynamic instability. During the dissection of the common carotid artery, manipulation and stimulation of the carotid sinus can stretch the baroreceptors' nerve endings, leading to an increase in discharge that produces bradycardia and hypotension. Treatment includes cessation of surgical stimulation, administration of an anticholinergic, and infiltration of the carotid sinus with 1% lidocaine to block impulses from the baroreceptors.

Hypertension is common in the postoperative period as a result of baroreceptor dysfunction. As a result of stripping of sensory nerve endings from the arterial lumen, the reflex is essentially denervated, leading to decreased afferent input and therefore efferent vagal output. The hypertension that results is usually temporary, peaks in the first 48 hours after surgery, and may last for several hours or days after surgery. Although this is a temporary phenomenon and persistence of hypertension is quite rare, an increase in blood pressure and its variability 12 weeks after surgery has recently been demonstrated and characterized as *baroreflex failure syndrome*.

Postoperative hypotension occurs less frequently than hypertension after carotid endarterectomy. It is thought that carotid sinus baroreceptor hypersensitivity or reactivation likely plays an important role. If baroreceptors are intact after the removal of plaque, they are now exposed to a much higher perfusion pressure than they were used to, and therefore discharge at a much higher rate, leading to an exaggerated response.

Microcirculation

Eric Chiang, MD, and Tricia Desvarieux, MD

Microcirculation can be defined structurally as blood vessels less than 150 μm in diameter and encompasses the arterioles, capillaries, and venules. Structurally, capillaries consist of a single layer of epithelium along with a basement membrane. The parenchymal cells are arranged in close proximity to at least one capillary to ensure an adequate oxygen supply through passive diffusion.

Physiologically, microcirculation can be defined as the part of circulation where oxygen, nutrients, and waste products are exchanged, and vessels respond to changes in internal pressure with changes in lumen diameter. This physiologic definition highlights the critical role that microcirculation plays in oxygenation and hemodynamic stability.

NORMAL FUNCTIONS

The two primary functions of microcirculation are: (1) to optimize nutrient and oxygen supply and (2) to reduce large hydrostatic pressure fluctuations. Microcirculation is the important interface between supply that the circulation provides and demands of the parenchymal cells. The pathway for oxygen begins after release from oxyhemoglobin, through the interstitium, into parenchymal cells, and ending with mitochondrial oxidative phosphorylation in which cellular ATP is generated. The cardiovascular system must provide sufficient blood flow to the capillaries of an organ to support the diffusional fluxes of solutes across the capillary walls to meet metabolic needs. Autoregulation and vasomotor changes occur in the microvasculature to maintain adequate and stable blood flow. Thus, from the end-organ perspective, the main determinants of tissue perfusion are oxygen concentration and capillary blood flow.

FICK'S PRINCIPLE

The transcapillary flux of solutes can be calculated using Fick's equation, which is based on the Law of Conservation of Mass. The arteriovenous difference of a solute multiplied by the blood flow through the capillary gives the flux of that solute across the capillary wall. Thus, increasing the oxygen concentration or blood flow will influence solute flux to meet the metabolic demands of the cells.

$$\text{Transcapillary Flux of X (Fx)} = BF \times ([X]a - [X]v)$$
$$Fx = BFa \times [X]a - BFv \times [X]v$$

Fx = flux of solute X across the capillary wall (mass/min)
BFa = blood flow entering capillary (mL/min)
BFv = blood flow leaving capillary (mL/min)
[X]a = concentration of X in arterial blood (mass/mL)
[X]b = concentration of X in venous blood (mass/mL)

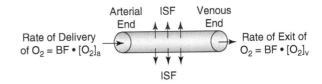

METHODS TO ASSESS MICROCIRCULATION FLOW

To accurately assess microcirculation, information regarding the oxygen tension and blood flow is needed. Microelectrodes are used to study oxygen tension in the interstitial fluid and mitochondria. Optical technologies such as the orthogonal polarization spectral and sidestream dark-field imaging methods are used to determine microcirculatory network through detecting erythrocyte movements. Clinically, mixed venous saturation and cardiac output are used as surrogates to determine adequacy of oxygen balance and microvasculature flow. Hemodynamic flow affects shear-sensitive mechanisms and responses by the microvasculature results in changes to vascular resistance and flow.

REGULATORS OF MICROVASCULATURE

Regulation of the microvasculature also hinges on the local mediators and blood flow. The main mediators that affect the microvasculature are nitric oxide N_2O and oxygen. N_2O is closely related to oxygen and has the ability to affect oxygen supply by controlling arteriolar caliber and oxygen demand through influencing mitochondrial oxygen consumption in parenchymal cells. N_2O is released from vascular endothelial cells and relaxes the smooth muscles through increasing cGMP. Oxygen also plays a role in regulation as increasing oxygen supply to peripheral tissue results in vasoconstriction of the resistance vessels and decreasing oxygen supply leads to vasodilation. The shear stress mechanism affects ATP-sensitive K^+ channels, while cGMP inhibit Ca^{2+} influx to activate K^+ channels to hyperpolarize and relax the smooth muscles, resulting in vasodilation.

MICROCIRCULATION AND DISEASE

In hypertension, microcirculation is altered both functionally and structurally. First, there is change to the regulation of vasomotor tone, resulting in enhanced vasoconstriction and reduced vasodilator responses. Second, there are changes structurally to individual precapillary resistance vessels, leading to an increase in the wall-to-lumen ratios. Lastly there is a change to the microvascular network with a reduction in density within a vascular bed.

Microcirculation in sepsis displays a heterogeneous distribution of blood flow where certain microcirculatory units become underperfused and other areas show normal or even high blood flow. This phenomenon is thought to be due to autoregulatory dysfunction of N_2O synthase, which is largely responsible for regulating microcirculation. In sepsis, smooth muscles also lose their adrenergic sensitivity and tone, and erythrocytes aggregation increases.

MICROCIRCULATION AND ANESTHESIA

The effects of intravenous and volatile anesthetics on the hemodynamics of microcirculation have been studied in the experimental settings using animal models. Propofol at higher doses led to significant reduction in renal, myocardial, and large-intestinal blood flow. Desflurane was associated with significant increase to gut blood flow when compared with isoflurane. Desflurane, isoflurane, and sevoflurane were found to not alter renal blood flow. Epidural anesthesia increased gastrointestinal blood flow and improved perfusion at the microcirculatory level.

SUGGESTED READING

Turek Z, Sykora R, Matejovic M, Cerny V. Anesthesia and the Microcirculation. *Semin Cardiothorac Vasc Anesth*. 2009;13:249-258.

Regional Blood Flow

Michael J. Savarese, MD and Tricia Desvarieux, MD

The human body self-regulates its internal environment to maintain homeostasis during stress, injury, or disease. Various organs in the body regulate blood flow to maintain perfusion during otherwise ischemic conditions.

Blood flow through a vessel can be approximated by **Poiseuille's law:**

$$Q = \frac{\pi P r^4}{8\eta l}$$

Q = flow rate; P = pressure; r = radius; η = fluid viscosity; l = length of tubing.

Blood flow through a vessel is directly proportional to the pressure difference but proportional to the fourth power of the radius. This law underscores how regulation of regional blood flow occurs throughout the body.

CORONARY BLOOD FLOW

The heart continually exercises, with "resting" cardiac blood flow approximately 250 mL/min (5% of CO). The heart's O_2 extraction ratio is 75%-80%, and is therefore dependent on increased blood flow to sustain oxygenation during stress. Myocardial O_2 consumption (MVo_2) is determined by the rate of force development (dP/dt) and the left ventricular wall tension (T). T is related to the left ventricle (LV) diameter and LV pressure by **LaPlace's law:**

$$T \propto Pr$$

During systole, the LV and right ventricle (RV) pump blood to systemic, high-pressure circulation and pulmonary, low-pressure circulation, respectively. The LV needs to achieve such a high pressure so that LV myocardial blood flow occurs only during diastole. Right and left coronary arteries originate from the aorta just distal to the aortic valve, so aortic diastolic pressure is the driving force for cardiac perfusion. Blood flow to the myocardium can be approximated by the equation:

Coronary perfusion pressure (CPP) = DBP_{Aorta} − LVEDP

Blood flow through the right coronary artery (RCA) to the RV is not interrupted during systole due to lower RV pressures and less extravascular compression. Blood flow through the coronary sinus is maximal during late systole, secondary to extravascular compression and minimal right atrial pressure.

The LV subendocardium is exposed to higher pressures during systole than the subepicardium, and is therefore more susceptible to ischemia. Disease states such as coronary artery disease (CAD) (decreased vessel radius), pressure overload hypertrophy (increased LVEDP), severe tachycardia (decreased diastolic period), or aortic insufficiency (decreased aortic diastolic pressure) expose LV subendocardium to ischemia.

Regulation of cardiac blood flow is controlled by neural and metabolic factors. Both the sympathetic and parasympathetic nervous system influence cardiac blood flow. Sympathetic vascular tone results from a feed-forward, beta adrenergic induced vasodilation of small arterioles. The parasympathetic system controls heart rate via the vagus nerve to the SA node. Decreased parasympathetic activity allows HR elevation with minimal direct effect on blood flow.

Metabolic factors considered to influence coronary blood flow include nitric oxide (NO), K_{atp}, Ca^{2+}, pH, O_2 and CO_2 tension, and prostaglandins. Adenosine increases cerebral blood flow (CBF) during hypoxia.

CORONARY RESERVE

Coronary reserve is the difference between resting and maximal coronary blood flow. The coronary blood flow in normal individuals increase 4-5 times during stress. In diseased states such as CAD, coronary arteries are already maximally dilated, so flow optimization and myocardial oxygen demand reduction are essential.

CORONARY STEAL

Coronary steal occurs in critically stenosed vessels and contributes to myocardial ischemia. Critically stenosed blood vessels will not vasodilate during periods of stress or exercise.

During periods of increased O_2 consumption, nearby vessels with dilatory reserve respond with dilation. Blood is shunted away from the stenosed vessel, resulting in paradoxical ischemic insult.

PULMONARY BLOOD FLOW

The pulmonary vascular system is a low-pressure system that receives 100% of CO. The blood volume held by the lung is approximately 900 mL, and in cases of hypovolemia or hemorrhage, this blood can be utilized via sympathetically mediated vasoconstriction of pulmonary vasculature. Both the sympathetic and parasympathetic nervous systems affect the alveolar and bronchial smooth muscles. Parasympathetic (muscarinic) receptor signals are transmitted via the vagus nerve and cause bronchoconstriction. Sympathetic (beta-2 adrenergic) signals are transmitted from thoracic plexi and cause bronchodilation. Overall, despite rich innervation, neural control of pulmonary blood flow is secondary to metabolic factors such as O_2 tension.

The lung can be thought of as having three zones with varying degrees of ventilation (V) and perfusion (Q):

Zone 1

Zone 1 is the upper third of the lung, which has more ventilation relative to perfusion (V/Q >1), and contributes to dead space ventilation. In Zone 1, pulmonary alveolar pressure (P_A) > pulmonary artery pressure (P_a), resulting in arteriole and capillary collapse.

Zone 2

Zone 2 is the middle third, where ventilation and perfusion are matched (V/Q ~ 1). In Zone 2, pulmonary artery pressure > alveolar pressure > pulmonary venous pressure, and blood flow is dependent on the pressure gradient between the pulmonary arterial and alveolar pressure.

Zone 3

In Zone 3, gravity pulls blood toward dependent lung fields, resulting in greater perfusion than ventilation (V/Q <1). In this zone, pulmonary artery pressure > pulmonary venous pressure > alveolar pressure, and blood flow becomes dependent on the pressure gradient between the arterial and venous systems. Since in Zone 3, blood flow is independent of alveolar pressure, shunting can develop. Atelectasis in this region will not inhibit blood flow, resulting in shunt. In the supine position, this effect is amplified due to V/Q mismatches at lower pressure gradients. Overall, the V/Q ratio in the normal lung is approximately 0.9. Also see Chapter 137 for additional discussion of lung zones.

To maintain optimal V/Q matching, the lung enacts **hypoxic pulmonary vasoconstriction (HPV)**. Pulmonary

endothelial O_2 sensors → decreased outward K^+ current → increased Ca^{2+} influx → vasoconstriction. In the setting of chronic hypoxia, pulmonary hypertension results from proliferation of vascular smooth muscle. Other metabolic factors such as epinephrine, NO, angiotensin, and prostaglandins decrease pulmonary vascular resistance to improve blood flow.

CEREBRAL BLOOD FLOW

The brain is dependent on continuous blood flow for O_2 and glucose supply. The brain is 2% of total body weight, but receives 15% of CO. Cerebral blood flow (CBF) is directly coupled to cerebral metabolic rate ($CMRO_2$). Motor and sensory stimulation activate neuronal tissue, increasing $CMRO_2$ and local metabolic factor (CO_2, H^+, lactate, adenosine, NO, K^+, Ca^{2+}) production, which increases CBF.

Under normal conditions, cerebral vasculature autoregulates CBF between an MAP of 50 and 150 mm Hg. Beyond these limits, blood flow and perfusion are dependent on pressure:

Cerebral perfusion pressure (CPP)
  = mean arterial pressure (MAP) – intracranial pressure (ICP)
  or central venous pressure (CVP) (whichever is higher)

Chronic hypertension shifts the range of autoregulation to the right, resulting in impaired cerebral perfusion at "normal" MAPs. Volatile anesthetics and hypercarbia directly inhibit cerebral autoregulation, making careful blood pressure and ventilatory control imperative under anesthesia. CBF increases by 1-2 mL/100 g tissue/min for each 1 mm Hg increase in $Paco_2$. Hyperventilation beyond a $Paco_2$ of approximately 25 mm Hg does not continue to reduce CBF. The brain senses $Paco_2$ as extracellular H^+ ions. The blood-brain barrier is impermeable to H^+ ions; hence, metabolic acidosis does not affect ICP as compared to respiratory acidosis. Sedatives should be avoided in patients with increased ICP because hypoventilation will cause a respiratory acidosis, further increasing the ICP and decreasing CPP.

RENAL BLOOD FLOW

The kidney regulates electrolyte and acid–base balance, assists in production of red blood cells, regulates plasma volume, and filters toxins and metabolic wastes. Tight regulation of renal blood flow (RBF) ensures proper function.

The kidney autoregulates blood flow via regulatory feedback mechanisms to maintain a relatively constant RBF and glomerular filtration rate (GFR) from SBP approximately 80 to 200 mm Hg. The **myogenic reflex** theory suggests that increased afferent renal artery pressure activates stretch receptors that cause reflex constriction to decrease RBF and perfusion pressure. Additionally, low systemic arterial BP causes a reflex dilation of the afferent renal artery, increasing RBF and perfusion. **Tubuloglomerular feedback** is a mechanism by which RBF is regulated in the kidney by chemical sensors in the juxtaglomerular apparatus. When RBF decreases, the juxtaglomerular apparatus senses less Cl^- filtration, which causes afferent arteriolar dilation and increased RBF and GFR. Additionally, the decreased Cl^- stimulates renin release, activating the renin–angiotensin–aldosterone axis. Angiotensin II causes constriction of the efferent arterioles, increasing glomerular perfusion pressure.

Several hormones control RBF. Antidiuretic hormone (ADH) released from the posterior pituitary in response to hypernatremia or hypovolemia causes H_2O retention to increase systemic perfusion. During stress, ADH induces renal cortical vasoconstriction, shifting renal blood from the cortex to the less vascular, ischemic-prone medulla. Atrial natriuretic peptide is released by the atria with stretch, increasing GFR via afferent arteriole dilation. Nitric oxide, produced by the renal endothelium, directly dilates renal vessels and increases perfusion. Stress-induced production of renal prostaglandins cause dilation of renal arterioles.

HEPATIC BLOOD FLOW

The liver is responsible for biosynthesis, metabolism, and toxin clearance. It accounts for approximately 2.5% of total body weight but receives 25% of CO, 800-1200 mL/min. The liver has dual afferent blood supply, arising from the hepatic artery and portal vein, each contributing 50% to hepatocyte oxygenation. The portal vein supplies approximately 75% of the hepatic blood flow, while the hepatic artery supplies 25%.

Hepatic blood flow is regulated by intrinsic and extrinsic mechanisms to maintain a constant flow rate. The portal vein is not directly regulated, and its flow is determined by systemic blood pressure. The hepatic artery is controlled by intrinsic mechanisms, which include the myogenic response and hepatic arterial buffer response (HABR). The myogenic response results in a reflex hepatic artery constriction in response to increased arterial pressures. HABR is mediated by adenosine and causes modulation of hepatic artery tone to compensate for portal vein flow changes.

Extrinsically, systemic blood pressure and splanchnic vascular resistance determine hepatic blood flow. The hepatic perfusion pressure (HPP) = (MAP or portal vein pressure) − hepatic vein pressure. Splanchnic vasculature receives sympathetic innervation in response to pain, hypoxemia, and stress, increasing resistance and decreasing hepatic blood flow. Some beta-blockers, such as propranolol decrease hepatic blood flow. Positive pressure ventilation and hepatic congestion (CHF, fluid overload, or cirrhosis) decrease blood flow by decreasing the HPP.

Regulation of Circulation and Blood Volume

Michael J. Savarese, MD and Tricia Desvarieux, MD

Human circulation is a closed system that can be thought of as two separate components connected in series. The arterial system is under high pressure and consists of low capacitance vessels. The venous system is a lower pressure system with high capacitance vessels. One can also classify the circulation as either systemic circulation or pulmonary circulation. Forward flow of blood relies on the heart to actively pump blood from venous to arterial system. Blood travels from the Heart → Arteries → Arterioles → Capillaries → Venules → Veins → Heart.

Without the heart, the vascular system would rely on vascular mechanics to determine where blood pools. Due to the high capacitance of the venous system, the majority of the blood would be in the venous circulation. Mean circulatory filling pressure (MCFP), 7 mm Hg, is the mean pressure that exists within the vascular system if pressure is allowed to redistribute in the absence of cardiac output (CO). It is a measure of vascular fullness and elastic recoil, the energy stored in vessel walls. The difference between the MCFP and central venous pressure (CVP) or right atrial pressure, is an important determinant of venous return to the right heart (preload).

Cardiac output and vascular fullness are coupled in the cardiovascular system. CO is both a determinant of, and dependent on preload and afterload, which is a function of vascular tone.

$$CO = HR \times SV = \text{pressure/resistance}$$

HR = heart rate; SV = stroke volume.

The **Frank–Starling** law of the heart states that increasing ventricular end-diastolic volume (preload) results in increased force production and higher stroke volumes. It is derived from the myocyte's ability to increase force production by starting at a longer sarcomere length due to increased affinity of troponin C for Ca^{2+} and more actin–myosin cross-bridges. Stretching sarcomeres further than optimal decreases contractility, secondary to decreased thick and thin filaments overlap (ie, volume overload heart failure). Less sarcomere stretching (decreased preload) diminishes Ca^{2+} affinity, thereby weakening contractions.

BLOOD VOLUME

The human body contains a total blood volume of approximately 7 mL/kg of blood, or 5 L for a 70 kg man, with women having slightly less. Blood contains two major components: plasma and cellular structures. Plasma consists of H_2O, proteins (albumin), and electrolytes (Na^+, K^+, Ca^{2+}, and glucose). Cellular structures include white blood cells, red blood cells, and platelets. Of the total body water, two-third remains intracellular, and one-third is extracellular; of the extracellular water, one-third is intravascular and two-third is interstitial. The net movement of fluid between the intravascular and interstitial compartment is governed by the **Starling equation**:

$$J_v = K_f([P_c - P_i] - \sigma[\pi_c - \pi_i])$$

J_v is the net fluid movement between compartments; P_c is the capillary hydrostatic pressure; P_i is the interstitial hydrostatic pressure; π_c is the capillary oncotic pressure; π_i is the interstitial oncotic pressure; K_f is the filtration coefficient; σ is the reflection constant. Both σ and K_f are constants, which are tissue-specific.

Under normal conditions, the net driving force in the capillaries is positive (flow out of the intravascular space). Excess capillary fluid leakage becomes interstitial fluid, and is returned to the circulation via lymphatics. Increased capillary permeability (ie, sepsis) can allow small osmotically active substances (proteins) to diffuse out of the intravascular space, increasing the outward driving force of H_2O and resulting in interstitial edema. Increasing the oncotic pressure of the intravascular space by increasing osmolarity, or the addition of oncotically active colloids such as albumin can shift fluid from the interstitial space into the vasculature.

BLOOD RESERVOIRS

Certain organ systems have the capacity to hold blood within their vasculature, mitigating the effects of increased blood volume (fluid overload, congestive heart failure [CHF]) or utilization in times of hypovolemia or hemorrhage to support circulation. Blood volume shifts from reservoir organs to systemic circulation direct pressure forces and stimulation of sympathetic vasomotor tone. The lung, liver, and skin act as the major blood reservoirs.

Hepatic

The hepatic vasculature normally holds 25-30 mL blood/100 g liver weight, or 400-500 mL, and accounts for approximately 10% of total blood volume (TBV). Large capacitance vessels (hepatic vein, portal vein, and hepatic artery) hold 40% of the hepatic reserve, while the sinusoids hold 60%. In addition to passive hemodynamic forces, the liver can actively expel stored blood via norepinephrine release, which decreases hepatic vascular capacitance via activation of alpha-adrenoreceptors.

Pulmonary

The lung's compliant vasculature allows it to mitigate pressure changes at varied COs. At rest, the pulmonary vascular network is not fully perfused. In increased CO, vessel recruitment accommodates increased blood volumes. Resting pulmonary blood volume is 450 mL, or 9% TBV. During hypovolemia or hemorrhage, pulmonary blood reserves are utilized via sympathetically mediated vasoconstriction of pulmonary vasculature to boost preload and circulating blood volume.

Epidermal

At rest, the skin receives 450 mL/min of blood, or 9% of CO. The skin contains large, subcutaneous venous plexuses that act as blood reservoirs. Additionally, arteriovenous (AV) anastomoses connecting arterioles directly to venules bypass capillary circulation, and are vasoconstricted at rest. The AV anastomoses are controlled by sympathetic tone via epinephrine and norepinephrine. During stress, skin AV anastomoses undergo further sympathetic vasoconstriction to increase circulating blood volume.

RENAL CONTROL OF BLOOD VOLUME

The kidney is integral for controlling blood volume, which it achieves through pressure, osmotically, and hormonally mediated mechanisms. The kidney maintains blood volume by regulating excretion and absorption of H_2O and electrolytes in the nephron. **Pressure natriuresis** is a phenomenon by which increased renal perfusion pressure results in increased excretion of Na^+ and H_2O, and diminished absorption of Na^+. **Osmotic diuresis** is a result of osmotically active solutes (ie, glucose, mannitol) in the renal tubules causing increased oncotic pressure in the tubule and increased H_2O excretion.

Renin release by afferent arterioles is stimulated by hypotension, which stimulates production of angiotensin II. Angiotensin II causes efferent arteriolar constriction, raising renal perfusion and glomerular filtration rate (GFR). Angiotensin II also stimulates the posterior pituitary to release antidiuretic hormone (ADH), which increases Na^+ reabsorption by the proximal tubule and stimulates aldosterone release by the adrenal gland. Aldosterone enhances the absorption of Na^+ and H_2O from the distal convoluted tubule and collecting duct, expanding plasma volume. Aldosterone release is additionally stimulated directly by sympathetic innervation. Further, ADH and aldosterone induce renal cortical vasoconstriction, shifting RBF to the renal medulla.

The posterior pituitary releases ADH in response to angiotensin II stimulation, hypernatremia, increased osmolarity, arterial baroreceptors, and atrial stretch receptors when they detect a diminished intravascular volume. ADH increases collecting duct and distal tubule H_2O permeability via aquaporin upregulation, resulting in increased H_2O retention and urine concentration.

THIRST MECHANISM

With the other mechanisms of blood volume control mentioned, the body compensates for lost volume by shifting fluids between compartments or preventing further loss. However, this does not return the body fluid level to the normal state. The thirst mechanism, arising from the hypothalamus, stimulates replenishment of lost fluid volume.

Thirst drive is stimulated by low H_2O volume, and inhibited by signals of increased volume. Cerebral osmoreceptors, which are located in the anterior wall of the third ventricle, sense intravascular volume depletion when the extracellular osmolarity is elevated. Renin and angiotensin II, which are released in response to hypovolemia and hypotension, have been demonstrated to produce thirst. Finally, ANP inhibits thirst.

Mixed Venous Oxygen Saturation

Ronak Patel, MD, and Katrina Hawkins, MD

Mixed venous oxygen saturation (Svo_2) can provide useful information regarding a patient's clinical condition. As such, there continues to be an interest in this value as a clinical predictor of outcomes. Svo_2 is measured at the level of the pulmonary artery. It reflects the oxygen saturation of the blood returning from the body to the heart. To obtain a true measurement, a blood sample is drawn from the distal tip of a pulmonary artery catheter. This allows the blood to be a true mixture of superior and inferior vena cava as well as coronary sinus blood (venous return from all parts of the body). More sophisticated monitoring exists whereby mixed venous oxygenation is displayed continuously via specialized pulmonary artery catheters. This technology allows for early changes in clinical status to be detected, though it has not been proven to be superior to periodic measurement via a standard pulmonary artery catheter.

Normal Svo_2 is 70%, with a range of 60%-80%. The absolute number is an indicator of the percentage of reduced hemoglobin left after the body's organs and tissues have extracted oxygen.

The Fick equation is vital to understanding mixed venous oxygen saturation. It states that:

$$Svo_2 = Sao_2 - Vo_2/(CO \times 1.34 \times Hb)$$

In this equation, Svo_2 is the mixed venous oxygen saturation, Sao_2 the arterial oxygen saturation, Vo_2 the oxygen consumption, CO the cardiac output, and Hb the hemoglobin. This equation shows that Svo_2 decreases as oxygen utilization increases. If tissues extract or utilize more oxygen, less is returned to the heart, thus a lower Svo_2. If Svo_2 is low due to increased tissue utilization of oxygen, one must increase oxygen delivery to meet the body's needs. Oxygen delivery is dependent on CO and oxygen content of blood. The oxygen content of blood is largely determined by hemoglobin level and oxygen saturation of arterial blood. To improve oxygen delivery, one must either improve CO, correct anemia, or improve oxygen saturation. Alternatively, a high Svo_2 may indicate problems as well. High Svo_2 can signify a decrease in tissue oxygen delivery (inadequate CO) or a decrease in tissue oxygen extraction (adequate CO) (Figure 161-1).

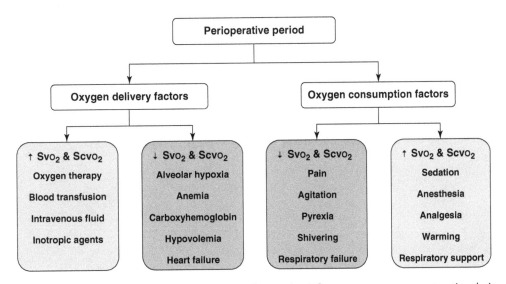

FIGURE 161-1 Common physiologic, pathologic, and therapeutic factors that influence venous oxygen saturation during the perioperative period. (Reproduced with permission from Shepherd S, Pearse, Rupert M. Role of central and mixed venous oxygen saturation measurement in perioperative care, *Anesthesiology.* 2009;111(3):649-656.)

LIMITATIONS

Svo_2 is a value obtained from the entire body's venous return, and hence can be misleading. This number does not indicate the status of specific organ perfusion. Intracardiac shunting, liver failure, severe sepsis, or focal ischemia (any etiology where blood is shunted) may give a falsely high value. Special care must be taken when drawing blood samples as well. A strong, negative force on a syringe can cause pulmonary capillary blood to be sampled. This blood has already received oxygen from the lungs and when drawn back will produce a falsely high value. Once blood is drawn, a cooximetry, via spectrophotometry, which senses the difference in light absorption between oxyhemoglobin and deoxyhemoglobin allows for the oxygen saturation of hemoglobin to be calculated. While Svo_2 can be a useful tool, it must be correlated with other clinical factors.

Using Svo_2 for Management

Properly derived and understood, Svo_2 can be used to guide therapy. It is a tool that gauges how much oxygen is being extracted from the blood to the tissues to meet metabolic demand. Svo_2 can be used to adjust ventilator settings and optimize oxygen delivery. Positive end expiratory pressure (PEEP) can be adjusted to balance high arterial oxygen saturation with low Svo_2. A high fraction of inspired oxygen (Fio_2) may increase Svo_2 even though extraction has not decreased. Fio_2 does not affect the difference of oxygen content between arterial and venous sides because both are proportionally affected. For illustration, an equation for oxygen extraction is:

$$O_2 \text{ extraction} = Cao_2 - Cvo_2/Cao_2$$

where C = content. Normal values range from 24% to 28%.

Complications from surgery as a result of diminished cardiopulmonary reserve are a major cause of morbidity and mortality. Problems with impaired microvascular flow may be the etiology. Fluids and inotropic therapy are used to increase oxygen delivery. Additionally, the use of Svo_2 to guide therapy may be helpful. Shivering or pain, causing a decrease in Svo_2, may increase postoperative oxygen consumption. Anesthetic drugs that reduce metabolic demand may increase Svo_2. These medications include benzodiazepines, opioids, and propofol.

The use of a central mixed venous gas ($ScVO_2$) can also be used and is becoming more common. As opposed to blood drawn from the pulmonary artery, blood is drawn from the superior vena cava, thus lacking coronary sinus and inferior vena cava blood. Since patients often have central lines without a pulmonary catheter, this option is being utilized more. $ScVO_2$, however, only reflects venous drainage from the upper body and is generally 2%-5% less than Svo_2 (venous drainage from the kidneys is oxygen rich). In times of shock, when blood is diverted away from the kidneys and splanchnic circulation to the upper body, $ScVO_2$ may be greater than Svo_2. Overall, there are many factors that influence an Svo_2 value, but along with a clinical correlation, it can guide therapy in critically ill patients.

SUGGESTED READING

Shepherd SJ, Pearse R. Role of central and mixed venous oxygen saturation measurement in perioperative care. *Anesthesiology* 2009;111:649-656.

Cardiac Anatomy

Caleb A. Awoniyi, MD, PhD

In humans, blood circulates within a closed system of blood vessels. The system is said to be closed because arteries and veins are connected with each other through small vessels. This requires the action of a pump, which is provided by the heart. The heart is composed of four chambers, right atrium and ventricle, and the left atrium and ventricle. The right and left atria receive blood from the venous system and the left atrium and ventricles pumps blood into the arterial system.

Atrioventricular valves separate the atria and ventricles (mitral valve on the left and tricuspid valve on the right). The right atrium and ventricle is separated from the left atrium and ventricle by a septum. Deoxygenated blood returns from the body via the great veins, superior and inferior vena cava, to the right atrium and then passes through the tricuspid valve into the right ventricle. From the right ventricle, blood is pumped through the pulmonary valve into the pulmonary artery—the only artery in the body that carries deoxygenated blood—and into the pulmonary capillaries in the lung. In the lungs, carbon dioxide is removed from the blood and the blood is oxygenated.

Blood returns to the left side of the heart via the pulmonary veins—the only vein in the body that carries oxygenated blood—and into the left atrium. The blood that returns to the left atrium by way of pulmonary veins is, therefore, enriched with oxygen and partially depleted of carbon dioxide. The path of blood from the heart (right ventricle), through the lungs, and back to the heart (left atrium) completes one circuit—the pulmonary circulation. Oxygen-rich blood in the left atrium enters the left ventricle (LV) via the mitral valve and is pumped out of the LV into the systemic circulation via the aorta. The arterial branches from the aorta supply oxygen-rich blood to all the organ systems and thus the systemic circulation.

CORONARY ARTERIES

Like all organs, the heart is made of tissue that requires a steady supply of oxygen and nutrients. Although its chambers are full of blood, the heart does not receive nourishment from this blood. The heart receives its own supply of blood from a network of arteries, called the coronary arteries. There are two major coronary arteries (left and right) that provide blood supply to the heart and both these arteries originate from the beginning (root) of the aorta, immediately above the aortic valve.

The left and right coronary arteries originate at the base of the aorta from openings called the coronary ostia, located behind the aortic valve leaflets. These two major vessels provide blood flow to different regions of the heart and because their branches lie on the surface of the heart they are sometimes called the epicardial coronary vessels. The left and right coronary arteries further branch into arterioles, and the arterioles branch into numerous capillaries that lie adjacent to the cardiac myocytes. A high capillary-to-cardiomyocyte ratio and short diffusion distances ensure adequate oxygen delivery to the myocytes and removal of metabolic waste products from the cells (eg, CO_2 and H^+).

LEFT CORONARY ARTERY

The left coronary artery (LCA) arises from the aorta above the left cusp of the aortic valve as the left main coronary artery. The left main artery typically runs for a few millimeters (~1-25 mm) and then bifurcates into the left anterior descending (LAD) artery and the left circumflex artery (LCX). If an artery arises from the left main between the LAD and LCX, it is known as the ramus intermedius. The ramus intermedius occurs in 37% of the general population, and is considered a normal variant. The LAD runs down the anterior interventricular groove and reaches the apex of the heart in 78% of cases. It supplies the anterolateral myocardium, apex, and interventricular septum. The LAD typically supplies 45%-55% of the LV.

The LAD gives off two types of branches: septals and diagonals. Septals originate from the LAD at 90 degrees to the surface of the heart, perforating and supplying the intraventricular septum. Diagonals run along the surface of the heart and supply the lateral wall of the LV and the anterolateral papillary muscle. The LCX runs across the left atrioventricular groove. It gives off obtuse marginal (OM) branches. The LCX supplies the posterolateral LV and the anterolateral papillary muscle. It also supplies the sinoatrial nodal artery in 38% of people. It supplies 15%-25% of the LV in right-dominant systems. If the coronary anatomy is left-dominant, the LCX supplies 40%-50% of the LV.

Right Coronary Artery

The right coronary artery (RCA) originates above the right cusp of the aortic valve. It travels down the right atrioventricular groove, toward the crux of the heart. At the origin of the RCA is the conus artery. In addition to supplying blood to the right ventricle, the RCA supplies 25%-35% of the LV. In 85% of patients, the RCA gives off the posterior descending artery (PDA). In the other 15% of cases, the PDA is given off by the LCX. The PDA supplies the inferior wall, ventricular septum, and the posteromedial papillary muscle. The RCA also supplies the SA nodal artery in 60% of patients. Forty percent of the time, the SA nodal artery is supplied by the LCX.

The artery that supplies the PDA and the posterolateral artery (PLA) determines the *coronary dominance*. If the RCA supplies both these arteries, the circulation can be classified as "right-dominant." If the LCX supplies both these arteries, the circulation can be classified as "left-dominant." If the RCA supplies the PDA and the LCX supplies the PLA, the circulation is known as "codominant." Approximately 70% of the general population are right-dominant, 20% are codominant, and 10% are left-dominant.

Although there is considerable heterogeneity among people, Table 162-1 and Figure 162-1 indicate the regions of the heart that are generally supplied by the different coronary arteries as well as measurement by electrocardiography. This anatomic distribution is important because these cardiac regions are assessed by 12-lead ECGs to help localize

ischemic or infarcted regions, which can be loosely correlated with specific coronary vessels; however, because of vessel heterogeneity, actual vessel involvement in ischemic conditions needs to be verified by coronary angiograms or other imaging techniques.

CONDUCTION SYSTEM

Sinoatrial Node

The dominant pacemaker in the human heart is the sinoatrial (SA) node. It is a subepicardial structure located at the junction of the right atrium and superior vena cava. The SA nodal cells depolarize and produce action potentials almost synchronously. The SA node is located superiorly in the right atrium at the junction of the crista terminalis, a thick band of atrial muscle at the border of the atrial appendage, and the superior vena cava. Histologic studies showed that the sinus node has a crescent-like shape with an average length of 13.5 mm. While it appears that the electrical signals from the sinus node to the atrial periphery can exit randomly, there appears to be preferential pathways of conduction from the sinus pacemaker cells to the atrium. The conduction velocity within the sinus node is very slow compared with nonnodal atrial tissue. This is a result of poor electrical coupling arising from the relative paucity of gap junctions in the center of the node compared to the periphery.

The blood supply to the SA node is commonly from the RCA in about 55% of patients. Whereas the SA nodal artery (from the RCA) may take one to six different routes, two or more branches to the node may be present in about 54% of patients. This suggests that collateral blood supplies are common, hence reason of rarity.

The SA node is innervated by the parasympathetic and the sympathetic nervous systems, and the balance between these systems controls the pacemaker rate. The vagal parasympathetic nerves slow the SA nodal pacemaker and are dominant at rest, while increased activity of the sympathetic nervous system as well as the adrenal medullary release of catecholamines increases the sinus rate during exercise and stress.

Atrioventricular Node

The atrioventricular (AV) node is an area of specialized tissue between the atria and the ventricles of the heart, specifically in the posteroinferior region of the interatrial septum near the opening of the coronary sinus, which conducts the normal electrical impulse from the atria to the ventricles. It is located at the center of Koch's Triangle—a triangle enclosed by the septal leaflet of the tricuspid valve, the coronary sinus, and the membranous part of the interatrial septum. A wave of excitation spreads out from the SA through the atria along specialized conduction channels to activate the AV node. Functions of the AV node include: (1) delayering of the cardiac impulses from the SA node for approximately 0.12 seconds to allow the

TABLE 162-1   Coronary Blood Flow Distribution

Coronary Artery	Cardiac Anatomic Region
Right coronary	Posterior, inferior
Left coronary	Anterior, septum (anteroseptal)
Circumflex	Anterior, lateral (anterolateral)

I	AVR	V1	V4
II	AVL	V2	V5
III	AVF	V3	V6

Blue   : I, V5, V6   = Circumflex (Lateral wall)
Yellow : II, III, AVF = RCA (Inferior wall)
Red   : V1-V4   = LAD (Anterior septum)

FIGURE 162-1 Relationship between ECG leads and coronary blood flow distribution.

atria to contract and empty their contents first, and (2) relaying cardiac impulses to the AV bundle. The delay in the cardiac impulse from the SA node to the AV node is extremely important. It ensures that the atria have ejected their blood into the ventricles first before the ventricles contract. This also protects the ventricles from excessively fast rate response to atrial arrhythmias.

An important property that is unique to the AV node is decremental conduction in which the more frequently the node is stimulated the slower it conducts. This is the property of the AV node that prevents rapid conduction to the ventricle in case of rapid atrial rhythms, such as atrial fibrillation or atrial flutter. The blood supply of the AV node can be from (1) the posterior interventricular, or posterior descending, artery (which is a branch of the RCA in right-dominant individuals (70%)) or (2) the posterior interventricular artery (which is a branch of the LCX (10%)); the coronary circulation in these individuals is considered left-dominant.

Digitalis

Brian S. Freeman, MD

INDICATIONS AND PHARMACOKINETICS

Digitalis is the genus of the foxglove plant group, a species from which cardiac glycosides are derived. Cardiac glycosides contain a primary sugar group (usually a polysaccharide) that is bound to a steroid nucleus. Digoxin is the most common form of digitalis used in cardiac patients today.

The primary indications for digoxin therapy are: (1) ventricular rate control of chronic atrial fibrillation or flutter, especially in patients with compromised myocardial contractility; (2) treatment of narrow-complex paroxysmal supraventricular tachycardia (PSVT); and (3) treatment of congestive heart failure. Because of improved outcomes with first-line drugs like ACE inhibitors and angiotensin receptor blockers, digoxin is used much less frequently today in patients with congestive heart failure due to left ventricular systolic dysfunction.

Digoxin can be given as 0.5-1 mg IV bolus. It has a 5-30-minute onset time, achieves peak effect in 1-3 hours, and has a 36-hour elimination half-life if renal function is normal. Digoxin undergoes minimal hepatic metabolism and is mostly excreted unchanged by the kidneys. Patients with chronic renal insufficiency should have reduced doses and digoxin plasma levels should be closely monitored.

PHARMACODYNAMICS

Digoxin's mechanism of action on myocardial cell membranes is complex. Digoxin binds to and inhibits the sodium–potassium adenosine triphosphate pump, leading to increased cytosolic sodium concentrations. Without the normal electrochemical gradient for sodium, the sodium–calcium transporter cannot remove calcium in exchange for sodium, resulting in increased free intracellular calcium. Higher levels of calcium release from the sarcoplasmic reticulum promote sarcomere contraction and enhance myocardial contractility. This nonadrenergic mechanism of positive inotropy makes digoxin a unique vasopressor. Unlike sympathomimetic drugs such as epinephrine and dopamine, digoxin will not precipitate tachydysrhythmias. Patients taking beta-blockers benefit from digoxin's independence from myocardial beta-1 receptors.

Digoxin directly affects cardiac pacemaker cells with negative chronotropy. In the atrioventricular (AV) node, inhibition of the Na^+/K^+ ATPase transporter alters the resting membrane potential, increases the absolute refractory period, and decreases action potential conduction velocity. Digoxin also increases vagal activity and enhances the AV node's response to acetylcholine. Heart transplant patients, who lack vagal innervation, do not respond to the rate control effects of digoxin. At therapeutic levels, digoxin decreases pacemaker cell automaticity by prolonging phase 4 spontaneous depolarization of the cardiac action potential. The primary ECG effects of therapeutic levels of digoxin are prolonged PR interval, ST segment depression, T-wave flattening or inversion, and increased U-wave amplitude.

TOXICITY

Digoxin has a narrow therapeutic index (0.5-2.5 ng/mL). Conditions which increase the risk of digoxin toxicity include hypoxemia, renal insufficiency, hypothyroidism, hypoglycemia, hypomagnesemia, and hypercalcemia. Since both digoxin and K^+ compete for the same binding site on the Na^+/K^+ ATP pump, hypokalemia will augment the effects of digoxin, leading to toxicity. Patients receiving diuretic therapy should have potassium levels closely monitored.

In an awake patient, the signs and symptoms of digoxin toxicity encompass multiple organ systems. Patients may report confusion, delirium, hallucinations, and other mental status changes. Headaches, syncope, seizures, and dizziness may also occur. Gastrointestinal manifestations include nausea, vomiting, abdominal pain, and anorexia. Patients may also report blurry or yellow-green vision.

Cardiac dysrhythmias are particularly concerning in patients with toxic concentrations of digoxin. Because of greater sympathetic nervous system activity and intracellular calcium overload, myocardial pacemaker cells have higher spontaneous rates of diastolic depolarization (phase 4) plus delayed afterdepolarizations. Lower threshold potentials can predispose the myocardium to develop ectopy and trigger dysrhythmias. The pathognomonic dysrhythmia associated with digoxin toxicity is paroxysmal atrial tachycardia with a 2:1 AV block. Other common rhythm disturbances include ectopic beats (premature ventricular contractions [PVCs] and ventricular bigeminy), junctional tachycardia, first-degree AV nodal block, and ventricular tachycardia. Sinus bradycardia, sinus arrest, and high degree AV nodal blocks are less common.

The treatment of digoxin toxicity starts with the management of cardiac dysrhythmias. Hemodynamically stable dysrhythmias may require little therapy aside from intensive monitoring until resolution. For malignant ventricular dysrhythmias, the preferred antidysrhythmic drug is phenytoin, which decreases automaticity, increases the fibrillation threshold and conduction through the AV node. Lidocaine is an alternative agent to phenytoin. Magnesium may be helpful to suppress ventricular irritability. Electrical cardioversion is a therapy that is used as last resort. It may induce intractable ventricular fibrillation and should be used with caution (low energy doses of 10-25 J). Digoxin-induced bradydysrhythmias should be treated with atropine and cardiac pacing.

Digoxin toxicity can lead to severe, life-threatening hyperkalemia. Massive inhibition of the Na^+/K^+ ATPase pump prevents the normal intracellular transport of potassium. Acute digoxin toxicity correlates more closely with potassium levels better than serum digoxin levels. Treatment includes immediate administration of glucose, insulin, sodium bicarbonate, potassium resin binders, and hemodialysis. Hyperkalemia due to digoxin toxicity should probably not be treated with calcium. Administration of calcium chloride or gluconate can lead to increased incidence of ventricular dysrhythmias.

Anti-digoxin immunotherapy is available as an antidote for life-threatening digoxin toxicity. Purified Fab antibody fragments bind and remove digoxin from tissue-binding sites, usually within 1 hour of administration. Indications for the antibody fragments are ventricular dysrhythmias, hemodynamically significant bradydysrhythmias unresponsive to standard therapy, and hyperkalemia greater than 5.5 mEq/L.

ANESTHETIC CONSIDERATIONS

Patients should take their prescribed digoxin dose on the day of surgery.

- Routine measurement of digoxin levels is not necessary unless there is clinical suspicion for noncompliance or evidence of toxicity.
- Serum potassium levels should be measured prior to surgery. Potassium supplement should be administered, if necessary.
- Serum potassium levels may fluctuate in the surgical patient due to ventilation, pH changes, fluid shifts, and concurrent drugs.
- Any cardiac dysrhythmia that occurs in a patient taking digoxin should be considered a sign of toxicity.
- Digoxin-induced cardiac dysrhythmias are difficult to treat.
- Use diuretics with caution (hypokalemia predisposes patients to digoxin toxicity).
- Beta-blockers and calcium channel blockers may increase the risk of AV nodal block.
- If inotropy is needed, consider using other drugs (dobutamine, norepinephrine) that are less toxic and reversible than digoxin.

Inotropes

Amanda Hopkins, MD, and Jeffrey S. Berger, MD, MBA

Inotropes are agents that affect cardiac contractility. Positive inotropes, or inotropes that increase contractility, augment cardiac output, thereby enhancing end-organ perfusion. The pharmacology of inotropes varies not only with drug class, but also with drug dosage. Inotropic therapy routinely treats a wide variety of cardiovascular disease processes, including cardiogenic shock complicating acute myocardial infarction, acute decompensated heart failure, cardiopulmonary arrest, right ventricular infarction, and bradyarrhythmias. In perioperative medicine, inotropes frequently support patients with low cardiac output syndrome while weaning from cardiopulmonary bypass and during recovery.

CATECHOLAMINES

Several frequently used inotropic agents are sympathomimetics, drugs which mimic the effects of endogenous catecholamines (Table 164-1). The primary adrenergic receptors utilized by these agents are alpha-1, beta-1, beta-2, and the dopaminergic receptors, D1 and D2.

Activation of beta-1 receptors, found exclusively in cardiac muscle, is chiefly responsible for the inotropic effect of sympathomimetics. The beta-1 receptor mediates the intracellular formation of cyclic adenosine monophosphate (cAMP); with increased activation, cAMP is increased, producing a greater release of Ca^{2+} from the sarcoplasmic reticulum. Ca^{2+} facilitates the binding of troponin C to the actin–myosin complex, producing forceful muscular contraction.

TABLE 164-1 Summary of Catecholaminergic Inotropes and Their Receptor Selectivities

Catecholamine	Receptor Selectivity
Epinephrine	Low dose (<0.04 µg/kg/min): β_1, β_2 Moderate dose (0.04-0.12 µg/kg/min): β_1 High dose (>0.12 µg/kg/min): α_1
Norepinephrine	$\alpha_1 > \beta_1$
Dopamine	D1=D2 > β > α
Dobutamine	$\beta_1 > \alpha_1 = \beta_2$
Isoproterenol	$\beta_1 = \beta_2$ (no α)

In addition to increased inotropy, activation of the beta-1 receptor results in increased chronotropy (heart rate), increasing myocardial oxygen demand, which may be associated with new or worsening ischemia. Beta agonists also increase cardiac arrhythmia risk, attributable either to increased conductance through the sinoatrial node or ectopy. These effects are dose-limiting, meaning that at some drug level, serious side effects prevent further escalation of dosing.

Though an agent's activation of other receptor subtypes does not directly contribute to inotropic action, the relative drug-receptor selectivity plays an important role in drug selection. The alpha-1 receptor is found primarily on vascular smooth muscle cells, and its activation results in vasoconstriction, increasing systemic vascular resistance. The beta-2 receptor functions as the counterbalance to alpha-1, decreasing intracellular Ca^{2+} bioavailability, and encouraging vasodilation. Lastly, the dopaminergic receptors, found in the renal and splanchnic vasculature, produce renal and mesenteric vasodilation.

Epinephrine

Epinephrine, an analog to the adrenaline produced by the adrenal medulla, interacts with alpha-1, beta-1, and beta-2 receptors. Its interaction with receptors is dose-dependent. At lower doses (<0.04 mcg/kg/min), the beta-adrenergic effects dominate, resulting in positive inotropy and vasodilation. Moderate doses (0.04-0.12 µg/kg/min) produce mixed alpha and beta effects, with alpha-mediated vasoconstriction overshadowing beta-induced vasodilation. Finally, high doses of epinephrine (>0.12 µg/kg/min) produces potent vasoconstriction and negligible beta-mediated effects.

Norepinephrine

Endogenous norepinephrine is a neurotransmitter released by postganglionic adrenergic nerves. It is primarily an alpha-1 receptor agonist with some beta-1 activity, making it a potent vasoconstrictor with less forceful effects on cardiac contractility. Similar to epinephrine, the alpha-adrenergic activity of norepinephrine increases with increasing dosages. Typical dosages are 0.02-0.25 µg/kg/min.

Dopamine

The effect of dopamine is also dose-dependent. At low doses (0.5-3 µg/kg/min), dopamine stimulates D1 and D2, increasing renal and mesenteric blood flow through vasodilation. At low doses, dopamine can be used to encourage diuresis and, theoretically, help preserve kidney function through increased renal blood flow. This indication may be important for patients at high risk for acute renal failure. At moderate doses (3-5 µg/kg/min), dopamine activates beta-1 receptors, and at high doses (5-20 µg/kg/min), dopamine's primary effect is alpha-1-mediated vasoconstriction.

Dobutamine

Dobutamine has a high affinity for beta-1 receptors. Though it also acts on alpha-1 and beta-2 receptors, dobutamine has roughly equivalent affinity for each receptor subtype, resulting in no net effect on vascular tone. As would be expected for a beta-1 agonist, dobutamine is dose-limited by tachycardia and increased ventricular response rate in patients with atrial fibrillation, as it increases conduction through the sinoatrial node.

Isoproterenol

Isoproterenol is a nonselective beta-agonist with no appreciable alpha receptor affect. Its beta-1 activation increases stroke volume and, thus, increases systolic blood pressure. Simultaneously, its beta-2 activation vasodilates, causing decreased diastolic and mean arterial pressure. The net result is a markedly increased heart rate and cardiac output without compensatory enhancement in coronary blood flow; this mismatch in myocardial oxygen supply and demand commonly results in myocardial ischemia. For this reason, isoproterenol is only indicated in patients with bradyarrhythmias.

PHOSPHODIESTERASE INHIBITORS

Phosphodiesterase inhibitors (PDIs) augment cardiac output via increased inotropy and improved lusitropy (myocardial relaxation). Similar to the catecholamines, PDIs produce increased intracellular Ca^{2+} levels. Endogenous phosphodiesterase degrades cAMP; PDIs block this degradation, increasing concentrations of cAMP, resulting in higher cytoplasmic Ca^{2+} levels. Because PDIs also block degradation of cAMP in smooth muscle cells, these agents result in profound vasodilation, sometimes necessitating concurrent use of vasoconstrictors to maintain vascular tone. These agents decrease pulmonary vascular resistance, thus improving right ventricular outflow. Examples of PDIs include milrinone, amrinone, and enoximone.

INVESTIGATIONAL INOTROPES

Several new inotropic agents are currently under investigation. Though a complete review of these investigatory agents is beyond the scope of this discussion, one class in particular is worth noting, as it has already been approved for use in over 50 countries and is expected to be available in the United States in the coming years. Levosimendan is the prototype agent in the class of myofilament Ca^{2+} sensitizers. The class demonstrates dual mechanisms of action. First, Ca^{2+} sensitizers increase contractility by enhancing the Ca^{2+} binding to troponin C, thereby increasing cardiac contractility without increasing cytoplasmic Ca^{2+} concentration. Second, they open ATP-dependent K^+ channels on vascular smooth muscle, resulting in arteriolar and venous vasodilation, which may provide some benefit in reducing risk for myocardial ischemia. Increased cytoplasmic Ca^{2+} is associated with greater myocardial energy expenditure and an increased risk of arrhythmia. Therefore, by avoiding this concern, the Ca^{2+} sensitizers may provide a survival benefit over sympathomimetics and PDIs, though proof is still lacking.

SUGGESTED READINGS

Metra M, Bettari L, Carubelli V, Dei Cas L. Old and new intravenous inotropic agents in the treatment of advanced heart failure. *Prog Cardiovasc Dis.* 2011;54:97-106.

Overgaard CB, Dzavik V. Inotropes and vasopressors: review of physiology and clinical use in cardiovascular disease. *Circulation* 2008;118:1047-1056.

Phosphodiesterase Inhibitors

Johan P. Suyderhoud, MD

Phosphodiesterase inhibitors (PDEI) are a broad category of drugs that act to prevent the hydrolysis of cyclic 3,5 adenosine monophosphate (cAMP) and 3,5 guanosine monophosphate (cGMP) by phosphodiesterases. Phosphodiesterases (PDEs) are a heterogeneous group of at least 11 isoenzymes, with over 50 isoforms, present in a wide variety of tissues, and their actions are important in regulating intracellular levels of cAMP and cGMP, both important components of intracellular second messenger systems. Inhibition of phosphodiesterases will lead to an increase in intracellular cyclic nucleotides and amplify their actions in various organ beds. The main clinical interest of anesthesiologists resides with the direct effects of PDEIs in cardiac and vascular tissue mediated by the PDEI type III (3) isoenzyme. Other PDEIs have clinical applications in treating primary pulmonary hypertension, persistent pulmonary hypertension of the newborn, and erectile dysfunction (PDEI type 5); this will be discussed briefly at the conclusion of this chapter. PDEI, primarily type 4, may also prove to be of benefit in treating inflammatory (eg, reactive airway disease) and some neoplastic disease states (where cAMP levels have been found to be reduced).

Hydrolysis of cAMP is caused by the action of PDE, yielding a monophosphate and a free hydroxyl moiety. Clinically, relevant drugs that inhibit PDE and thus improve contractility are the biguanides, amrinone and milrinone, and the imidazoline-derived enoximone (which is not available in the United States). For all intents, milrinone has supplanted amrinone in clinical practice in the United States.

Figure 165-1 illustrates the mechanism of myocardial contraction at the myocyte and how PDEI type 3 promotes contractility. Inhibiting the action of PDE will lead to amplification of the adrenergic-initiated generation of cAMP from the G protein-linked adenylyl cyclase, and thus increase intracellular Ca^{2+} and the force of contraction. Activation of protein kinase A (PKA) by cAMP will not only cause release of Ca^{2+} through L-type calcium channels, but also through its ability to phosphorylate regulatory proteins involved with contraction, phospholamban, and calmodulin. These, in turn, will promote the release of Ca^{2+} from the sarcoplasmic reticulum, independent of L-type calcium channel Ca^{2+} release, and this is felt to be a more important feature of PDEI action than via catecholamine-mediated stimulation of L-type channels.

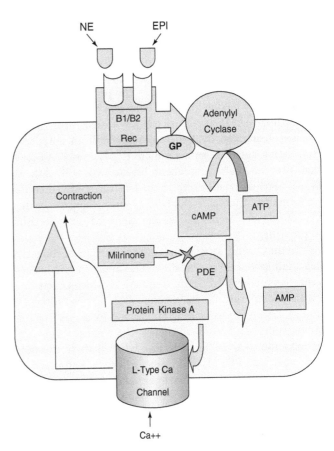

FIGURE 165-1 Schematic drawing of myocyte showing mechanism of action for contraction and the effects of PDEI type 3 inhibitors like milrinone. Adrenergic receptor activation by norepinephrine and epinephrine will lead to generation of cAMP via G protein (GP)-linked adenylyl cyclase, which will in turn activate PKA and lead to both stimulation of the L-type Ca^{2+} channel (Ca^{2+} influx) and phosphorylation of contractile proteins to enhance contractility. Milrinone will prevent the breakdown of cAMP by PDE and thus amplify cAMP-mediated inotropic activity.

PDEI type 3 also exert their action on vascular smooth muscle. Activation of beta-2 adrenergic receptors will also produce a rise in intracellular cAMP via G protein complex-mediated adenylyl cyclase activity and subsequent activation of PKA. However, in contradistinction to cardiac cells, activation of PKA in smooth muscle will result in a reduction in intracellular Ca^{2+} by activating calcium channel pumps to sequester calcium out of the cell, thus promoting relaxation and vasodilation. PDEI type 3 has affinity for arterial and venous smooth muscles, in addition to cardiac muscle; PDEI type 5 drugs such as sildenafil are active on corpus cavernosum-specific PDE type 5 isozymes, leading also to vascular relaxation and penile erection.

Together, PDEI type 3 drugs promote enhanced cardiac performance by both increasing cardiac inotropy while at the same time reducing afterload by reducing vascular resistance. As such, they are termed "inodilators" in view of their dual mechanism of actions. These make them ideal candidates in treating patients with congestive heart failure, either in the acute or chronic setting. In the acute setting, however, monotherapy with PDEI type 3 drugs may often lead to excessive vasodilation and hypotension without corresponding increases in cardiac output. In acute heart failure, such as that which occurs after cardiac surgery, the primary mechanism for failure may be due to lack of sufficient cAMP generation. Intracellular cAMP levels are too low to receive inhibition. In these instances, dual therapy with both an adrenergic-stimulating agent to generate more cAMP and PDEI drugs that prevent their subsequent breakdown will shift the Frank–Starling relationship to the left for improved cardiac performance. Thus, at normal therapeutic dosing levels, there is greater vascular relaxation and afterload reduction than improvements in inotropy.

In the chronic setting, the pathophysiology of congestive heart failure (CHF) is a bit different. Failure in this instance generates further adrenergic stimulation, which begets myocardial adrenergic desensitization and further adrenergic output, leading to worsening failure and increases in vascular resistance and afterload (hence, the paradoxical benefits of moderate beta-1 blockade in CHF). In these instances, treatment with PDEI type 3 agents will reduce afterload and improve cardiac performance by enhancing myocyte calcium cycling and promoting vascular smooth muscle relaxation, and thus decreasing vascular resistance. This will lead to improvements in left ventricular performance and an increase in the ejection fraction (EF). Decreases in vascular resistance may lead to compensatory increases in heart rate and may limit their usefulness. In addition, long-term treatment with these agents has been associated with decreased survival, and hence, has fallen out of favor as a chronic treatment modality. They remain useful, however, for treating acute episodes of decompensated CHF, in combination with other agents such as diuretics, ACE inhibitors, and beta blockers, as well as digoxin.

In the acute setting of either the operating room or the ICU, milrinone is given as a bolus followed by continuous infusion. Steady-state levels are achieved in 6-12 hours, and the terminal elimination half-life is approximately 2.5 hours. Milrinone is primarily excreted by the kidney, and thus needs to be adjusted in patients with renal impairment. In studies of patients undergoing cardiac surgery, milrinone will reliably reduce systemic vascular resistance, pulmonary capillary wedge pressure, and central venous pressure, all by 15%-40%, which will reduce myocardial wall stress and oxygen consumption, and lead to increases in EF of approximately 30%. The most common side effect may be ventricular arrhythmias, occurring up to 10 or more percent (which, given the setting of heart failure, is quite common).

As mentioned earlier, the type 5 isoform of PDE is found in the corpus cavernosum of the penis and in vascular smooth muscle. This enzyme is responsible for breaking down cGMP that forms in response to increased nitric oxide generated by the endothelium. Increased intracellular cGMP inhibits calcium entry into the cell, thereby decreasing intracellular calcium concentrations and causing smooth muscle relaxation. PDEI type 5 specific agents may have a role in reducing pulmonary vascular resistance as well, in patients with primary pulmonary hypertension and in persistence pulmonary hypertension of the newborn. For patients using PDEI type 5 drugs for erectile dysfunction, concomitant reduction in systemic vascular resistance may result and lead to hypotension, angina, and headaches, especially when taken in combination with other vasodilating medications.

SUGGESTED READINGS

Boswell-Smith V, Spina D, Page CP. Phosphodiesterase inhibitors. *Brit J Pharmacol.* 2006;147:S252-S257.

Feneck R. Phosphodiesterase inhibitors in and the cardiovascular system. *Continuing Education in Anesthesia, Critical Care, and Pain* 2007;7:203-207.

166

Antidysrhythmic Drugs

Johan P. Suyderhoud, MD

Antidysrhythmic agents, which are also known as antiarrhythmic agents, are a broad category of medications that help ameliorate the spectrum of cardiac arrhythmias to maintain normal rhythm and conduction in the heart. Arrhythmias generally arise as a result of abnormal impulse generation or abnormal conduction, or a combination of the two. Abnormal impulse generation falls into one of two categories: abnormal automaticity or triggered activity. Abnormal automaticity is thought to occur due to reduced resting membrane potential, causing the membrane to be closer to the threshold for generating an action potential. Triggered activity, or after-depolarization, occurs during the early stages after depolarization, such as in phase 2 and 3, or in the later stage during phase 4. With either form, it requires a preceding triggering beat to create the abnormal depolarization. Abnormal conduction is usually due to conduction block or a reentry phenomenon, with the latter being the most common cause of dysrhythmias. Antidysrhythmics exert their effect on specific ion channels on the cardiac cell membrane which then alters the shape of the action potential, and thus have inotropic, chronotropic, and toxic actions as a result.

CLASSIFICATION

The most common classification system for antidysrhythmic agents is the Harrison modification of Vaughan Williams (Table 166-1). This system classifies each agent based upon its unique electrophysiologic and pharmacological properties. Vaughan Williams classification divides these agents in one of four groups, Class I, II, III, and IV. There is a further subdivision of Class I agents, the so-called sodium channel blockers, into IA, IB, and IC.

- *Class I agents* block the rapid inward sodium channel, slow the rate of rise of phase 0, and so decrease the rate of depolarization. The subgrouping of Class I agents allows for differentiating their electrophysiologic effects. *Class IA* drugs (quinidine, procainamide, and disopyramide) prolong the repolarization and the refractoriness of isolated myocardial tissue as well as block the inward sodium current. They also have potassium channel blocking properties, and so increase action potential duration and the effective refractory period. *Class IB*

TABLE 166-1 Classification of Antidysrhythmic Agents

Vaughan Williams Classification	Electrocardiographic Effect	Membrane/Ion Channel	Examples of Agents
IA	↑QRS and Q-T intervals	Blocks fast Na^+ and intermediate K^+	Quinidine/procainamide/disopyramide
IB	↓ →Q-T interval	Fast sodium channel blocker	Lidocaine/tocainide/mexilitine
IC	↓ QRS Interval	Sodium channel blocker	Flecainide/propafanone
II	↓ HR; ↑P-R interval	β adrenergic receptor blockade	Propranolol/esmolol/metoprolol
III	↑ Q-T interval	K^+ channel blocker	Amiodarone/sotalol/ibutilide/dronedarone
IV	↓ HR; ↑ P-R interval	L-type Ca^{2+} channel blocker	Verapamil/diltiazem
Digoxin	↑ P-R interval; ↓ Q-T interval	Na^+/K^+ ATPase inhibitor	
Adenosine	↓ HR; ↑ P-R interval	Purinergic A_1 receptor agonist	

drugs (lidocaine, tocainide, and mexiletine) produce only modest inhibition of the rapid inward sodium current and so shorten the refractory period, and reduce the action potential duration. In *Class IC* agents (flecainide and propafenone), these sodium channel inhibitors increase the QRS interval more than the other Class I drugs, slow the conduction velocity but have little effect on either action potential duration or the refractory period.

- *Class II agents* include the beta-1 selective adrenergic blocking agents, such as metoprolol, atenolol, and bisoprolol, in addition to the nonselective agents such as propranolol, labetalol, carvedilol, and nadolol. These agents block adrenergic stimulation through sympathetic activity and thus decrease conduction velocity.

- *Class III agents* block potassium channels and thus delay repolarization of the action potential during phase 3. They also increase both the effective refractory period and the action potential duration. Drugs in this class include amiodarone, sotalol, ibutilide, and bretylium.

- *Class IV agents* are the calcium channel blocking agents which exert their effects on L-type channels. Calcium channel blockers that are effective agents in slowing atrioventricular (AV) nodal conduction, and to a lesser degree sinoatrial (SA) nodal conduction, are from the benzothiazepine class, such as diltiazem and verapamil. Dihydropyridine calcium channel blockers, such as amlodipine, nifedipine, and isradipine, have virtually no antiarrhythmic effect and work primarily to relax vascular smooth muscle.

- Both digoxin and adenosine do not have a Vaughan Williams classification. Digoxin is useful as a rate control medication for atrial fibrillation and flutter, as well as for its positive inotropic actions in patients with congestive heart failure. Adenosine acts by inhibiting the influx of calcium through L-type channels as well as reduces the slope of the uprise in phase 4 of the pacemaker cell current. It also reduces conduction through the AV node.

SIDE EFFECTS

Toxicity is a major concern with nearly all of the antidysrhythmic agents and limits their usefulness.

Class IA agents were, for many years, mainstays in arrhythmia therapy but have been supplanted by newer and less toxic agents. Quinidine has significant gastrointestinal side effects, can cause hemolytic anemia and hepatitis, and precipitate torsade de pointe, a variant of polymorphic ventricular tachycardia. Procainamide can cause agranulocytosis and a lupus-like syndrome, as well as show proarrhythmic activity, and its major metabolite, *n*-acetyl procainamide, has Class III activity.

Class IB agents, particularly mexiletine, was associated with greater mortality than placebo in long-term trials, probably because of its proarrhythmic effects.

Class IC agents are current options to maintain rhythm in atrial and ventricular tachydysrhythmias but have moderate beta blocking activity and conduction pathway suppression, and hence should not be used in patients with significant structural heart disease or baseline conduction abnormalities.

Class II agents, while a mainstay of therapy for all types of patients with cardiovascular pathology, carry the usual precautions with their use, especially in patients with advanced left ventricular dysfunction.

Class III agents exhibit significant overlap with other Vaughan Williams characteristics. For example, sotalol has Class II beta blockade activity as well as Class III, and amiodarone exhibits the effects of all four classes. Amiodarone has significant extracardiac toxicities, among them are ocular, thyroid, and pulmonary. Of these, amiodarone-induced pulmonary toxicity (APT) is the most serious and results in a diffuse interstitial pneumonitis that, if the drug is not discontinued and treated with corticosteroid, can result in irreversible pulmonary fibrosis. Pulmonary toxicity correlates with both total cumulative dose and daily dose; patients taking less that 400 mg daily (current recommendations) have a 1.6% incidence of APT versus earlier, higher doses above 400 mg daily, with an incidence of between 5% and 15%. Of note, approximately 10% of patients who develop APT can progress to irreversible pulmonary fibrosis. Thus, anesthesiologists caring for patients on long-term amiodarone therapy should be aware of potential coexisting thyroid and pulmonary pathophysiology.

INDICATIONS

Table 166-2 outlines the broad indications for antidysrhythmic therapy and the specific agents that can be used. In treating atrial dysrhythmias, particularly atrial fibrillation and flutter, recent studies that examine long-term outcome have shown less benefit of chemical conversion and maintenance of sinus rhythm, and more on rate control alone, in combination with appropriate anticoagulation, particularly now with the advent of new direct thrombin inhibitors and drugs like them that reduce the risk of thromboembolic disease and warfarin-related complications. In younger patients who may be intolerant of the hemodynamic effects of atrial fibrillation and flutter, rhythm control may still be preferred over simple heart rate control, whereas in older patients (with already diminished ventricular function) rate control and avoiding toxicity of the antidysrhythmic agents appear to be superior in outcome. As with ventricular tachydysrhythmias (see Table 166-2), atrial tachydysrhythmias are more aggressively being treated with electrophysiologic therapies such as ablation.

Patients who have recurrent ventricular tachydysrhythmias have benefited tremendously from implantable defibrillating devices (now termed cardiac implantable electrical devices [CIED]) and so rely less on pharmacological suppression. Patients with CIEDs are on concurrent antidysrhythmic

TABLE 166-2   Indications for Antidsyrhythmic Therapy

Indication	Drugs
Sinus tachycardia	Metoprolol, propranolol
Sinoatrial reentrant tachycardia	Metoprolol, propranolol, verapamil
AV nodal reentrant tachycardia	
Termination	IV diltiazem, IV verapamil
Prevention	Verapamil, propranolol, metoprolol, flecainide, sotalol, propafanone
Atrial fibrillation or flutter	
Termination	IV amiodarone, IV metoprolol, IV diltiazem, IV verapamil, IV propranolol, IV digoxin, IV procainamide
Prevention	Quinidine, flecanide, sotalol, propafanone, amiodarone, dofetilide, dronedarone
Ventricular tachycardia	
Termination	IV lidocaine, IV amiodarone
Prevention	Amiodarone, sotalol, carvedilol, metoprolol, bisoprolol

therapy, about 50% of the time. A majority of these patients with CIEDs will exhibit some degree of ventricular failure as a primary cause of their dysrhythmias, and so specific pharmacological therapy is now targeted more in treating the underlying heart failure as a means to treat the dysrhythmias. Current guidelines recommend the use of beta blockers, ACE inhibitors, and aldosterone inhibitors, along with amiodarone, for prophylaxis in patients who have both ventricular tachydysrhythmias and reduced cardiac performance.

Torsade de pointe, a particular variant of polymorphic ventricular tachycardia, deserves brief mention because of the approach to treating it. Torsade has a strong association with prolonged Q-T interval, and occurs in response to an early afterdepolarization trigger, probably due to abnormal K^+ channel activity in phase 3. Drugs that prolong the Q-T interval, of which there are many (Class IA and some Class III agents, antihistamines, mycin-class of antibiotics, antifungal agents, antiemetics, etc) can precipitate torsade, as can hypomagnesemia and hypokalemia. Removing the offending agents as well as correcting any underlying metabolic abnormality is the treatment of choice, and cardioversion is reserved as a last resort since torsade is frequently paroxysmal. Magnesium therapy can be considered, as well as agents that increase an underlying bradycardia.

SUGGESTED READINGS

Compton SJ. Ventricular tachycardia.http://emedicine.medscape.com/article/159075-overview. Accessed December 5, 2013.

Crossley GH. Perioperative management of cardiac implantable electrical devices. Cardiac Rhythm Management /Cardiosource.org. Accessed December 5, 2013.

Fuster V, Ryden L, Cannom D, et al. 2011 ACCF/AHA/HRS focused updates incorporated into the ACC/AHA/ESC 2006 guidelines for the management of patients with atrial fibrillation: a report of the American College of Cardiology foundation/ American Heart Association task force on practice guidelines. *Circulation* 2011;123:e269-e367.

Kowey PR. Pharmacologic effect of antiarrhythmic drugs: review and update. *Arch Intern Med*. 1998;158:325-332.

Vasodilators

Brian S. Freeman, MD

Perioperative hypertension can increase afterload and decrease left ventricular systolic function. Poorly controlled blood pressure can also result in increased bleeding and increased risk of cerebral and myocardial ischemia. For these reasons, intravenous vasodilator therapy is necessary to manage hypertension caused by increased systemic vascular resistance.

Vasodilator drugs reduce the contraction of vascular smooth muscle cells through two general mechanisms, both of which reduce intracellular calcium concentrations. One, vasodilator drugs modulate the sympathetic nervous system by either decreasing the central sympathetic activity or by blocking peripheral adrenergic receptors. Two, they can also directly relax vascular smooth muscle. The magnitude of systemic blood pressure decrease by vasodilator therapy depends on preload, myocardial contractility, and compensatory reflexes.

Systemic vasodilators, whether arterial or venous, have a number of potential physiologic side effects. Decreases in systemic vascular resistance and mean arterial pressure activate the baroreceptor reflex leading to tachycardia. To blunt this response, vasodilators are often administered concurrently with beta adrenergic receptor antagonists. Inhibition of hypoxic pulmonary vasoconstriction may cause hypoxemia in patients with underlying pulmonary disease or receiving one-lung ventilation. Coexisting pulmonary hypertension combined with systemic vasodilation may shunt blood through a patent foramen ovale and cause arterial hypoxemia. Dosing of vasodilators should be carefully titrated. Short-acting agents are preferable. Hypotension due to vasodilation may be aggravated by concurrent intraoperative hypovolemia or sympathectomy from regional anesthesia.

DRUGS THAT BLUNT SYMPATHETIC NERVOUS SYSTEM ACTIVITY

Alpha Adrenergic Receptor Antagonists

Nonselective alpha adrenergic antagonists are most often used to manage hypertensive crises, such as that associated with pheochromocytomas. Blockade of the alpha-2 adrenergic receptor prevents increases in intracellular calcium, which

then enables vascular smooth muscle relaxation in both arterioles and venules. *Phentolamine* is a reversible competitive antagonist of both alpha-1 and alpha-2 adrenergic receptors. Unlike phentolamine, which is given in IV form only, *phenoxybenzamine* is an oral alpha adrenergic antagonist used to manage pheochromocytoma-induced hypertension prior to resection. It has an elimination half-life of 18-24 hours. The vasodilation may cause reflex tachycardia, orthostatic hypotension, and nasal congestion.

Alpha-2 Adrenergic Receptor Agonists

Activation of presynaptic alpha-2 adrenergic receptors in the locus coeruleus results in decreased sympathetic outflow. The mechanisms include inhibition of adenylate cyclase, reduction in cyclic adenosine monophosphate (cAMP) levels, decreased intracellular calcium concentrations, and cellular hyperpolarization. Lower levels of catecholamines such as norepinephrine lead to peripheral arterial vasodilation. Parasympathetic, or vagal, activity predominates.

Clonidine is a nonselective alpha adrenergic receptor agonist which is given orally and transdermally to manage preoperative hypertension. It preferentially binds to alpha-2 receptors but can still activate alpha-1 receptors. In contrast, *dexmedetomidine* is a much more selective alpha-2 agonist (1600:1) than clonidine, leading to a profound decrease in plasma catecholamines. It is an intravenous drug that has an elimination half-life of 1.5 hours and a more rapid onset (<5 minutes). Dexmedetomidine is used as a sedative-hypnotic, not an antihypertensive, although its sympatholytic properties may be helpful to reduce peripheral vascular resistance.

DRUGS THAT RELAX VASCULAR SMOOTH MUSCLE

Calcium Channel Blockers (CCB)

Calcium channel antagonists decrease systemic vascular resistance by inhibiting the influx of calcium ions into smooth muscle cells. The extracellular targets are L-type voltage-gated calcium channels located within the smooth muscle of arterial resistance vessels. The venous capacitance vessels have few of these channels. These drugs also blunt the intracellular calcium release in response to depolarization.

Nicardipine is a dihydropyridine which preferentially induces peripheral vasodilation. It has little to no inotropic or chronotropic effects. Unlike the nitrovasodilators, cardiac preload is minimally affected. As a result, cardiac output often increases with the reduction in vascular tone. Nicardipine causes potent coronary and cerebral vasodilation. It is the only titratable intravenous CCB and can be given as an infusion. Nicardipine causes mild reflex tachycardia, causes no increase in ICP, and has positive lusitropic effects. It may reduce coronary vasospasm. *Clevidipine* is a relatively new dihydropyridine CCB with a short half-life and easy titratability.

In contrast, **verapamil** is a phenylalkylamine with mild vasodilating effects. Verapamil primarily inhibits calcium channels in myocardial cells, causing significant negative inotropic and chronotropic (phase 4 depolarization) effects. It is used as third-line therapy for the treatment of supraventricular tachydysrhythmias.

Diltiazem is a benzothiazepine CCB with intermediate actions. It inhibits calcium influx into both vascular smooth muscle and myocardial cells. However, its effects are primarily vasodilatory in nature rather than negative inotropy.

Nitroglycerin

Nitroglycerin directly relaxes the smooth muscle of venous vessels more than arterial resistance vessels. This drug becomes metabolized into nitric oxide which then stimulates the enzyme guanylate cyclase, increases intracellular cGMP levels, and activates kinases that relax the smooth muscle. The resultant pooling of blood in the capacitance vessels decreases venous return and preload. Myocardial oxygen demand decreases due to the subsequent reduction in ventricular end-diastolic classes. Heart rate is typically unchanged. Selective vasodilation of the coronary arteries can relieve coronary vasospasm. Nitroglycerin also dilates the pulmonary arterial vasculature.

Nitroglycerin is commonly administered in 50 µg IV bolus doses or infusions (50-100 µg/min). Onset occurs within 1 minute; half-life is 1-3 minutes. Toxicity can cause methemoglobinemia due to production of nitrite from reductive hydrolysis in the liver. Long-term use can lead to tachyphylaxis. Glass containers and special intravenous tubing are recommended to reduce absorption by polyvinylchloride.

Sodium Nitroprusside

Sodium nitroprusside (SNP) is an intravenous peripheral vasodilator that acts primarily on arterial resistance vessels (with mild effects on the venous circulation). Its mechanism is a result of both direct and indirect guanylate cyclase activation via the production of nitric oxide. Increased intracellular cGMP induces peripheral vasodilation. Decreased vascular resistance leads to a decrease in systemic blood pressure. Cardiac output is minimally affected; but may increase in patients with impaired cardiac ejection due to high afterload.

Within erythrocytes, SNP interacts with oxyhemoglobin to form methemoglobin and an unstable radical that spontaneously breaks down into five cyanide ions and nitric oxide. Cyanide can bind to methemoglobin to form cyanomethemoglobin, to thiosulfate to form thiocyanate, and to tissue cytochrome oxidase, causing tissue hypoxemia. Nitroprusside toxicity results from an accumulation of cyanide due to high rates (>10 µg/kg/min) or prolonged infusions. Signs include acute tachyphylaxis to increasing doses, metabolic acidosis, dysrhythmias, and increased venous oxygen content. In addition to ventilation with 100% oxygen, treatment includes administration of sodium thiosulfate (to provide a sulfur group necessary for cyanide metabolism), sodium nitrate (to oxidize hemoglobin into methemoglobin), or hydroxycobalamin (to bind cyanide and form cyanocobalamin, or vitamin B_{12}).

Aqueous solutions of SNP require opaque coverings because of photodegradation. The potency of SNP necessitates the use of continuous intraarterial blood pressure monitoring. SNP has an extremely rapid onset (<a minute) and short duration (1-2 minutes). It is typically administered as an infusion (0.5-10 µg/kg/min). Acute discontinuation of SNP may result in rebound hypertension.

Hydralazine

Hydralazine is a direct-acting arterial vasodilator. It has multiple cellular actions: hyperpolarization of vascular smooth muscle by K^+ ion efflux, activation of intracellular guanylate cyclase, and inhibition of calcium release from sarcoplasmic reticulum. It has a slow onset time (15 minutes) and a long elimination half-life (3 hours). Typical doses to manage perioperative hypertension are 5 mg IV boluses up to 20 mg total. Hydralazine may cause reflex tachycardia necessitating concurrent administration with beta-blockers to blunt adverse compensatory effects in patients with coronary artery disease. Hydralazine also has potent vasodilatory effects in the cerebral circulation. It disrupts cerebral autoregulation and causes increased cerebral blood flow and intracranial pressure.

ACE Inhibitors and Angiotensin Receptor Blockers

Brian S. Freeman, MD

RENIN–ANGIOTENSIN–ALDOSTERONE SYSTEM

Renin, angiotensin, and aldosterone are three peptide hormones which have an important role in the long-term regulation and homeostasis of blood pressure, intravascular volume, and electrolyte composition. The renin–angiotensin–aldosterone (RAA) system essentially involves the kidney, lungs, and adrenal gland. Juxtaglomulerar (JG) cells within the renal afferent arterioles secrete renin in response to systemic (and afferent arteriolar) hypotension, hypovolemia, and sympathetic nervous system activation of beta-1 receptors. Lower pressures in the afferent arteriole decrease glomerular filtration rate (GFR), which increases sodium reabsorption. Macula densa cells within the distal tubules sense the lower NaCl filtrate concentration and lower the filtrate flow rate and respond by stimulating the JG cells to renin release. In the plasma, renin catalyzes the cleavage of the circulating inactive peptide *angiotensinogen* (synthesized and secreted by the liver) into the new decapeptide *angiotensin I*. In the lung capillaries, endothelial angiotensin converting enzyme (ACE) further cleaves angiotensin I into the octapeptide *angiotensin II*.

The new peptide product angiotensin II has several important and potent vasoactive physiologic effects. Angiotensin II has two receptor subtypes (AT1 and AT2), but it is the AT1 receptor that yields its multiple clinical effects, which include:

1. Direct vascular smooth muscle contraction, which rapidly increases the systemic vascular resistance (SVR) and mean arterial pressure (MAP).
2. Enhancement of peripheral sympathetic nervous system synaptic transmission (increases norepinephrine release and decreases its reuptake).
3. Increases sodium reabsorption and water retention in the proximal convoluted tubule.
4. Stimulates antidiuretic hormone (ADH) release from the posterior pituitary, which acts on the distal convoluted tubule to increase water reabsorption.
5. Stimulates central thirst centers, thereby increasing blood volume.
6. Stimulates cardiac and vascular hypertrophy, and remodeling due to increased cardiac afterload and vascular wall tension as well as increased production of growth factors and ECM proteins.
7. Stimulates aldosterone synthesis and secretion from the zona glomerulosa of the adrenal cortex. Aldosterone stimulates the distal renal tubules to increase sodium and water reabsorption (in exchange for potassium excretion) to maintain intravascular volume.

ACE inhibitors (ACEIs) and angiotensin receptor blockers (ARBs) are two classes of drugs which act to suppress the function of the RAA system at different sites (Figure 168-1). These forms of drug therapy act on this system for the treatment of hypertension, congestive heart failure, and to decrease post-myocardial infarction (MI) mortality. Both ACEIs and ARBs are used to decrease arterial pressure, afterload, blood volume, and hence ventricular preload, as well as inhibit and reverse cardiac and vascular hypertrophy.

ACE INHIBITORS

a. ***Commonly used drugs***—Lisinopril, benazepril, enalapril.
b. ***Mechanism***—ACEIs affect the RAA system by suppressing the function of ACE, thereby decreasing the formation of angiotensin II. Since ACE is also involved in the destruction of the peptide bradykinin, ACEIs increase levels of bradykinin which leads to additional peripheral vasodilation.
c. ***Clinical effects***—Lower levels of angiotensin II and higher levels of bradykinin reduce mean blood pressure through peripheral arteriolar dilation and a decrease in systemic vascular resistance. Reflex tachycardia is generally absent. Due to the myocardial afterload reduction, stroke volume and cardiac output usually increase. In the renal vasculature, ACEIs vasodilate both afferent and efferent arterioles, leading to an increase in renal blood flow but without an increase in the GFR.
d. ***Therapeutic uses***—ACEIs are a mainstay in the pharmacological treatment of hypertension. Patients with a history of congestive heart failure who have left

459

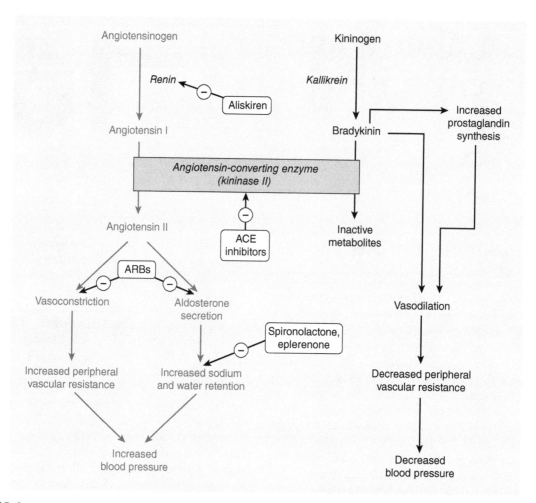

FIGURE 168-1 Sites of action of drugs that interfere with the renin–angiotensin–aldosterone system. ACE, angiotensin-converting enzyme; ARBs, angiotensin receptor blockers. (Reproduced with permission from Katzung BG, Masters SB, Trevor AJ. *Basic and Clinical Pharmacology*, 12th ed. McGraw-Hill; 2011.)

ventricular systolic dysfunction should take ACEIs, which have been shown to prevent or delay the progression of heart failure and myocardial ischemia. ACEIs can also prevent or delay the progression of renal disease in patients with type I diabetes and diabetic nephropathy. It is thought that ACEIs reduce glomerular injury from high capillary pressures by decreasing MAP, dilating the efferent arterioles, and attenuating mesangial cell growth.

e. **Side effects**:
- *Cough*—ACEIs can cause dry cough, sometimes with wheezing. It is thought that increased levels of mediators like bradykinin and substance P within the bronchiolar endothelium cause this refractory problem.
- *Hyperkalemia*—Patients with renal insufficiency, diabetes, or those taking K+-sparing diuretics or potassium supplements are at higher risk for ACEI-induced hyperkalemia.

- *Acute renal failure*—Lower levels of angiotensin II means that the efferent renal arteriole is more dilated. In patients with low baseline renal perfusion pressures (bilateral renal artery stenosis, unilateral renal artery stenosis to a single remaining kidney, CHF, hypovolemia), this can lead to acute renal failure. Patients may develop orthopnea, dyspnea, and peripheral edema.
- *Angioedema*—A small percentage of patients may experience rapid mucosal swelling of the lips, face, tongue, pharynx, glottis, or larynx. The angioedema usually disappears within hours of discontinuing the ACEI. However, a compromised airway necessitates emergent treatment with epinephrine, diphenhydramine, hydrocortisone, and endotracheal intubation.
- *Teratogenic risk*—ACEIs are strictly contraindicated during pregnancy. Exposure may lead to an increased fetal malformation, fetal hypotension, anuria, and renal failure.

ANGIOTENSIN RECEPTOR BLOCKERS

a. *Commonly used drugs*—Losartan, olmesartan, valsartan.

b. *Mechanism*—ARBs competitively inhibit the binding of angiotensin II to angiotensin-1 (AT1) receptor with high affinity. These drugs are highly selective for the AT1 receptor over the AT2 receptor. AT1 receptors are G-protein-coupled receptors located in the vascular endothelium, heart, kidney, lung, and adrenal cortex. Compared to ACEIs, ARBs decrease activation of AT1 receptors more efficaciously and more selectively block the effects of angiotensin II. ARBs have no effect on bradykinin metabolism; therefore, bradykinin levels are normal.

c. *Clinical effects*—ARBs are selective inhibitors of the physiologic effects of angiotensin II. They lead to increased venous pooling of blood, arterial hypotension, and decreased cardiac output.

d. *Therapeutic uses*—Angiotensin receptor blocker drugs are safe, effective, and a good alternative for patients who cannot tolerate the side effects of ACEIs. They have excellent efficacy in controlling blood pressure. ARBs also have similar protective effects as ACEIs for patients with diabetes, chronic renal insufficiency, and congestive heart failure. In hypertensive patients, ARBs can lead to a reduction of left ventricular hypertrophy, an improvement in filling, and a decrease in ventricular dysrhythmias.

e. *Side effects*—ARBs are much better tolerated drugs than ACEIs, particularly because of their lack of adverse effects due to no extra bradykinin production. Cough and angioedema are very uncommon. Hyperkalemia in at-risk patients (renal disease, potassium-sparing diuretics) may occur. Similar to ACEIs, acute renal failure in patients with compromised renal perfusion may occur. ARBs also should not be used during pregnancy.

ANESTHETIC CONSIDERATIONS

Renin–angiotensin–aldosterone antagonists are associated with a variable incidence of severe hypotension during the initial 30 minutes after induction of anesthesia in noncardiac surgery patients. This drop in blood pressure is often refractory to conventional treatment with vasopressors (ephedrine, phenylephrine), intravascular volume loading, and a decrease in volatile anesthetic concentration. ARBs are highly protein bound, which may act as a reservoir to release some of the bound fraction to maintain equilibrium as the unbound drug is metabolized and excreted. ARB-induced hypotension is typically resistant to alpha adrenergic agonists like phenylephrine,

norepinephrine, and ephedrine. This is due to the chronic AT1 blockade, which reduces the vasoconstrictor response.

The treatment of choice after conventional measures for ACEI or ARB-induced refractory hypotension is vasopressin. Systemic arterial blood pressure is maintained and regulated by three neurohumoral mechanisms: the sympathetic nervous system, the RAA system, and the arginine vasopressin system. These three systems are synergistic and also act to compensate when another component is inhibited. Patients taking RAA antagonists will have a depressed RAA system, and general or neuraxial anesthesia typically blunts the influence of sympathetic nervous system on vascular tone. To support vascular tone, it becomes necessary to supplement the vasopressin system with exogenous vasopressin because of an increased reliance on this system. Vasopressin acts on V1 receptor to cause arterial vasoconstriction, and an increase in SVR and mean arterial blood pressure. The recommended starting dose is a 0.5-1 unit bolus of vasopressin with a subsequent infusion of 0.03-0.04 U/min if necessary. Potential side effects include decreased cardiac output, decreased renal blood flow, splanchnic vasoconstriction, and ischemic skin necrosis if there is peripheral infiltration.

Although these hypotensive episodes have not been linked to any significant postoperative complications or an increase in mortality, questions still remain regarding the timing for discontinuing these medications. There are no existing national or international guidelines supporting the withdrawal or continuation of ACEIs or ARBs in the preoperative setting. Patients taking ACEIs and ARBs are typically advised to take their usual dose on the day of surgery. This is true for all antihypertensive drugs. Some, however, advocate holding the morning dose to reduce the incidence and severity of intraoperative hypotension. Sometimes holding the ARB for greater than 24 hours prior to surgery may be necessary. Renin–angiotensin–aldosterone antagonists in the perioperative period have been linked to postoperative acute renal failure, secondary to the intraoperative hypotension and use of vasopressors. Patients taking RAA system antagonists should be assessed for evidence of renal insufficiency. Although it is not necessary to check preoperative potassium levels on all patients taking these drugs, they should be monitored for any signs of hyperkalemia in the correct clinical context.

SUGGESTED READING

Auron M, Harte B, Kumar A, Michota F. Renin-angiotensin system antagonists in the perioperative setting: clinical consequences and recommendations for practice. *Postgrad Med J*. 2011;87:472-481.

Nonadrenergic Vasoconstrictors

Brian S. Freeman, MD

VASOMOTOR PHYSIOLOGY

Vasoconstrictors comprise a class of endogenous compounds and vasopressor drugs which increase arterial blood pressure by two mechanisms: (1) increasing systemic vascular resistance (SVR) in the high resistance, low capacitance arteries and arterioles, and (2) increasing venous pressure and preload in the low resistance, high capacitance veins and venules (Table 169-1).

Vascular tone is mediated by multiple receptor subtypes located on smooth muscle cells, the most significant being the adrenergic receptors. The sympathetic nervous system regulates vascular tone by releasing catecholamines which bind to adrenergic receptor targets. Of the four main adrenergic receptors (alpha and beta subtypes), the alpha-1 receptor is responsible for peripheral vasoconstriction. In fact, it is the most predominant receptor subtype located on vascular smooth muscle. Binding of adrenergic vasoconstrictors such as phenylephrine to the alpha-1 receptor initiates a G-protein-coupled signal transduction cascade that leads to vascular smooth muscle contraction, particularly of cutaneous and mesenteric beds. Activation of adenylate cyclase and phospholipase C second messenger systems promote calcium release from the sarcoplasmic reticulum. Intracellular calcium–calmodulin complexes then stimulate kinases which phosphorylate myosin, allow actin and myosin to interact, and cause muscle contraction.

Although the sympathetic nervous system has the most predominant role in vasoconstriction, there are also nonadrenergic cellular mechanisms responsible for maintaining vascular tone.

TABLE 169-1   Vasoconstrictor Drugs

Adrenergic	Nonadrenergic
Ephedrine	Vasopressin
Phenylephrine	Methylene blue
Norepinephrine	Angiotensin II
Epinephrine	
Dopamine	

1. Vascular smooth muscle contains **vasopressin V1 receptors** which serve as targets for the endogenous hormone, arginine vasopressin (AVP) or antidiuretic hormone (ADH). Activation of the V1 receptor leads to smooth muscle contraction through the phospholipase C system.
2. **Nitric oxide** (NO) released from vascular endothelial cells diffuses into the smooth muscle and activates guanylate cyclase, the enzyme which synthesizes cyclic guanosine monophosphate (cGMP) from guanosine triphosphate (GTP). High cGMP levels inhibit calcium influx, activate K^+ channels, and hyperpolarize the muscle cell, leading to vasodilation.
3. Vascular smooth muscle contains **angiotensin II (AT) receptors**, the most important being subtype 1 (AT1). Binding of angiotensin II to the AT1 receptor causes vasoconstriction through the G-protein-phospholipase C pathway.

VASOPLEGIA

Pharmacological vasoconstriction is often necessary to correct states of low SVR, such as anesthetic-induced vasodilation. First-line adrenergic drugs (eg, phenylephrine, norepinephrine) are usually effective. *Vasoplegia*, or vasoplegic syndrome, describes the vasodilatory shock state when vascular tone is profoundly decreased and unresponsive to traditional sympathomimetic drugs. This syndrome is characterized by severe hypotension refractory to adrenergic vasoconstrictors and fluid resuscitation, very low SVR, tachycardia, high cardiac output, and low cardiac filling pressures (Table 169-2). In the differential diagnosis of hypotension, vasoplegia is often a diagnosis of exclusion.

The mechanisms underlying this vasodilatory shock state are multifactorial: increased release of nitric oxide and other cytokines which promote cGMP production; cellular hyperpolarization via ATP-gated potassium channels; downregulation of adrenergic receptors; endothelial cell dysfunction; relative vasopressin deficiency.

Vasoplegic syndrome can occur during any type of surgical procedure. It has been most well described in cardiac surgical patients who have just separated from cardiopulmonary bypass. Other conditions associated with vasoplegia include septic shock, anaphylaxis, hemorrhagic shock, post-reperfusion

TABLE 169-2 **Vasoplegic Syndrome**

MAP ↓ (< 50 mm Hg)	SVR ↓↓ (<800 dyn·s/cm⁵)
HR ↓	RAP ↓ (<5 mm Hg)
PAP ↓	LAP ↓ (<10 mm Hg)
PCWP ↓	CI ↑ (>2.5 L/min/m²)
PVR ↓	

liver transplant recipients, post-pheochromocytoma resection, and postinduction refractory hypotension in patients taking chronic angiotensin converting enzyme (ACE) inhibitor or angiotensin II receptor blocker therapy. In all of these cases, the nonadrenergic vasoconstrictors used to treat vasoplegic syndrome are vasopressin and methylene blue.

VASOPRESSIN

Vasopressin, or AVP, is a peptide hormone synthesized in the hypothalamus and released from the posterior pituitary. As ADH, vasopressin regulates extracellular osmolarity and urine concentration. AVP promotes water reabsorption in the kidney by binding to vasopressin type 2 (V2) receptors located within collecting duct cells and increasing their permeability. AVP also regulates systemic blood pressure by causing potent arterial vasoconstriction through the effect of vasopressin type 1 (V1) receptors located within vascular smooth muscle. Vasoconstriction primarily occurs within the arterioles of the skin, splanchnic, renal, and coronary circulatory beds. Interestingly, in the cerebral and pulmonary circulations, AVP promotes vasodilation via the release of nitric oxide. The hypothalamus produces additional vasopressin in shock states to maintain SVR.

Vasopressin is most commonly used as a nonadrenergic vasoconstrictor in cardiac arrest patients receiving advanced cardiac life support (ACLS). Epinephrine, the gold standard vasopressor, may be less effective in prolonged cardiac arrest due to hypoxemia and severe metabolic acidosis. Compared to epinephrine, vasopressin produces a greater increase in coronary perfusion pressure but lower myocardial oxygen demand and fewer postresuscitation dysrhythmias. Cerebrovascular dilation may lead to better cerebral perfusion and improved neurologic outcomes. Whether used as a first-line vasopressor or in combination with epinephrine, vasopressin has not yet been shown to affect arrest outcomes (return of spontaneous circulation, survival rates, or neurologic outcomes) compared to epinephrine. Therefore, ACLS algorithms only recommend the option of replacing the first or second dose of epinephrine with a single bolus of vasopressin (40 units IV/IO) for patients in cardiac arrest regardless of the initial rhythm. Vasopressin may possibly lead to better outcomes for patients in asystole or with persistent ventricular fibrillation after multiple defibrillation attempts.

Vasopressin is also useful in clinical practice as a second-line vasoconstrictor in states of extremely low SVR or

vasodilatory shock. In severe sepsis, the vasculature can become unresponsive to catecholamine therapy. Vasopressin levels are often inappropriately deficient. Infusions of vasopressin result in higher SVR, higher mean arterial blood pressures, and lower norepinephrine requirements. Boluses of vasopressin analogs are also useful in treating hypotension refractory to catecholamines in patients chronically treated with ACE inhibitors or angiotensin receptor blockers. Vasopressin has been shown to be helpful in reversing other vasoplegic states, such as shock after cardiopulmonary bypass, anaphylaxis, and severe hemorrhagic shock.

Compared to norepinephrine, vasopressin better preserves mesenteric blood flow and has a significantly lower incidence of tachydysrhythmias. However, increasing arterial pressure with powerful vasoconstriction may come at a cost. Increasing the afterload may reduce cardiac output and lead to myocardial oxygen-demand imbalance and ischemia. Other side effects include postoperative hypertension and a higher risk of thrombosis from platelet aggregation. The antidiuretic effects may cause water intoxication and hyponatremia. Extravasation of vasopressin through an infiltrated peripheral intravenous line may lead to ischemic skin lesions.

Dosing of AVP for the treatment of refractory hypotension needs further study. Advanced cardiac life support protocols call for a single 40 unit dose for patients in cardiac arrest. To raise the mean arterial pressure in vasoplegic states, bolus doses should start at 0.5-1 units. Patients in septic shock receive infusions between 0.01 and 0.04 U/min.

METHYLENE BLUE

Methylene blue is the recommended treatment for methemoglobinemia. In the perioperative setting, methylene blue more commonly serves as a tracer dye in various procedures. After intravenous administration, rapid excretion of the leucomethylene blue metabolite in urine allows for a visual assessment of urinary tract integrity. For mastectomies, methylene blue is injected into the breast to trace the lymphatic system visually and help identify the sentinel lymph node. Chromoendoscopy involves spraying colonic tissues with methylene blue for dysplasia surveillance in patients with inflammatory bowel disease. Abnormal tissue (inflamed or dysplastic) will not absorb the dye, producing a pattern that helps with tissue localization for biopsy.

Like vasopressin, methylene blue produces vasoconstriction through a nonadrenergic mechanism. It competes directly with nitric oxide in the vascular endothelial cell for the soluble enzyme, guanylate cyclase. Methylene blue binds to the iron heme-moiety of guanylate cyclase and effectively inhibits the enzyme. Decreased levels of cGMP effectively end the intracellular cascade which would eventually lead to vascular smooth muscle relaxation. The vasculature is no longer responsive to vasodilator mediators like nitric oxide.

Methylene blue is useful as last resort nonadrenergic vasoconstrictor in patients with vasoplegia after separating from cardiopulmonary bypass. Due to contact activation from the bypass run, patients can develop extremely low SVR refractory to prolonged norepinephrine therapy. A single dose of methylene blue can rapidly increase SVR, decrease the dose of norepinephrine, stabilize hemodynamics, and even decrease the serum lactate levels. Preoperative use of methylene blue in patients at risk for developing vasoplegia may reduce its incidence, morbidity, and mortality.

Side effects are dose dependent and include transient dysrhythmias, increased pulmonary vascular resistance, coronary vasoconstriction, decreased mesenteric and renal blood flow, hyperbilirubinemia, and gas exchange abnormalities. Methylene blue can precipitate acute hemolytic anemia in patients with glucose-6-phosphate dehydrogenase deficiency. In high doses, methylene blue can actually oxidize hemoglobin causing methemoglobinemia. Neurologic dysfunction, especially in patients taking serotonin reuptake inhibitors, may result from the production of oxygen free radicals. Due to renal elimination, this drug is contraindicated in patients with severe renal insufficiency. Intravenous administration may interfere with light transmission in pulse oximetry and cause spuriously false readings of arterial desaturation. Patients can develop a blue-green discoloration of the urine or skin.

Methylene blue is formulated in a 10 mg/mL solution. Due to lack of widespread use, dosing is not well defined. Clinical practice and studies use 1-2 mg/kg IV bolus dose over 20 minutes infusion time, then 0.25 mg/kg/h infusion for 48-72 hours. The drug is reduced to leucomethylene blue and eliminated in the urine and bile.

SUGGESTED READINGS

Fischer G, Levin MA. Vasoplegia during cardiac surgery: current concepts and management. *Semin Thorac Cardiovasc Surg.* 2010;22:140-144.

Lavigne D. Vasopressin and methylene blue: alternate therapies in vasodilatory shock. *Semin Cardiothorac Vasc Anesth.* 2010;14:186-189.

Neumar RW, Otto CW, Link MS, et al.Part 8: Adult Advanced Cardiovascular Life Support: 2010 American Heart Association Guidelines for Cardiopulmonary Resuscitation and Emergency Cardiovascular Care. *Circulation* 2010;122:S729-S767.

Shanmugam G. Vasoplegic syndrome—the role of methylene blue. *Eur J Cardiothorac Surg.* 2005;28:705-710.

Treschan TA, Peters J. The vasopressin system: physiology and clinical strategies. *Anesthesiology* 2006;105:599-612.

Electrolyte Abnormalities: Cardiac Effects

170

Jeannie Lui, MD, and Katrina Hawkins, MD

Electrolyte homeostasis is the foundation of physiology. Even slight abnormalities in the concentration of any electrolyte can have significant effects on cardiovascular function. The management of electrolyte abnormalities is directed to prevent and treat life-threatening complications, to diagnose and treat the underlying cause, and if needed, to correct the electrolyte imbalance by repletion or removal of the unbalanced electrolyte. The severity of the electrolyte derangement should dictate the urgency of therapy but one should also remember that rapid correction of electrolytes might be detrimental.

POTASSIUM

Potassium, the major intracellular cation, exists in greater concentrations inside the cell as compared to the extracellular space. It is this difference in concentration that plays a crucial role in membrane potentials. In addition to its role in membrane potential, potassium also plays a role in neuromuscular excitability and cardiac rhythmicity. The normal range for serum potassium concentration is 3.5-5.5 mEq/L. The degree and duration of deviation in serum potassium concentration from this range is proportionate to the severity of the clinical manifestations of hypo- or hyperkalemia.

Hypokalemia

Hypokalemia, simply defined as a serum potassium level less than 3.5 mEq/L, can be due to three main processes: (1) inadequate potassium intake, (2) altered potassium distribution

between the intracellular compartment and the extracellular space, and (3) loss of potassium from the body. This loss can occur from the skin, gastrointestinal tract, or kidneys.

In most cases, mild hypokalemia (levels between 3.0 and 3.5 mEq/L) are asymptomatic. Clinically significant hypokalemia is generally defined as a serum potassium level less than 3.0 mEq/L. This increases the resting membrane and increases both the duration of the refractory period and the duration of the action potential, the former to a greater degree. This impairs the ability of the myocardial cell to depolarize and contract appropriately, potentially leading to arrhythmias. In addition, hypokalemia increases the resting membrane potential (hyperpolarization), which also leads to arrhythmias. The presence of other factors such as ischemic heart disease, preexisting arrhythmias, concurrent use of digitalis, increased beta adrenergic activity and hypomagnesemia can exacerbate hypokalemia and further the development of arrhythmias.

A wide range of arrhythmias may be seen in patients with hypokalemia, including premature atrial and ventricular contractions, atrial fibrillation, junctional tachycardia, ventricular tachycardia, and ventricular fibrillation.

Hypokalemia also produces characteristic electrocardiogram changes: ST segment depression, T wave depression, and prominent U waves, which are most often seen in the lateral precordial leads V_4 to V_6 (Figure 170-1). In addition, hypokalemia prolongs the QT interval. This is particularly significant in those patients with a preexisting genetic predisposition to long QT syndrome or those patients who are

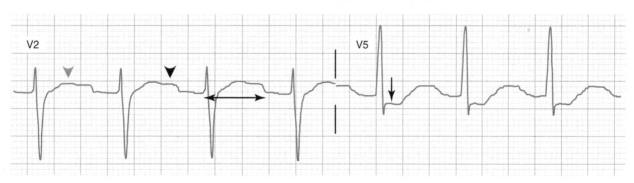

FIGURE 170-1 Prominent U waves seen in hypokalemia. (Reproduced with permission from Knoop KJ, *Atlas of Emergency Medicine*, 3rd ed. New York: McGraw-Hill; 2010.)

concomitantly ingesting medications that prolong the QT interval as this can potentially trigger torsades de pointes.

Treatment of hypokalemia begins with diagnosing and treating the underlying cause. Repletion of potassium is the mainstay of treatment. The route and rate of administration are dependent on the severity of the hypokalemia and the rate of decline of the serum potassium level. In instances of cardiac effects due to hypokalemia, potassium should be repleted rapidly. Oral potassium should begin with 40 mEq. Potassium can also be given IV at the rate of 10-20 mEq/h while monitoring levels closely and keeping the patient on telemetry.

Hyperkalemia

Hyperkalemia, defined as a serum potassium level greater than 5.5 mEq/L, is also due to three main mechanisms: (1) excessive potassium intake, (2) increased potassium release from cells, and (3) impaired excretion of potassium from the kidneys.

Clinical manifestations of hyperkalemia usually do not occur until plasma potassium concentration is greater than 7.0 mEq/L, though if the potassium concentration rises quickly and acutely, levels below 7.0 mEq/L can lead to potential cardiac toxicity. In particular, ischemic myocardium is especially vulnerable to cardiac effects of hyperkalemia, as local myocardial ischemia and cellular damage results in leakage of intracellular potassium with a subsequent local increase in myocardial interstitial potassium concentration.

The pathogenesis of the cardiac effects of hyperkalemia returns to potassium's fundamental physiologic role in the generation of an action potential. An increase in the serum potassium above normal alters the concentration gradient between the intracellular and extracellular compartments, making the resting potential less electronegative and thereby partially depolarizing the cell membrane. This will initially increase membrane excitability, but persistent depolarization or reduction in action potential eventually inactivates the fast sodium channels and electrical transmission is ultimately hindered. This translates to impaired cardiac conduction and contractility.

Hyperkalemia can be associated with several electrocardiogram changes, though several studies have noted that electrocardiogram changes are not sensitive and do not reflect the severity of serum potassium derangements. Nevertheless, hyperkalemia can manifest from initial symmetrically peaked T-waves with a shortened QT interval (Figure 170-2), to progressive lengthening of the PR interval and QRS complex, to the disappearance of P waves. If not treated, progressive widening of the QRS complex into a sinusoidal wave (Figure 170-3) will ensue and ultimately a flatline signifies ventricular asystole and lack of electrical activity. Hyperkalemia can be associated with a variety of arrhythmias and conduction abnormalities, including ventricular tachycardia, ventricular fibrillation, right and/or left bundle branch blocks, and atrioventricular block.

Treatment of hyperkalemia is aimed at three aspects: (1) prevent or minimize cardiotoxicity, (2) shift potassium, and

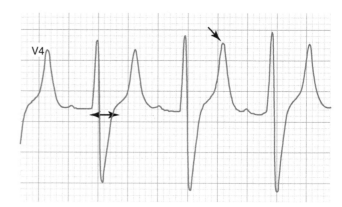

FIGURE 170-2 Peaked T-waves seen early in hyperkalemia. (Reproduced with permission from Knoop KJ, *Atlas of Emergency Medicine*, 3rd ed. New York: McGraw-Hill; 2010.)

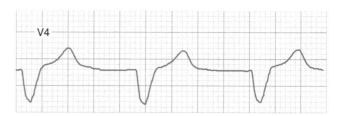

FIGURE 170-3 Wide QRS, near sinusoidal pattern, and peaked T-waves seen in more severe hyperkalemia. (Reproduced with permission from Knoop KJ, *Atlas of Emergency Medicine*, 3rd ed. New York: McGraw-Hill; 2010.)

(3) excrete potassium from the body via the gastrointestinal or renal route. To prevent the cardiotoxic effects of hyperkalemia, intravenous calcium should be infused which helps to stabilize the cardiac membrane while awaiting the effects of the shifting and binding agents. The next step in treating hyperkalemia is aimed at shifting potassium intracellularly. This is best achieved with intravenous insulin, given concomitantly with glucose to avoid hypoglycemia. Other agents that may help shift potassium into the cells are the beta adrenergic agonist, albuterol, and finally sodium bicarbonate. Lastly, there should be an aim to permanently excrete potassium from the body. This can be done via the gastrointestinal tract with potassium-binding resins such as sodium polystyrene sulfate or via the renal system with diuretics and ultimately dialysis.

CALCIUM

Total serum calcium concentration is comprised of the fraction of calcium that is bound to plasma proteins and the fraction of calcium that exists in the ionized state. It is the ionized calcium which is metabolically active as it can be freely transported in and out of cells. However, due to the added difficulty in measuring ionized calcium, most laboratories simply report total serum calcium concentrations with normal range from 8.5 to 10.5 mg/dL.

Calcium plays an essential role in cardiac function. It is involved in excitation–contraction coupling and in glycogenolysis where calcium is an integral substrate for the enzymes in the process, which result in breakdown of glycogen for fuel for cardiac muscle cells. Disturbances in calcium result in a plethora of electrocardiographic changes and conduction abnormalities but unlike potassium, arrhythmias due to hypo- or hypercalcemia are rare.

Hypocalcemia

Hypocalcemia, defined as a true serum calcium concentration of less than 8.5 mg/dL, can be divided into two major etiologies: (1) decreased entry of calcium into circulation such as hypoparathyroidism, severe hypomagnesemia, or vitamin D deficiency, and (2) increased loss of calcium from circulation such as hyperphosphatemia, pancreatitis, or chelation from rapid transfusion of citrated blood products.

A decrease in serum calcium concentration prolongs action potentials and as a result electrical transmission is slowed. This ultimately impairs cardiac conduction and contractility. Clinical cardiac manifestations of hypocalcemia include hypotension, which is especially common during massive transfusions of blood products containing citrate and in rare cases congestive heart failure. Other classic noncardiac clinical manifestations of hypocalcemia include signs of tetany, Trousseau sign (carpopedal spasm as induced by inflation of a sphygmomanometer above systolic blood pressure for 3 minutes), Chvostek sign (twitching and spasms of the ipsilateral facial muscles as induced by tapping the facial nerve just anterior to the ear), and seizures.

The characteristic electrocardiogram derangement in hypocalcemia is prolongation of the QT interval with an increased ST segment and normal T-wave (Figure 170-4). Hypocalcemia can also be associated with early after-depolarizations and promote torsades de pointes (though torsades de pointes is more often seen with hypomagnesemia and/or hypokalemia).

Myocardial dysfunction is reversible with calcium repletion. It is important to note that calcium levels must be corrected for serum albumin concentration so that overcorrection does not occur. If hypocalcemia is severe enough to

cause ECG changes, seizures or other symptoms, intravenous calcium should be administered. For asymptomatic patients, oral repletion is acceptable.

Hypercalcemia

Hypercalcemia is recognized as a true serum calcium concentration of greater than 10.5 mg/dL and though it can be caused by a variety of disorders, the vast majority of hypercalcemia is due to primary hyperparathyroidism or malignancy.

An elevation in serum calcium concentration shortens the myocardial action potential, causing increased myocardial excitability and contraction, leading to arrhythmias. In addition, chronic hypercalcemia can result in deposition of calcium on cardiac valves, coronary arteries, and myocardial fibers, causing hypertension and cardiomyopathies.

Electrocardiogram changes seen with hypercalcemia include shortening of the QT interval (due to a decrease in phase 2 of the myocyte action potential). There is also a decrease in the duration of the T-wave upstroke resulting in an abrupt upslope of the T-wave (Figure 170-4).

Treatment of hypercalcemia generally relies on the treatment of the underlying cause. However, for severe hypercalcemia (serum concentration > 14 mg/dL), intravenous saline should be administered as these patients are generally dehydrated. Short-term reduction in calcium can be achieved with calcitonin, while longer effects are achieved with bisphosphonates. Ultimately, if the calcium levels cannot be brought down and the patient is still symptomatic, dialysis can be employed to remove calcium.

MAGNESIUM

Magnesium is the second most common intracellular cation after potassium. Similar to the derangements in potassium, disturbances in magnesium concentrations also have profound cardiac consequences. The majority of intracellular magnesium is bound to organic matrices so levels of serum magnesium may reflect only a minute portion of the total magnesium source in the body. A normal range of serum magnesium is from 1.5 to 2.5 mg/dL, though recent studies have suggested that serum magnesium concentration above 2.0 mg/dL is cardioprotective.

Hypomagnesemia

Hypomagnesemia, defined as a serum magnesium concentration of less than 1.5 mg/dL, is a common occurrence in up to 10%-65% of hospitalized patients with increased incidence among those in the intensive care setting.

The mechanism underlying hypomagnesemia and arrhythmias has not been clearly elucidated. However, it is understood that magnesium is responsible for the regulation of several cardiac ion channels, such as the calcium channel and outward delayed rectifying potassium channel. Magnesium depletion will increase these outward currents of calcium and potassium, thereby shortening the action potential

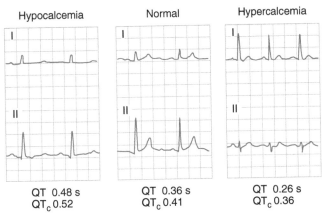

Hypocalcemia	Normal	Hypercalcemia
QT 0.48 s	QT 0.36 s	QT 0.26 s
QT$_c$ 0.52	QT$_c$ 0.41	QT$_c$ 0.36

FIGURE 170-4 Altered QT intervals due to changes in serum calcium levels. (Reproduced with permission from Longo DL, Harrison TR, *Harrison's Principles of Internal Medicine*, 18th ed. New York: McGraw-Hill; 2012.)

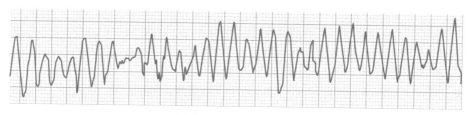

FIGURE 170-5 Torsades de pointes seen in cases of hypomagnesemia. (Reproduced with permission from Knoop KJ, *Atlas of Emergency Medicine*, 3rd ed. New York: McGraw-Hill; 2010.)

and potentially causing arrhythmias. Hypomagnesemia, like hypokalemia and hypocalcemia, also increases the risk of torsades de pointes (Figure 170-5). In addition, the incidence of ventricular arrhythmias is higher in those patients with hypomagnesemia and concurrent acute myocardial infarction.

Low serum magnesium is associated with higher carotid intima-medial thickness and serves as a risk factor for coronary disease. Hypomagnesemia is also associated with increased inflammation, exemplified by elevation of C-reactive protein and cytokine production with subsequent endothelial and platelet dysfunction.

Treatment of hypomagnesemia is simply the administration of magnesium. There are multiple formulations such as oral magnesium oxide and magnesium gluconate, or intravenous or intramuscular magnesium sulfate. Generally, intravenous magnesium sulfate is administered for severe hypomagnesemia. It has also been recommended for the management of torsades de pointes or refractory ventricular fibrillation.

Hypermagnesemia

Hypermagnesemia is a rare electrolyte disorder unless there is concomitant renal failure or excessive administration of magnesium. Mild elevation of serum magnesium between concentrations 4 and 6 mg/dL usually contributes to neuromuscular effects, including headache, lethargy, and diminished deep tendon reflexes. Cardiovascular effects are generally not seen until serum magnesium rises above 6 mg/dL when hypotension and bradycardia can occur. In circumstances of severe untreated hypermagnesemia, complete heart block and cardiac arrest can occur.

Electrocardiogram changes of hypermagnesemia are similar to those of hyperkalemia with comparable prolongation of the PR interval, increased duration of QRS complex, and increase in QT interval. In addition, because elevated concentrations of magnesium can inhibit parathyroid hormone secretion, promoting hypocalcemia, electrocardiogram findings associated with hypocalcemia may be concurrently seen.

Treatment of hypermagnesemia depends on the severity of elevation of magnesium. Mild hypermagnesemia in a patient with normal renal function is managed with supportive care and removal of the offending agent. More severe cases of hypermagnesemia may require loop diuretics or even dialysis to remove the excess magnesium. In emergency situations, while awaiting dialysis to be set up, intravenous calcium can be administered as a magnesium antagonist.

Hepatic Blood Flow

Jeffrey Plotkin, MD

The liver is a large organ (around 1500 grams in the normal adult). It receives approximately 25% of the cardiac output; meaning, about 1.2 L of blood flows through the liver per minute at rest. The liver also accounts for about 20% of resting total body oxygen consumption. This organ uniquely receives a dual blood supply from the hepatic artery and portal vein (Figure 171-1).

HEPATIC ARTERY

The hepatic artery accounts for 25% of the liver's blood supply and delivers oxygenated blood as an arterial branch off the celiac axis. In fact, 75% of the liver's oxygen supply comes from the hepatic artery. The biliary system and connective tissue is supplied by the hepatic artery alone whereas the rest of the liver receives the dual supply. The hepatic artery also has both alpha- and beta-adrenergic receptors; therefore, flow through the artery is controlled, in part, by the splanchnic nerves of the autonomic nervous system.

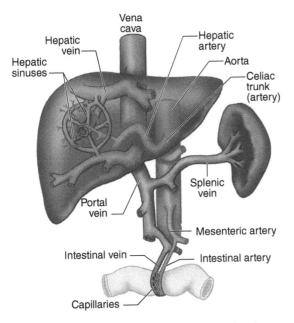

FIGURE 171-1 Hepatic blood flow. (Reproduced with permission from Butterworth JF, Mackey DC, Wasnick JD, *Morgan and Mikhail's Clinical Anesthesiology*, 5th ed. McGraw-Hill; 2013.)

PORTAL VEIN

In contrast, the portal vein accounts for 75% of the blood supply and 50% of the oxygen delivery. It is formed as a confluence of the splenic and superior mesenteric veins. Unlike most veins, the portal vein has no valves. It delivers blood low in oxygen but high in nutrients directly from the stomach, spleen, pancreas, and small intestine, thus giving the liver first exposure to nutrients absorbed through the gastrointestinal tract. Like the hepatic artery, portal vein blood flow is under control of the autonomic nervous system; however, it has only alpha adrenergic receptors. Normal portal venous pressures range from 5 to 10 mm Hg. Portal hypertension is defined as pressures greater than 12 mm Hg.

HEPATIC VEINS AND SINUSOIDS

Blood entering the liver parenchyma from terminal branches of the hepatic artery and portal vein mixes as it enters the hepatic sinusoids. These sinusoids are distensible vascular channels lined with endothelial cells and Kupfer cells, and bounded circumferentially by hepatocytes. These sinusoids then form the central vein of each hepatic lobule. Ultimately these central veins coalesce into the three main hepatic veins (right, left, and middle) which drain directly into the vena cava.

DETERMINANTS OF LIVER BLOOD FLOW

Portal vein blood flow is controlled primarily by the arterioles in the preportal splanchnic organs and by the resistance within the liver. Hepatic venous resistance, primarily at the level of the lobular venules (postsinusoidal), is regulated largely by the sympathetic nervous system through alpha adrenergic receptors. Hepatic arterial resistance resides primarily in the hepatic arterioles. The smooth muscle in these arterioles is affected predominantly by local and intrinsic mechanisms that adjust arterial flow to compensate for changes in portal blood flow. This autoregulation is known as the "hepatic arterial buffer response."

Total liver blood flow is affected by arterial and portal pressures on the afferent side and by hepatic venous pressure on the efferent side. Therefore, factors such as cardiac output, hypoxia, hypercarbia, and catecholamine release affect inflow. Factors that elevate hepatic venous pressure, such as congestive heart failure, volume overload, or positive pressure ventilation, will decrease the total hepatic blood flow.

Chronic liver disease is also associated with decreased liver blood flow. The scarring that occurs with cirrhosis completely destroys the architecture of the liver parenchyma, obstructs blood flow, and leads to portal hypertension. Surgical stimulation, when combined with the effects of anesthetics, can decrease total hepatic blood flow by as much as 30%-40%. The greatest decrease occurs during intraabdominal operations. Lower perfusion pressures, positive pressure ventilation, volume status, and activation of the endocrine stress response to surgery (catecholamines, antidiuretic hormone, renin, angiotensin, aldosterone), all contribute to lower total hepatic blood flow.

Hepatic Function

Jeffrey Plotkin, MD

The liver has numerous functions, including glucose homeostasis, protein metabolism, bilirubin formation and excretion, carbohydrate and lipid metabolism, blood filter, blood reservoir, drug metabolism, and excretion.

GLUCOSE HOMEOSTASIS

The liver is the major site for glucose formation from lactate, amino acids (mainly alanine), and glycerol (derived from fat metabolism). Hepatic gluconeogenesis is primarily responsible for maintaining a normal blood glucose concentration. It should be noted that gluconeogenesis is inhibited by general anesthesia.

Glucose absorbed following a meal is stored in the liver as glycogen. When the liver's capacity to store glycogen is exceeded, excess glucose is converted into fat. Insulin enhances glycogen synthesis, while epinephrine and glucagon enhance glycogenolysis. Normal glycogen stores about 65 g/kg of liver tissue in total. Average daily glucose consumption is 150 g/day, so glycogen stores are depleted within 48 hours of fasting.

PROTEIN METABOLISM

The liver is responsible for four primary aspects of protein metabolism: (1) deamination of amino acids, (2) formation of urea to eliminate the ammonia, (3) interconversion between nonessential amino acids, and (4) formation of plasma proteins. Deamination occurs via enzymes (usually transaminases) as part of the metabolic process of converting excess amino acids into carbohydrates and fats. The deamination of alanine is critically important to hepatic gluconeogenesis. Ammonia is formed as a byproduct of deamination and is highly toxic to tissues. The liver combines two molecules of ammonia with CO_2 to form urea which is then excreted by the kidneys.

Virtually all plasma proteins, with the exception of immunoglobulins, are formed by the liver. The most important of these proteins is albumin. Roughly, 10-15 g of albumin per day are synthesized by the liver to maintain the plasma albumin concentration between 3.5 and 5.5 g/dL. Albumin is responsible for maintaining plasma oncotic pressure as well as serving as the principal binding and transport protein for drugs and hormones. In fact, when plasma albumin concentration falls below 2.5 g/dL, there is increased drug sensitivity. In addition, the liver produces nearly all coagulation factors (I, II, and V-XIII) as well as plasma cholinesterase, antithrombin III, alpha-1 antitrypsin, transferrin, haptoglobin, and ceruloplasmin.

CARBOHYDRATE AND LIPID METABOLISM

When carbohydrate stores are saturated, the liver converts excess ingested carbohydrates (and proteins) into fat, as well as storing fat. In addition, the liver is responsible for the synthesis of all lipoproteins which are used for the transport of lipids in the blood. Further, the liver is responsible for the synthesis of cholesterol and phospholipids, necessary components of cellular membranes.

BILIRUBIN METABOLISM AND EXCRETION

Bilirubin is formed in the reticuloendothelial system from the breakdown of hemoglobin and then bound to albumin for transport to the liver. The liver then conjugates bilirubin with glucuronic acid via glucuronyl transferase into a water-soluble form where it is excreted into the bile canaliculi along with bile salts, cholesterol, and phospholipids. These canaliculi ultimately form the common bile duct which empties into the duodenum and also communicates with the gallbladder, the principal site of bile storage. Hepatocytes continually form bile up to 500 mL/ day. Bile is important for fat absorption as well as the excretion of bilirubin and many drugs. In the intestine, bilirubin is reduced by bacteria to urobilinogen, most of which is excreted in the stool. There is a very small fraction of conjugated bilirubin that is reabsorbed into the bloodstream and ultimately excreted in the urine.

RETICULOENDOTHELIAL FUNCTION

The liver is the largest organ in the reticuloendothelial system. Kupffer cells, which line the sinusoids, phagocytose antigens, and colonic bacteria are absorbed through the gastrointestinal tract. These cells act as a filter for the systemic circulation.

RESERVOIR FUNCTION

Normal hepatic blood volume is about 450 mL but may expand up to 1 L. Sympathetic stimulation of the hepatic veins and sinuses, such as that occurring during hemorrhage, can discharge up to 350 mL into the circulation.

Hepatic Drug Metabolism and Excretion

Andrew Winn and Brian S. Freeman, MD

The liver is the primary organ involved in drug metabolism. Under normal conditions, it receives approximately 1.2-1.4 L of blood per minute, which is roughly 25% of cardiac output. Seventy five percent of blood arriving to the liver is from the portal vein, whereas the remaining 25% is from the hepatic arteries.

The route of administration of a drug has significance with regard to its metabolism. When medications are given by mouth, they are absorbed by the gut, enter the hepatic portal system, and are transported to the liver where they undergo metabolism before entering the systemic circulation. This process sharply decreases the concentration of drug that is available to enter the systemic circulation, a phenomenon called the *first pass effect*. Other routes of administration such as intravenous, intramuscular, inhalation, transdermal, and sublingual undergo significantly less of a first pass effect because they enter the systemic circulation before arriving at the liver. Two related terms, *bioavailability* and *hepatic extraction ratio*, can be viewed as quantitative descriptors of the first pass effect.

Bioavailability refers to the fraction of drug administered that reaches the systemic circulation. When a drug is administered intravenously, its first pass effect is minimal, and its bioavailability is often close to 100%. The *hepatic extraction ratio* is the fraction of drug that is removed from the blood by the liver. It is calculated by dividing the rate at which the liver removes drug from the plasma by the rate at which the drug arrives at the liver. The hepatic extraction ratio is dependant on many factors, including hepatic blood flow, liver disease, the induction and/or inhibition of metabolizing enzymes by other drugs, genetic predisposition, and protein binding. Generally, if a drug has a high liver extraction ratio, it will have a high first pass effect and low bioavailability. Conversely, if the drug has a low extraction ratio, it will have a low first pass effect and a high bioavailability.

Most active drugs are lipophilic, enabling them to cross cell membranes and exert their effect by binding to active sites. It can be difficult for the body to excrete lipophilic compounds. When they are filtered at the glomerulus of the kidney and enter tubular fluid, lipophilic compounds easily diffuse out of the renal tubules, into capillaries lining the nephron, and return to systemic circulation. A fundamental concept and purpose of drug metabolism by the liver is the *biotransformation of lipophilic compounds into water-soluble compounds*. Water solubility enables excretion from the body via urine and bile.

BIOTRANSFORMATION REACTIONS

The smooth endoplasmic reticulum of hepatocytes contains microsomal enzymes (cytochrome P-450 system) which are responsible for conversion of lipid-soluble drugs into more water soluble and pharmacologically less active metabolites. These chemical reactions are classified as phase I reactions in which reactive chemical groups are modified through mixed function oxidases or the cytochrome P-450 system, and phase II reactions, which involve conjugation with ultimate excretion in the urine or bile.

Phase I Reactions

In the first phase of biotransformation, *phase I reactions* modify compounds in the liver through the processes of oxidation, reduction, and hydrolysis. Approximately 90% of phase I reactions are oxidation reactions whereby electrons are removed from a compound in a series of reactions involving NADPH. The removed electrons are accepted by oxygen. The result is the formation of water (H_2O) and a hydroxyl group (OH^-) ion. The hydroxyl group is added to the substance to render it more polar and reactive. Reduction reactions, which occur in the absence of oxygen, involve the addition of electrons to the drug, increasing its reactivity in preparation for phase II metabolism. Hydrolysis, involving amidases and esterases, involves the addition of water to a drug, leading to instability and splitting of the compound.

Phase I reactions are catalyzed predominantly by the enzymes of the cytochrome P450 monooxygenase system, with a minority of the reactions catalyzed by nonmicrosomal enzymes. Cytochrome P-450 (CYP450) enzymes are genetically determined, and their function is affected by age and liver disease. They are a group of enzymes located in the smooth endoplasmic reticulum of hepatocytes that enable the body to metabolize many compounds.

Drugs can affect the function of CYP450 enzymes and thereby plasma levels of other drugs taken concomitantly. For example, phenytoin, tobacco, and chronic alcohol use act as *inducers* of CYP450 enzymes, leading to an increased rate of drug metabolism. St John's wort, a herbal remedy commonly used to treat depression, is an inducer of CYP3A4. Many other marketed medications are also metabolized by CYP3A4, and a higher dose may be necessary to achieve therapeutic levels when taking St John's wort.

Drugs can also act as *inhibitors* of CYP450 enzymes, leading to a decreased rate of drug metabolism. Cimetidine, bupropion, and ciprofloxacin are all CYP450 inhibitors. When taking cimetidine, the dose of other administered medications may have to be decreased to prevent build up of levels in the blood. Other factors, including toxins, infections, cancer, and hepatic congestion can alter the function of CYP450 enzymes, requiring a prescribing physician to be aware of changes in metabolism when dosing medications.

Other than CYP450 enzymes, nonmicrosomal enzymes account for a small fraction of phase I metabolism. Such enzymes catalyze the process of conjugation, hydrolysis, oxidation, and reduction. They are located in liver, plasma, and gut and do not undergo induction. An example of nonmicrosomal enzymes is nonspecific esterases. In summary, phase I metabolism modifies compounds, rendering them more reactive.

Phase II Reactions

Phase II reactions are conjugation reactions. They involve coupling of a drug with a polar chemical group to increase the water solubility of the compound. Amino acids, acetate, glucuronic acid, methyl groups, sulfates, and glutathione are all compounds used in conjugation reactions. Phase II conjugation results in compounds such as phenols, alcohols, and carboxylic acids. After phase II metabolism, compounds are generally prepared for excretion.

The main excretory organ in humans is the kidney. Other organs such as the liver, lungs, salivary glands, and lacrimal glands also play a role in excretion. Each of these organs use routes termed *elimination pathways* as a way to remove substances from the body. Some of these elimination pathways are urine, bile, perspiration, saliva, tears, milk, and feces.

Compounds are water soluble after phase I and/or phase II metabolism. The kidney plays a major role in the excretion of such water-soluble compounds. In contrast to lipophilic molecules, water-soluble molecules, once filtered at the glomerulus into tubular fluid, are unable to diffuse across tubular epithelium and regain access to the systemic circulation. Rather, they travel through the nephron and accumulate with other waste products and are expelled from the body in urine. In contrast, some drugs, once metabolized, are not filtered by the glomerulus, often due to their large size. These compounds, including some heavy metals, can become toxic if they are allowed to accumulate in the body. Once they have undergone metabolism, they are excreted by the liver into bile, which is released into the intestines to be eventually expelled from the body in feces.

EFFECTS OF DISEASE

Alterations in hepatic structure and function can markedly change the metabolism of drugs and hence their effects. Chronic liver disease (cirrhosis) yields decreased numbers of functional hepatocytes, thus leading to decreases in the enzymatic clearance of drugs with a low extraction ratio. Decreased hepatic blood flow which accompanies cirrhosis may decrease the clearance of drugs with a high hepatic extraction ratio (lidocaine, propranolol, morphine, etc). Drug effects are also influenced by altered plasma binding that occurs with low albumin levels as well as by increases in the volume of distribution that occurs with cirrhosis. Finally, decreased production of plasma cholinesterase will decrease the ester linkage hydrolysis needed for the metabolism of drugs such as succinylcholine and ester local anesthetics.

Renal Physiology

Elvis W. Rema, MD

The kidney is a complex network of approximately two million nephrons that are involved in several regulatory and homeostatic functions. Each nephron consists of a glomerulus and a tubule that empties into a collecting duct. Urine is formed by glomerular ultrafiltration, and tubular reabsorption and secretion. The nephron regulates hormones that contribute to fluid homeostasis, bone metabolism, and hematopoiesis.

THE NEPHRON

The **glomerulus** is composed of capillaries that feed into the Bowman's capsule. Blood enters through the afferent arteriole and is drained by the efferent arteriole. The endothelial cells and epithelial cells provide an effective filtration barrier for large molecular weight substances and negatively charged molecules due to the net negative charge of the barrier. Therefore, the filtration barrier is both size selective and charge selective. Mesangial cells contain contractile proteins and respond to various stimuli and regulate filtration.

The main function of the **proximal tubule** is the reabsorption of Na^+ by active transportation. Water and Cl^- usually follow Na^+ passively. About 65%-75% of Na^+, water, and Cl^- are reabsorbed. Na^+ reabsorption is also coupled with the secretion of hydrogen ions and reabsorption of 90% of filtered bicarbonate ions. Glucose and amino acids are completely reabsorbed. The proximal tubule also secretes organic cations, such as creatinine.

About 25%-35% of the ultrafiltrate reaches the **loop of Henle**. Here 15%-20% of the filtered Na^+ is reabsorbed. Some Ca^{2+} and Mg^{2+} reabsorption also takes place here.

The **distal tubule** has very tight junctions and is comparatively impermeable to water and Na^+. The distal tubule is the major site of parathyroid hormone-regulated Ca^{2+} reabsorption. The latter end of the distal tubule, unlike the proximal part, participates in aldosterone-mediated Na^+ reabsorption.

The **juxtaglomerular apparatus** is a specialized area of the afferent arteriole and the ascending segment of the loop of Henle, the macula densa. Juxtaglomerular cells contain renin and are innervated by the sympathetic nervous system. Release of renin depends on beta adrenergic stimulation, changes in afferent arteriolar wall pressure, and changes in Cl- flow past the macula densa. Renin acts on angiotensinogen, produced in the liver to form angiotensin I. This is converted in the lungs by angiotensin converting enzyme to form angiotensin II that is responsible for blood pressure regulation and aldosterone secretion. Collectively, this mechanism is termed the **renin–angiotensin system**.

RENAL BLOOD FLOW

The volume of blood delivered to the kidney is approximately 20%-25% of cardiac output. This amounts to 1.1-1.5 L/min in a 70 kg man. When determining renal blood flow (RBF), clearance is often calculated. The clearance of a substance is the volume of blood that is completely cleared off that substance per unit time. P-aminohippurate (PAH) clearance is utilized in the measurement of RBF and is as follows:

RPF = [Concentration on PAH in urine/concentration of PAH in plasma] × Urine flow

RBF = RPF/(1 − hematocrit)

Regulation of Renal Blood Flow

A. Autoregulation

Autoregulation of RBF occurs between mean arterial pressures of 80-180 mm Hg. This process occurs mainly through the intrinsic myogenic response of the afferent arteriole to changes in blood pressure. Therefore, within this range, RBF can be kept relatively constant.

B. Tubuloglomerular Feedback

Tubuloglomerular feedback mechanisms also play a role in maintaining constant glomerular filtration rate (GFR) over a wide range of perfusion pressures. The macula densa can exert effects on the afferent arteriole tone as well as the permeability of the glomerular capillary itself.

C. Hormonal Regulation

Hormonal regulation via angiotensin II can cause generalized arteriolar vasoconstriction and reduce RBF. Both afferent and efferent arterioles are constricted, but due to the smaller caliber of the efferent arteriole, its resistance is greater than that of the afferent arteriole, thereby preserving GFR. Epinephrine and norepinephrine increase afferent arteriole tone, but GFR does not decrease by much due to angiotensin-mediated prostaglandin synthesis. Inhibitors of prostaglandin synthesis, such as NSAIDs, block this mechanism. Atrial natriuretic peptide (ANP) is another hormone released mainly in response to atrial distention. ANP is a smooth muscle dilator and antagonizes the effects of norepinephrine and angiotensin II. It preferentially dilates the afferent arteriole and increases GFR.

GLOMERULAR FILTRATION RATE

Glomerular filtration rate is approximately 20% of renal plasma flow. GFR is the volume of fluid filtered from the renal glomerular capillaries into the Bowman's capsule per unit time. GFR can be calculated by measuring clearance of inulin, a fructose polysaccharide that is completely filtered and is not secreted or reabsorbed. Normal values for GFR are 120 ± 25 mL/min in men and 95 ± 20 mL/min in women. A more practical but less accurate method to measure GFR is to calculate the creatinine clearance. This can overestimate GFR as some creatinine is secreted by the kidney tubules. Creatinine clearance is calculated as follows:

$$\text{Creatinine clearance} = \frac{(\text{Urine creatinine}) \times (\text{Urinary flow rate})}{\text{Plasma creatinine}}$$

Renal Function Tests

175

Michael Rasmussen, MD

The human kidney is responsible for many vital homeostatic processes throughout the body. Since proper kidney function is essential to life, the anesthesiologist must be able to recognize, diagnose, and properly treat kidney dysfunction. An important step in managing perioperative renal physiology is familiarity with basic renal function tests (RFTs).

INULIN CLEARANCE TEST

The gold standard for measuring glomerular filtration rate (GFR) is the inulin clearance test, which involves intravenous injection of inulin (a polyfructose sugar), and measurement of urinary inulin excretion over time. Inulin is completely filtered from the blood by the glomerulus, and is not secreted or reabsorbed by the renal tubules. Therefore, its clearance from the body into the urine is an accurate indicator of GFR and renal function. However, its use is limited in clinical practice because it is labor intensive and requires strict attention to detail. Thus, other methods for assessing renal function are generally used.

SERUM CREATININE

Creatinine is an end product of skeletal muscle ATP energy production. It is cleared from the blood by the kidneys through glomerular filtration, and then excreted in the urine. Creatinine production in the body depends on many factors, such as skeletal muscle mass, dietary protein intake, physical activity, and catabolism, and can vary from one person to another, but is usually stable on an individual basis.

A common pitfall in interpreting creatinine levels is not accounting for muscle mass. Although a creatinine of 1.2 mg/dL may be normal in a muscular 25 year-old man, it likely indicates significant renal dysfunction in a frail, elderly woman. The serum creatinine level represents the balance between muscle creatinine production and creatinine excretion by the kidneys. Thus, all else being equal, a change in an individual's serum creatinine level reflects a linear change in GFR and proper kidney function. For example, an increase in creatinine from 0.8 to 1.6 mg/dL indicates a 50% reduction in GFR.

The Acute Kidney Injury Network defined acute kidney injury (AKI) as one or more of the following occurring within a 48-hour time period:

- An absolute increase in the serum creatinine of 0.3 mg/dL or more.
- A 50% or more increase in serum creatinine.
- A reduction in urine output to less than 0.5 mL/kg/h (for more than 6 hours).

However, monitoring serum creatinine levels will not detect acute changes in GFR because it takes hours for serum creatinine levels to rise in response to decreased GFR. Conversely, serum creatinine levels may be elevated for a time even though GFR is recovering or has normalized.

CREATININE CLEARANCE

Much like the clearance of inulin, creatinine clearance (CrCl) can be used to measure GFR by comparing urinary and plasma creatinine levels over time (usually 24 hours). However, in addition to filtration through the glomeruli, some creatinine is also secreted from the blood into the urine through the walls of the renal tubules (unlike inulin), thus, CrCl actually overestimates GFR by 10%-20%.

Two formulas (Table 175-1) used in clinical practice to gauge a patient's baseline GFR are the Cockcroft–Gault

TABLE 175-1 Calculation of Glomerular Filtration Rate

Cockcroft–Gault Equation:

Creatinine clearance (mL/min)

$$= \frac{(140 - age) \times wt\ (kg)}{Serum\ creatinine\ (mg/dL) \times 72} (\times 0.85\ for\ women)$$

Modification of Diet in Renal Disease Equation:

Glomerular filtration rate (mL/min/1.73 m²) = 170
× [serum creatinine (mg/dL)]$^{-0.999}$ × [age]$^{-0.176}$
× [urea nitrogen (mg/dL)]$^{-0.170}$
× [albumin (g/dL)]$^{+0.318}$ × (0.762 if woman)
× (1.180 if black)

equation and the Modification of Diet in Renal Disease (MDRD) equation, both of which were developed using nomograms based on population studies. After a baseline GFR is established, these equations can be used to monitor changes over time for a given patient. Much like creatinine and CrCl, these formulas are not accurate during acute changes in renal function.

BLOOD UREA NITROGEN

Blood urea nitrogen (BUN) is formed through the breakdown of nitrogenous waste products, such as ammonia during the urea cycle in the liver; urea then travels to the kidneys for excretion. Although urea is rapidly cleared from the blood through glomerular filtration, it is not a good marker of GFR because some urea is reabsorbed back into the blood by the renal tubules. BUN levels can also be altered by intravascular volume changes, diet changes, liver disease, pregnancy, gastrointestinal bleeding, hematoma reabsorption, and many other conditions.

Blood Urea Nitrogen/Creatinine Ratio

The ratio of serum BUN to serum creatinine (BUN/Cr) can be useful in the diagnosis of AKI, specifically prerenal azotemia (Table 175-2). A ratio of 20:1 or greater indicates a prerenal process. However, the utility of the BUN/Cr ratio is limited by the same factors that limit the interpretation of the individual BUN and creatinine levels.

URINE OUTPUT

Measuring urine output is a simple, inexpensive marker of kidney function and volume status. Normal urine output should be between 0.5 and 1 mL/kg/h, however, urine output can vary

greatly during the perioperative period even in the absence of renal dysfunction. For example, pneumoperitoneum during abdominal laparoscopic surgery can cause oliguria without adversely altering postoperative renal function. Additionally, normal urine output does not guarantee proper renal function, as illustrated by the fact that nonoliguric renal failure is the most common manifestation of perioperative AKI.

URINE SODIUM, SPECIFIC GRAVITY, AND OSMOLALITY

Evaluating urine color (dark vs light) is quick and easy, and may be an indication of the kidney's ability to concentrate urine, which is a very sensitive indicator of renal tubular function. A more precise way to evaluate the concentration of urine is to measure urine sodium, urine specific gravity, and urine osmolality. Various primary or secondary renal problems can affect the way the kidney concentrates urine. For example, in hypovolemic states, the kidney attempts to retain water by reabsorbing sodium, causing an osmolar gradient for water to follow. The resulting urine will have low sodium, high specific gravity, and high osmolality (Table 175-2). However, in acute tubular necrosis (ATN) when renal tubules are damaged and become necrotic and dysfunctional, the kidney loses its ability to concentrate urine, and specific gravity will be identical to the specific gravity of the glomerular filtrate, which is 1.010. Assessing the ratio of urine osmolality to serum osmolality can also be helpful (Table 175-2).

FRACTIONAL EXCRETION OF SODIUM

Building on the evaluation of urinary sodium is an assessment called the fractional excretion of sodium (FeNa). FeNa expresses sodium clearance as a percentage of creatinine clearance, or rather the percentage of the sodium filtered by the kidney that is excreted in the urine. It is useful in differentiating a prerenal versus intrarenal cause of AKI (Table 175-2). However, since sodium levels in the urine and plasma are used in the calculation of the FeNa, a patient's use of diuretic agents (eg, furosemide) will invalidate the calculation of the FeNa as these agents affect normal renal sodium transfer. In these circumstances, a different test can be used, such as determining the fractional excretion of urea.

FRACTIONAL EXCRETION OF UREA

Since diuretic medications skew the results of the FeNa, a different yet similar test can be used in patients taking diuretic medications, namely the fractional excretion of urea nitrogen (FeUrea). This test functions similar to the FeNa, but uses urea instead of sodium (Table 175-2). The FeUrea is inaccurate during concomitant use of acetazolamide or osmotic diuretics such as mannitol, which prevent proximal tubule water reabsorption.

TABLE 175-2   Determination of Prerenal versus Intrarenal AKI

Renal Function Test	Prerenal	Intrarenal (Acute Tubular Necrosis)
Urinary sodium	< 20 mEq/L	> 35 mEq/L
Urinary osmolality	> 500 mOsm	< 350 mOsm
Urinary specific gravity	> 1.015	1.010-1.015
BUN/Cr ratio	> 20:1	< 10:1
Fractional excretion of sodium	< 1%	> 2%
Fractional excretion of urea	< 35%	> 50%
Urine/plasma urea ratio	> 20:1	< 10:1
Urine/plasma creatinine ratio	> 40:1	< 10:1
Urine/plasma osmolality	> 1.5:1	< 1:1

URINE-TO-PLASMA CREATININE RATIO

The urine-to-plasma creatinine ratio (U/P Cr ratio) represents the proportion of water reabsorbed by the distal tubule. The urine should normally contain a much higher concentration of creatinine than the serum because most of the water passing through the kidneys is reabsorbed, while creatinine is excreted. In prerenal states, such as dehydration, the U/P ratio exceeds 40:1, whereas in times of tubular dysfunction, such as acute tubular necrosis, it is less than 10:1. A similar test is the urine to plasma urea ratio (U/P urea ratio), which can also be helpful in assessing renal tubular function (Table 175-2).

CYSTATIN C

A relatively new marker of potential importance is cystatin C (CysC), a protease inhibitor released into circulation by all nucleated cells in the body. It is completely filtered by the glomerulus and not secreted or reabsorbed by the tubules; its levels are also unaffected by age, muscle mass, race, or gender. Thus, CysC could be more accurate than creatinine as an indicator of low GFR states; however, studies have shown that CysC levels may be confounded by patient factors such as cigarette smoking, inflammation, and immunosuppressive therapy.

SUGGESTED READINGS

Kellen M, Aronson S, Roizen MF, Barnard J, Thisted RA. Predictive and diagnostic tests of renal failure. *Anesth Analg.* 1994;78:134-142.

Mehta RL, Kellum JA, Shah SV, et al. Acute Kidney Injury Network: report of an initiative to improve outcomes in acute kidney injury. *Crit Care.* 2007;11:R31.

Regulatory Functions of the Kidney

Elvis W. Rema, MD

The kidneys serve several essential regulatory roles. They are essential in the regulation of electrolytes, maintenance of acid-base balance, and regulation of blood pressure. They serve the body by filtering blood to remove wastes that are diverted to the urinary bladder for excretion. The kidneys excrete wastes such as urea and ammonium, and are also responsible for the reabsorption of water, glucose, and amino acids. Furthermore, the kidneys also produce hormones, including calcitriol, erythropoietin, and the enzyme renin.

REGULATION OF SODIUM AND WATER

There are three major hormones that are involved in regulating Na^+ and water balance in the body at the level of the kidney. **Antidiuretic hormone** (ADH) from the posterior pituitary acts on the kidney to promote water reabsorption, thus preventing its loss in urine. The most important variable in regulating ADH is plasma osmolarity. Reduced volume of extracellular fluid promotes secretion of ADH, but is a less sensitive mechanism. Other stimuli for ADH secretion include decrease in systemic arterial blood pressure, stress, nausea, hypoxia, pain, and mechanical ventilation. **Aldosterone** from the adrenal cortex of the adrenal gland acts on the kidney to promote Na^+ reabsorption. It acts mainly on the distal tubules and the collecting ducts of the nephron. Water follows Na^+, thereby increasing intravascular volume. K^+ levels are the most sensitive stimulator of aldosterone secretion. **Atrial natriuretic hormone** (ANH) from the atrium of the heart acts on the kidney to promote Na^+ excretion to decrease intravascular volume. The main stimulus for ANH secretion is atrial distention.

REGULATION OF BLOOD PRESSURE

The renin-angiotensin system (RAS) is a hormone system that regulates blood pressure and fluid balance. A decrease in mean arterial pressure induces juxtaglomerular cell secretion of renin. Renin is responsible for converting angiotensinogen to angiotensin I. Angiotensin converting enzyme (ACE) in the lungs converts angiotensin I to angiotensin II. Angiotensin II is a potent vasoconstrictor resulting in increased blood pressure. It also stimulates aldosterone release from the adrenal cortex that increases Na^+ and water reabsorption, increasing total effective circulatory volume.

pH REGULATION

The metabolism of amino acids in proteins produces acids referred to as nonvolatile acids that are rapidly buffered, producing CO_2 and ammonium salts. The lungs excrete the CO_2, whereas the kidneys excrete the ammonium salts. In the process of excreting ammonium, bicarbonate is generated and returned to the blood to replace the bicarbonate lost in titrating the nonvolatile acid. About 85%-90% of the filtered bicarbonate is reabsorbed in the proximal tubule. Cells of the distal tubule and collecting ducts reabsorb the rest. The major factors that control bicarbonate reabsorption are luminal bicarbonate concentration, arterial CO_2, and angiotensin II. An increase in any of these factors can cause an increase in bicarbonate reabsorption.

Ca²⁺ REGULATION

Calcitriol is the hormonally active form of vitamin D that is produced in cells of the nephron's proximal tubule. The enzyme vitamin D alpha-hydroxylase is responsible for the conversion of calcifediol to the active calcitriol. The activity of this enzyme is dependent on parathyroid hormone activity and is an important step in Ca^{2+} homeostasis. Calcitriol increases serum Ca^{2+} levels by promoting the absorption of dietary Ca^{2+} from the gastrointestinal tract and increasing renal tubular reabsorption of Ca^{2+}. It also stimulates release of Ca^{2+} from bone by its action on osteoblasts and osteoclasts. Finally, calcitriol inhibits the release of calcitonin, a hormone that reduces serum Ca^{2+} by inhibiting Ca^{2+} release from bone.

ERYTHROPOIETIN REGULATION

Erythropoietin (EPO) is a glycoprotein hormone responsible for red blood production by promoting the proliferation and differentiation of erythrocytic progenitors. Initially produced in the liver in the fetus, renal production predominates in the adult. Regulation is mainly dependent on blood oxygenation. EPO production may increase up to a thousandfold in situations of anemia or hypoxia.

Distribution of Water and Electrolytes

Elvis W. Rema, MD, and Adam W. Baca, MD

FLUID COMPARTMENTS

Fluid in the body is distributed between intracellular and extracellular compartments. Total body water (TBW) is the sum of the intracellular and extracellular compartments. In a 70-kg adult male, it comprises 60% of body weight or about 42 L. This value can vary with age, gender, and with the amount of adipose tissue versus lean muscle present in the body, as the latter has higher water content.

The extracellular fluid compartment (EFC) is equal to approximately one-third of the TBW or about 14 L in a 70-kg adult male. The extracellular compartment is subdivided into vascular, interstitial fluid, and transcellular compartments. The vascular compartment accounts for about 5% of total body weight or 3.5 L. The interstitial fluid compartment accounts for about 15% of total body weight or 9 L. The interstitial fluid tends to be low in protein and thus has a low oncotic pressure as compared to the vascular compartment. The intracellular fluid compartment accounts for two-third of TBW or about 28 L in a 60-kg adult male.

ELECTROLYTES

Sodium

Sodium is the major cation found in the ECF. Its normal concentration in serum is 135-145 mmol/L. Sodium concentration plays a large role in governing the ECF volume through osmotic forces. Additionally, sodium plays an important role in the ability of neuronal and cardiac tissue to generate an action potential.

The main factors that control sodium balance in the body are renal function (glomerular filtration rate), renin-angiotensin-aldosterone system, antidiuretic hormone (ADH), and atrial natriuretic peptide. Changes in serum sodium concentration largely have to do more with imbalances of TBW rather than sodium itself.

Hyponatremia is largely due to an excess of water relative to sodium in the setting of increased ADH secretion, either due to hypovolemia, decreased effective atrial volume, or inappropriate secretion of ADH (SIADH). Hyponatremic patients can present with symptoms, including vomiting,

weakness, mental status changes, seizures, and coma. The severity of these symptoms is related to acuity of the changes in serum sodium concentration. In asymptomatic patients, sodium concentration should be corrected slowly with a rate of no greater than 0.5 mEq/L/h using isotonic fluids such as normal saline or lactated ringers. Correcting at too rapid a rate can cause fluid shifts from the intracellular compartment to the extracellular compartment, potentially leading to central pontine myelinolysis. In symptomatic patients, the rate of sodium correction should be faster, with a goal of 2 mEq/L/h for the first 2-3 hours, until symptoms begin to improve. Treatment for hyponatremia can vary depending on the etiology. In patients with hypovolemic hyponatremia, normal saline infusion will provide volume resuscitation, removing the stimulus for ADH secretion and allowing the kidneys to remove excess free water. In patients with SIADH, fluid restriction and treatment of the underlying cause is most effective. With hypervolemic hyponatremic, patients require loop diuretics to mobilize excess water and sodium.

Hypernatremia is defined as a deficit of water relative to sodium, which usually occurs in patients with impaired access to water such as the elderly, those with altered mental status, or intubated patients. Symptoms include fever, nausea, vomiting, mental status changes, and focal neurologic changes. Treatment generally involves calculating the patient's free water deficits: ([Serum sodium concentration] − [target serum sodium concentration, usually 140]/[target serum sodium concentration]) × TBW, and infusing 1/2 normal saline to replace free water and intravascular volume. As with hyponatremia, the rate of correction should not exceed 0.5 mEq/L/h to avoid brain edema.

Potassium

Potassium is found primarily in the intracellular compartment, which accounts for approximately 98% of total body potassium. Intracellular distribution of potassium is maintained by the sodium-potassium ATP pump located in cell membranes throughout the body. Acute changes in serum potassium levels are usually due to transcellular shifts. Common causes of transcellular potassium shifts include: (1) pH disturbances (pH and serum K being inversely related); (2) insulin which stimulates the sodium-potassium ATP pump, resulting in an intracellular shift of potassium; (3) tissue necrosis during which the lysis of cells releases potassium into the extracellular compartment; (4) catecholamine release stimulates the sodium-potassium ATP pump; and (5) digoxin inhibition of the sodium-potassium ATP pump, causing hypernatremia.

Hypokalemia is defined as a serum concentration less than 3.5 mmol/L and can present clinically with nausea, vomiting, weakness, flaccid paralysis, hyporeflexia, myalgias, and ileus. Causes of hypokalemia include: decreased pH, excess insulin, excess catecholamines, hypothermia, mineral corticoid excess (hyperaldosteronism), renal losses such as in renal tubular acidosis types I and II, and diuretic use, specifically thiazide and loop diuretics. ECG changes seen include flattening of T-waves or the presence of U-waves as well as prolongation of the QT interval. Treatment is repletion of potassium either orally or intravenously at a rate of 10 mEq/h.

Hyperkalemia is defined as a serum concentration greater than 5.0 mmol/L and can present clinically with symptoms of weakness, dysrhythmias, paresthesias, palpitations, and cardiac conduction abnormalities. Common causes of hyperkalemia include decreased pH, diabetic ketoacidosis, cellular necrosis, such as in ischemic injury or rhabdomyolysis, hemolysis, packed red blood cell transfusions, and with succinylcholine administration. Abnormalities seen on ECG begin with peaking of T-waves and progresses to prolongation of the PR interval, flattening of P-waves, and prolongation of the QRS complex leading to ventricular arrhythmias. Treatment of hyperkalemia consists of calcium gluconate administration to stabilize cell membranes, regular insulin accompanied with glucose to shift potassium into cells, sodium bicarbonate which increases pH and drives potassium into cells, beta-2 agonists, kayexalate (onset 1-2 h), or dialysis, if necessary.

Magnesium

Primarily in the intracellular compartment, magnesium is found in high amounts in bone and muscle. Magnesium plays a role in DNA and protein synthesis, as a cofactor in many enzymatic reactions, and for proper cardiac function.

Hypomagnesemia is defined as serum magnesium less than 1.7 mg/dL. For cardiac patients, it is generally recommended to keep magnesium levels greater than 2.0 mg/dL as a hypomagnesemic state is thought to be arrhythmogenic. Hypomagnesemia can be caused by decreased absorption from the gastrointestinal tract or through renal losses that can occur with diuresis or disorders of the renal tubules. Clinically, hypomagnesemia can present with neuromuscular excitability, seizures, cardiac arrhythmias as a deficiency in magnesium can lead to prolongation of the QT interval. Magnesium can be repleted intravenously through the administration of magnesium sulfate.

Hypermagnesemia is considerably less common than hypomagnesemia. Patients tend to be asymptomatic until levels greater than 5 mg/dL are reached in the serum. Presentation includes hyporeflexia, weakness, and somnolence. Hypomagnesemia can result in neuromuscular junction abnormalities, including decreased release of presynaptic acetylcholine and changes in receptor sensitivity to acetylcholine.

Calcium

Calcium is highly protein bound in the body. Serum levels can fluctuate with varying amounts of plasma proteins such as albumin, although the free calcium levels may stay relatively unchanged. Regulation of serum calcium levels involves endocrine feedback regulation through parathyroid hormone and calcitonin.

Hypocalcemia is defined as serum calcium levels less than 8.5 mg/dL. It is important to take into account serum albumin concentration, as measured serum calcium needs to be corrected to determine actual calcium levels. Actual calcium levels = measured calcium + 0.8 (4.0 − measured serum albumin). Causes of hypocalcemia include magnesium depletion, sepsis, alkalosis, and blood transfusions due to citrate binding to calcium, pancreatitis, or parathyroid hormone deficiency. Symptoms can present as neurologic signs, including paresthesias, perioral numbness, tetany, and seizures. Treatment options include intravenous repletion of calcium or with oral supplementation.

Hypercalcemia is defined as serum concentration of calcium greater than 10.2 mg/dL. Common causes include endocrine dysfunction such as hyperparathyroidism, vitamin D toxicity, thiazide diuretics, Paget disease, malignancy, multiple myeloma, and renal failure through secondary hyperparathyroidism. Symptoms include cognitive dysfunction, abdominal pain, nausea, vomiting, bone pain, and nephrolithiasis. Initial treatment is through hydration with fluids. ECG changes seen include prolonged PR interval, widened QRS complex, and shortened QT interval.

Diuretics

Elizabeth E. Holtan, MD

Diuretics are a class of medications that increase urine output by decreasing the reabsorption of water and sodium. They are used to treat conditions of intravascular volume overload, particularly in those patients refractory to fluid and salt restriction. Common indications include hypertension, congestive heart failure, pulmonary edema, and cerebral edema. Diuretics target receptors on cell membranes within the renal tubule. They are typically categorized by their primary site of action in the nephron (Figure 178-1).

CARBONIC ANHYDRASE INHIBITORS

In the lumen of the proximal convoluted tubule, secreted protons (H^+) combine with bicarbonate (HCO_3^-) to form carbonic acid (H_2CO_3). Catalyzed by the enzyme carbonic anhydrase, H_2CO_3 breaks down to form water (H_2O) and carbon dioxide (CO_2).

$$H^+ + HCO_3^- \leftrightarrow H_2CO_3 \xrightarrow[\text{anhydrase}]{\text{Carbonic}} H_2O + CO_2$$

When carbonic anhydrase is inhibited, H_2CO_3 is unable to form into H_2O and CO_2, so H_2CO_3 is converted back into H^+ and HCO_3^-.

H^+ ions that accumulate in the tubule are then reabsorbed in exchange for Na^+ ions. H_2O follows Na^+, enabling diuresis. Accumulation and excretion of bicarbonate, plus H^+ reabsorption, results in alkaline urine.

Acetazolamide and methazolamide are the most commonly prescribed carbonic anhydrase inhibitors. Despite blocking sodium reabsorption, carbonic anhydrase inhibitors are considered weak diuretics. Subsequent reabsorption of sodium distally in the nephron limits their effectiveness. These drugs are often used to improve excretion of acidic substances (eg, salicylate overdose) through urine alkalinization. Inhibition of carbonic anhydrase in the ciliary body decreases intraocular pressure in open-angle glaucoma by decreasing aqueous humor production. Other indications include increasing respiratory drive in patients who suffer from central sleep apnea and treating altitude sickness. Hyperchloremic

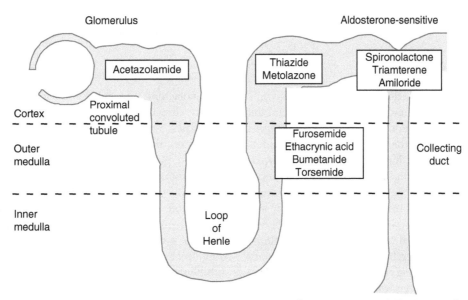

FIGURE 178-1 Diuretics—tubular sites of action. (Reproduced with permission from Fuster V, *Hurst's The Heart,* 13th ed. New York: McGraw-Hill; 2011.)

metabolic acidosis and possible sedation are possible side effects of carbonic anhydrase inhibitors.

OSMOTIC DIURETICS

Once filtered through the renal glomerulus, osmotic diuretics enter the proximal convoluted tubule where they are either poorly reabsorbed or not absorbed at all. The presence of the diuretic increases intraluminal oncotic pressure, thereby decreasing passive water reabsorption and leading to increased urinary excretion of water. In higher doses, osmotic diuretics may increase excretion of sodium, potassium, and magnesium. Massive diuresis can result in hypovolemia and hypernatremia (due to greater water loss relative to sodium).

Mannitol, a sugar with six carbons, is the most commonly used osmotic diuretic. The usual dose is 0.25-1 mg/kg IV given over 30 minutes. In patients with elevated intracranial pressure from cerebral edema, mannitol decreases intracranial volume within 30 minutes and lasts for nearly 6 hours. Mannitol enhances renal blood flow (RBF) and dilutes the tubular filtrate to prevent tubular obstruction. Of note, mannitol is also a free radical scavenger. For these reasons, mannitol may also be effective for prophylaxis against acute renal failure due to acute tubular necrosis. Patients undergoing cadaveric kidney transplant, cardiac, aortic, or renal artery surgery, or patients with rhabdomyolysis or hemolytic reactions, have higher risk of developing renal failure. Lastly, mannitol can be used to decrease intraocular pressure.

Mannitol may have adverse cardiovascular effects. As a hypertonic diuretic, mannitol initially increases plasma osmolality, causing an increase in intravascular fluid. Patients with decreased cardiac ejection fraction or with poor renal function may not tolerate the sudden increase in volume load. Higher renal blood flow may also limit renal concentrating ability. It can also result in hyponatremic, hyperkalemic metabolic acidosis.

LOOP DIURETICS

Examples of loop diuretics include furosemide, ethacrynic acid, bumetanide, and torsemide. These diuretics inhibit sodium and chloride reabsorption at the $Na^+-K^+-2Cl^-$ channel in the thick ascending limb of the loop of Henle. Loop diuretics are the most potent class of diuretics; they excrete approximately 15% of filtered sodium. The nephron has reduced ability to dilute or concentrate the filtrate, but the urine is usually hypotonic. Loop diuretics increase renal blood flow and alter the normal blood flow between the renal medulla and cortex. They are primarily used to treat sodium and volume overload in patients with congestive heart failure, pulmonary edema, nephrotic syndrome, and end stage liver disease. These diuretics can also lower calcium levels in patients with acute hypercalcemia refractory to intravenous fluid therapy.

Side effects include hyponatremia, hypochloremic metabolic alkalosis, hypocalcemia, and hypomagnesemia. Hypercalciuria may lead to nephrolithiasis. Hypokalemia is also a common side effect of loop diuretics. For patients who are also treated with digoxin, caution must be taken as hypokalemia can potentiate digoxin toxicity. If diuresis is too significant, prerenal azotemia may result. Ototoxicity is also possible but usually reversible. All loop diuretics, with the exception of ethacrynic acid, are contraindicated in patients with a sulfa allergy.

THIAZIDE DIURETICS

Hydrochlorothiazide is the most commonly used thiazide diuretic. Others include metolazone, chlorthalidone, indapamide, and quinethazone. Thiazide diuretics inhibit sodium reabsorption by competing with chloride at the Na^+-Cl^- channel in the distal convoluted tubule (DCT). They are considered less potent than loop diuretics. Thiazide diuretics can only excrete less than 5% of filtered sodium because a portion of the sodium load is reabsorbed distally in the collecting tubules. This class of diuretics notably enhances calcium reabsorption in the DCT.

The most common indication for thiazides is first-line treatment of hypertension. Other indications include treatment of nephrogenic diabetes insipidus and nephrolithiasis due to hypercalciuria. Notable side effects are hypokalemic metabolic alkalosis, hypercalcemia, hyperglycemia, hyperuricemia, and hyperlipidemia.

POTASSIUM-SPARING DIURETICS

Potassium-sparing diuretics block sodium reabsorption in the cortical collecting tubules. They are considered weak diuretics that only excrete 1%-2% of the filtered sodium because of their site of action in the distal nephron. Therefore, they are often used as an adjunct to diuretics that cause hypokalemia.

Aldosterone Antagonists

Spironolactone and eplerenone inhibit the hormone aldosterone directly in the collecting duct. Aldosterone normally stimulates sodium reabsorption and potassium excretion. Therefore, aldosterone antagonists promote sodium excretion and potassium retention. They are useful in patients with secondary hyperaldosteronism, especially for those with intractable volume overload secondary to cirrhosis. The antiandrogenic effect of spironolactone may help in the treatment of hirsutism. Since aldosterone antagonists may cause hyperkalemia, it should be used with caution in patients with renal conditions or those taking angiotensin-converting enzyme inhibitors and beta-blockers. Other possible side effects include metabolic acidosis, diarrhea, gynecomastia, fatigue, and decreased libido.

Noncompetitive Potassium-Sparing Diuretics

Amiloride and triamterene inhibit the opening of sodium channels in the collecting duct, which blocks sodium reabsorption and potassium secretion. These drugs are most commonly used to treat hypertension in conjunction with hydrochlorothiazide. They also are combined with loop diuretics to treat congestive heart failure. Side effects include hyperkalemic metabolic acidosis, as well as nausea and vomiting, diarrhea, and renal insufficiency.

179

Dopaminergic Drugs

Brian S. Freeman, MD

THE DOPAMINERGIC SYSTEM

Dopamine is one of several endogenous catecholamines that serve as neurotransmitters within the central and autonomic (sympathetic) nervous systems. Dopamine is synthesized in neurons of the central nervous system, particularly the substantia nigra and the ventral tegmental area, and the adrenal medulla. Dopamine is derived from its precursor, L-dihydroxyphenylalanine (L-DOPA), by the enzyme DOPA decarboxylase. Dopamine then becomes a precursor in the synthesis of norepinephrine and epinephrine, two very important catecholamines. It does not cross the blood-brain barrier. Endogenous dopamine has a half-life of one minute. It is rapidly metabolized into inactive metabolites by the enzymes monoamine oxidase (MAO) and catechol-*o*-methyl transferase (COMT). Homovanillic acid, the primary metabolite, is excreted into the urine.

Of the five known subtypes of peripheral dopamine (DA) receptors, DA1 and DA2 receptors are physiologically most important. Vascular DA1 receptors are located on the smooth muscle of most arterial circulations (especially mesenteric, renal, and coronary) and mediate vasodilation through adenylate cyclase signal transduction pathways. These effects are greatest in the renal vasculature. Stimulation of the DA1 receptor increases vasodilation, renal blood flow distribution, and glomerular filtration rates. DA1 receptors in the renal proximal tubules also mediate natriuresis (by inhibiting the Na^+/H^+ exchanger and Na^+/K^+ ATPase pump) and diuresis. The DA2 receptor is located on the presynaptic terminal of postganglionic sympathetic neurons and autonomic ganglia. Like alpha-2 adrenergic receptors, stimulation of the DA2 receptor inhibits the release of norepinephrine from presynaptic vesicles.

The dopaminergic system has multiple roles in the central and autonomic nervous systems. In the brain, dopamine has important functions related to mood, behavior, reward, learning and memory, and attention. Central dopamine receptors (DA2) may mediate nausea and vomiting. In systemic circulation, dopamine has an integral role in endogenous vasodilation, natriuresis, and the maintenance of normal blood pressure. It particularly helps to improve blood flow through the renal and splanchnic circulations. Dopamine can also bind to alpha and beta adrenergic receptors to promote inotropy and vasoconstriction.

Dopamine Receptor Agonists

A. Synthetic Dopamine

Exogenous dopamine can be used as a vasopressor to treat severe hypotension in vasodilatory shock states like sepsis, and as an inotrope in low cardiac output states. It can supplement normal circulatory function in situations of induced hypertension, such as for the treatment of cerebral vasospasm after subarachnoid hemorrhage. Since dopamine cannot cross the blood-brain barrier, synthetic dopamine will not affect the central nervous system. When used in dosages to support blood pressure and cardiac output, dopamine, like any vasopressor, may become harmful. Tachycardia combined with vasoconstriction can decrease oxygen delivery, increase myocardial oxygen demand, and may trigger myocardial ischemia.

Synthetic dopamine is administered in a continuous intravenous infusion without a loading dose. The physiologic effects are dose-dependent. At low doses (1-3 µg/kg/min), dopamine stimulates the DA1 receptors. The net effect is dilation of the mesenteric, coronary, cerebral, and renal vascular beds, which lowers diastolic blood pressure and increases renal perfusion. There is minimal effect on heart rate and cardiac output. It was once thought that dopamine infusions could "protect" the kidney by increasing renal blood flow and inducing diuresis and natriuresis. However, routine use of "renal dose" dopamine in shock states is controversial. Dopamine has been shown to have little beneficial effect in preventing acute renal failure in shock patients.

At intermediate doses of 4-10 µg/kg/min, dopamine is a beta-1 receptor agonist (with only mild effects on beta-2 receptors). It increases heart rate, myocardial contractility, and cardiac output, leading to a sustained increase in blood pressure. The higher infusion rates also promote the release of endogenous norepinephrine and inhibit norepinephrine reuptake in presynaptic nerve terminals. The result is a mild increase in systemic vascular resistance. Since dopamine can induce tachydysrhythmias at this dose, it is a good choice for vasodilatory shock states associated with bradycardia.

At higher infusion rates (10-20 µg/kg/min), dopamine stimulates alpha-1 adrenergic receptors in addition to beta-1 receptors. The prominent alpha-1 mediated vasoconstriction, especially in skeletal muscle beds, will raise systemic arterial pressure.

However, the intense vasoconstriction may eliminate the renal dilation and natriuretic effects, and could also compromise extremity circulation. At the highest doses (>20 µg/kg/min), only the alpha-1 adrenergic effects predominate.

B. Fenoldopam

Fenoldopam is a selective peripheral DA1 receptor agonist. The primary effect is systemic arteriolar vasodilation leading to afterload reduction. Although fenoldopam also improves renal blood flow, diuresis, and natriuresis, it remains unclear whether the drug can actually preserve renal function in susceptible patients. Like dopamine, fenoldopam is poorly lipid soluble and therefore does not cross the blood-brain barrier. The drug has a rapid onset and short duration with a 5-minute elimination half-life.

Intravenous fenoldopam is indicated for the short-term management of severe perioperative hypertension and hypertensive emergencies. Fenoldopam is a useful alternative to sodium nitroprusside. It causes fewer episodes of hypotension, lacks the potential for toxicity (cyanide or thiocyanate toxicity), and is not degraded by light. Bolus doses should not be given. The initial infusion rate is 0.1 µg/kg/min, and the maximum recommended dose is 1.6 µg/kg/min. Potential side effects are usually related to arterial vasodilation: headache, flushing, reflex tachycardia, and increases in intraocular pressure. Patients with sulfa sensitivities may have life-threatening allergic reactions to the sodium metabisulfite preservative found in fenoldopam solutions.

Dopamine Receptor Antagonists

A. Antipsychotics

Psychiatric diseases such as schizophrenia and bipolar disorder are associated with excessive dopamine transmission in the central nervous system. Patients who present for surgery may be taking antipsychotics, or neuroleptics, that competitively antagonize central dopamine DA2 receptors. The "typical" antipsychotics like *chlorpromazine* and *haloperidol* have a high affinity for DA2 receptors and can cause Parkinson-like extrapyramidal side effects such as akinesia, spasticity, and rigidity. The "atypical" antipsychotics (*risperidone, quetiapine*, and *olanzapine*) have less affinity for blocking DA2 receptors and therefore cause fewer extrapyramidal side effects. These drugs tend to inhibit DA3 and DA4 receptors.

B. Antiemetics

Dopamine mediates feelings of nausea by binding to DA2 receptors located on neurons within the medullary chemoreceptor trigger zone of the fourth ventricle. Several antiemetic drugs used in the perioperative period act by antagonizing the dopaminergic input. The three most commonly used intravenous antiemetics which inhibit central DA2 receptors are *prochlorperazine* (a phenothiazine), *metoclopramide* (also a prokinetic gastric motility agent), and *droperidol* (also an antipsychotic). These dopamine receptor antagonists have an extensive side effect profile that includes sedation, orthostatic hypotension, neuroleptic malignant syndrome, and dystonic extrapyramidal symptoms such as tardive dyskinesia and akathisia. Droperidol has been associated with prolongation of the QT interval and an increased risk of sudden cardiac death due to torsades de pointes.

SUGGESTED READING

Murphy MB, Murray C, Shorten GD, et al. Fenoldopam: a selective peripheral dopamine-receptor agonist for the treatment of severe hypertension. *NEJM* 2001;345:1548-1557.

Anticoagulants

Vinh Nguyen, DO

When tissue injury occurs, platelets gather around the injured site to form the primary hemostatic plug. This step in turn activates other platelets and releases additional cellular and humoral components of hemostasis. Furthermore, exposed tissue factors promote thrombin generation during the coagulation phase of hemostasis to stabilize the weak platelet hemostatic plug. This process leads to a cascade of protease activation that foster the formation of a fibrin clot localized to the injury (Figure 180-1). Further fibrin clot formation is limited due to a series of inhibitors balancing out the coagulation. Normal hemostasis is a balance between procoagulant and anticoagulant mechanism. When there is an imbalance, a hypercoagulable state can lead to unwanted arterial of venous thrombosis. This can

give rise to devastating injury and leave the patient disabled with an increase in mortality.

UNFRACTIONATED HEPARIN

Unfractionated heparin (UFH) is a sulfated polysaccharide that binds to its cofactor, antithrombin III or simple antithrombin (AT), to accelerate the rate of anticoagulant activity. The enhanced antithrombin activity inhibits clotting cascade proteins—in particular, thrombin and Factor Xa. Unfractionated heparin has a unique pentasaccharide sequence that is found on one-third of the chains of commercial heparins that is highly specific for AT. Subsequently, this "AT-Heparin"

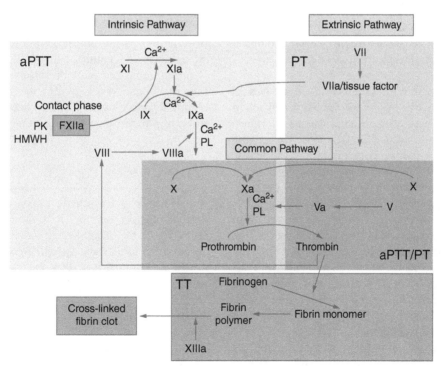

FIGURE 180-1 Coagulation cascade and associated laboratory tests. (Reproduced with permission from Longo DL, Harrison TR, *Harrison's Principles of Internal Medicine*, 18th ed. New York: McGraw-Hill; 2012.)

complex promotes a conformational change to enhance the rate of inhibition to thrombin and Factor Xa. UFH requires at least an addition of 18 saccharides downstream to tightly bring the two proteins together to enzymatically form a stable covalent "Heparin-AT-Thrombin" complex. This binding promotes a suicidal effect to thrombin but the heparin molecule is able to dissociate unchanged. In contrast, inhibition of Factor Xa requires that heparin bind to AT to enhance anticoagulant activity without a suicidal effect. Generally, UFH affects the intrinsic pathway, but at higher level it may stimulate the release of tissue factor plasma inhibitor (TFPI) and limit the formation of the prothrombinase complex with FXa via the extrinsic pathway. Heparin can directly affect platelet itself and subsequently disrupt aggregation.

Hemorrhage is one complication that can occur with intravenous heparin therapy. The risk is greatest with concomitant administration, with other drugs affecting hemostasis such as antiplatelet or fibrinolytic therapy. On the other hand, it is rarely seen with prophylactic use for DVT. Approximately up to 30% of patients who suffer from anticoagulant-induced hemorrhage may have preexisting lesion that goes undetected. The incidence of major life-threatening bleeding is about 5%. In such a case, protamine sulfate can be given to neutralize heparin. Protamine sulfate, a polypeptide isolated from salmon sperm, binds with high affinity to heparin. This inactive complex is eventually removed from circulation by the kidney, thus removing any heparin activity.

The biggest concern with heparin therapy is heparin-induced thrombocytopenia (HIT). The incidence can range from 1% to 2% for those on continuous intravenous therapy but rarely prophylactic use. UFH not only bind to clotting proteins but also interact with platelets factor 4 (PF4). This particular interaction exposes a neoantigen that can trigger IgG mediated-antibody specific to the heparin-platelet 4 complex. There are two distinct clinical syndromes associated with HIT: type 1 (mild) and type 2 (severe). Type 1 causes mild thrombocytopenia and recovers within a few days even in the presence of heparin. The hypothesis mechanism of action may be due to a mild platelet aggregator. Patients are generally asymptomatic and do not require treatment. Unlike type 2, a progressive thrombocytopenia can drop levels as low as 50×10^9/L. Platelets will recover after discontinuation but recur when heparin is restarted. The autoantibody produces two opposing effects on coagulation. First, autoantibody binding to the "heparin-PF4 complex" can be eliminated from circulation by the reticuloendothelial system thus, causing severe thrombocytopenia and ultimately significant bleeding. Secondly, these "heparin-PF4 complex" once bound forms circulating microparticles. They are procoagulant and can lead to a hypercoagulant state. This phenomenon is less seen with low molecular weight heparin (LMWH) but never seen with fondaparinux or direct thrombin inhibitors.

Another concern with long-term intravenous heparin therapy is the development of osteoporosis. Heparin can alter the activity of osteoclast and osteoblast cells. Studies have shown that heparin causes bone resorption by decreasing bone formation and augmenting bone resorption.

LOW MOLECULAR WEIGHT HEPARIN

Low molecular weight heparin (LMWH) (mean molecular weight 4500-5000 Da) is a truncated version of heparin. The biological fragmented molecule improves the specificity for Factor Xa. LMWH houses the required pentasaccharide sequence for AT binding but lacks the extended saccharide arm to fully bridge thrombin with AT. However, this sequence causes a conformation change that is highly specific to Factor Xa. One benefit of using LMWH is that it is more susceptible to inactivation by platelet factor 4 and lacks protein binding. These features limit its side effect profile compared to UFH. Due to greater bioavailability and longer half-life, anti-Xa levels are two to four times greater than that achieved with UFH. LMWH administration occurs once or twice a day. There is no need to monitor patient on LMWH, but if monitoring is necessary, antifactor Xa level can be measured.

With its truncated fragment, LMWH shares a similar but less extensive side effect profile compared to UFH. There is a lower incidence of osteoporosis with long-term therapy. Since LMWH has minimal binding affinity to platelets, less PF4 is exposed as a neoantigen, therefore reducing the risk of HIT. However, some cross-reactivity does exist between LMWH and heparin-dependent antibody, so caution must be taken if patient has a history of previous HIT. Like heparin, bleeding with LMWH is a concern especially with combined anticoagulant therapy. The disadvantage of LMWH is the lack of an exclusive antidotal therapy. Protamine is selective for UFH because of its specificity to the extended long peptide chain. Since LMWH is manufactured as a mixture of various truncated fragment length, there will be limited neutralization of antithrombin and partial reversal of antifactor Xa activity. Patients at high risk for bleeding should be treated with intravenous heparin instead of LMWH because of its short half-life and complete reversal with protamine.

FONDAPARINUX

Fondaparinux is a synthetic analog of the pentasaccharide sequence for AT binding. It is about one-third the size of LMWH, with factor Xa specific activity (about 300 times) but no thrombin inhibition. As well, there is no known effect on platelet function. It has 100% bioavailability and a 17 hour half-life. Due to its predictable anticoagulant response, the drug is given once daily. Fondaparinux is marketed for prophylaxis venous thromboembolism, and treatment of deep venous thrombosis. Its side effect profile is favorable with no development of HIT or cross-reactivity of HIT antibodies to fondaparinux. There is a lower incidence of bleeding compared to UFH or LMWH.

WARFARIN

Warfarin inhibits vitamin-K dependent coagulation proteins such as factors II, VII, XI, X as well as regulatory factors protein C and S. Normal coagulation requires vitamin-K dependent prozymogens to be carboxylated at the glutamic acid by the catalysis of gamma-glutamyl carboxylase, to form gamma-carboxyglutamic acid zymogen. This modification is essential to allow the activated coagulation protein to bind to the phospholipid surfaces such as platelets and propagate the coagulation cascade. The oxidized vitamin K is recycled back to the reduced form by vitamin K epoxide reductase (VKOR). This enzyme can be interfered by warfarin, thus limiting the reduced form of vitamin K and allowing prozymogen carboxylation.

Warfarin has a long half-life and requires one dose daily. It is a unique drug that requires special attention due to its mechanism and pharmacokinetics. Since protein C and S (the anticoagulant inhibitors) are vitamin K-dependent, the initial therapy can become temporarily biased toward thrombus formation. In this case, warfarin should be coadminstered with heparin until warfarin becomes therapeutic for around 3-4 days. Although the international normalized ratio (INR) will immediately be prolonged with the loading dose (rapid decline of Factor VII), it may take several days for full antithrombin effect because of the long half-life of prothrombin (about 60 hours). The therapeutic effect only affects newly synthesized factors and not circulating coagulation factors. Since warfarin is metabolized by the liver P450, warfarin can be influenced by other drug interaction, dietary vitamin K intake, disease states, or liver injury. Because of the myriad problems and narrow therapeutic range, frequent anticoagulation monitoring is crucial to prevent devastating complications. Prothrombin time has been utilized as a laboratory monitor. The test includes a reagent, thromboplastin to determine the time for clot formation. Since the sensitivity of the reagent varies, the INR was established to circumvent the prothrombin time assay. For most clinical therapy, an INR range between 2.0 and 3.0 is the most desired target.

The most common side effect, like all anticoagulants, is hemorrhage. Patients are at a greatest risk if the INR is outside its therapeutic range. This can lead to life-threatening intracranial hemorrhage, blood in urine and stool, hemoptysis, or mucosal bleeding leading to epistaxis. Vitamin K can be given for minor to moderate bleeding but those with serious bleeding may require more aggressive therapy such as fresh frozen plasma or prothrombin complex concentrates. A rare but serious complication of warfarin is skin necrosis which occurs a few days after initiation of therapy. This effect is historically seen in those with protein C and S deficiency. These proteins are important in the anticoagulant balance. The addition of warfarin will eliminate all existing protein C and S, and promote a procoagulant state, thus triggering vascular thrombosis that manifests as skin necrosis or limb gangrene. Warfarin is contraindicated during pregnancy because of the placenta transmission leading to fetal abnormalities or bleeding. The risk of embryopathy is highest during the first trimester but is avoided entirely.

DIRECT THROMBIN INHIBITORS

Intravenous preparation such as lepirudin (hirudin derivative), bivalirudin, and argatroban binds directly to thrombin and prevents the interaction with other substrates for coagulation. Unlike heparin and LMWH, they require a plasma cofactor, antithrombin, for activity. The greatest clinical benefit using these direct thrombin inhibitor is the alternative treatment for HIT therapy. Argatroban is a univalent inhibitor that targets the active site of thrombin. Similarly, the divalent inhibitors, hirudin derivative and bivalirudin, bind to the active site of thrombin but also to exosite 1, the substrate binding site. Argatroban is metabolized by the liver and is an alternative to patient with HIT therapy and kidney dysfunction, while hirudin derivative and bivalirudin is better tolerated in patients with hepatic dysfunction because of its excretion by the kidney. The oral form includes ximelagatran, which has been withdrawn from the market due to elevated hepatic enzymes. The other oral preparation is dabigatran, which is approved and used as an alternate to vitamin K antagonists for prevention of stroke with atrial fibrillation.

Antithrombotic Drugs

Vinh Nguyen, DO

Obstruction of arterial or venous blood flow to vital vessels can have a dramatic impact on mortality and morbidity. Prior to thrombolytic agents, open surgical procedures were preformed to restore vessel patency and preserve vital organs. Antithrombotic agents are currently the mainstay therapy for achieving fibrinolysis during an acute ischemic event. Indications include acute myocardial infarction, ischemic stroke, deep venous thrombosis, pulmonary embolism, limb ischemia, and central line occlusion. Therefore, antithrombotic agents are used to target these blood clots directly using a catheter-directed thrombolysis or a systemic approach to dissolve the existing obstruction.

The ideal thrombolytic agent would include a high fibrin specificity while still remaining affordable. It should allow easy administration and rapid lysis response time with a limited side effect profile. It should be able to monitor drug level and its fibrinolysis effectiveness to predict potential hemorrhagic complications. Plasminogen activators were initially discovered from biological sources (streptokinase and urokinase). Later, genetically produced recombinant forms were developed (alteplase, reteplase, tenecteplase). The direct-acting thrombolytic drugs (alfimeprase, human plasmin) are a growing area of recent research. A new wave of novel plasminogen activators (staphylokinase, desmoteplase) are not yet commercially available.

MECHANISM OF ACTION

Plasminogen is the inactive precursor form of the enzyme plasmin, which is the primary catalyst for fibrinolysis. Plasminogen activators such as tissue plasminogen activators (t-PA) or urokinase plasminogen activators (u-PA) activate the initial stage for fibrin degradation. Likewise, it is highly regulated at two different levels. These include plasminogen activator inhibitors (PAI-1), which prevent excessive activation of plasminogen. Second, when plasmin is generated, it is further regulated by a competitive inhibitor, alpha-2 antiplasmin, to prevent the breakdown of fibrin. To override this system, large amount of plasmin conversion can outcompete alpha-2 plasmin for fibrinolysis. This endogenous balance ensures a counterbalance between excessive fibrin crosslinking and fibrin degradation.

The inactive protein, plasminogen, exists in the bloodstream as a circulating plasminogen and fibrin-bound plasminogen. Activation of the circulating plasminogen results in unopposed plasmin to degrade fibrinogen and clotting factors. This will trigger a "systemic lysis state," reducing the hemostatic potential of blood but increasing the risk of bleeding. These are considered *nonspecific* activators, which include streptokinase, urokinase, and anistreplase. Activation of fibrin-bound plasminogen begins the *specific* phase of fibrinolysis commonly seen with alteplase. A tertiary complex is assembled when plasminogen and t-PA specifically bind to fibrin. This complex generates large amount of bound plasmin, which is relatively shielded away from the inactivation of alpha-2 antiplasmin. This sequence promotes efficient plasminogen activation and propagation. The fibrin degradation exposes itself to more binding sites for additional plasminogen and t-PA, which amplifies the fibrinolytic process.

The fibrin specificity of plasminogen activators reflects their capacity to distinguish between fibrin-bound and circulating plasminogens, which depends on their affinity for fibrin. Plasminogen activators with high affinity for fibrin preferentially activate fibrin-bound plasminogen. This results in the generation of plasmin on the fibrin surface. Fibrin-bound plasmin, which is protected from inactivation by alpha-2 antiplasmin, degrades fibrin to yield soluble fibrin degradation products. In contrast, plasminogen activators with little or no affinity for fibrin do not distinguish between fibrin-bound and circulating plasminogens. Activation of circulating plasminogen results in systemic plasminemia and subsequent degradation of fibrinogen and other clotting factors.

ROUTE OF ADMINISTRATION

Thrombolytic agents have been widely used in clinical practice. The route of administration is important for certain clinical situation to decrease or avoid complications. Intravenous route has been the therapy of choice for acute myocardial infarction or acute ischemic stroke. The use of catheter-directed thrombolysis (CDT) provides a more direct mean for thrombolysis, thus avoiding systemic bleeding complications. Catheter-directed thrombolysis is best used for obvious occlusion such as AV graft occlusion, DVT, or limb ischemia. Furthermore, newer agents in development are inactivated with systemic infusion, thus making CDT the best delivery method.

PLASMINOGEN ACTIVATORS

Streptokinase

The first report on the "fibrinolysin" property of the bacteria beta-hemolytic *Streptococci* was submitted in the 1930s. The active agent was streptokinase (SK), which had similar property to t-PA. Due to this discovery, Group C *Streptococci equisimilis* was chosen because of its lack of production of erythrogenic toxin and rapid growth to produce streptokinase. Unlike other plasminogen activators, SK is not an enzyme. Streptokinase binds to plasminogen to form a 1:1 stoichiometric SK-plasminogen complex. This will cause a conformation change and expose a proteolytic active site of both circulating and fibrin-bound plasminogens (nonspecific). The potential disadvantage for clinical use is its antigenicity. Patients with prior *streptococci* infection or previous exposure to SK can mount an antibody response and limit its effectiveness. Minor hypersensitivity reaction can manifest as rash, fever, chills, or rigors. Transient hypotension may be seen with each administration due to plasmin-mediated release of bradykinin, while life-threatening anaphylaxis is rare.

Urokinase

Urokinase (UK) exists in human plasma as urine plasminogen activator (u-PA). It can be detected in low quantity in plasma and urine. It is endogenously produced by kidney cells and isolated for commercial use. The naturally occurring protein exists as an inactive single chain urokinase plasminogen activator (scu-PA). In the presence of fibrin, the plasminogen-bound fibrin causes a favorable conformation change that allows the plasmin to cleave the scu-PA. In turn, a two-chain UK plasminogen activator (tcu-PA) or a truncated low molecular weight form are produced which has catalytic property. Unlike SK, u-PA will enzymatically cleave plasminogen to plasmin and amplify the fibrinolytic system. Compared to SK, UK lacks the antigenicity due to its low quantity and fibrin specificity. Urokinase is manufactured as the active tcu-UK and currently approved for pulmonary embolism.

RECOMBINANT PLASMINOGEN ACTIVATORS

Alteplase

Alteplase (rt-PA) is the recombinant form of endogenous tissue plasminogen activator. Its structure is genetically identical to t-PA, which consists of five functional domains. The fibronectin (F) and the two-kringle domains (K1, K2) assist in binding to fibrin. Epidermal growth factor (EGF) domain will determine the elimination of the plasminogen activator in general because the domain assists in liver binding. The fifth domain is the protease domain (P), the site of enzymatic activity.

Tenecteplase, Reteplase

Although alteplase is the prototype, other genetically engineered variants were developed to potentially extend the half-life of rt-PA, improve fibrin-specific binding, or evade plasminogen activator inhibitors (PAI-1). *Tenecteplase* has two specific differences from the prototype. Amino substitutions within the K1 domain allows the removal of one glycosylation site, but the addition of another. This in turn decreases the clearance and prolongs its half-life. The other significant change would be the addition to four alanine amino acids in the protease domain, position 296-299. This increases the specificity of fibrin but more importantly renders the molecule resistant to PAI-1. *Tenecteplase*'s clinical profile demonstrates an 80-fold resistance to PAI-1, a 14-fold enhanced fibrin specificity, and about fivefold increase in half-life. *Reteplase* is the highly truncated variant that lacks finger, EGF, and K1 domains. A lack of EGF and carbohydrates side chain decreases the clearance from the liver and increases its half-life. Although the finger domain was eliminated, the K2 domain still gives it some fibrin/fibrinogen specificity.

DIRECT-ACTING THROMBOLYTIC AGENTS

Recombinant t-PA and biologically extracted proteins, SK and UK, use an "indirect" approach to activate plasminogen to plasmin. Therefore, direct-acting thrombolytic would eliminate the potential systemic side effects and are highly effective via a catheter-directed administration. During preclinical trials, *alfimeprase* produced promising results for occluded central venous catheters and peripheral arterial occlusion, but failed advanced clinical trials. On the other hand, *human plasmin*, the active form, has shown better clinical results. It is extracted from donors and given as a catheter infusion for ischemia of the lower extremity. Due to its potential blood-borne pathogen administration, gamma-plasmin, a recombinant plasmin, has been developed and is currently in preclinical development.

NOVEL PLASMINOGEN ACTIVATORS

Since the discovery of SK, scientists have looked into other bacterium for similar plasminogen activator. *Staphylococcus aureus* was found to have some thrombus activity by isolating its key component, staphylokinase. It has the same mechanism of action compared to SK, except that the staphylokinase-plasminogen complexes in circulation are greatly inhibited by alpha-2 plasminogen. Compared to SK, it has a much shorter half-life and a high susceptibility to antigenicity. Genetically modified staphylokinase variant has provided a longer half-life, decreased antigenicity, and maintained fibrin-specific thrombolytic potential. Another novel plasminogen activator, desmoteplase, was isolated from the saliva of vampire bat. The molecular structure contains all the necessary structure compared to t-PA, except for only one kringle domain. Desmoteplase's unique feature is the dependency on the presence of fibrin to be active. It is resistant to PAI-1 and has a longer half-life. Although these two novel plasminogen activators can potentially benefit patient thrombotic state, intracranial bleeding has complicated the small clinical trials.

COMPLICATIONS

The most devastating complication using thrombolytic is an intracerebral hemorrhage. Other sites that may cause an increased morbidity and mortality if undetected include retroperitoneal or gastrointestinal hemorrhage. Hypersensitivity reactions, from minor mild skin rashes to life-threatening anaphylaxis, the antigen of the extracted component from bacteria such as SK have been reported. Catheter-directed thrombolysis can cause minor local bleeding around the puncture site and also major vascular injury such as artery dissection and pseudoaneurysm during catheter removal. Embolic phenomenon can occur during thrombolysis therapy due to distal fragment dislodgement. This can lead to PE during DVT therapy or worsening limb ischemia.

Antiplatelet Drugs

Vinh Nguyen, DO

The hemostatic system is composed of vascular endothelium, platelets, and the coagulation and fibrinolytic system. An injury to the vessel sets off a chain reaction of events which prevent excessive bleeding but maintains a balance with blood fluidity. An imbalance can cause thrombosis, such as stroke, myocardial infarction, or pulmonary embolus.

Platelets make up the initial response for adequate hemostasis during vascular injury via three steps: adhesion, amplification, and aggregation. The initial injury attracts circulating platelets to adhere to the subendothelial matrix as the primary hemostasis phase. Platelets express a series of receptors (GPVI, GPIbα, GPIIb/IIIa) that are exposed on its surface for collagen and von Willebrand factors (vWF) to dock at the injured site. The adhesion produces a signaling pathway that activates platelets, causing a conformational shape change and release of mediators to recruit additional platelets during the amplification phase. These mediators are synthesized through the COX-1 and COX-2 pathways to generate thromboxane A_2, a potent vasodilator, and ADP. Both molecules locally activate ambient platelets. In the final step of thrombus formation, the GP IIb/IIIa receptors of activated platelets bind to free floating fibrinogen and vWF. Bound fibrinogen then bridges adjacent platelets to form linkages. Antiplatelet agents target different receptors to limit the adhesion, activation, and aggregation.

INHIBITORS OF PLATELET ADHESION

Platelets binding to vascular collagen require the interaction of glycoprotein (GP) Ib/IX/V on the platelets with the collagen receptors ($α_2β_1$ and GPVI). Therefore, antagonizing GPIb or collagen binding would interfere with platelet activation and secretion of modulators, which in turn prevent possible restenosis. Different categories of GP1b antagonists have been utilized ranging from the purification of snake venom protein to isolated recombinant peptides specific to the GPIb docking protein. Although the *in vitro* use of snake venom toxin has antiplatelets effect, its *in vivo* use causes serious thrombocytopenia limiting clinical approval.

On the other hand, antagonized recombinant peptides to the GPIb-mediated platelet adhesion receptor cause the lack of adhesion and minimal bleeding in various animal studies. The drawback is the short plasma half-life of the peptide thus requiring a continuous infusion. The newest therapy to emerge is the use of monoclonal antibodies to GPIb. Specifically, humanized Fab fragment of 6B4 has demonstrated promising preliminary results in animal model with no effect on platelet count or bleeding time.

INHIBITORS OF PLATELET ACTIVATION AND AMPLIFICATION

Activation of platelets causes the release of thromboxane A_2 (TXA_2) and other mediators to allow recruitment at the vascular injury site. *Aspirin*, the most widely used antiplatelet drug, blocks TXA_2 synthesis by irreversible acetylating amino acid of arachidonate cyclooxygenase (COX-1, COX-2). This ultimately reduces TXA_2 synthesis by 98%. A small dose of 30 mg is effective and there does not seem to be any additional benefit on platelet activity at doses greater than 300 mg.

Activation of purinergic receptors ($P2Y_1$, $P2Y_{12}$) is required for normal ADP-induced platelet activation. ADP is released from damaged vessels, red blood cells, and platelets stimulated by other agonists. Purinergic activation causes a G-protein response to activate GIIb/IIIa. Therefore, these receptors have become a recent target for drug development (Table 182-1). *Ticlopidine* is the prototype of all the thieno-pyridines, which also includes clopidogrel and prasugrel. These compounds are prodrugs that require metabolism via the P-450 pathway to its active metabolite. They cause

TABLE 182-1 **Purinergic Receptor Antagonists**

	Clopidogrel	Prasugrel	Cangrelor	Ticagrelor
Prodrug	Yes	Yes	No	No
Administration	Oral	Oral	Intravenous	Oral
Half-life	6 h	8 h	1.5-3 min	6-12 h
Reversible	No	No	Yes	Yes
Time to recovery of platelet aggregation	5 days	7 days	60-90 min	24-48 h

TABLE 182-2   **The Comparison Between GPIIb/IIIa Inhibitors**

	Chemistry	Inhibitor	Plasma Half-life	Clearance
Abciximab	Fab fragment monoclonal abs	Noncompetitive	10 min	Reticuloendothelial system
Tirofiban	Peptidomimetic	Competitive	2 h	Renal
Eptifibatide	Cyclical KGD-containing heptapeptide	Competitive	2.5 h	Renal

irreversible covalent bridging to the $P2Y_{12}$ receptor that lasts for the lifetime of the platelet.

Clinically, ticlopidine has been replaced by *clopidogrel* due to its more toxic side effect (neutropenia, skin rash) and bleeding concerns. Clopidogrel has a much safer profile and shorter half-life but is being challenged by prasugrel, which shows more consistent antiplatelet response. *Prasugrel* has been used as an alternative to nonresponder clopidogrel with greater inhibition of platelet aggregation. Direct-acting reversible inhibitors, intravenous *cangrelor,* and oral *ticagrelor* have emerged in the market as the newest drugs today but are still in clinical trials for efficacy.

Dipyridamole is the prototype antiplatelet drug used for prevention of stroke and transient ischemic attacks. Dipyridamole increases levels of cAMP in platelets by blocking the reuptake of adenosine, thereby increasing the concentration of adenosine available to bind to the adenosine A2 receptor and by inhibiting phosphodiesterase-mediated cAMP degradation. By promoting calcium uptake, cAMP reduces intracellular levels of calcium. This effect inhibits platelet activation and aggregation.

INHIBITORS OF PLATELET AGGREGATION

GPIIb/IIIa is the most abundant receptor protein on the platelet surface. These receptors are utilized at the final step of thrombus formation. After the platelets activation phase, a signal pathway causes the platelet to change shape, thus triggering conformational activation of the receptor for affinity to fibrinogen and vWF. Once activated, fibrinogen and vWF are utilized as a bridge for adjacent platelets to promote aggregation. Attractive strategies for antiplatelet therapy target GPIIb/IIIa to prevent aggregation (Table 182-2).

Abciximab is a chimeric monoclonal antibody that targets GPIIb/IIIa by a noncompetitive approach. It prevents the platelets from binding to vWF and fibrinogen. It has an extremely short half-life in plasma due to uptake with the receptor. However, its high affinity will not return platelet aggregation within 12-24 hours following discontinuation.

Eptifibatide is a cyclic heptapeptide derived from snake venom. It contains a lysine-glycine-aspartic acid sequence that is specific for the IIb/IIIa receptor. *Tirofiban* is a specific nonpeptide antagonist of GPIIb/IIIa that mimics the GPIIb/IIIa recognizing peptide RGD. Both engineered drugs are competitive inhibitors with longer half-lives but shorter platelet-bound half-lives. Consequently, the return to normal platelet function takes about 4-8 hours after drug discontinuation (compared to abciximab, which requires 24-48 hours).

SUGGESTED READINGS

De Meyer S, Vanhoorelbeke K, Broos K, et al. Antiplatelet drugs. *Br J Haematol.* 2008;142:515-528.

Hall R, Mazer D. Antiplatelet drugs: a review of their pharmacology and management in the perioperative period. *Anesth Anal.* 2011;112:292-318.

Immunosuppressive and Antirejection Drugs

Brian S. Freeman, MD

CONCEPTS OF IMMUNOSUPPRESSION

Patients who receive organ transplants from a donor who is genetically different must receive immunosuppressive drug therapy to prevent or treat rejection of the transplanted organ. These agents dampen the immune response triggered by the foreign antigen. Graft rejection reactions are classified according to the time course after transplantation: within the first 24 hours (hyperacute), in the first few weeks (acute), or months to years later (chronic).

Immunosuppressive therapy consists of three phases:

1. Induction: the set of drugs administered prior to transplantation
2. Maintenance: a combination of drugs for long-term efficacy
3. Antirejection: new drugs or higher dose agents to treat rejection

Immunosuppressive therapy is tailored to the patient. The first order of importance is the specific organ transplanted. Different organs have special pharmacological requirements. The characteristics of the recipient are also important. Patients who are presensitized or receive an organ incompatible with their blood group will require much more aggressive therapy. A number of immunosuppressant drugs are combined to maximize synergy while minimizing side effects and toxicity.

Unfortunately, no therapy currently exists that is completely effective in preventing rejection. While progress has been made in reducing the incidence of acute rejection, the rates of long-term organ survival are improving but at a slower pace. Furthermore, because these patients have to receive multiple nonspecific immunosuppressants, they are now predisposed to malignant and infectious complications. In fact, cancer now has assumed significant morbidity and mortality in this patient population.

In the perioperative period, patients should continue taking their immunosuppressive drugs. Since there is an increased risk of adverse drug interactions, all transplant patients should receive a detailed preoperative review of their medications with a focus on potential side effects and drug interactions. These immunosuppressive drugs can have significant implications for anesthetic management.

SPECIFIC IMMUNOSUPPRESSANTS

Inhibition of T-Cell Interaction

A. Steroids (Prednisolone)

With their broad anti-inflammatory effects, glucocorticoids are a major component of all phases of immunosuppressant therapy. They are particularly helpful, however, in the prevention and treatment of acute rejection. The specific mechanisms of action are somewhat unknown. Steroids suppress the proliferation and activation of T-lymphocytes by downregulating expression of cytokines (such as IL-1, IL-2, and IL-6) in macrophages. They also reduce plasma antibody levels, decrease capillary permeability, and promote a transient decrease in peripheral lymphocyte counts.

Oral prednisone, usually less than 5 mg per day, is the most common regimen. High doses of intravenous methylprednisolone are used to treat acute rejection. The chronic use of steroids can have serious side effects, including Cushing disease, poor wound healing, bone disease (avascular necrosis, osteopenia), glucose intolerance, cataracts, hypertension, hyperglycemia, and increased infection risk. The combination of glucocorticoids with other agents such as calcineurin inhibitors has enabled lower doses and therefore a decrease in morbidity.

B. Muromonab-CD3 (OKT3)

Muromonab-CD3 is a monoclonal murine antibody that binds to the CD3 receptor of T-lymphocytes and inhibits their activation. This drug is primarily used for induction therapy for patients undergoing solid organ transplantation, especially kidney. Adverse effects carry a high incidence and include pulmonary edema, anaphylactic reactions, and cytokine release syndrome (fever, headache, bronchospasm, tachycardia, hypotension). Pretreatment with steroids, acetaminophen, and diphenhydramine may prevent this syndrome. Seizures and hypertension can also occur.

Inhibitors of Cytokine Synthesis

Calcineurin is a protein phosphatase that is important in normal T-cell intracellular signal transduction pathways. Calcineurin activates T cells by dephosphorylating a cytoplasmic transcription factor (NFAT) that migrates to the nucleus and induces transcription and upregulation of IL-2 expression. IL-2 then stimulates growth and differentiation of the T-cell response to antigenic stimulation. By targeting this pathway, calcineurin inhibitors blunt signal transduction in T lymphocytes, which eventually suppresses T-cell proliferation and the response of helper T lymphocytes.

A. Cyclosporine

This agent is used for induction and maintenance immunosuppression. Derived from fungi, cyclosporine combines with cyclophilin, a cytoplasmic binding protein, and promotes its interaction with calcineurin to block phosphatase activity in helper T cells. IL-2 production is now reduced. Cyclosporine also increases expression of transforming growth factor (TGF), a potent inhibitor of IL-2–stimulated T-cell proliferation and generation of cytotoxic T lymphocytes.

Because of its adverse effects, monitoring of plasma levels is essential. The primary concerns are hypertension and nephrotoxicity. In fact, most patients on cyclosporine therapy develop renal dysfunction, a major reason for modifying or stopping therapy. Multiple drug interactions are possible with agents affecting the cytochrome P-450 system. Any drug that affects microsomal enzymes, especially CYP3A, may impact cyclosporine blood concentrations. Cyclosporine seems to enhance the effects of neuromuscular blockade. If doses of nondepolarizing muscle relaxants are not reduced, the recovery time may be prolonged.

B. Tacrolimus (FK-506)

In addition to maintenance immunosuppression, tacrolimus is often used as rescue therapy for patients with acute rejection of a liver transplant that is refractory to other agents. Tacrolimus is a macrolide antibiotic that combines with FK-binding protein 12 (FKBP-12), an intracellular binding protein, and enables it to interact with calcineurin to block its phosphatase activity. Unlike cyclosporine, tacrolimus also inhibits the expression of tumor necrosis factor (TNF-β). It is also highly protein-bound, particularly with albumin or alpha-1 glycoprotein.

Blood levels need to be closely monitored. Renal dysfunction is a major concern, especially when administered with other potentially nephrotoxic drugs like aminoglycoside antibiotics. Hypertension can be treated with calcium channel blockers. Neurotoxicity is also problematic and may manifest as headaches, tremors, and seizures. Perioperative mechanical ventilation should avoid excessive hyperventilation which could trigger seizures in patients with an already decreased seizure threshold. Other complications include glucose intolerance and diabetes mellitus due to the inhibitory effect of tacrolimus on pancreatic islet cells. Caution should be taken with drugs that can inhibit the CYP3A enzyme, such as calcium channel blockers and metoclopramide, or induce the enzyme, such as anticonvulsants, which is responsible for tacrolimus metabolism.

C. Sirolimus

Used primarily in maintenance therapy, sirolimus is typically combined with other drugs to avoid permanent renal damage in patients at high risk for calcineurin inhibitor-associated nephrotoxicity or glucocorticoid side effects. Sirolimus is a macrolide antibiotic that also binds to immunophilin, an FKBP-12. This complex, however, does not affect calcineurin. Instead, it inhibits a protein kinase known as "targets of rapamycin" (TOR), which slows down cellular division and proliferation of T cells. Its major adverse effects are myelosuppression (leukopenia, anemia, thrombocytopenia) and hyperlipidemia (cholesterol and triglycerides). Because of its extremely long half-life, multiple drug interactions are possible. Caution must be taken with any drug that can induce or inhibit CYP3A4, the enzyme which metabolizes sirolimus.

D. Monoclonal Anti-CD25 Antibodies

Basiliximab (Simulect) and daclizumab (Zenapax) are antimonoclonal antibodies that target the IL-2 receptor. Both agents are used for induction therapy. They are given immediately before transplantation and are not useful for treating acute rejection. They may delay the need for adding calcineurin inhibitors to an immunosuppressant regiment.

Inhibitors of DNA Synthesis

A. Azathioprine

Maintenance regimens often include azathioprine, but this drug has little efficacy for treating acute organ rejection. Azathioprine is a derivative of 6-mercaptopurine. This purine antimetabolite analog undergoes conversion to additional metabolites that inhibit purine synthesis (thus decreasing DNA and RNA synthesis). It functions to inhibit lymphocyte proliferation. Significant side effects include myelosuppression (leukopenia, thrombocytopenia, anemia), hepatic dysfunction, and pancreatitis. In patients with renal failure, azathioprine has been shown to produce transient antagonism of nondepolarizing muscle blockade.

B. Mycophenolate Mofetil

Mycophenolate is used for maintenance and chronic rejection. It is an ester prodrug that becomes rapidly hydrolyzed to the active drug, mycophenolic acid (MPA). Mycophenolic acid is a selective, noncompetitive, reversible inhibitor of inosine monophosphate dehydrogenase (IMPDH), an important enzyme for purine synthesis. This inhibition leads to impairment of B- and T-cell activity and proliferation. Major toxicities of MPA are hematologic (leukopenia, anemia, thrombocytopenia) and gastrointestinal (diarrhea, vomiting). Because of the risk of myelosuppression, mycophenolate should never be used in combination with azathioprine.

Inhibitors of Adhesion Molecules: Antithymocyte Globulin/Thymoglobulin (ATG)

Thymoglobulin is used for induction therapy and for treating acute rejection of transplanted kidneys. It is a purified product obtained from the serum of rabbits immunized with human thymocytes. Antithymocyte globulin contains cytotoxic antibodies that bind to a variety of antigen markers on the surface of human T cells, including CD2, CD3, CD4, CD8, CD44, and HLA class I molecules. The result is an inhibition of T-cell function and depletion of circulating lymphocytes. Anaphylaxis and leukopenia are significant concerns. Other side effects include fever, nausea, chills, and hypotension. These reactions can be minimized by slow infusion and premedication with antihistamines, acetaminophen, and corticosteroids.

SUGGESTED READINGS

Kostopanagiotou G, Smyrniotis V, Arkadopolous N, et al. Anesthetic and perioperative management of adult transplant recipients in nontransplant surgery. *Anesth Analg.* 1999;89: 613-620.

Blood Preservation and Storage

John Yosaitis, MD

The volume of a unit of blood is approximately 1 pint (450-500 mL). Units of blood collected from donors are separated into multiple components, such as packed red blood cells, platelets, and plasma. Red blood cells may be stored for a maximum of 42 days. Older blood is less effective. It has been clear for some time that stored blood degrades before the 42-day limit, and some research suggests that this degradation may be harmful to patients who receive older blood. In fact, 75% of red blood cells should survive posttransfusion to be classified as a successful transfusion.

There are three areas of concern during the preservation and storage of red blood cells:

1. **Red blood cell metabolism**—*The function of red blood cells* is to transport oxygen. However, erythrocytes do not have mitochondria, which is the site of aerobic respiration. Instead, red blood cells produce ATP anaerobically by the breakdown of glucose, thus not using any of the oxygen for its own metabolism. Anaerobic metabolism allows red blood cells to deliver 100% of the oxygen to the organ sites.
2. **Red blood cell membrane function**—A recent study has shown that increased duration of erythrocyte storage is associated with decreased cell membrane deformability. Furthermore, these changes are not readily reversible after transfusion. The decreased deformability is the result of damage over time. Changes in red blood cell morphology occurred as quickly as 22 days. This alteration can be harmful because red blood cells are similar in size to the diameter of small capillaries; therefore, red blood cells have to change shape to get through the capillaries.
3. **Hemoglobin function**—2,3-diphosphoglycerate (DPG) is a carbon molecule important in erythrocyte metabolism. It binds to deoxygenated hemoglobin and increases oxygen off-loading from hemoglobin into the tissues. As erythrocyte storage time increases, the levels of 2,3-DPG decrease. Transfusion of 2,3-DPG-depleted blood may shift the oxygen–hemoglobin dissociation curve to the left. As a result, red blood cells will have difficulty in unloading oxygen from hemoglobin into the issues.

PRESERVATION SOLUTIONS

Anticoagulants

Citrate–phosphate–dextrose (CPD), an anticoagulant solution, is the mainstay of blood preservation. Citrate works as an anticoagulant by binding to and inhibiting the function of calcium (factor IV). Phosphate stabilizes pH which maintains proper levels of 2,3-DPG. The dextrose component is necessary for red blood cell ATP production. If adenine, a purine nucleotide, is added to CPD (CPD-A), storage time jumps from 21 days to 35 days. Adenine assists in the production of ATP.

Red Blood Cell Additive Solutions

Additive solutions replace nutrients lost when the plasma is removed from red blood cells. When additive solutions are added, red blood cell's storage time can be increased from 35 days to 42 days. Two of the solutions (Adsol, Optisol) contain adenine, glucose, saline, and mannitol. Mannitol prevents hemolysis in the stored red blood cells. Another solution, Nutricel, contains adenine, glucose, saline, citrate, and phosphate

PLATELET PRESERVATION AND STORAGE

Platelets for transfusion are available in two forms: pools of platelet concentrates and apheresis platelets. Platelet concentrates are prepared from units of donated whole blood and contain a minimum of 5.5×10^{10} platelets. The usual quantity transfused to adults is a pool of six units containing a total of 250-300 mL of plasma. Apheresis platelets are collected from a single donor and contain a minimum of 3×10^{11} platelets (equivalent to five or six platelet concentrate units) suspended in 250-300 mL of plasma.

Platelets are stored for a maximum of 5 days at room temperature. After 5 days, the risk of bacterial contamination and platelet quality degradation is high. At this point, platelets are discarded. After a bag of platelets is opened, it must be transfused within 4 hours.

Most platelets are stored in plasma. There is currently one approved platelet additive solution in the United States. This solution helps improve platelet survival, decreases the amount of plasma transfused, and decreases bacterial contamination.

If platelets are refrigerated, the viability time decreases to 18 hours. The lower temperature causes platelets to change from their normal discoid shape to a spherical shape. This change in shape is not reversible. A similar conformational change can also be seen when the pH drops to 6.2 or below. This decrease in pH may be avoided by using gas permeable containers which allow for oxygen transport and escape of carbon dioxide. Continuous agitation is also used to facilitate gas transport.

FRESH FROZEN PLASMA PRESERVATION AND STORAGE

Plasma is separated from the red blood cells and platelets. The plasma is also mixed with anticoagulants such as CPD or CPD-A. Fresh frozen plasma (FFP) can be stored for 1 year at $-18°C$ or 7 years at $-65°C$. Once FFP is thawed it must be refrigerated and used within 5 days.

SUGGESTED READING

Frank S. Decreased erythrocyte deformability after transfusion and the effects of erythrocyte storage duration. *Anesth Analg.* 2013;57(6):277-278.

Blood Transfusion: Indications

John Yosaitis, MD

RED BLOOD CELLS

Red blood cell (RBC) transfusions are indicated for patients who need an increase in oxygen carrying capacity. However, determining which patients need more oxygen carrying capacity can be difficult. It is recommended that the anesthesiologist perform a clinical assessment of tissue perfusion prior to initiating erythrocyte transfusions. In a conscious patient, the signs of inadequate tissue perfusion include:

- Respiratory rates above 30 per minute
- Heart rates above 100 beats per minute
- Weakness
- Angina
- Altered mental status

The body has several compensatory mechanisms for anemia:

1. Blood volume is maintained by increasing plasma volume.
2. Increased cardiac output: Systemic vascular resistance (SVR) is decreased by decreasing vascular tone and viscosity of blood (from hemodilution). The decrease in SVR results in increased stroke volume and therefore, cardiac output and blood flow to tissues.
3. Blood flow is redistributed to the brain and heart.
4. Tissues compensate by increasing the oxygen extraction ratio in multiple tissue beds, leading to an increase in the total body oxygen extraction ratio and a decrease in mixed venous oxygen saturation.
5. The oxyhemoglobin dissociation curve is shifted to the right. Now hemoglobin has decreased affinity for the oxygen molecule and releases oxygen to the tissues at higher partial pressures. Since this shift occurs only after increased 2,3-DPG, it occurs only with chronic anemia.

A unit of whole blood or packed red cells will raise the hematocrit by 3% and the hemoglobin by 1 g/dL. However, the American Society of Anesthesiologist recommends not using the hemoglobin or hematocrit as a "trigger" for transfusion.

In 2006, a Task Force on transfusion practices from the American Society of Anesthesiologists produced the following recommendations:

1. A close watch on assessment of blood loss during surgery and assessment of tissue perfusion should be maintained.
2. Transfusion is rarely indicated when the hemoglobin concentration is greater than 10 g/dL, and is almost always indicated when it is less than 6 g/dL.
3. For intermediate hemoglobin concentrations (6-10 g/dL), justifying or requiring RBC transfusion should be based on the patient's risk for complications of inadequate oxygenation.
4. Use of a single hemoglobin "trigger" for all patients and other approaches that fail to consider all important physiologic and surgical factors affecting oxygenation are not recommended.
5. When appropriate, preoperative autologous blood donation, intraoperative and postoperative blood recovery, acute normovolemic hemodilution, and measures to decrease blood loss (deliberate hypotension and pharmacologic agents) may be beneficial.
6. The indications for transfusion of autologous RBCs may be more liberal than for allogeneic RBCs because of the lower risks associated with autologous blood.

PLATELET TRANSFUSIONS

Low platelet levels frequently do not lead to clinical signs. Thrombocytopenia is usually found on a routine complete blood count. If clinical signs are seen, they may include bleeding gums, nosebleeds, easy bruising, petechia, and purpura. Significant spontaneous bleeding does not usually occur until the platelet count falls below 5000/μL.

Indications for platelet transfusions include documented thrombocytopenia with clinical symptoms (bleeding) or platelet function disorders (hereditary or acquired). Prophylactic platelet transfusions may be given before an invasive procedure when there is a significant risk for platelet-related bleeding. The target platelet count for thrombocytopenic patients who are to have an invasive procedure is controversial.

For patients on antiplatelet agents, platelets should not be transfused prophylactically, but only to those patients with abnormal bleeding thought to be related to the effects of antiplatelet therapy.

In adults, a pool of six platelet concentrates, or a single apheresis unit should increase the platelet count by 20 000-60 000/μL. Commonly, the platelet count is raised to at least 50 000/μL,

FRESH FROZEN PLASMA

Fresh frozen plasma (FFP) contains all of the coagulation factors, both procoagulant and anticoagulant. Fresh frozen plasma is indicated to correct deficiencies of coagulation factors for which no specific factor concentrates are available. Factor concentrates are used before FFP in cases of single-factor deficiencies. Factor concentrates carry far less infectious disease risk than FFP. Warfarin should be reversed with vitamin K if surgery is not an emergency. Fresh frozen plasma can be used for the patient on warfarin who is actively bleeding or appropriate time (4-24 h) is not available.

For patients with more than one factor deficiency and active bleeding, such as liver failure patients, FFP is indicated. It is not uncommon that 4-5 units of FFP are required to control bleeding.

ABO compatibility is required between donor and recipient, however, Rh compatibility is not required.

SUGGESTED READINGS

American Society of Anesthesiologists. Practice guidelines for perioperative blood transfusion and adjuvant therapies. *Anesthesiology* 2006;105:198-208.

Lecompte T, Hardy JF. Antiplatelet agents and perioperative bleeding. *Can J Anaesth* 2006;53:S103-S112.

O'Shaughnessy DF, Atterbury C, Bolton Maggs P, et al. Guidelines for the use of fresh-frozen plasma, cryoprecipitate and cryosupernatant. *Br J Haematol* 2004;126:11-28.

Synthetic and Recombinant Hemoglobins

Chris Potestio, MD, and Brian S. Freeman, MD

No blood substitutes are available in the United States today. However, many substances have been synthesized and studied over the years in an attempt to mimic the oxygen carrying capacity of hemoglobin, including several products that are in phase II and III trials in the United States. Products under development lack many of the ideal properties of a synthetic oxygen carrier (Table 186-1).

HEMOGLOBIN-BASED OXYGEN CARRIERS

The majority of synthetic oxygen carriers aim to alter or encapsulate actual human hemoglobin molecules to take advantage of its cooperative binding. Unfortunately, free hemoglobin molecules in solution have many shortcomings as an oxygen carrier:

1. **Rapid renal excretion**—Normally, the 64 kDa hemoglobin molecule is filtered by the glomerulus and does not cause tubular damage. However, these molecules often degrade into 32 kDa dimers that bypass glomerular filtration and cause renal tubular damage. In addition, these dimers lose the cooperative binding effect of the hemoglobin tetramer.

TABLE 186-1   Ideal Characteristics of Blood Substitute

Oxygen carrying capacity greater than or equal to donated blood
Volume expansion
Universal compatibility
Pathogen free
Minimal toxicities
Stable at room temperature
Long shelf-life
Increased availability compared to donated blood
Cost efficient

They have a much higher p50 for oxygen and release O_2 only at very low oxygen concentrations.

2. **Reduced P50**—Free hemoglobin in plasma has a lower P50 than hemoglobin contained in RBCs. Functionally, the difference can be thought of as a left shift in the hemoglobin dissociation curve, where free hemoglobin "holds more tightly" to oxygen at a given O_2 tension and will only release O_2 if the O_2 tension is very low. Hemoglobin contained in RBCs has a P50 of 26-28 mm Hg. Hemoglobin-based oxygen carriers (HBOCs) have reduced P50 of 10-16 mm Hg. Hemoglobin dimers, which are spontaneous split products of free hemoglobin, lose the cooperative binding properties of the hemoglobin tetramer. These dimers have a hemoglobin dissociation curve similar to that of myoglobin, and will only release oxygen at O_2 tensions as low as 5 mm Hg.

3. **Nitrous oxide scavenging**—Hemoglobin contained in RBCs is a known nitrous oxide (NO) scavenger, so it is not surprising that HBOCs exhibit NO binding capacity. However, HBOCs free in plasma are free to cross through the vascular endothelium, allowing them to bind a greater amount of NO. Nitrous oxide scavenging leads to vasoconstriction and subsequent hypertension and pulmonary hypertension, so this is a major drawback of HBOCs. Nitrous oxide present at the endothelium mediates smooth muscle relaxation by preventing the conversion of pro-endothelin to endothelin, which is a potent vasoconstrictor. The NO scavenging with HBOCs causes increased levels of endothelin. Many other side effects of HBOCs can be linked to NO scavenging. Reported side effects of HBOC administration include esophageal spasm, abdominal discomfort, pain, nausea, and vomiting. Nitrous oxide has smooth muscle relaxation effect in the gut as well, so NO scavenging is implicated in these symptoms. Nitrous oxide scavenging also promotes platelet aggregation with possible activation of the complement system and the coagulation cascade.

4. **Free radical production**—Hemoglobin breaks down spontaneously in plasma to form free heme and iron. Both breakdown products, as well as hemoglobin itself, produce oxygen free radicals and cause free radical injury. In addition, the oxidative potential of HBOCs leads to an increase

TABLE 186-2   Effect of HBOC on Laboratory Values

Inaccuracy	No Effect
Hematocrit	Total hemoglobin
Bilirubin	Other hematology
Alkaline phosphatase, gamma-glutamyltransferase	Blood gases
Lactate, lactate dehydrogenase	Electrolytes
Creatinine	
Coagulation studies	

in methemoglobin concentration. Neither animal nor human HBOC trials have shown pathologic levels of free radicals or methemoglobin.

5. **Interference w/labwork**—Laboratory studies, especially photometric lab tests, are skewed by free hemoglobin (Table 186-2). HBOC administration leads to the presence of plasma hemoglobin and hemoglobinuria which would most certainly interfere with the diagnosis of any hemolytic condition, including transfusion reactions.

Much of the research on synthetic O_2 carriers aims at developing strategies to overcome these multiple deficits. Early attempts at preparing the hemoglobin molecule contained stroma lipids. These stroma lipids contained end toxins which also caused nephrotoxicity, so more advanced preparations were designed. Recent biochemical strategies include intramolecular cross-linking of hemoglobin molecules, polymerization of hemoglobin molecules, and conjugation of hemoglobin molecules with polyethylene glycol (pegylation). Each of these efforts attempts to stabilize the hemoglobin molecules at a molecular weight high enough to prevent it from rapid filtration through the glomerulus. Other strategies such as encapsulation of the hemoglobin molecule within a synthetic lipid membrane and synthesis of recombinant hemoglobin molecules have also been employed.

PRODUCTS WITH LINEAR BINDING KINETICS (PERFLUOROCARBONS)

The other group of synthetic oxygen carriers under investigation is perfluorocarbons (PFCs). Perfluorocarbons achieve oxygen delivery by using organic chemicals with high gas solubility. Unlike hemoglobin's cooperative binding, PFCs bind to oxygen with linear binding kinetics. These products have many unique characteristics that separate them from HBOCs.

- **Hydrophobic molecules**—PFCs do not mix with blood, therefore they must be suspended in emulsions.
- **Very small particles**—PFC particles are about 1/40 the size of the diameter of a red blood cell. In theory, this will allow the particles to penetrate damaged, blood-starved tissue that RBCs cannot reach or transplanted organ tissue. Another possible advantage of these pervasive molecules is their ability to augment tumor oxygenation to render cancerous tissue more sensitive to chemotherapy and radiation. Their small size also leads to rapid renal excretion. Intravascular half-life is around 9-10 hours for Oxygent, a PFC is in clinical trials in the United States currently.
- **Inefficient O_2 carrier**—A PFC solution has much greater O_2 carrying capacity than plasma; however, when compared to hemoglobin and HBOCs, PFCs are far inferior O_2 carriers on a per volume basis. Therefore, significantly more PFC must be used compared to PRBCs or HBOCs. The fact that PFC solutions absorb about 50 times more O_2 than plasma is interesting, in that it may be effective in dissolving air emboli.

Transfusion Reactions

John Yosaitis, MD

ACUTE INTRAVASCULAR HEMOLYSIS

Acute Hemolytic Transfusion Reaction

Acute transfusion reactions usually occur within minutes. The most common cause of an acute hemolytic transfusion reaction (AHTR) is a transfusion of incompatible red cells. The recipient must have antibodies to an antigen on the transfused cells. Most often the reaction is due to ABO incompatible blood; however, other antibodies may also be responsible.

During these reactions, the lysis of erythrocytes results in hemoglobinemia and hemoglobinuria. Other laboratory findings with AHTR are decreased hematocrit, increased lactate dehydrogenase (LDH), increased serum bilirubin, and decreased haptoglobin.

Clinical symptoms of AHTR include abdominal, chest, flank, or back pain, hypotension, bronchospasm, pulmonary edema, shock, renal failure, and disseminated intravascular coagulation (DIC). There are several important steps in its management (Table 187-1).

Acute Hemolysis Induced by Cell Trauma

There are multiple causes of trauma to red blood cells that can result in hemolysis. Common causes of trauma include severe cardiac valve disease, prosthetic cardiac valves, vascular grafts,

TABLE 187-1 Management of Acute Intravascular Hemolysis

If a transfusion reaction is expected, a transfusion reaction workup includes the following:–
• Stop transfusion immediately.
• IV fluids to maintain urine output, blood pressure, and CVP.
• Maintain urine output—urine output should be > 1.5 cc/kg/h. Use diuretics such as mannitol, if necessary. It may also be beneficial to alkalinize the urine with bicarbonate to prevent the precipitation of hematin in the kidneys.
• Bronchodilators if indicated for bronchospasm.
• Clerical check: review the records for patient identification, blood component labels, type, and crossmatch data.
• Hemolysis check—visually check the urine for signs of free hemoglobin—pink or red colored plasma.
• Direct antiglobulin test (DAT). The DAT is used to demonstrate the presence of antibodies or complements bound to red blood cells.

TABLE 187-2 Drugs, Food and Conditions that cause Hemolysis in G6PD

Infections
Severe stress
Certain foods (fava beans)
Antimalarial drugs
Aspirin
Nitrofurantoin
Nonsteroidal anti-inflammatory drugs (NSAIDs)
Quinidine
Quinine
Sulfa drugs

intraaortic balloon pumps, ventricular assist devices. In addition, the mixing of packed red blood cells with hypotonic solution or excessive warming of packed red blood cells can result in hemolysis. Severe burns can also cause hemolysis to exposed red blood cells.

Glucose-6-Phosphate Dehydrogenase Deficiency

A glucose-6-phosphate dehydrogenase (G6PD)-deficient patient lacks the ability to protect red blood cells against oxidation. Numerous drugs, infections, and metabolic conditions have been shown to cause acute hemolysis of red blood cells in the G6PD-deficient patient (Table 187-2). Management of this reaction involves blood transfusions for hemolysis. Occasionally, dialysis is needed for acute renal failure. When a blood transfusion is given, the transfused red cells are generally not G6PD-deficient and will live a normal lifespan in the recipient's circulation. Most commonly there is spontaneous recovery from a hemolytic episode due to G6PD.

DELAYED HEMOLYTIC TRANSFUSION REACTIONS

After transfusion, transplantation, or pregnancy, a patient may produce antibodies to the red cell antigens that have been transfused. If the patient is later exposed to a red cell transfusion which expresses this antigen, a delayed hemolytic transfusion reaction (DHTR) may occur. Less potent antigens than A or B are usually responsible. The clinical severity of a DHTR depends on the immunogenicity or dose of the antigen. Antibodies associated with DHTRs are commonly the Kidd, Duffy, Kell, and MNS types.

Delayed hemolytic transfusion reactions do not result in intravascular lysis. There is extravascular cell destruction in the reticuloendothelial system.

Patients with DHTRs present between 24 h and 14 days after transfusion of a red cell component. Signs include fever, anemia, and jaundice. Laboratory studies reveal elevated bilirubin, elevated LDH, reticulocytosis, spherocytosis, a positive antibody screen, and a positive direct antiglobulin test.

Most delayed hemolytic reactions have a benign course and require no treatment. However, life-threatening hemolysis with severe anemia and renal failure may occur in which case the same treatment as for acute hemolytic reactions is used.

FEBRILE NONHEMOLYTIC TRANSFUSION REACTIONS

When these reactions occur during red blood cell transfusion, the patient has an increase in temperature by at least 1°C. The rise in temperature is an acute reaction, usually occurring during or up to 30 minutes after the transfusion. Often times the temperature increase is accompanied by an increase in blood pressure and/or heart rate.

Cytokines released by white cells during storage (also seen in platelet units) is the most common cause of febrile nonhemolytic transfusion reactions (FNHTRs). Prestorage leukodepletion has reduced this risk. FNHTR is also caused by recipient antibodies (formed from previous transfusions or pregnancies) attacking donor human leukocyte antigens or other antigens on donor lymphocytes, granulocytes, or platelets.

Acetaminophen and diphenhydramine have been used in treatment, and leukoreduction of future transfusions is effective in prevention.

GRAFT VERSUS HOST DISEASE

Graft versus host disease is a rare complication of blood transfusion, in which the donor T lymphocytes mount an immune response against the recipient's tissue. It is usually only seen in the immunocompromised patient. Graft versus host disease occurs because the recipient's immune system is not able to destroy the donor lymphocytes. The incidence in the immunocompromised patient receiving a blood transfusion is less than 1.0%. Prevention includes radiation of the lymphocyte-containing blood products and the use of leukoreduction blood filters.

Complications of Transfusions

Alan Kim, MD, and Hannah Schobel, DO

A total of 30 million blood components are transfused in the United States every year. These components may be separated into the individual components of packed red blood cells, platelets, and fresh frozen plasma. Infrequently, they can be transfused as whole blood as well. Complications vary with the type and amount of components that are transfused. To designate a transfusion as a cause of a complication, the complication must be temporally linked. Generally, it must occur during, or within 24 hours of a transfusion. There are two significant exceptions to this rule that may present weeks to a month after the initial transfusion.

Regardless of the category of complication (immune, nonimmune, and infectious), the most common cause of complications is administrative. These complications occur because of the administration of the wrong blood product, usually incorrectly matched, to a patient.

IMMUNE-RELATED COMPLICATIONS

There is a wide range of immunologic reactions. These reactions range from a mild urticaria to anaphylaxis. As mentioned before, the most likely cause of these reactions is an administrative error, in which a blood product is mislabeled or misread, and subsequently given to the wrong patient. However, even when the correct blood is given to the correct patient, immunologic reactions can occur.

The most common of these reactions is the *urticarial allergic reaction*. It occurs between 1% and 3% of all transfusions, resulting in urticaria and pruritus. The airway is not usually involved in such a mild reaction. If awake, the patient may complain of increasing itchiness. While under general anesthesia, the patient will present with urticarial rashes that develop after the administration of a blood product. Treatment with Benadryl is often adequate to curb the reaction, and the transfusion may be continued as needed. If affiliated with any cardiovascular or pulmonary instability, the product should be stopped and supportive care initiated.

The next most common reaction is a *febrile nonhemolytic reaction*. It occurs at an incidence of 0.2%. Antibodies in the donor blood react with the recipient's white blood cells, activating the inflammatory cascade, causing fever and chills.

Antibodies increase with a greater number of transfusion exposures. As such, a patient with a history of chronic transfusions is at greater risk of this reaction. The transfusion needs to be stopped if this reaction is detected.

Graft versus host disease can occur when whole blood is given. The underlying pathology involves donor white blood cells attacking host cells. This is a life-threatening complication that generally affects patients who are already immunocompromised. Like the delayed febrile hemolytic reaction, this reaction occurs a while after the initial transfusion. Often it presents a month after the transfusion as fever, diarrhea, and rash. Its incidence can be reduced by pretreating donor white blood cells with irradiation, or by running them through third or fourth generation leukoreduction filters.

The most severe reaction occurs in patients with *underlying IgA deficiencies*. These reactions occur at a frequency between 1 in 20 000 and 1 in 50 000. Anaphylaxis is associated with bronchoconstriction, cardiovascular collapse, and hemolysis. The offending transfusion must be stopped immediately. Airway protection via intubation, ventilator support, cardiovascular support with volume and vasopressors, histamine reaction mediation, and bronchodilatory therapy are among the potential interventions that may be required to resuscitate a patient. Early recognition and intervention are key to addressing this process.

TRANSFUSION-RELATED ACUTE LUNG INJURY

Transfusion-related acute lung injury (TRALI), has a 0.04%-0.1% incidence across all cases of transfused blood components. However, it is the leading cause of death after a transfusion. The mortality of those afflicted by TRALI ranges between 5% and 10%. It is most closely associated with fresh frozen plasma (FFP) transfusion, but also occurs with packed red blood cells (PRBCs).

The underlying etiology is not clear. One hypothesis states that TRALI is caused by blood donor anti-HLA or anti-HNA antibodies present within the plasma. These antibodies activate the complement cascade, resulting in neutrophil recruitment to the pulmonary vasculature, and subsequent activation. Neutrophil activation leads to endothelial damage and capillary leak, the basis for pulmonary edema.

An alternative hypothesis involves a two-hit model. The first hit involves neutrophil sequestration in the lungs due to a trigger (surgery, massive transfusion, infection). Upon receiving a transfusion with donor antibodies against HLA or HNA subtypes, the antibodies activate the sequestered neutrophils causing neutrophil-mediated lung injury. The initial hit is associated with some degree of pulmonary compromise as well.

A TRALI reaction meets the following criteria:

- An acute onset of hypoxemia within 6 hours of transfusion.
- Bilateral pulmonary infiltrates on chest X-ray.
- No cardiogenic cause of the pulmonary edema (pulmonary capillary wedge pressures <18 mm Hg).
- No preexisting lung injury.

Treatment is supportive. Oxygen supplementation, positive pressure ventilation as well as cardiovascular support via fluid boluses or vasopressor support may be needed. Diuretic use is not indicated, and can have a detrimental effect. Steroid therapy may help ameliorate the degree of inflammatory response.

TRANSFUSION-ASSOCIATED CIRCULATORY OVERLOAD

The incidence of transfusion-related circulatory overload (TACO) is difficult to assess. First, there is no consensus regarding its criteria. Second, its clinical picture is similar to TRALI and is difficult to diagnose. Third, its incidence seems to vary significantly depending on the population that is involved; the range is wide and varies between 1% and 10%. At-risk populations (critically ill, advanced cardiac disease, advanced renal disease, infants, and the elderly) are all at the upper end of that incidence range, while others are at the lower end of the spectrum.

Superficially, the clinical presentation is similar to that of TRALI. However, there are a few notable differences. Patients present with an acute onset of dyspnea, tachypnea, peripheral edema, increased jugular venous distention (JVD), and hypertension within a few hours of receiving a transfusion. The signs of volume overload with increased JVD, peripheral edema, and hypertension can be used to distinguish between TRALI and TACO.

Identification of at-risk populations and subsequent slower administration of blood products can be helpful in reducing the occurrence of TACO. Treatment consists of diuretics and oxygen supplementation. For those with intrinsic cardiac disease, inotropic support or afterload reduction may be needed to support the patient. Most cases are self-limiting once the initial fluid burden is redistributed or removed.

TRANSFUSION-RELATED IMMUNOMODULATION

Nonimmune related reactions, including transfusion of a massive volume of blood products can lead to transfusion-related immunomodulation (TRIM). This response was first noted in kidney transplant recipients who had received allogeneic blood transfusions prior to transplant. There was a higher rate of kidney transplant survival in this population than those who had not received the transfusion.

Blood donor leukocytes are thought to play a significant role in this process. Regardless of the exact mechanism of effect, the following were noted effects of blood transfusion. Natural killer cell function and macrophage phagocytosis decreased. Lymphocyte production was suppressed and effective antigen presentation was impaired. Theoretical risks of immunosuppression include an increased risk of cancer recurrence, postoperative infection and short-term mortality rates. Studies investigating these concerns have had conflicting results without any definitive conclusions.

COMPLICATIONS RELATED TO MASSIVE TRANSFUSION

Large volume transfusions are affiliated with several significant complications. The introduction of a significant volume of non-physiologic blood component into a tightly regulated ecosystem results in hemostatic and metabolic derangements. When this volume exceeds 10 units within a 24-hour period, it is considered to be a massive transfusion. Patients who receive five units over 3 hours are also at risk for the same complications associated with massive transfusion. The combination of acidosis, hypothermia, and coagulopathy associated with a massive transfusion can be associated with a high mortality rate.

Red blood cells are preserved in a medium that has a low pH, low bicarbonate levels, and high glucose. A rapid infusion can lead to a profound acidemia. Additionally, hyperglycemia can result from elevated glucose levels. Over a period of time, once red blood cells exhaust their cycle duration and are broken down, iron levels can increase. As little as 10 transfusions are associated with this complication. Chelation therapy may be necessary when iron levels are excessive.

Dilutional coagulopathy is caused by a reduction in coagulation factor or platelet concentration. Below a threshold concentration, the coagulation cascade and clot strength are both impaired. In massive transfusion protocols, a set 1:1 ratio of PRBCs to FFP or platelets, has been suggested to avoid falling below this critical level.

Without fluid warmers, a profound hypothermia can occur because all blood components except platelets are refrigerated. Even platelets, which are kept at room temperature, are still substantially below physiologic temperatures. Routine use of blood warmers is recommended when rapidly transfusing blood components (with the exception of platelets).

Electrolyte imbalances are also another significant concern. Citrate in preservative solution binds calcium, causing hypocalcemia. Calcium levels should be checked regularly during high volume transfusion and supplemented accordingly. Hyperkalemia can occur when older or irradiated blood, both of which have increased potassium levels, are transfused. Infants and children are especially sensitive to this complication due to their overall lower total blood volumes. Small transfusion volumes can cause relatively exaggerated imbalances and hence, frequent monitoring is needed.

INFECTION-RELATED COMPLICATIONS

Viral Infections

Viral infection transmission risks of blood transfusions have markedly fallen after the institution of standardized blood screening. The introduction of nucleic acid amplification testing in 1999 has been particularly helpful in this regard. However, transmission risks are still present, given that the screening tests are not a 100% infallible. Transmission of viral infections via false negative blood components occur at the rates given in Table 188-1.

Cytomegalovirus (CMV) transmission is particularly concerning in immunocompromised recipients of transfusions. Given that it is generally a latent infection, only at-risk immunocompromised patients require CMV negative transfusions.

Bacterial Infections

Bacterial infections are most likely to present with platelet transfusions. This increased risk is due to the storage of platelets at room temperature. Roughly 1 in 5000-15 000 transfused units of platelets are associated with a sepsis response. Signs of sepsis can present very acutely, within a few hours of a contaminated transfusion.

In 2004, blood banks began to routinely test platelets for bacterial contamination prior to releasing them. As a result,

TABLE 188-1 Viral Transmission Rates

Viral Infection	Risk
Hepatitis A	1 in 1 000 000
Hepatitis B	1 in 200 000-500 000
Hepatitis C	1 in 1 150 000-1 400 000
HIV 1, HIV 2	1 in 1 500 000-2 000 000
Human T-lymphocytic virus 1 and 2 (HTLV-1, HTLV-2)	1 in 2 000 000-3 000 000
Babesia	<1 in 4 000 000
Syphilis	<1 in 4 000 000
West Nile Virus	None observed since screening
B19 Parvovirus	1 in 20 000-50 000

the risk of transfusing bacteria-contaminated blood components decreased. This risk can be further reduced by platelet apheresis, reducing the amount of potential medium for bacterial growth.

Initial treatment needs to be instituted quickly due to the rapid onset of symptoms to avoid progression to septic shock. Treatment entails a combination of pulmonary and cardiovascular supportive therapy and the early administration of broad-spectrum antibiotics. Once the offending organism is identified, the antibiotics should be tailored to its antibiotic sensitivities.

Creutzfeldt–Jakob Disease

Creutzfeldt–Jakob disease (CJD) is a prion disease, which differs from conventional microorganisms such as bacteria and viruses. So far there are no clinically effective treatments for any prion disease, including CJD. These diseases in general, have long incubation periods and are characterized by severe and irreversible damage to the central nervous system, resulting in death. A blood test for CJD infection is not yet available for screening blood products.

Blood Type, Screen, and Crossmatch

John Yosaitis, MD

BLOOD TYPE

The leading cause of death from hemolytic transfusion reactions is transfusion of the incorrect ABO group blood. The ABO system is by far the most significant of all the antigen–antibody groups in transfusion practice. The ABO classification is the only blood group system in which patients have antibodies to antigens that have never been present in their system. In other blood group systems there needs to be an exposure to the antigen through prior transfusion or pregnancy.

Patients are categorized into an ABO blood group (Table 189-1). The system is comprised of four groups (O, A, B, and AB) and four components (two antigens and two antibodies). If the patient has blood group A, they have A antigens on the surface of their red blood cells and B antibodies in their plasma. If the patient has blood group B, they have B antigens on the surface of their red blood cells and A antibodies in their plasma. If the patient has blood group AB, they have both A and B antigens on the surface of their red blood cells and no A or B antibodies in their plasma. If the patient has blood group O, they have neither A nor B antigens on the surface of their red blood cells but they have both A and B antibodies in their plasma. Table 189-2 illustrates the possible combinations of antigens and antibodies with the corresponding ABO type.

The Rh system classifies blood groups according to the presence or absence of the Rh antigen in the red blood cells. Rh positive blood given to a Rh negative patient can be dangerous. Symptoms may not occur the first time Rh-incompatible blood is given. Rh antibodies are IgG antibodies which are acquired through exposure to Rh-positive

TABLE 189-1   ABO Frequencies in the United States

Blood Group	Whites (%)	African American (%)
O	45	50
A	40	26
B	11	20
AB	4	4

TABLE 189-2   Plasma Composition of ABO Blood Types

ABO Blood Type	Antigen A	Antigen B	Antibody Anti-A	Antibody Anti-B
A	+	−	−	+
B	−	+	+	−
O	−	−	+	+
AB	+	+	−	−

blood (commonly through pregnancy or transfusion of blood products). If the patient is exposed to Rh-positive blood after the antibodies form, antibodies will attack the foreign red blood cells, causing hemolysis.

A person with type O blood is said to be a universal donor. A person with type AB blood is said to be a universal recipient. In an emergency, type O Rh negative blood can be given because it is most likely to be accepted by all blood types.

When it comes to platelet and cryoprecipitate transfusions, the same ABO type as the patient is preferred. However, any ABO and Rh type may be transfused.

Recipients can receive fresh frozen plasma of the same blood group, but otherwise the donor–recipient compatibility for plasma is the *reverse* of that of red blood cells (Table 189-3).

TABLE 189-3   Blood Types and Compatability

ABO Group	Compatible Red Blood Cells	Compatible Plasma
O	O	O A B AB
A	A O	A AB
B	B O	B AB
AB	AB A B O	AB

For instance, type AB plasma can be given to patients in any blood group. Patients in blood group O can receive plasma from any blood group. Type O plasma can be used only by type O recipients.

ANTIBODY SCREEN

A blood type with antibody screen is ordered when the likelihood of the patient needing a blood transfusion is low. A type and screen involves typing the patient's red blood cells for ABO and Rh type, and performing an antibody screen. The type and screen process takes about 15 minutes. It uses a panel of commercially prepared type O red blood cells containing antigens for those most common and clinically significant antibodies. The patient's serum is mixed with these donor erythrocytes to check for agglutination. The antibodies tested for in the patient's serum are potentially capable of causing red cell destruction if the patient received a transfusion of incompatible red cells. The incidence of unexpected antibodies in the patient population is between 0.5% and 2%.

If the antibody screen is negative, units will not be cross-matched until a request is received for blood. A patient receiving blood after a type and screen that is negative has less than a 1/50 000 chance of having an antibody that might cause a significant hemolytic reaction.

CROSSMATCH

A type and crossmatch is ordered when the possibility of a red blood cell transfusion is high. When a type and cross is ordered, the blood bank performs a type and screen, and crossmatches the number of units requested. This process mixes the patient's serum with the donor's red blood cells in a centrifuge. Positive hemolytic reactions occur when there is agglutination in the test tube. A full type and crossmatch takes about 45 minutes to 1 hour.

In the blood bank, properly matched units will be set aside for the patient for immediate availability. If the type and screen is negative and no significant antibodies are found in the serum, an electronic or computer generated crossmatch can be performed. If the type and screen shows significant antibodies, a classic antiglobulin crossmatch (anti-IgG) will be carried out before releasing the blood, also known as the Coombs test. The antiglobulin crossmatch will require an additional 45 minutes to complete. This additional time is necessary for the blood bank to crossmatch the appropriate antigen-negative red blood cells for the patient.

Alternatives to Blood Transfusion

Caleb A. Awoniyi, MD, PhD

Blood transfusions have inherent risks and associated costs. For example, blood transfusions have been associated with an increase in mortality, length of stay in the hospital, and multiorgan system dysfunction, as well as continued increase in blood cost. In addition, potential known and unknown risks such as transmission of blood-borne pathogens are still a concern. Because of religious practices or personal preferences, some patients may seek alternative to a blood transfusion. Therefore, anesthesiologists should be familiar with the various effective strategies to minimize the use of allogeneic blood and alternatives to allogeneic blood transfusion.

VOLUME EXPANDERS

Because normal human blood has significant excess oxygen transport capability that is only used in cases of great physical exertion, patients can safely tolerate very low hemoglobin levels (about one-third in normal healthy patient). As such, a volume expander can be used to provide volume during surgical blood loss and can help prevent shock; the remaining red blood cells can still oxygenate body tissue. Crystalloids and colloids are the two main types of volume expanders. Crystalloids are aqueous solutions of mineral salts or other water-soluble molecules. The most commonly used crystalloid fluid is normal saline (0.9% NaCl solution). Others include Lactated Ringer's and plasmaLyte. Colloids contain large insoluble molecules, such as gelatin; blood itself is a colloid. Colloid volume expanders include hydroxyethyl starch (hetastarch), albumin, dextran, and gelofusine. Limitations to the use of colloids include their cost, potential allergic reaction, and their effect on coagulation. Dextran can decrease platelet adhesiveness, depress von Willebrand factor (vWF) level, and can cause anaphylactoid reaction; it is rarely used as volume expander. Hetastarch can decrease fibrinogen, vWF, and factor VIII levels as well as decrease platelet function. Recent concerns about hetastarch will probably limit its use as volume expander.

AUTOLOGOUS BLOOD SALVAGE

This method is also known as autologous blood transfusion or cell salvage (cell saver). The technique involves recovering

blood lost during surgery and reinfusing it into the patient. It is a major form of autotransfusion. This alternative to blood transfusion eliminates the need and associated risk of giving a patient blood collected through blood donation of an unknown person. It is also a useful method in patients whose religious belief (eg, Jehovah Witness) prohibits them from receiving allogeneic blood transfusion. Some of these patients may accept the use of autologous blood salvaged during surgery to restore their blood volume and homeostasis. Autologous blood salvage is frequently used in cardiothoracic and vascular surgery, or in other surgeries in which blood loss is anticipated to be high. It is generally restricted to clean surgical fields and nononcologic procedures because of the risk of reinfusing bacteria or tumor cells into the patients. Several medical devices have been developed to assist in salvaging the patient's own blood in the perioperative setting. The final product—which is devoid of plasma, clotting factors, or platelets—is a collection bag of red blood cells having a hematocrit of 50%-70% that is ready for immediate reinfusion after about 3 minutes of processing time.

AUTOLOGOUS BLOOD DONATION

Autologous blood donation is the process of donating one's own blood prior to an elective surgical or medical procedure to avoid or reduce the need for an allogeneic blood transfusion. With this technique, blood may be collected up to 42 days before the date of use, but no later than 7 working days prior to the date of anticipated use. Patient's health status and red blood count (hemoglobin or hematocrit) determine whether they can donate. Current blood banking guidelines require predonation hemoglobin of at least 11 g/dL, donations no more frequently than 3 days, and no donations in the 72 hours before surgery. It is also recommended that patient donating autologous blood should receive iron supplement because depleted iron stores frequently limit red blood cell recovery.

Autologous blood donation has several advantages. This technique prevents transfusion-transmitted diseases, prevents red cell alloimmunization, decreases the number of banked allogeneic units needed, and provides compatible blood for patients with alloantibodies. It also prevents some adverse transfusion reactions, and provides reassurance to patients concerned about blood risks. Some disadvantages of autologous donation include its higher cost compared to allogeneic blood and the wastage of blood that is not transfused. Autologous blood donation may subject patients to perioperative anemia, which increases the likelihood for transfusion and delayed recovery.

ACUTE NORMOVOLEMIC HEMODILUTION

In this technique, blood is collected prior to operative blood loss with simultaneous replacement with a cell-free solution (eg, normal saline) to maintain intravascular volume. The benefit of acute normovolemic hemodilution includes reduced need for allogeneic blood transfusion and its associated risks, while at the same time providing a source of fresh whole blood for autologous transfusion. In addition, there is reduction in blood loss because intraoperative blood loss is at a diluted or reduced hematocrit value. By collecting blood before operative blood loss, fresh autologous blood is available for later reinfusion after surgical blood is complete. Because blood collected is stored at room temperature in the operating room and is reinfused to patient within 8 hours, platelets and coagulation factors remain functional. Normally, blood is reinfused in the reverse order of collection because the first unit collected and the last unit transfused has the highest concentration of red blood cells, coagulation factors, and platelets. This method can be used in selected clinical setting, such as in patients with preoperative hemoglobin levels undergoing surgical procedure with expected high blood loss.

PHARMACOLOGICAL STRATEGIES

The goal of using pharmacological agent as an alternative to blood transfusion is geared toward either reducing or stopping the bleeding, or reducing the likelihood of transfusion by raising the hemoglobin level. Agents that have been used include desmopressin (1-desamino-8-D-arginine vasopressin; DDAVP), antifibrinolytic agents, erythropoiesis-stimulating agents, and recombinant activated factor VII.

1. **Antifibrinolytic agents**—These agents are used to reduce blood loss in patients undergoing complex surgeries, such as cardiac, major vascular, major spine, or orthopedic cases. An antifibrinolytic inhibits the physiologic fibrinolytic pathway, which is responsible for limiting and dissolving clot. Aminocaproic acid and tranexamic acid are lysine analogs that inhibit fibrinolysis—the endogenous process by which fibrin clots are broken down. Aprotinin is a serine protease inhibitor that has been shown to be effective in diminishing blood loss after cardiopulmonary bypass. However, aprotinin was removed from the market in 2007 after some studies suggested an association with increased mortality when compared with other antifibrinolytics. The antifibrinolytics in a randomized trial study (Blood Conservation Using Antifibrinolytics in a Randomized Trial—BART study) and other data have led to a reversal of this decision and there are plans to reintroduce aprotinin in Canada and Europe. A recent Cochrane review concluded that antifibrinolytics provide reduction in blood loss and allogeneic transfusion.

2. **Desmopressin (DDAVP)**—Desmopressin is a synthetic analog of vasopressin, the hormone that reduces urine production. It also induces the release of stored factor III and vWF from endothelial cells. It has been shown to be effective in controlling and preventing bleeding in patients with platelet disorders (hemophilia A, vWF disease) and platelet dysfunction (renal failure). In addition, it is particularly effective in decreasing blood loss in patients undergoing cardiac surgery who received aspirin up to the time of operation, and thus decreasing the need for allogeneic blood transfusion. However, because DDAVP has not been shown to provide significant reduction in perioperative blood loss or need for transfusion in critically ill patient without specific bleeding disorder, it may not be effective in improving homeostasis in all bleeding situations. It should be noted also that DDAVP is associated with rare thrombotic events, acute cerebrovascular thrombosis, and myocardial infarction particularly in patient with hypercoagulable states.

3. **Recombinant activated factors VII (rFVII)**—This product is known to enhance thrombin generation and has been approved specifically for patients with factor VII deficiency (hemophilia). However, there has been off-label use of rFVII in providing homeostasis in various other clinical situations, including obstetrical, trauma, and cardiac bleeding. Because of this increase in off-label use, a consensus panel developed recommendation for appropriate clinical use to include close space (intracranial) and surgical bleeding, as well as other situations, such as trauma, postpartum, and active gastrointestinal bleeding.

4. **Erythropoiesis-stimulating agents (ESAs)**—Erythropoietin is a circulating glycosylated protein hormone that is the primary regulator of RBC formation. Majority of erythropoietin is produced in the kidney, although it is also made in lower amounts in the liver and brain. Successful cloning of the human erythropoietin gene allowed for production of recombinant human erythropoietin, and later approval to treat patients with low hemoglobin in humans. Recombinant human erythropoietin is an ESA that now serves several therapeutic purposes, including treatment of anemia associated with kidney disease, chemotherapy in cancer, and blood loss following surgery or trauma. Thus, ESAs can be used to raise hemoglobin levels and reduce blood transfusion requirements. The currently approved ESAs by the US FDA are epoetin alfa and darbepoetin alfa. The major difference between these two is that darbepoetin alfa has a longer half-life and lower binding affinity than epoetin alfa *in vitro*, taking 3-5 times longer

to reach peak serum concentrations. The ESA dose, dose frequency, rate of rise of hemoglobin, as well as target hemoglobin levels are carefully monitored and controlled to maximize benefit while at the same time minimizing possible risk associated with polycythemia.

5. **Blood substitutes**—Artificial oxygen carriers such as hemoglobin-based oxygen carriers (HBOCs) and perfluorocarbons (PFCs) such a Fluosol-DA, are developed as blood substitutes capable of carrying oxygen to improve oxygen delivery in patients with acute blood loss, or in patients needing an urgent demand of oxygen delivery. Emulsions of Fluosol-DA dissolve high concentrations of oxygen that can then be extracted by oxygen-deprived tissues. Both HBOCs and PFCs have been tested in humans, but currently offer limited applicability of oxygen transport *in vivo*. They do not respond to 2,3-DPG so they are less effective in oxygenation when compared to PRBC. In addition, they both have significant side effects. Hemoglobin-based oxygen carriers promote vasoconstriction and can increase blood pressure, decrease cardiac output, and can cause malaise and abdominal pain. Perfluorocarbons can cause back pain, malaise, and transient fever.

SUGGESTED READINGS

Elliott S. Review: erythropoiesis-stimulating agents and other methods to enhance oxygen transport. *Brit J Pharmacol.* 2008;154:529-541.

Porte RJ, Leebeek FW. Pharmacological strategies to decrease transfusion requirements in patients undergoing surgery. *Drugs* 2002;62:2193-2211.

Shander A. Blood conservation strategies. *Adv Stu Med.* 2008;8:363-368.

Shander A, Goodnough L. Why an alternative to blood transfusion? *Crit Care Clin.* 2005;25:261-277.

Spahn DR, Goodnough L. Alternatives to blood transfusion. *Lancet* 2013;381:1855-1865.

Endocrine Physiology

Alan Kim, MD

The endocrine system plays a vital role in maintaining cell integrity. It consists of a series of ductless glands that secrete chemical messengers (hormones) into the bloodstream to act on distal locations. Although these hormones vary in structure and function, together their effects maintain a stable environment that can adapt to stressors. These effects include managing the production, storage and utilization of energy, development and growth, and maintenance of intravascular volume status.

HORMONES

Hormones can be divided into four groups based on their chemical structure: amino acids, polypeptides, steroids, and eicosanoids. Amino acids are structurally modified from their base amino acid structures, allowing participation in signaling. Polypeptide hormones consist of chains of amino acids that are further modified by adding carbohydrates. Steroidal hormones are cholesterol-derived lipids that generally cross the cell membrane to enact their effects. Eicosanoids are also plasma membrane phospholipid-based messengers. These hormones are secreted to the surrounding interstitial spaces or travel into the bloodstream to distal sites.

There are two main signaling mechanisms based on the hormone's solubility characteristics:

- Lipid-soluble hormones cross the cell membrane and bind to cytoplasmic proteins. The hormone–protein complex promotes the transcription of a target DNA segment, stimulating the production of enzymes to enact the hormone's effect.
- Water-soluble proteins bind membrane receptors on the target cells. The receptor–hormone complex triggers the production of a secondary messenger in the cytoplasm. This second messenger cascade has a variety of effects, but ultimately results in the upregulation of target enzymes as well.

Hormone regulation occurs via neural regulation or feedback mechanisms. Direct neural regulation can be seen in catecholamine release, where preganglionic sympathetic nerve fibers synapse directly on the adrenal medulla to stimulate catecholamine release.

When the body senses changes to its equilibrium, the endocrine system acts to restore it. These changes can be an aberrant glucose level, an abnormal temperature, or a sudden physical stressor. Hormone production is upregulated when its effects are needed. When the body senses that the intended physiologic effect exceeds what is necessary, an inhibitory signal is sent to halt production of the messengers via a negative feedback loop. Positive feedback loops, however, are rare. One notable exception is that of oxytocin during labor. Once a threshold level of oxytocin is reached, oxytocin production is further increased, until labor occurs.

HYPOTHALAMUS AND PITUITARY GLAND

The hypothalamus and pituitary gland are distinct from the other members of the endocrine system. They act as the control center of the endocrine system with a wide arsenal of hormones to enact their effects. This tiered system of control offers two main benefits. First, it allows an amplification of the initial signal to generate a more significant end effect. Second, it provides multiple targets for feedback loops, offering layers of control.

The hypothalamus is located near the corpus callosum above the pituitary gland. It regulates the activity of the pituitary gland with a number of hormones, such as thyrotropin releasing hormone (TRH), growth hormone releasing hormone (GHRH), prolactin releasing hormone (PRH), gonadotropin releasing hormone (GnRH), and corticotropin-releasing hormone (CRH).

The pituitary gland consists of two main lobes with distinct functions:

1. **Adenohypophysis (anterior lobe)**—The anterior pituitary gland produces, stores, and releases eight hormones: luteinizing hormone (LH), follicle-stimulating hormone (FSH), thyroid stimulating hormone (TSH), growth hormone (GH), insulin-like growth factor (IGF), prolactin (PRL), adrenocorticotropic hormone (ACTH), melanocyte-stimulating hormone (MSH).

2. **Neurohypophysis (posterior lobe)**—The posterior pituitary only stores the two hormones (oxytocin and vasopressin) that are produced in the hypothalamus, and releases them in response to upstream signaling. Oxytocin is produced by magnocellular neurosecretory neurons of the supraoptic nucleus and the paraventricular nucleus that reside in the hypothalamus. Oxytocin serves to intensify uterine contractions as well as trigger lactation. Vasopressin is produced by both magnocellular and parvocellular neurosecretory neurons of the supraoptic and paraventricular nuclei. Vasopressin has a key role in the maintenance of intravascular volume homeostasis. Both hormones are packaged in vesicles after being formed and delivered to the posterior pituitary to await a trigger for release.

THYROID

The thyroid gland is a bilobar gland sitting anterior to the larynx. It consists of two main cell types: follicular and parafollicular cells. Follicular cells produce two hormones: thyroxine (T4) and 3,3′,5 triiodothyronine (T3). Their primary purpose is to increase basal metabolic rate. Parafollicular cells are responsible for calcitonin production. Calcitonin is produced in response to high serum calcium levels. Calcitonin reduces intravascular calcium concentration, by inhibiting calcium absorption in the intestines, inhibiting osteoclast activity in the bones, and inhibiting calcium and phosphate reabsorption in the kidneys. It shifts calcium from the bloodstream into the bones, reinforcing them. This action is directly opposed by parathyroid hormone (PTH).

The thyroid gland is regulated by upstream components, by both the hypothalamus and the anterior pituitary gland. The hypothalamus releases TRH, triggering TSH release from the anterior pituitary, which in turn stimulates the thyroid gland to produce and release T3 and T4. Negative feedback occurs at the hypothalamus and the pituitary gland when there is an excess of T4. TSH levels are stimulated by cold exposure and blunted by somatostatin, excessive glucocorticoids, and sex hormones.

Dietary iodine is absorbed and incorporated into tyrosine residues to form monoiodotyrosine and diiodotyroisine. These are combined by thyroid peroxidase to T3 and T4. These hormones are bound to thyroglobulin protein and stored in the gland until further signaling. T3 is the physiologically active version and when needed T4 is mono-deiodinated to T3. This conversion may produce rT3 which is a biologically inactive conformation of T3, but does so at a low rate. The bulk of this conversion (80%) takes place outside of the thyroid gland with the remainder occurring in the thyroid gland itself.

The bulk of the circulating hormones are bound to thyroxine-binding globulin, with less bound to albumin and thyroid-binding prealbumin. A very small percentage (<0.1%) remains as free, unbound hormone. The normal plasma level is between 5 and 12 μg/dL of T4 and 80 and 220 ng/dL of T3. The half-life of T4 is between 6 and 7 days in circulation. T3 has a shorter half-life of 24-30 hours.

PARATHYROID

The parathyroid glands consist of four small glandular tissues that rest on the thyroid gland consisting of two types of cells: oxyphil and chief cells. Oxyphil cells have no known function. Chief cells produce PTH. The parathyroid gland responds to the calcium concentration found in the extracellular fluid surrounding these glands. Low calcium concentrations trigger PTH release.

Parathyroid hormone works antagonistically against calcitonin to increase serum calcium levels. It targets bone, kidneys, and the GI system. It enhances bone resorption, stimulating osteoclast activity, leading to calcium release into the bloodstream. Kidneys reabsorb more calcium in the renal tubules. It reduces reabsorption of phosphate, increasing the fraction of unbound calcium. It promotes the synthesis of biologically active vitamin D, 1,25-dihydroxycholecalciferol, which in turn allows a greater degree of GI absorption of dietary calcium.

ADRENALS

The two triangular adrenal glands sit atop their respective kidneys. Each gland is divided into two main regions: the cortex and the medulla. The cortex comprises 80%, while the medulla comprises 20% of the organ mass. The primary purpose of these glands is to mobilize various mechanisms to adequately endure outside stressors. A secondary purpose is the production of sex hormones.

The adrenal medulla produces and releases catecholamines, primarily epinephrine. This response is a short-lived response to stress. Catecholamine release reinforces the sympathetic tone of the autonomic system. Preganglionic sympathetic nerve fibers directly synapse on the adrenal medulla, entirely bypassing the ganglia that act as intermediaries in other organs. The direct connection emphasizes the importance of tightly regulating catecholamine levels. Additionally, the adrenal medulla also produces and releases androgens. These androgens serve as the main source of androgenic activity in women, while serving a relatively minor role in men.

The adrenal cortex produces several classes of hormones: glucocorticoids, mineralocorticoids, and androgens. All three are derived from a cholesterol precursor. These hormones moderate a prolonged response to stress. The cortex is divided into three zones: glomerulosa, fasciculata, and reticularis. The zona glomerulosa is responsible for the production of aldosterone, fasciculata for the production of glucocorticoids, reticularis also for glucocorticoids and androgens.

Glucocorticoids

Glucocorticoids include cortisol aka hydrocortisone, corticosterone, and cortisone. These hormones mobilize energy by promoting gluconeogenesis, assist in the metabolism of energy sources (protein, fat, and carbohydrates), delay bone formation, and mitigate the inflammatory cascade.

Glucocorticoid production increases in response to ACTH release from the hypothalamus, which in turn responds to

CRH from the hypothalamus. The secretion of these factors is primarily governed by three components: glucocorticoid levels, sleep–wake cycle, and stress. High glucocorticoid levels will directly inhibit the release of ACTH, to maintain a physiologic level. Cortisol levels are highest immediately after awakening. Psychological or physical stressors, such as trauma, surgery, and exercise can trigger ACTH release.

Daily endogenous cortisol production is 20 mg in a normal patient. In response to stressors, this amount can increase to 150-300 mg. Most of the secreted cortisol is bound to alpha globulin transcortin, with only a small fraction being responsible for its systemic activity. It is inactivated by the liver and cleared by the kidneys. Cortisol production is decreased in the elderly; however, the decreased rate of cortisol inactivation and clearance leads to relatively stable serum levels with aging.

Mineralocorticoids

Mineralocorticoids regulate the fluid balance of the body by controlling the salt concentration. Aldosterone has the greatest potency among the mineralocorticoids, which also includes 11-deoxycorticosterone. Aldosterone levels are regulated by the renin–angiotensin–aldosterone (RAA) cascade, in response to fluid status and serum potassium levels.

The juxtaglomerular apparatus produces renin when it senses low perfusion pressures or is triggered by an increased sympathetic tone. Renin converts angiotensinogen to angiotensin I, which is further converted to angiotensin II in the lungs by angiotensin converting enzyme (ACE). Angiotensin II is a very potent vasoconstricting agent that increases blood pressure. Furthermore, it leads to aldosterone production, increasing intravascular volume. Other triggers of aldosterone production include hyperkalemia and to a lesser extent, hyponatremia, ACTH, and prostaglandin E.

Aldosterone acts on the distal convoluted tubule (DCT) and the collecting duct (CD), conserving sodium concentrations at the cost of potassium excretion. Aldosterone also acts outside of the kidney on the distal colon and sweat glands to further preserve sodium levels. Sodium retention leads to increased fluid retention, buffering the intravascular volume in times of stress.

Androgens

Adrenal androgens consist of DHEA and androstenedione. They have weak androgenic activity. When they reach the testes, they can be converted into the more potent testosterone. In men, the testosterone production in the testes makes the contributions from adrenal androgens clinically irrelevant. However, in women, the adrenal androgens are the primary source. As a result, aberrant adrenal androgen production can lead to a virilization of the female patient.

PANCREAS

The pancreas serves a dual role as both an endocrine and an exocrine gland. Its exocrine role revolves around its role in the GI system. It produces digestive enzymes that function in the breakdown of proteins, fats, and carbohydrates. The organ sits in the peritoneum, posterior to the stomach. It has a conduit to the duodenum at the sphincter of Oddi and serves as a conduit for bile that is released from the gall bladder.

Its endocrine role relies on its islet cells that are divided into alpha, beta, and delta subtypes. Alpha cells produce glucagon, beta cells produce insulin, and delta cells produce somatostatin. Glucagon and insulin act in direct opposition to each other. By modifying the relative levels of each hormone, the pancreas regulates plasma glucose levels.

These hormones enter the portal vein, coursing through the liver first. Glucagon promotes liver glycogenolysis, gluconeogenesis, and ketogenesis to increase serum glucose levels. Glucagon acts by promoting intracellular cAMP levels. Insulin decreases cAMP levels. Insulin has a wide range of functions. It promotes glucose transport across the cell membrane, reducing serum glucose levels. It promotes glucose oxidation, promotes glycogen formation, inhibits lipolysis, fatty acid utilization, hepatic and muscle ketogenesis, and increases amino acid and protein synthesis in muscles. The net effect is to promote energy conservation.

Somatostatin is secreted by the delta cells, intestine, and stomach to affect the digestive tract. In the stomach, it causes the parietal cells to reduce acid secretion, decreases gastric emptying, and suppresses pancreatic hormone release. It also acts to inhibit GI hormone production, such as gastrin, cholecystokinin, secretin, motilin, vasoactive intestinal peptide, gastric inhibitory peptide, enteroglucagon, and histamine. Lastly, it serves to retard the exocrine function of the pancreas. Its net effect is to impede digestion.

THYMUS

The thymus is located in the anterior, superior mediastinum; anterior to the heart, and posterior to the sternum. The thymus is mainly active in the neonatal and preadolescent periods. The thymus gland is the primary site educating T lymphocyte cells in establishing immunity. It helps to educate the T cells in recognizing a wide range of antigens. It also plays a key role in developing central tolerance. By the early teens, the gland begins to atrophy and convert to adipose tissue, although residual T cell lymphopoiesis persists throughout life.

PINEAL (EPIPHYSIS)

The pineal gland is a pea-sized midline structure centrally located in the brain. It is composed of parenchymal and neuroglial cells. It is responsible for melatonin production. Melatonin's primary function is in the establishment of a native circadian rhythm. It induces drowsiness and lowers body temperature in anticipation of sleep. Melatonin production peaks at nighttime and is inhibited by the presence of light on the retina. These triggers are processed through the hypothalamus, which releases MSH.

Carbohydrate Metabolism

Matthew de Jesus, MD

Metabolism is the series of chemical reactions within the body required to sustain life. It is typically divided into two broad categories. Catabolism is the breakdown of organic matter resulting in the release of energy. Anabolism uses energy to synthesize complex organic materials such as tissues and enzymes.

The oxidation of biological food substrates (carbohydrates, proteins, fats) produces carbon dioxide, water, and energy. The energy is used to form adenosine triphosphate (ATP), the energy currency of the body.

The unit of energy is calorie, defined as the amount of energy required to raise one gram of water (1 mL) by 1°C. A kilocalorie or dietary calorie is equal to 1000 calories, and is used in nutritional context. The kilocalorie is commonly referred to as a calorie in lay terminology. According to the International System of Units, the unit of energy is joule. One calorie is equal to 4.2 joules.

BASAL METABOLIC RATE

Basal metabolic rate (BMR) is the amount of energy expended at rest. This energy is sufficient for vital organ function. Basic metabolic rate can be calculated using the Harris—Benedict equation:

For men: BMR = (13.7 × weight in kg) + (5 × height in cm) − (6.76 × age in years) + 66

For women: BMR = (9.6 × weight in kg) + (1.8 × height in cm) − (4.7 × age in years) + 655

Since 1919, various alternatives for calculating BMR have been formulated. Today, metabolic rate can be calculated using methods of direct or indirect calorimetry. Metabolic rate increases with increased lean body mass, muscle exertion, food digestion, thermogenesis, temperature extremes, growth, reproduction, lactation, increased thyroid activity, and increased stress. Both sepsis and burns can drastically increase BMR.

RESPIRATORY QUOTIENT

Respiratory quotient (RQ) is the ratio of volume of carbon dioxide eliminated to oxygen consumed in a steady state.

A pure carbohydrate diet will result in an RQ = 1. Fats have an RQ = 0.7, and proteins have an RQ = 0.82. When eating a balanced diet, the RQ = approximately 0.8. In critically ill patients, such as in sepsis and burns, the body will shift to fat and protein breakdown, and an RQ of 0.6-0.7. These patients will require fat and protein supplementation in addition to carbohydrates in their diets or total parental nutrition.

ABSORPTION

Ingested carbohydrates are divided into two groups, simple and complex. Simple carbohydrates are composed of single (monosaccharide) or double (disaccharide) sugar units. Monosaccharides include glucose, fructose, and galactose. Disaccharides are lactose, maltose, and sucrose. Complex carbohydrates have structures consisting of three or more sugars. Digestive enzymes breakdown complex carbohydrates, while simple carbohydrates can absorb freely into the bloodstream.

Once in the bloodstream, glucose uptake into cells occurs via two methods, facilitated diffusion and secondary active transport. Once intracellular, glucose is phosphorylated into glucose-6-phosphate via two enzymes, hexokinase in muscle and fat or glucokinase in liver. The energy cost is one ATP and magnesium is also required. Glucose-6-phosphate cannot easily cross cell membranes and thus it stays intracellular. Liver tissues also contain the enzyme glucose-6-phosphatase, which converts glucose-6-phosphate back into glucose. Since liver tissue is able to transform glucose to and from glucose-6-phosphate, it is able to help act as a glucose regulator, accepting glucose from the bloodstream during hyperglycemia, and releasing it when hypoglycemic.

Glucose $\xrightarrow{\text{ATP + hexokinase (in muscle)}}$ Glucose-6-phosphate

Glucose $\xrightarrow{\text{ATP + glucokinase (in liver)}}$ Glucose-6-phosphate

Glucose-6-phosphate $\xrightarrow{\text{H}_2\text{O + glucose-6-phosphatase (in liver)}}$ Glucose

GLYCOLYSIS

Glycolysis is a series of 10 reactions that converts glucose into pyruvate. Free energy released during this process is used to ultimately form 2 ATP, 2 NADH, 2H$^+$, and 2 H$_2$O. Pyruvate dehydrogenase will irreversibly convert pyruvate into two acetyl-CoA molecules. The acetyl CoA is then fed into the citric acid cycle for further energy utilization.

CITRIC ACID CYCLE

The citric acid cycle, also known as the Krebs cycle or tricarboxylic acid cycle, is the common metabolic pathway for intermediaries from carbohydrate, protein, and fat substrates. The first step of the citric acid cycle has acetyl-CoA transferring its two carbon acetyl group to oxaloacetate, a four carbon moiety, forming citrate. This is the rate limiting step of the citric acid cycle. Electrons are released as citrate and transformed through various steps. NAD^+ accepts these electrons to form 3 NADH for each acetyl-CoA. At the end of the process, oxaloacetate is reformed, which can then repeat the process with a new acetyl-CoA.

Oxidative phosphorylation forms ATP in the cell's mitochondria, which can then be used as energy in the body. H^+ ions from NADH are shifted into the mitochondrial intermembranous space, creating an H^+ gradient. This gradient drives ATP synthase to generate ATP. The process requires ADP and oxygen.

LACTIC ACID CYCLE

The lactic acid cycle, or Cori cycle, functions under anaerobic conditions such as intense muscular activity. In the process, two ATP and two lactate molecules are generated from glucose. The ATP can be used as an energy source for the muscle. Lactate is transferred to the liver where, at the cost of 6 ATP, it can be converted back into glucose. Thus, the energy burden is lifted from the muscle, but now shifted onto the liver.

GLUCONEOGENESIS

Gluconeogenesis is the process of generating glucose from sources such as pyruvate, lactate, some amino acids, and some fatty acids. Gluconeogenesis occurs in the liver and is upregulated by fasting, low carbohydrate diets, and intense exercise.

GLYCOGEN

Glycogen is a multi-branched polysaccharide of glucose that is the main form of glucose storage in the body. Glucose intake causes an elevation in the blood glucose level. The increase in blood glucose level stimulates the pancreatic beta islet cells to secrete insulin. Insulin activates glycogen synthase to form glycogen. Glycogen can be quickly mobilized to meet glucose needs via glycogenolysis. The enzyme glycogen phosphorylase is the primary enzyme associated with glycogen breakdown. It is stimulated by glucagon.

INSULIN

Insulin is an anabolic peptide hormone secreted by the beta islet cells of the pancreas. Insulin is secreted in response to an elevation in blood sugar. It promotes the absorption of glucose from the bloodstream into various tissues, including muscle, fat, and liver. The glucose can then be used as an energy source as previously described. Insulin-activated storage processes, such as glycogen synthesis, fatty acid synthesis inhibit proteolysis, lipolysis, and gluconeogenesis. Insulin inhibits the effects of glucagon described below. Insulin also shifts serum potassium intracellularly, and is used as therapy for hyperkalemia.

GLUCAGON

Glucagon is a catabolic peptide hormone secreted by the pancreas that generally opposes the effects of insulin. Its release occurs during hypoglycemia or during a stress response via epinephrine. Glucagon promotes stored energy breakdown and mobilization via glycogenolysis, gluconeogenesis, and lipolysis to raise blood glucose levels.

Protein Metabolism

Matthew de Jesus, MD

Proteins are biological molecules that serve various functions, including muscle structure and contraction, molecular transportation, enzymatic reactions, and as an energy source. Proteins form three-fourth of the total body solids and are the second most abundant molecule in the body after water. Amino acids are the building blocks of proteins. Amino acids contain an acidic group and a nitrogen-containing amino group. There are 20 different amino acids found in proteins of the human body. Of these amino acids, 10 are termed essential amino acids, which cannot be synthesized, and thus must be ingested. Sources of protein include meats, eggs, milk, nuts, legumes, whole grains, and various fruits and vegetables.

As proteins are digested, the component amino acids are absorbed into the bloodstream. These free amino acids in the blood act as a small reservoir for the various intracellular locations of protein utilization. There is a reversible equilibrium between plasma amino acids and intracellular proteins. A low concentration of plasma amino acids will cause intracellular protein catabolism and release of amino acids back into the bloodstream.

Amino acids enter into cell via either facilitated diffuse or active transport, as they are too large to passively diffuse through cellular membranes. Once inside of a cell, the amino acids are combined via cellular machinery to form intracellular proteins with various functions. The liver is a primary location for synthesis of plasma proteins which are released into the bloodstream. Examples include albumin, fibrinogen, and globulins. Albumin provides colloid osmotic pressure, retaining plasma in the capillaries. Failure to produce albumin (malnutrition, liver disease) or inability to retain albumin (renal disease) can result in hypoalbuminemia.

Once the body's protein stores are maximized, excess amino acids can be broken down for energy or converted into storage entities like fat or glycogen. Protein release 4.1 kcal/g when oxidized. A byproduct of protein breakdown is ammonia, which is converted into urea by the liver. Urea is then excreted via the kidneys to remove nitrogenous waste. Liver failure can cause a decreased ability to convert ammonia into urea, leading to excess ammonia levels, ultimately resulting in hepatic encephalopathy.

The human body has a basal metabolic rate of approximately 20 grams of protein per day. Nitrogen balance is the measure of nitrogen intake minus nitrogen output. A positive nitrogen balance is required in times of growth (birth through adolescence, pregnancy) or to balance out losses. A negative nitrogen balance occurs during malnutrition or excessive wasting states, such as in septic or burn patients.

The body's primary choice for energy under normal circumstances is carbohydrates. In a fasting state, stored energy sources of glycogen and fat are used. Once stores are depleted, proteins become a final source of energy. Degradation of proteins leads to rapid deterioration of cellular function and impending morbidity.

Protein metabolism is under multifactorial hormonal control. Anabolic hormones include growth hormone, insulin, and testosterone. Growth hormone promotes an increase in tissue proteins and inhibits tissue protein breakdown. Insulin facilitates the transport of amino acids into cells. Without insulin, protein synthesis halts. Testosterone increases protein deposition throughout the body, namely the contractile proteins of muscle. Estrogen also causes some protein deposition, but much less than testosterone. Glucocorticoids, secreted from the adrenal cortex, promote tissue protein breakdown and an increase in plasma amino acids.

The metabolic response to injury or sepsis is catabolism and hypermetabolism. The magnitude of a stress response is dependent on the magnitude of injury, total operative time, amount of intraoperative blood loss, and degree of postoperative pain. The result is accelerated proteolysis of skeletal muscle which can provide substrate for gluconeogenesis. Nitrogen is lost in proportion to the degree of stress. In the case of severe burns, protein breakdown and amino acid losses can double. Catabolic factors include cortisol, TNF-alpha, IL-1, IL-6, and interferon-gamma, all of which are increased during a stress response. In addition to the stress response, skeletal muscle weakness and wasting occurs with prolonged bed rest.

Lipid Metabolism

Matthew de Jesus, MD

The general category of lipids in the body is composed of *triglycerides*, phospholipids, and cholesterol. The basic building blocks of triglycerides and phospholipids are long chain hydrocarbon organic acids known as fatty acids. Cholesterol does not contain fatty acids, but its sterol ring is synthesized from fatty acids, and thus it shares many similarities with the other lipids. Lipids serve various bodily functions, but primarily act as an energy source. Phospholipids and cholesterol are key components in cellular membranes.

ABSORPTION OF FATS

Fats in the diet are mainly absorbed from the intestines into the intestinal lymph. In the intestines, the majority of triglycerides are split into monoglycerides and fatty acids via pancreatic lipase. After passing through intestinal epithelial cells, they are re-synthesized into new triglycerides, and then enter into the lymphatic system as small droplets called chylomicrons. The chylomicrons travel through the thoracic duct and are emptied into the bloodstream at the juncture of the jugular and subclavian veins. The chylomicrons are removed from the circulation in the capillaries of tissues containing lipoprotein lipase, namely adipose, skeletal muscle, liver, and heart tissue. Lipoprotein lipase hydrolyzes the chylomicron triglycerides, releasing fatty acids that diffuse into the cells, where they can act as a fuel source or regenerated into intracellular triglycerides.

A small amount of ingested fat, in the form of short-chain fatty acids, are directly absorbed through intestinal mucosal villi, and transported via the portal vein with the aid of lipid carrier proteins to the liver. The liver has multiple roles in fat metabolism, including fatty acid breakdown for energy, triglyceride synthesis from carbohydrates as well as proteins, and synthesis of functional lipids, that is cholesterol, phospholipids.

LIPOLYSIS

Fats are the primary storage source for energy in the human body, and yield 9 kcal/g, compared to 4 kcal/g for carbohydrates. Lipolysis is the first step in utilizing a triglyceride for energy. Lipases hydrolyze triglycerides into glycerol and free fatty acids. Free fatty acids diffuse into the bloodstream, attach to plasma albumin for transport to their destination tissue. Once in the cytosol, fatty acids are transported into the mitochondria with the assistance of the carrier protein carnitine. Inside of the mitochondria, fatty acids are processed into the two carbon moiety acetyl-CoA, which enters the citric acid cycle to produce NADH and FADH2. NADH and FADH2 are then used in the electron transport chain to create ATP.

KETOSIS

Excess accumulation of acetyl-CoA can result in the formation of acetoacetic acid, which can then be converted to beta-hydroxybutyric acid and acetone. These three compounds, known as ketone bodies, are acids and can cause an extreme metabolic acidosis. Most commonly occurring in insulin-depleted diabetics, the body's cells do not absorb glucose from the bloodstream. The body shifts into starvation mode and catabolizes fatty acids, resulting in ketone body formation. Acetone, a volatile substance, can be detected on the breath of a patient in diabetic ketoacidosis (DKA), as it smells sweet and fruity, or like nail polish remover.

LIPOGENESIS

Triglycerides can be synthesized when carbohydrate stores are maximized. Acetyl-CoA produced from glycolysis is polymerized into fatty acids with the intermediates malonyl-CoA and NADPH. Fatty acid chains grow to 14-18 carbon entities which are combined with glycerol to form a triglyceride. During this process, some energy is lost in the form of heat. Triglycerides are the body's preferred form of energy storage, as the yield of energy is 9 kcal/g compared to 4 kcal/g for carbohydrates. Some amino acids can be converted to acetyl-CoA and so excess protein can also be converted into fat stores. Essential fatty acids must be ingested as they cannot be synthesized in the human body. In humans, and under normal metabolic conditions, there are two essential fatty acids: alpha-linolenic acid and linoleic acid.

HORMONAL CONTROL

In addition to an excess or paucity of carbohydrates, lipid metabolism is under hormonal control. Insulin is a primary anabolic hormone and promotes lipogenesis. As mentioned earlier, a lack of insulin will stimulate lipolysis and may lead to ketone body accumulation, ketosis, and ultimately ketoacidosis. The stress response of epinephrine and norepinephrine activates a hormone-sensitive triglyceride lipase in fat cells, leading to fatty acid mobilization. Corticotropin and glucocorticoids, elevated in a stress response or in Cushing syndrome, also activate lipases that elevate free fatty acids, and may lead to ketosis. Growth hormone has a similar effect to corticotropin and glucocorticoids albeit weaker. Thyroid hormone increases the body's metabolic rate and can cause lipolysis.

CHOLESTEROL

Cholesterol is a structural component of cellular membranes. It is also a precursor for the synthesis of cholic acid, a bile salt which promotes the absorption of fats. Cholesterol is used to form various hormones, including glucocorticoids, mineralocorticoids, estrogen, progesterone, and testosterone, as well as vitamin D.

C H A P T E R

195

Physician Impairment

Caleb A. Awoniyi, MD

Physician impairment is an important issue that needs to be identified and rectified early. If not treated, it poses significant problems for the patients, physician himself, colleagues, and hospital staff. Detrimental effects of an impaired physician may include loss of license, dissolution of marriage, family problems, health problems, and even death. Therefore, early identification and treatment is imperative. Fortunately, once identified and treated, physicians often do better after recovery than others, and typically can return to a productive career and a satisfying personal and family life. Unfortunately, disciplinary action and stigma are powerful disincentives to physicians referring their colleagues or themselves. However, physicians have an ethical responsibility to act proactively with regards to impaired colleagues not only to help them, but also to protect patients.

Illness is sometimes equated with impairment. However, these entities are distinct, and it is important to draw a distinction between illness and impairment. For example, addiction is a potentially impairing illness. Individuals with an illness may or may not have evidence of impairment. Typically, addiction that is untreated progresses to impairment over time. Hence, in addressing physician impairment, it makes sense to identify illness early and offer remedial measures prior to the illness becoming impairment.

WHO IS AN IMPAIRED PHYSICIAN?

According to the American Medical Association, an impaired physician is one who is "unable to practice medicine with reasonable skill and safety to patients because of physical or mental illness, including deterioration through the aging process

or loss of motor skill, or excessive use of alcohol or abuse of drugs including alcohol." Virtually, any significant medical problem that affects the physician's judgment and inability to fulfill professional or personal responsibilities can be classified as physician impairment. This chapter focuses on substance abuse and dependence leading to physician impairment.

It is a fact that many physicians possess a strong drive for achievement, exceptional conscientiousness, and a tendency to deny personal problems. These attributes are advantageous for "success" in medicine, ironically, however, they may also predispose to impairment. Impaired physicians may face some obstacles in accepting that they have an illness and should seek help. Some of these obstacles may include denial, aversion to being a patient, practice coverage, stigma, fear of disciplinary action, to mention just a few. When early referrals are not made, physicians afflicted by illness often remain without treatment until overt impairment manifests in the workplace.

COMMON CAUSES OF PHYSICIAN IMPAIRMENT

Data from state physician programs have shown that alcohol or opiates are the drug of choice for physicians enrolled for substance abuse disorders. The exact number of impaired physicians in the United States is unknown and hard to estimate. Reasons for difficulty in getting an accurate estimate include the fact that most impaired physicians self-report, and many that sought help and entered treatment did so confidentially without being part of the statistics. A 2001 data estimates that approximately 15% of physicians are impaired. Among health professionals that were followed by several state treatment programs, alcohol was the drug of choice for 47%-57%, opioids for 30%-32%, cocaine for 3%-7%, and for all other 9%-16%. Physicians often begin using alcohol and other drugs to self-medicate their own stress. In addition, social use of drugs and alcohol often begin in college and continues in medical school and beyond. Some physicians also come from families with a history of alcoholism and drug dependence, which can potentially contribute to their use and dependence. Other factors include easy access to alcohol and prescription drugs, physician's overconfidence in their belief that they can maintain "control" over drugs and alcohol, and misbelief that addiction is only a problem of "street people."

Preferential use of substances by physicians from various specialties leading to impairment also exists. Whereas oral medications, such as mood stabilizing drugs are available to all physicians, parenteral narcotics such as Demerol are much more accessible to physicians engaged in medical or surgical interventions. Likewise, fentanyl, a potent mind-altering anesthetic with high dependence potential, is readily available to anesthesiologists.

IDENTIFYING IMPAIRMENT

Physicians are skillful in concealing many signs and symptoms of substance abuse and often exhibit severe compromise before their problem is detected. The key to detection of physician impairment is recognition of subtle changes in behavior and performance. Although work is often the last area to be affected, there may be other clues such as marital and family problems. Some of the warning signs that may exist among impaired physicians are as follows:

General red flags:

- Heavy drinking at social functions
- Embarrassing behavior at social functions
- Driving under the influence (DUI), or arrests for DUIs
- Frequent or unusual accidents
- Outburst of anger and increased irritability
- Isolation or withdrawal
- Deterioration of personal hygiene or appearance
- Wearing long sleeves in warm weather

Red flags at work:

- Frequent and unexplained work absences
- Frequently late, absent, or getting ill
- Frequent trips to the restroom
- Inaccessible ("locked door syndrome")
- Lack of, or inappropriate, responses to pages or calls
- Desire to work alone, or refusing work relief
- Decreasing quality of performance or patient care
- Poor judgment, poor memory, confusion
- Inappropriate conversations with patients

ADDRESSING AND TREATING IMPAIRMENT

Ignoring the problem of physician impairment is really not an option. In fact, the Joint Commission on Accreditation of Healthcare Organizations requires health-care organizations to develop a systematic approach to physician impairment. Nationwide programs are available from the Federation of State Physician Health Programs and the Federation of State Medical Boards. Most state licensing boards have assumed the responsibility of supervising the evaluation and treatment of impaired physician through the establishment of the Physician Health Programs. These programs provide nondisciplinary, confidential assistance to physicians, residents, medical students, and physician assistants experiencing problems from stress, emotional, substance abuse, and other psychiatric disorders. They not only provide support and referrals to those participating in the program, but also to those calling in with concerns about physicians, including healthcare coworkers, colleagues, and family members. Punitive measures such as reporting physicians to the medical board usually are not pursued unless the individual does not comply with treatment and monitoring guidelines.

Addressing Impairment

Addressing cases of physician impairment will depend on whether there is suspicion, or whether the physician is caught in the act. An openness to accept the possibility of impairment is required before assistance is possible. When a colleague is suspected of being impaired, one should tactfully confront him/her to seek professional help. Usually the typical initial response will be that of denial. Initial approach to help might simply include further discussions and encouragement to seek help from a counselor or mental health professionals. However, if the impairment is job or performance related, more immediate measure is mandated because one has a moral and ethical responsibility to protect patients and others. All information should be treated confidentially to the extent allowed by law and all good faith reports of possible impairment can be made without fear of retaliation. Hospital staff should be knowledgeable about the procedure they should follow if a physician is suspected of being impaired. The following are the usual courses of action:

- Immediately notify the administrator on duty.
- The administrator will promptly investigate and determine if:
  - suspicion is legitimate
  - drug testing is appropriate
  - the physician should relinquish clinical responsibilities
  - privileges should be suspended
- There should be thorough documentation of all actions, observations, statements, and other pertinent facts.
- If the physician is unruly or disruptive, hospital security staff should be notified.

- Determination will be made regarding mandatory reporting to the law enforcement and drug enforcement agency or the licensing board.

Treating Impairment

Treatment should be geared toward, and unique to, addressing the specific impairment. Treatment plans could involve a variety of inpatient and outpatient services for detoxification, rehabilitation, and psychiatric issues, in addition to attendance at self-help or peer support groups. Several programs around the country specialize in treatment of addiction among physicians and other professionals. Many of these programs offer intensive evaluation to determine the nature of addiction as well as any other comorbid psychiatric conditions that may affect both treatment and outcomes. Impaired physicians should also enroll in their state medical board and allow them to be monitored long term without any board action and public notification. Once engaged in treatment programs, the prognosis for physicians is better than that for members of the general population. The reasons for this include high level of education, motivation, and possession of a professional career that provides financial resources that can support and sustain treatment and recovery. After treatment, a physician under the supervision of the state physician health program is usually guided by a signed contract for 5 years or longer. This will often include the following:

- required attendance at 12-step meetings and other support groups;

- a worksite monitor that regularly works with the physician and reports to the oversight program;
- regular appointments with a primary care physician;
- follow-up with a therapist or psychiatrist, if indicated;
- random drug and alcohol screening.

RISK OF RELAPSE

Despite the success of many state programs in treating impaired physicians and returning them to clinical practice, some will relapse. The risk of relapse with substance abuse has been reported to increase in physicians who use major opioids or have a coexisting psychiatric illness, or a family history of substance abuse disorder. It also appears that the presence of more than one of these risk factors further increase the likelihood of relapse. Additionally, a variety of other psychological factors such as persistent denial, failure to accept the disease, dishonesty, stress, overconfidence, and withdrawal can also contribute to risk of relapse.

SUGGESTED READINGS

Boisaubin EV, Levine RE. Identifying and assisting the impaired physician. *Am J Med Sci.* 2001;322:31-36.

Carinci AJ, Christo PJ. Physician impairment: is recovery possible? *Pain Physician* 2009;12:487-491.

Domino KB, Hornbein TF, Polissar NL et al. Risk factors for relapse in health care professionals with substance use disorders. *JAMA* 2005;293:1453-1460.

Professionalism and Licensure

Brian S. Freeman, MD

Professionalism is an essential characteristic of every anesthesiologist. The American Board of Anesthesiology places a high value on professionalism. In fact, a resident deemed deficient in professionalism must receive an unsatisfactory semiannual evaluation—despite satisfactorily meeting the requirements of the other core competencies.

DEFINING PROFESSIONALISM

Professionalism is a difficult competency to measure, particularly when the physician has neither success nor failure in this area. All types of physicians should adhere to the four basic components of professionalism:

1. **Ethics**—Physicians should demonstrate the highest standards of moral behavior. They should have integrity, character, and honesty.
2. **Accountability**—Physicians should always place the needs of the patient over their self-interest. They should be committed to providing excellent clinical care, a strong sense of duty, and altruism.
3. **Humanism**—Humanism underlies the successful physician–patient relationship. An understanding of diversity is essential for having tolerance and respect for all human beings. Physicians should demonstrate compassion, dependability, and collegiality.
4. **Physician Well-Being**—Throughout their careers, physicians should not forget the importance of their own physical and mental health, as well as that of their colleagues. They should be aware of issues like substance abuse and depression, both of which could lead to physician impairment.

For most physicians, professionalism comes naturally. Failure to act professional, whether in residency training or in practice, can occur for many reasons, such as:

- Abuse of authority
- Lack of patient confidentiality
- Egotism
- Dishonesty
- Impairment
- Poor work ethic
- Conflict of interest
- Wasting of resources
- Fraud (research, billing)

THE PROFESSIONALISM CORE COMPETENCY

As defined by the American Council on Graduate Medical Education, every resident training to be anesthesiologist should:

- demonstrate integrity and ethical behavior
- accept responsibility and follow through on tasks
- admit mistakes
- put patient needs above own interests
- recognize and address ethical dilemmas and conflicts of interest
- maintain patient confidentiality
- be industrious and dependable
- complete tasks carefully and thoroughly
- respond to requests in a helpful and prompt manner
- practice within the scope of his/her abilities
- recognize limits of his/her abilities and ask for help when needed
- refer patients when appropriate
- exercise authority accorded by position and/or experience
- demonstrate care and concern for patients and their families regardless of age, gender, ethnicity, or sexual orientation
- respond to each patient's unique characteristics and needs

PROFESSIONALISM IN ANESTHESIOLOGY

Interaction with Patients

As consultants to surgeons, anesthesiologists have brief relationships with their patients. Professionalism in the preoperative

539

period includes thorough knowledge of the patient's medical history, ideally prior to meeting the patient for the first time. The anesthesiologist should assess and allay the patient's anxiety while at the same time obtain informed consent. In the operating room, the anesthesiologist should always attend to the patient, not the monitors. He/she should respect the patient's autonomy and dignity, and maintain strict patient confidentiality at all times. In the postoperative period, the anesthesiologist must be prepared to handle a dissatisfied patient. When dealing with an angry or hostile patient, the anesthesiologist should handle the criticism with a neutral response and empathy.

Interaction with Surgeons and Operating Room Staff

The successful anesthesiologist must have the ability to work with all members of the operating room and anesthesia care team. Anesthesiologists are consultants and surgeons are the primary physicians, so conflicts may arise over patient management in the perioperative setting, leading to confrontation. As the perioperative medicine expect, the anesthesiologist is uniquely prepared to facilitate patient care for the surgical patient through risk assessment, optimization, and postsurgical patient care. As patient safety advocates, the professional anesthesiologist maintains the patient's needs above all others, even when the surgeon's remarks may be inappropriate. Sometimes maintaining silence in the face of a surgeon's criticism is the most professional way of handling the situation. Proper vigilance may be affected by intraoperative conflict. Since many anesthesiologists serve as OR directors and manage the OR schedule, professional courtesy is essential in dealing with surgeons' demands.

Interaction with Colleagues

Being an anesthesiologist means being part of a team. Professional behavior within a team requires meeting the high standards of being an anesthesiologist. In the everyday work life, an anesthesiologist should be dependable, punctual, and honest. Professionalism means sharing the workload and having the willingness to help each other out. In the average workday, the anesthesiologist should respect the support members (eg, anesthesia technicians), respect the equipment, and seek to avoid waste when it comes to supplies and drugs. Professionalism in anesthesiology also requires awareness of substance abuse and the signs of physician impairment in one's colleagues. When it comes to the dissemination of information to colleagues through research, the anesthesiologist must understand the rules of research and avoid conflicts of interests. When reviewing and sharing scientific literature, it is important to identify flawed methodology or influence of commercial industry.

LICENSURE

Professionalism for the anesthesiologist requires a commitment to lifelong learning and continuing education. The American Board of Medical Specialties requires all specialty boards to assure the public that its board certified physicians continue to demonstrate commitment to clinical outcomes and patient safety. Since 2000, all new diplomates of the American Board of Anesthesiology must participate in the Maintenance of Certification in Anesthesiology (MOCA) program.

New board certificates are valid for 10 years. Each MOCA cycle is a 10-year program of continual self-assessment and lifelong learning, along with periodic assessment of professional standing, cognitive expertise, and practice performance and improvement. To avoid expiration of certification, all MOCA requirements must be completed within the 10-year period. Participation in MOCA by non-time-limited diplomates (those certified before 2000) is voluntary and encouraged.

The specific requirements of the MOCA program include:

1. **Professional Standing Assessment**—All American Board of Anesthesiology (ABA) diplomates must hold an active, unrestricted license to practice medicine in at least one jurisdiction of the United States or Canada.
2. **Lifelong Learning and Self-Assessment**—ABA diplomates should continually seek to improve the quality of their clinical practice and patient care through self-directed professional development. The cornerstone of this requirement includes 250 credits of Category 1 continuing medical education (CME). Effective 2013, no more than 60 CME credits may be completed in the same calendar year. For diplomates certified in 2010 and later, the ABA requires 90 Category 1 credits in ABA-approved self-assessment activities. For diplomates certified in 2008 and later, the ABA requires completion of 20 Category 1 credits of Patient Safety CME.
3. **Cognitive Expertise Assessment**—Diplomates who participate in MOCA must demonstrate their cognitive expertise by passing a computerized ABA examination. Diplomates may satisfy the examination requirement no earlier than the seventh year of their 10-year MOCA cycle and they must have completed half of the total CME requirement.
4. **Practice Performance Assessment and Improvement**—ABA diplomates should be continually engaged in a self-directed program of Practice Performance Assessment and Improvement. The requirement consists of three activities: (1) case evaluation; (2) simulation education course; and (3) attestation (professional references).

SUGGESTED READING

Tetzlaff JE. Professional in anesthesiology. *Anesthesiology* 2009;110:700-702.

Ethical Issues

Brian S. Freeman, MD

BASIC PRINCIPLES OF MEDICAL ETHICS

When making decisions regarding patient care, the anesthesiologist, as the provider of medical care, should demonstrate respect and honesty for the patient. The ethical practice of anesthesiology is based on the following guiding principles:

1. **Nonmaleficence**—Anesthesiologists abide by the doctrine of "do no harm" to their patients. However, sometimes a treatment, such as providing general anesthesia for an operation, can unintentionally lead to harm, such as cardiac arrest due to hypoxemia, when the intention was for good. Successful application of this principle may be difficult.
2. **Autonomy**—The patient is an independent being who can make fully informed decisions regarding his or her own health care. They have the right to accept or refuse diagnostic or therapeutic interventions. A full informed consent is necessary for the competent patient to understand risks and benefits, and to achieve autonomy. Coercion is unethical, even if the patient's decision may not be in his or her best medical interest.
3. **Justice**—Anesthesiologists should be fair when providing their services to surgical patients. All members of society deserve to receive medical resources, no matter how scarce. When considering the principle of justice, physicians should evaluate a patient's legal rights as well as possible conflicts with local laws.
4. **Beneficence**—While the principle of nonmaleficence is based on "do no harm," beneficence requires physicians to "do good" for the patient in every situation. Anesthesiologists should evaluate each patient's individual situation and not apply the same blanket decision for everyone. To do so, physicians must maintain their skills and update their medical knowledge on a regular basis.

GUIDELINES FOR THE ETHICAL PRACTICE OF ANESTHESIOLOGY

The American Society of Anesthesiologists (ASA) has published a set of guidelines for the ethical practice of anesthesiology. Revised in 2011, they can be found on the ASA website at http://www.asahq.org/For-Members/Standards-Guidelines-and-Statements.aspx. Although this document outlines important principles, every anesthesiologist should make individualized decisions for each patient. The basic guidelines are as follows:

Anesthesiologists have Ethical Responsibilities to Their Patients

1. The patient–physician relationship involves special obligations for the physician that include placing the patient's interests foremost, faithfully caring for the patient and being truthful.
2. Anesthesiologists respect the right of every patient to self-determination. Anesthesiologists should include patients, including minors, in medical decision making that is appropriate to their developmental capacity and the medical issues involved. Anesthesiologists should not use their medical skills to restrain or coerce patients who have adequate decision-making capacity.
3. Anesthetized patients are particularly vulnerable, and anesthesiologists should strive to care for each patient's physical and psychological safety, comfort, and dignity. Anesthesiologists should monitor themselves and their colleagues to protect the anesthetized patient from any disrespectful or abusive behavior.
4. Anesthesiologists should keep confidential patient's medical and personal information.
5. Anesthesiologists should provide preoperative evaluation and care, and should facilitate the process of informed decision making, especially regarding the choice of anesthetic technique.
6. If responsibility for a patient's care is to be shared with other physicians or nonphysician anesthesia providers, this arrangement should be explained to the patient. When directing nonphysician anesthesia providers, anesthesiologists should provide or ensure the same level of preoperative evaluation, care, and counseling as when personally providing these same aspects of anesthesia care.
7. When directing nonphysician anesthesia providers or physicians in training in the actual delivery of anesthetics, anesthesiologists should remain personally and

541

continuously available for direction and supervision during the anesthetic; they should directly participate in the most demanding aspects of the anesthetic care.

8. Anesthesiologists should provide for appropriate postanesthetic care for their patients.
9. Anesthesiologists should not participate in exploitive financial relationships.
10. Anesthesiologists should share with all physicians the responsibility to provide care for patients irrespective of their ability to pay for their care. Anesthesiologists should provide such care with the same diligence and skill as for patients who do pay for their care.

Anesthesiologists have Ethical Responsibilities to Medical Colleagues

1. Anesthesiologists should promote a cooperative and respectful relationship with their professional colleagues that facilitate quality medical care for patients. This responsibility respects the efforts and duties of other care providers, including physicians, medical students, nurses, technicians, and assistants.
2. Anesthesiologists should provide timely medical consultation when requested and should seek consultation when appropriate.
3. Anesthesiologists should cooperate with colleagues to improve the quality, effectiveness, and efficiency of medical care.
4. Anesthesiologists should advise colleagues whose ability to practice medicine becomes temporarily or permanently impaired to appropriately modify or discontinue their practice. They should assist, to the extent of their own abilities, with the re-education or rehabilitation of a colleague who is returning to practice.
5. Anesthesiologists should not take financial advantage of other physicians, nonphysician anesthesia providers, or staff members. Verbal and written contracts should be honest and understandable, and should be respected.

Anesthesiologists have Ethical Responsibilities to the Health-Care Facilities in Which They Practice

1. Anesthesiologists should serve in health care facility or specialty committees. This responsibility includes making good faith efforts to review the practice of colleagues and to help develop departmental or health-care facility procedural guidelines for the benefit of the health-care facility and all of its patients.
2. Anesthesiologists share with all medical staff members the responsibility to observe and report to appropriate authorities any potentially negligent practices or conditions which may present a hazard to patients or health-care facility personnel.
3. Anesthesiologists personally handle many controlled and potentially dangerous substances and, therefore, have a special responsibility to keep these substances secure from illicit use. Anesthesiologists should work within their health-care facility to develop and maintain an adequate monitoring system for controlled substances.

Anesthesiologists have Ethical Responsibilities to Themselves

1. The achievement and maintenance of competence and skill in the specialty is the primary professional duty of all anesthesiologists. This responsibility does not end with completion of residency training or certification by the American Board of Anesthesiology.
2. The practice of quality anesthesia care requires that anesthesiologists maintain their physical and mental health, and special sensory capabilities. If in doubt about their health, then anesthesiologists should seek medical evaluation and care. During this period of evaluation or treatment, anesthesiologists should modify or cease their practice.

Anesthesiologists have Ethical Responsibilities to Their Community and to Society

1. An anesthesiologist shall recognize a responsibility to participate in activities contributing to an improved community.
2. An anesthesiologist who serves as an expert witness in a judicial proceeding shall possess the qualifications and offer testimony in conformance with the ASA's Guidelines for Expert Witness Qualifications and Testimony.

PATIENTS WITH DO-NOT-RESUSCITATE ORDERS

Patients with orders for do-not-resuscitate (DNR) may present to the operating room requiring surgery. Communication is an essential component of the preoperative evaluation. A DNR patient maintains the right of autonomy and should be an active participant in the decision-making process. Institutional policies that automatically suspend the DNR directive for the operating room do not allow for patient self-determination. A complete discussion should be undertaken with the patient or their designated surrogate or power of attorney. This communication allows for patients to direct care according to their known goals and values.

The practice of anesthesiology involves various forms of "routine" resuscitation during a case, such as endotracheal intubation, administration of intravenous fluid, and use of vasopressors. Clarification of these issues is necessary with all parties involved with the case. The patient or surrogate may then decide to proceed with complete suspension of the DNR directive for the entire perioperative period. Another option involves allowing a limited attempt at resuscitation by consenting to specific measures (eg, intubation) but not others (eg, chest compressions). Some patients or surrogates may simply allow for the surgical team to use their clinical judgment in deciding on the appropriate interventions during surgery. This approach is more common when addressing adverse events (eg, hypotension, hemorrhage) that are reversible, rather than chronic problems (eg, prolonged ventilator dependence). It is important to clarify when the original DNR order should be reinstated, such as arrival in the ICU or PACU.

It is imperative for the anesthesiologist to document these discussions and modifications in the patient's medical record prior to the start of surgery. All members of the patient care team—surgeon, anesthesiologist, intensivist, or primary care physician—should concur. The primary responsibility of discussing the operation's risk and benefits lies with the surgeon.

Informed Consent

Hiep Dao, MD

HISTORY OF INFORMED CONSENT

The 1957 case of *Salgo vs Leland Stanford Jr. University Board of Trustees* brought to the forefront the current concept of informed consent. After a lumbar aortography, Mr. Salgo suffered permanent paralysis, a known risk of such a procedure, but of which he was never informed. The judge, in stating his judgment, said, "A physician violates his duty to his patient and subjects himself to liability if he withholds any facts which are necessary to form the basis of an intelligent consent by a patient to a proposed treatment." In other words, having a patient agree to the procedure without knowledge of the relevant risks and benefits is inappropriate.

Another landmark case was witnessed with the 1972 case of *Canterbury vs Spence*. Mr. Canterbury underwent a cervical laminectomy and subsequently became a paraplegic. The surgeons did not inform the patient of this unlikely risk. The courts held that the disclosure was insufficient without extenuating circumstances and suggested basing the extent of the disclosure on what is important to the patient's decision and not customary local practice. This established the "reasonable person standard," which requires disclosure of all material information to the extent that would satisfy a reasonable person.

OBTAINING INFORMED CONSENT

A signed legal document does not necessarily mean that patient has given informed consent. Patients may sign documents they do not understand. Anesthesiologists need to achieve informed consent in two senses: the legal sense and the ethical sense. Components of informed consent include an ability to participate in care decisions, to understand the pertinent issues, and to be free from control by others in making decisions.

Decision-making Capacity

Decision-making capacity should be assessed by anesthesiologists and other clinicians. Evidence that a person can make a decision includes the ability to understand the current situation, to use relevant information, and to communicate a preference supported by reasons. Anesthesiologists meet patients with limited decision-making capacity in three situations. The first is the patient who does not have decision-making authority (nonadult). These patients should be allowed to make decisions commensurate with their capacity and other further decisions should be made by their legal surrogate. The second situation is the patient who can usually make their own decisions but whose decision-making capacity is temporarily altered by preoperative sedation or pain medications. The anesthesiologist must then decide whether a patient can consent to anesthesia. The third situation is the patient who appears to have baseline difficulties in decision-making capacity. The anesthesiologist may wish to seek assistance from colleagues in ethics, psychiatry, and law in deciding whether the patient is sufficiently competent to proceed without legal intervention.

There is difficulty in obtaining consent from a patient already under general anesthesia. Although as a general rule consent should be obtained from the patient only after the patient has awakened and recovered from the anesthetic, extenuating circumstances may exist. This decision requires balancing the principles of autonomy and beneficence. Although the patient's spouse or family members would have no legal authority to give consent in this situation, seeking their understanding and agreement would be advisable.

A more difficult situation may be when an anesthesiologist believes a surrogate is making a decision that is not fully in the patient's best interests. The physician should obtain help from other caregivers or ethics consultants by communicating with the surrogate or assessing the appropriateness of the surrogate's choice. The ultimate intervention is to ask for legal intervention to order a specific action or to have someone else assume surrogacy. The primary obligation is always to the patient, not the decision maker.

Disclosure

Anesthesiologists have the duty to disclose pertinent information to patients. Exceptions include patients who choose not to be informed, emergencies in which an informed consent cannot be obtained, and situations of therapeutic privilege (withholding information because the physician believes disclosure would be significantly injurious to the patient).

Negligence may occur if the anesthesiologist provides a disclosure that is insufficient to allow a patient to make an informed decision and an injury subsequently occurs, even if the injury was foreseeable and in the absence of a treatment error. If the disclosure did not meet standard of care, then it may be considered in breach of duty.

The informed consent discussion should occur in a setting conducive to decision making, giving the patient a chance to ask questions and consider answers. Talking to the patient as they are being wheeled into the operating room does not meet these criteria. Preprinted consent forms are also not sufficient to get true informed consent.

Informing a patient about a risk does not eliminate liability for its occurrence. Liability is based on negligence theory and depends mainly on whether the standard of care was met and if the failure to meet the standard of care was a cause of the injury. Determining what to disclose is part of the art of medicine. The depth of discussion should vary in part with the level of risk. When getting informed consent, the relevance of the information and not the rote citation of a list should guide disclosure. One definition of what constitutes relevant risks for a procedure is events that have a 10% incidence of temporary complication or a 0.5% incidence of permanent sequelae. Some consider whether a serious complication is likely enough to occur that a reasonable person might choose to refuse the procedure or seek an alternative.

Reports have indicated that patients younger than 50 years may prefer more information than older patients, whereas sex, socioeconomic status, and previous experience with anesthesia were less predictive of desires for disclosures. After initial statements about the more common risks, a phrase such as, "There are other less likely but dangerous risks to anesthesia. Would you be interested in hearing about them"? allows the patient to control the extent of disclosure. Some specific events should be included in the process, such as instrumentation of the airway and complications of invasive monitoring. Risks and benefits of each anesthetic option should be discussed, as well as the possible use of a secondary plan, such as general anesthesia for a monitored anesthesia case. The patient should be informed if personnel other than the interviewing physician will be providing anesthesia care.

Anesthesiologists must also be careful in explaining the terms they use. In one study, only 50% of patients knew what a nasogastric tube was and only 25% thought fasting referred only to solid foods. It is also helpful to discuss the patient's path to the operating room. Particularly important are realistic time estimates, especially for the patient's family members.

Autonomous Authorization

Only informed patients can rightly exercise their autonomy and the concept of informed consent must accept the possibility of informed refusal. Persuasion, the act of influencing through justifiable arguments, is a technique for educating patients. Coercion, the act of affecting behavior through the use of a credible threat, is not. The rules of medicine, ethics, and law state that a competent patient has the right to choose or refuse medical treatment. The issue becomes problematic when a patient's request conflicts with medical options. If a patient refuses a procedure without all the relevant information, the physician has not fulfilled the tenets of informed refusal and may be legally liable for injury resulting from lack of information. When a patient refuses a recommended procedure or technique, the anesthesiologist should err on the side of giving additional information to the patient about the consequences of rejection. An anesthesiologist follows the spirit of informed consent by asking the question, "Is this the plan you want to follow"? Even a nonverbal patient can show authorization with a tap of the finger or nod of the head.

The Patient–Physician Relationship

The anesthesiologist must be forthright about relevant risks, benefits, and concerns. Truth telling, however, does not equate to forcing information on patients. A patient may actively choose not to receive information if they so choose.

Patients have the right of confidentiality. Facts should not be shared with others without the patient's direct or implied consent. Anesthesiologists should be careful about casual conversation harming patient confidentiality, such as in hospital public areas. When a patient does not believe in a caregiver's ability to maintain confidentiality, the lack of trust can lead to suboptimal care.

Anesthesiologists must recognize the importance of supporting a patient's religious beliefs, the most apparent of which is that of Jehovah's Witnesses regarding blood product transfusions. Jehovah's Witnesses interpret Biblical Scripture to prohibit taking in blood because it holds the "life force" and "anyone who partakes of it shall be cut off from eternal life after death." Although this is strictly followed, Jehovah's Witnesses can have different interpretations about the prohibition of blood transfusions, and the physician must clarify precisely what the patient considers acceptable. Some Jehovah's Witnesses accept autologous banked blood or cell saver blood, and some accept blood removed at the beginning of surgery and returned in a closed loop. In these instances, it is important to precisely document what interventions are acceptable and clearly communicate the patient's desires and to provide legal documentation for the anesthesiologist. Furthermore, the anesthesiologist must be comfortable of fulfilling the patient's requests, otherwise they should not agree to provide anesthesia.

Non-pregnant adults are generally free to choose refusal of blood products. For patients who are pregnant, a minor, or a sole provider, the courts are more likely to intervene and mandate transfusion. This is based on the legal doctrine of *parens patriae*, the state's power of guardianship to protect the interests of incompetent patients, such as the child of a Jehovah's Witness who would be incompetent to refuse a blood transfusion.

Refusing to Provide Care

A physician can respect autonomy without giving into the patient's wishes. It would be difficult for an anesthesiologist, not in ethical or moral agreement with the patient, to provide such care. In a non-emergent situation, such an anesthesiologist should withdraw from or refuse patient care if he or she does not feel ethically or morally capable of providing care consistent with the patient's wishes. The anesthesiologist is then obligated to make a reasonable effort to find a competent and willing replacement.

The decision to ethically refuse to provide care can also be based on the anesthesiologist's perception that the patient prefers an anesthetic technique for which the risks so outweigh the benefits that the requested technique is not a reasonable option.

Emergency Situations

In general, it is assumed that patients would consent to treatment in emergency situations. The physician needs to use his or her good judgment, and obtain as much informed consent as deemed reasonable.

The second difficult situation occurs when treatment is urgently needed but there is incomplete evidence that the patient would want to refuse treatment. In general, the practitioner would provide life-saving interventions until shown otherwise. The refusal of life-sustaining treatment must be unambiguous, either on the basis of refusal by a patient with decision-making capacity or on grounds of a clear and valid advance directive.

SUGGESTED READINGS

Dornette WHL. Informed consent and anesthesia. *Anesth Analg.* 1974;53:832-837.

Foley HT, Dornette WHL. Consent and informed consent. In:Dornette WHL, ed. *Legal Issues in Anesthesia Practice.* Philadelphia, PA: FA Davis; 1991:81-89.

Faden RR, Beauchamp TL. *A History and Theory of Informed Consent.* New York NY: Oxford University Press; 1986:23-143.

Gild WM. Informed consent: a review. *Anesth Analg.* 1989;68:649-653.

Patient Safety

Johan P. Suyderhoud, MD

The concept of providing a safe clinical environment centered on the patient is not a new concept in the field of anesthesiology. In fact, the profession was the first medical specialty to both identify and embrace the concept of patient safety as a central tenant of its clinical and research mission. The terms "patient safety," "patient safety movement," and "no patient shall be harmed" all came from the founding moments that led, in 1985, to the establishment of the first specialty-specific organization dedicated to patient safety, the Anesthesia Patient Safety Foundation (APSF). This organization has been the model on which all subsequent efforts to improve patient safety throughout organized medicine have been based, including the establishment of the National Patient Safety Foundation in 1997. Anesthesiology's proximal role in patient safety was lauded by the Institute of Medicine's Quality of Care in America Committee, which published *To Err Is Human: Building a Safer Health System in 1999*, which singled out the work the specialty had performed, demonstrating a commitment to patient safety as the model for all other specialties to emulate. Today, patient safety is arguably the strongest driving force in medicine besides cost, and serves as the preeminent metric by which we measure clinical outcomes.

Originally, patient safety in anesthesia arose, in part, to address concerns raised in the lay press concerning hypoxic-mediated morbidity and mortality in the early 1980s. Efforts lead by Dr. Ellison "Jeep" Pierce, former president of the ASA and Chair of the Department of Anesthesia at the New England Deaconess Hospital, and others in the Harvard consortium of hospitals resulted in identifying anesthesia accidents and malpractice costs as having a common solution, which was to make the practice of anesthesia safer. These early efforts resulted in the formation of the ASA Committee on Patient Safety and Risk Management, and with it several innovations. First, monitoring standards were identified and mandated to promote technical solutions to provide safer care, such as the use of pulse oximetry and real-time analysis of end-tidal gas concentrations to address the dangerous conditions of unrecognized/inadvertent esophageal intubation/intraoperative loss of adequate ventilation. Second, the nascent field of human factor engineering began to be adapted by the practice of anesthesia by incorporating critical incident analysis from other professions, mainly aviation safety.

Together, these efforts resulted, along with issues raised by an international symposium on Preventable Anesthesia Mortality and Morbidity in 1984, in the formation of the APSF.

In the current era, the focus on anesthesia patient safety has led to a number of important safety initiatives and has helped in identifying clinical areas of risk. At the same time, ASA, the APSF, individual anesthesiologists, and the newly formed Anesthesia Quality Institute (AQI) have worked in concert with other patient safety organizations to promote safety initiatives across spectrums of patient care, especially in the OR environment. Some of these include:

- Establishment of the ASA Closed Claims Project (CCP) and its registries, which involves all closed legal proceedings involving anesthesiology as well as registries for specific clinical entities. This work serves to identify safety concerns in anesthesia, patterns of injury, and to develop strategies for prevention to improve patient safety. ASA CCP has highlighted strategies to care for low-risk patients who have cardiovascular collapse during neuraxial anesthesia, how monitoring standards have reduced respiratory-related events during anesthesia, causes of regional anesthesia-related morbidity, eye and peripheral nerve damage during surgery and what to do to prevent them, mitigating the causes of OR fires, highlighting the risks of anesthesia- and surgery-related morbidity and mortality in out-of-OR settings with regard to equipment, monitors and protocols, factors associated with intraoperative awareness, and factors associated with central venous access catheters. In addition, registries have been created to catalog and discern the factors involved for rare intraoperative events, such as neurologic injury after nonsupine shoulder surgery, postoperative visual loss, and awareness during anesthesia. Heightened vigilance (the watchword for the ASA) has led to a 20 or more reduction in purely anesthesia-related perioperative mortality over the past 30 years.
- Embracing the concept of surgical and procedure checklists and protocols to help prevent wrong patient/wrong site/wrong-sided surgery, and regional blocks, as promoted by the World Health Organization as part of a global attempt to improve surgical care. Use of the

standard surgical safety checklist worldwide is thought to be able to reduce perioperative surgical mortality by as many as 500,000 deaths per annum.

- Identifying factors that contribute to catheter-related bloodstream infections (CLABSI) from central line catheters (CVC) and how following protocols that mitigate infection risk throughout the care of a patient during placement and maintenance of CVC can eliminate the incidence of CLABSI. Use of ultrasound during placement of CVC has reduced some of the complications associated with access.

- Recognition of the risk of postoperative respiratory depression and working to identify technologies and protocols that reduce iatrogenic complication for every hospital patient's stay in a health-care environment, be it surgical or nonsurgical.

- Adoption of information technology platforms that record, track, and provide decision support of all monitoring modalities used during anesthesia through an anesthesia information management system (AIMS), the so-called automated anesthesia record. More than a recording device, these platforms will collect and help anesthesiologists make clinical decisions based on a combination of recorded information, patient-specific characteristics, and laboratory data from other parts of the patient's electronic health information records. In addition, these platforms will also use population-based analytics from large amalgams of patient data (such as being currently assembled by the AQI) to provide up-to-the minute data. Anesthesiologists will be able to deliver the safest and most reliable anesthetic for each patient, all while removing the rote tasks of manual data entry, an inherently unreliable process. True real-time, unvarnished data collection will usher in insights to physiologic measurements that should help make anesthetic care continually safer and more cost effective.

- Focusing on safe medication practices in the OR, such as labeling of all medication, automated labeling systems, adopting prefilled syringe drug delivery to reduce operator error (wrong drug/wrong concentration), standardized drug concentrations/infusions, barcoding of medications and barcoded-assisted drug administration, in-OR automated drug storage units, and smart pump technologies that drive IV infusion pumps for the perioperative environment are some of the modalities related to medication safety that the field has adopted.

- Adoption of the ASA Difficult Airway algorithm to guide best practices when dealing with the challenging patient airway, and discovering/enhancing and embracing technologies and practices that allow for the safest methods to secure a patient's airway and to promote their use for other medical specialists who are involved in airway management, such as video-assisted laryngoscopy and numerous supraglottic airway devices.

- Intra- and postoperative warming modalities to limit hypothermia-related perioperative morbidity, such as infection, wound healing, and coagulopathy.

- Adopting enhanced body imaging technologies to deliver safer anesthetics and to perform safer procedures, such as ultrasound-guided regional nerve block with peripheral nerve stimulation enhancement, or expanding the use of cardiac ultrasound beyond its traditional place in cardiac surgery for both noncardiac surgery, transesophageal echocardiography as well as intraoperative and postoperative transthoracic cardiac imaging.

These initiatives are but a sampling of the myriad ways that anesthesiologists are involved in promoting and advocating for each of their patient's safety and well being during every procedure, whether surgical or diagnostic.

SUGGESTED READINGS

American Society of Anesthesiologists Closed Claims, Project and Its Registries. http://depts.washington.edu/asaccp/. Accessed on December 5, 2013.

Taenzer AH, Blike GT. *Postoperative monitoring—the Dartmouth experience.* APSF Newsletter, Spring/Summer, 2012.

World Health Organization Safe Surgery Saves Lives.http://www.who.int/patientsafety/safesurgery/en/index.html. Accessed December 5, 2013.

Index

Note: Pages followed by *f* or *t* indicate figures or tables, respectively.